BSAVA M
Canine a
Anaesthesia and Analgesia

Second edition

Editors:

Chris Seymour
MA VetMB DVA MRCVS
9 Hillside Close, Shillington, Hitchin, Hertfordshire SG5 3NN, UK

and

Tanya Duke-Novakovski
BVetMed DVA DipACVA DipECVA
Department of Small Animal Clinical Sciences,
Western College of Veterinary Medicine, University of Saskatchewan,
52 Campus Drive, Saskatoon, Saskatchewan S7N 5B4, Canada

Published by:

British Small Animal Veterinary Association
Woodrow House, 1 Telford Way, Waterwells
Business Park, Quedgeley, Gloucester GL2 2AB

A Company Limited by Guarantee in England.
Registered Company No. 2837793.
Registered as a Charity.

Figures 10.3, 10.4, 10.5, 10.6, 10.7, 10.8, 10.9, 10.10, 10.11, 10.12, 10.13, 17.2, 17.7 and 18.1 were drawn by S. J. Elmhurst BA Hons (www.livingart.co.uk) and are printed with her permission.

A catalogue record for this book is available from the British Library.

ISBN-13 978 0 905214 98 6

Printed by: Lookers, Upton, Dorset, UK

Other titles in the BSAVA Manuals series:

Manual of Advanced Veterinary Nursing
Manual of Canine & Feline Abdominal Surgery
Manual of Canine & Feline Behavioural Medicine
Manual of Canine & Feline Clinical Pathology
Manual of Canine & Feline Dentistry
Manual of Canine & Feline Emergency and Critical Care
Manual of Canine & Feline Endocrinology
Manual of Canine & Feline Gastroenterology
Manual of Canine & Feline Haematology and Transfusion Medicine
Manual of Canine & Feline Head, Neck and Thoracic Surgery
Manual of Canine & Feline Infectious Diseases
Manual of Canine & Feline Musculoskeletal Disorders
Manual of Canine & Feline Musculoskeletal Imaging
Manual of Canine & Feline Nephrology and Urology
Manual of Canine & Feline Neurology
Manual of Canine & Feline Oncology
Manual of Canine & Feline Wound Management and Reconstruction
Manual of Exotic Pets
Manual of Ornamental Fish
Manual of Practical Veterinary Nursing
Manual of Psittacine Birds
Manual of Rabbit Medicine and Surgery
Manual of Raptors, Pigeons and Waterfowl
Manual of Reptiles
Manual of Small Animal Cardiorespiratory Medicine and Surgery
Manual of Small Animal Dermatology
Manual of Small Animal Diagnostic Imaging
Manual of Small Animal Fracture Repair and Management
Manual of Small Animal Ophthalmology
Manual of Small Animal Reproduction and Neonatology
Manual of Veterinary Care
Manual of Wildlife Casualties

For information on these and all BSAVA publications please visit our website: www.bsava.com

Contents

Contributors

Hatim Alibhai BVSc MVM PhD DipECVA ILTM
The Queen Mother Hospital for Animals, The Royal Veterinary College, Hawkshead Lane, North Mymms, Hatfield, Herts AL9 7TA, UK

Adam Auckburally BVSc CertVA MRCVS
Companion Animal Sciences, Institute of Comparative Medicine, Faculty of Veterinary Medicine, University of Glasgow, Bearsden Road, Glasgow G61 1QH, UK

Rachel C. Bennett MA VetMB CertVA MRCVS
New Bolton Center, School of Veterinary Medicine, University of Pennsylvania, 382 West Street Road, Kennett Square, PA 19348, USA

Shauna Cantwell DVM MVSc DipACVA CVSMT CVA
Department of Large Animal Clinical Sciences, College of Veterinary Medicine, University of Florida, PO Box 100136, Gainesville, FL 32610-0136, USA

R. Eddie Clutton BVSc DVA DipECVA MRCA MRCVS
Department of Veterinary Clinical Studies, University of Edinburgh, Easter Bush Veterinary Centre, Midlothian EH25 9RG, UK

Paul Coppens DVM DipECVA
University of Veterinary Medicine, Department of Companion Animals and Horses,
Clinic of Anaesthesiology and Perioperative Intensive Care, Veterinärplatz 1, A-1210 Vienna, Austria

Petro Dobromylskyj BSc BVetMed DVA DipECVA MRCVS
6 Westfields, Compton, Newbury, Berkshire RG20 6NX, UK

Tanya Duke-Novakovski BVetMed DVA DipACVA DipECVA
Department of Small Animal Clinical Sciences, Western College of Veterinary Medicine,
University of Saskatchewan, 52 Campus Drive, Saskatoon, Saskatchewan S7N 5B4, Canada

Christine Egger DVM MVSc CVA CVH DipACVA
University of Tennessee, College of Veterinary Medicine, Department of Small Animal Clinical Sciences, C247 Veterinary Teaching Hospital, Knoxville, TN 37996-4544, USA

Derek Flaherty BVMS DVA DipECVA MRCA MRCVS
Companion Animal Sciences, Institute of Comparative Medicine, Faculty of Veterinary Medicine, University of Glasgow, Bearsden Road, Glasgow G61 1QH, UK

Richard Hammond PhD DVA DipECVA BSc BVetMed ILTM MRCVS
University of Nottingham, Sutton Bonington, Leicestershire LE12 5RA, UK

Daniel Holden BVetMed DVA DipECVA CertSAM MRCVS
The County Veterinary Clinic, 137 Kingston Road, Taunton, Somerset TA2 7SR, UK

Lynne Hughes MVB DipECVA DVA FCARCSI MRCVS
School of Agriculture, Food Science and Veterinary Medicine, Veterinary Sciences Centre,
University College Dublin, Belfield, Dublin 4, Republic of Ireland

Craig Johnson BVSc PhD DVA DipECVA MRCA MRCVS
Institute of Animal, Veterinary and Biomedical Sciences, Massey University, Private Bag 11 222, Palmerston North, New Zealand

Ronald S. Jones OBE JP DVSc FRCA FRCVS
Emeritus Professor of Veterinary Anaesthesia, Merseyside, UK

Sabine B.R. Kästner PD Dr med vet MVSc DipECVA
Clinic for Small Animals, University of Veterinary Medicine Hannover, Foundation Bischofsholer Damm 15, 30173 Hannover, Germany

Carolyn Kerr DVM DVSc PhD DipACVA
Department of Clinical Studies, University of Guelph, Ontario N1H 1Y3, Canada

Elizabeth Leece BVSc CVA DipECVA MRCVS
European Specialist in Veterinary Anaesthesia, The Animal Health Trust, Lanwades Park, Newmarket, Suffolk CB8 7UU, UK

Kip A. Lemke DVM MS DipACVA
Atlantic Veterinary College, University of Prince Edward Island, 550 University Avenue, Charlottetown, PE C1A 4P3, Canada

Nora S. Matthews DVM DipACVA
Texas A&M University, College Station, TX 77843-4474, USA

Robert E. Meyer DVM DipACVA
Department of Clinical Sciences, College of Veterinary Medicine, Mississippi State University, PO Box 6100, MS 39762-6100, USA

Yves Moens DVM PhD PD DipECVA
University of Veterinary Medicine, Department of Companion Animals and Horses,
Clinic of Anaesthesiology and Perioperative Intensive Care, Veterinärplatz 1, A-1210 Vienna, Austria

Paula F. Moon-Massat DVM DipACVA
New England Veterinary Anesthesia Services, Winchester, Massachusetts, and Director,
Preclinical Research, Biopure Corporation, Cambridge, Massachusetts, USA

Joanna C. Murrell BVSc (Hons) PhD DipECVA MRCVS
Institute of Animal, Veterinary and Biomedical Sciences, Massey University, Private Bag 11 222, Palmerston North, New Zealand

Gina Neiger-Aeschbacher Dr med vet DipACVA DipECVA MRCVS
Department of Clinical Veterinary Medicine, Vetsuisse Faculty, University of Bern, PO Box 8466, 3001 Bern, Switzerland

Andrea Nolan MVB MRCVS DVA PhD DipECVA DipECVPT
Office of Vice Principal (Learning, Teaching and Internationalisation), The Cloisters, Gilbert Scott Building, University of Glasgow, Glasgow G12 8QQ, UK

Elizabeth J. Norman BVSc MVM MACVSc MRCVS
Institute of Veterinary, Animal and Biomedical Sciences, Massey University, Private Bag 11 222, Palmerston North 4442, New Zealand

Peter J. Pascoe BVSc DVA DACVA DipECVA MRCVS
Department of Surgical and Radiological Sciences, School of Veterinary Medicine, University of California, Davis, CA 95616, USA

Lysa P. Posner DVM DipACVA
Department of Molecular Biomedical Sciences, College of Veterinary Medicine,
North Carolina State University, 4700 Hillsborough Street, Raleigh, NC 27606, USA

Jill Price BVMS PhD CertVA DipECVA
Department of Veterinary Clinical Studies, Saint George's University, Grenada, West Indies

Sarah Thomson BVSc CertVA MRCVS
Davies Veterinary Specialists, Manor Farm Business Park, Higham Gobion, Near Hitchin, Herts SG5 3HR, UK

Foreword

This new edition of the *BSAVA Manual of Canine and Feline Anaesthesia and Analgesia* has undergone massive changes since the last edition. A full section of four chapters on pain management has been added, reflecting the increased importance with which this subject is now considered in both human and veterinary medicine. These chapters include not only the basic science behind mechanisms of pain relief but much practical information concerning, for example, techniques utilising local anaesthesia and consideration of alternative therapies of providing analgesia. Among the many expanded areas there are now three chapters relating to equipment, including one which provides a comprehensive description of automatic ventilators suitable and available for small animal use. All other sections have been rewritten and updated.

This current book is one of a series which commenced as a very slim volume in 1979 as the *BSAVA Manual of Anaesthesia of Small Animal Practice*, and which was intended to provide a simple guide for those working in general practice. It was not until the 1989 edition that analgesia was awarded a chapter of its own! Each edition has seen expansion, yet the intention of use has not changed – everything in the new edition could be of relevance on a day-to-day basis to those in practice. The fact that the expansion has been necessary is a tribute to the continually improving practice standards of veterinary anaesthesia and pain management. The authors, all well known as 'experts' in the field of veterinary anaesthesia, come from every corner of the globe, and the book has been written so as to be relevant to veterinary surgeons in many countries. The content of the book now not only fulfils the original purpose of the series, but will be a useful text book for veterinary surgeons wishing to advance their knowledge, and possibly obtain further qualifications in veterinary anaesthesia and analgesia.

I thank the Editors, their authors and the BSAVA team assisting them from behind the scenes for all their work and congratulate them on the final outcome.

K.W. Clarke MA VetMB DVetMed DVA DipECVA FRCVS
RCVS and European Specialist in Veterinary Anaesthesia
Senior Lecturer in Veterinary Anaesthesia
Royal Veterinary College

February 2007

Preface

The administration of safe and reliable anaesthesia is important for all veterinary surgeons, whatever their primary area of expertise. The development of anaesthesia has also made possible some types of surgical intervention that would hitherto have been either impossible or extremely hazardous. In addition, good control of pain after injury, either traumatic or surgical, is one of our most important ethical responsibilities.

In compiling this new edition, we have retained the original broad sections dealing with basic principles, pharmacology and anaesthetic management in specific clinical situations. A new section on pain assessment and management has also been added. Details of anaesthesia and analgesia in exotic species have been moved to the relevant BSAVA Manuals.

Anaesthetic equipment, patient monitoring and anaesthetic accidents and emergencies are covered in much greater detail than in the previous edition, and the chapters on pharmacology and specific patient management revised or completely rewritten. We have used recommended international non-proprietary names (rINN) throughout, in line with the *BSAVA Small Animal Formulary*.

As with the previous edition, this book is aimed primarily at veterinary surgeons and students, but nurses and technicians will also find a wealth of useful information. We also hope those studying for examinations in veterinary anaesthesia will find the book useful. We have used contributors from around the world and have tried to make the book as universal as possible.

We are extremely grateful to all contributors, a truly international team of experts in their field, for finding the time to share their expertise and knowledge; also to Marion Jowett, Sabrina Cleevely and Nicola Lloyd at BSAVA, without whose help this book might never have come to fruition.

Chris Seymour
Tanya Duke-Novakovski

February 2007

1

Legal and ethical aspects of anaesthesia

Ronald S. Jones

Introduction

It is a fundamental aspect of veterinary medicine and surgery that adequate provision is made for the health and welfare of patients that are entrusted to our care. One of the most important aspects of this care is to prevent pain and suffering. A considerable amount of attention has been paid to the subject of pain in humans, but there is still scope for improvement. In animals, the situation has improved dramatically over the past decade but there is still much to be done. Pain is a subjective experience to the individual and is dependent both on the mental and physical state of the patient and on the environment. In animals, the perception of pain has to be inferred as they lack an effective means of verbal communication with humans. There are, however, no anatomical or physiological grounds to assume that animals do not perceive pain in a similar manner to humans. There are certain differences in the manifestation and the responses, but these can be attributed to species variation. This is a basic aspect of pain in animals where, for example, different behavioural reactions are observed in the cat and horse in response to a given painful stimulus.

Aims of anaesthesia

In general the aims of anaesthesia are to:

- Prevent awareness of, and response to, pain
- Provide restraint and immobility of the animal and relaxation of skeletal muscles when this is required for a particular procedure
- Achieve both of the above without jeopardizing the life and safety of the animal before, during and after anaesthesia.

Until relatively recently it was considered that a single anaesthetic agent could achieve all of these aims and occasionally this is still true today. However, as surgery becomes more complex and prolonged, and as new agents become available and new techniques are developed, a combination of agents with specific actions is more likely to be used to produce safe and relatively trouble-free anaesthesia.

Indications for anaesthesia

Animals are anaesthetized for a number of different reasons:

- **Humanitarian considerations.** It is a basic requirement that every effort should be made to relieve both pain and suffering in animals by all means available. Gentle and sympathetic handling with minimal restraint should always be used to reduce fear and apprehension and to avoid undue struggling, which has the potential to lead to injury to both patient and personnel. Adequate analgesia must always be provided as and when necessary
- **Technical considerations.** In view of the potentially uncooperative nature of veterinary patients, deep sedation or anaesthesia may be required as a means of restraint for procedures that are not considered painful (e.g. radiography). Other diagnostic and investigative procedures are often facilitated by a reduction in muscle tone and/or by intermittent positive pressure ventilation. Other technical considerations include the protection of personnel from injuries such as bites and scratches and accidental injury from hypodermic needles or scalpel blades
- **Legal considerations.** There is legislation in virtually all western countries which governs the prevention of pain and suffering in animals during treatment and procedures involving pain. In the UK, a number of Acts of Parliament are applicable. These include the Protection of Animals Act 1911, the Veterinary Surgeons Act 1966, the Protection of Animals (Anaesthetics) Act 1964 and the Scientific Procedures Act 1986. In the USA, there are no Federal Laws governing this particular area. As each state is its own political entity, the laws are only relevant to that particular geographical area, but there is a great deal of similarity between states.

Choice of anaesthetic technique

The ideal anaesthetic agent has not been developed, although the properties of such an agent have been defined. These include:

- Independence of the detoxification mechanisms of the body for the agent's destruction and elimination
- Rapid induction, quick changes in the depth of anaesthesia and a rapid recovery

- Lack of depression of the respiratory and cardiac centres
- Non-irritant to tissues
- Inexpensive, stable, non-inflammable and non-explosive
- No requirement for expensive equipment for its administration.

A wide variety of factors influences the choice of a particular anaesthetic technique. These include:

- **Facilities.** If facilities are poor and likely to prejudice the outcome of the anaesthetic procedure, they should not be used. For example, a well administered intravenous technique may be much safer than an inhalation agent given with inferior equipment
- **Skill and experience** of the anaesthetist and the surgeon. These are extremely important in choosing a technique (particularly noticeable if they are used to working as a team)
- **Facilities for postoperative recovery and care.** This will be influenced by whether the animal is to be hospitalized or returned to its owner following anaesthesia (see legal aspects below). It is important to ensure that adequate postoperative analgesia is provided
- **Temperament of the patient.** This can have an important influence on the choice of technique. In animals of good temperament, a minimum of sedative premedication may be required before the intravenous induction of anaesthesia. Competent and sympathetic assistance in restraint can be of extreme value. Some cats may be so unruly that crush cages or inhalation anaesthetic induction chambers are needed. Vicious dogs may require heavy sedative premedication before anaesthesia, which can influence the subsequent doses of both induction and maintenance agents
- **Species and breed of animal.** These can influence the choice of technique. Some breeds respond adversely to some intravenous agents. Some Boxers are sensitive to acepromazine
- **Age.** This is an important factor influencing the choice of anaesthetic agents and the doses used. Doses may need to be reduced in both young and elderly animals. In puppies and kittens of a very young age, inhalation agents are the drugs of choice. Such patients are also very susceptible to hypothermia
- **State of health of the animal.** The state of health of the animal is an important factor in the choice of technique. The physical status of the patient is often classified according to the five categories of the American Society of Anesthesiologists for human patients (see Chapter 2). The categories are classified from 1 to 5, where 1 is a normal healthy patient and 5 is moribund. Toxaemia is one of the most important disease conditions as it is often accompanied by cardiac and hepatic problems. Extra care is needed in the administration of computed doses to such patients, who may require very much lower doses than normal animals. Toxaemic animals may have a slow circulation and if this is not appreciated then overdosing with intravenous agents may occur. The myocardium may also be affected, which may lead to cardiac failure. Problems with fluid balance should be corrected and diabetic patients stabilized before anaesthesia. It is important that animals are in optimal health before anaesthesia, even if this means deferring anaesthesia for some days
- **Site and nature of the surgery.** These influence the choice of technique. Operations on the head and neck require endotracheal intubation. Special care must be taken during oral, dental and pharyngeal surgery to prevent the accumulation of any foreign material that could be inhaled after the removal of the endotracheal tube. The use of an endoscope within the respiratory tract presents problems because of competition for the airway, and anaesthetic techniques need to be adapted to deal with the problem
- **Use of muscle relaxant drugs.** Intermittent positive pressure ventilation is essential when relaxant drugs are used as part of the anaesthetic technique, e.g. to provide profound muscle relaxation for surgery of the thorax and abdomen and some orthopaedic procedures
- **Anaesthesia for Caesarean section.** This requires special techniques as multiple lives are involved
- **Examination under anaesthesia.** Although this normally requires only short periods of anaesthesia, a high level of care is required. The old adage that 'there may be minor procedures but never minor anaesthetics' certainly applies
- **Proposed duration of surgery.** This must always be considered when selecting an appropriate anaesthetic technique. Short procedures can often be carried out with a single dose of thiopental and slightly longer ones with multiple doses of propofol. Even under these circumstances equipment must be readily available to carry out endotracheal intubation and intermittent positive pressure ventilation. In situations where procedures are likely to be prolonged it is important to ensure that proper inhalation anaesthetic techniques are used.

Legislation

Veterinary Surgeons Act 1966

In the UK, the practice of veterinary medicine and surgery is governed by the Veterinary Surgeons Act 1966 and under that Act no person may practise unless he or she is registered with the Royal College of Veterinary Surgeons. There are certain minor exceptions under Schedule 3, which refer to certain procedures that may be performed by trained lay personnel and by veterinary nurses. None of these exemptions applies to the induction and maintenance of anaesthesia in animals.

The Protection of Animals (Anaesthetics) Act 1964

The Protection of Animals (Anaesthetics) Act 1964 governs anaesthesia of animals in the UK. It basically states that the performance of any operation, with or without the use of instruments and involving interference with the sensitive tissues or bone structures of an animal, shall constitute an offence unless an anaesthetic is used in such a way as to prevent any pain to the animal during the operation. Some exceptions to this general rule are included in the Act. They include:

- Castration of farm animals up to certain ages (anaesthesia is always required for the castration of cats and dogs)
- Amputation of the dewclaws of a dog before its eyes are open
- Any minor operation performed by a veterinary surgeon, which by reason of its quickness or painlessness is customarily performed without the use of an anaesthetic
- Any minor operation (whether performed by a veterinary surgeon or by some other person) which is not customarily performed by a veterinary surgeon. Other procedures not covered in the previous sentence are listed in the Act but apply mainly to farm animals.

The Misuse of Drugs Act 1971

The Misuse of Drugs Act 1971 and its various regulations govern the use of several agents that are administered to cats and dogs to provide anaesthesia and analgesia. The regulations impose legal obligations on all veterinary surgeons (as well as doctors, dentists and pharmacists) prescribing, supplying and administering these drugs. Over 100 substances are listed and they are placed in four schedules, which relate mainly to potential for harm to, and abuse by, human subjects:

- Schedule 1 drugs (such as cannabis and LSD) have no veterinary use and veterinary surgeons have no authority to prescribe them
- Schedule 2 drugs include morphine, fentanyl and methadone. A record of their purchase and supply must be kept in a bound controlled drug (CD) register (see below). A handwritten requisition is required by a supplier/wholesaler before delivery is permitted
- Schedule 3 drugs include buprenorphine and barbiturates. These require a requisition but their purchase and use do not have to be recorded
- Schedule 4 drugs include the benzodiazepines and are exempt from most controls.

Separate registers must be kept for all Schedule 2 drugs that are used and supplied. It is also a requirement that these drugs are to be kept in a locked safe/cabinet that can be opened only by an authorized person or with an authorized person's consent. The cabinet should preferably be made of steel, with suitable hinges, fixed to a wall or the floor with rag bolts (these bolts should not be accessible from outside the cabinet). Ideally the safe/cabinet should be within a cupboard or in some other position to avoid easy detection by intruders. Also, the room containing the safe/cabinet should be lockable. A locked motor vehicle is *not* classed as a locked receptacle. It makes sense to lock *all* Schedule 3 drugs (with Schedule 2) in the CD cabinet.

The CD register must:

- Be a bound register with appropriately ruled and headed columns (there are commercially printed registers available of varying standards)
- Have the drugs to which the entries relate specified at the head of the page
- Show drugs obtained and drugs supplied. The name and address of the person or firm from whom they are received should be recorded, as well as the name and address of the owner and animal supplied
- Be kept on the premises and be available for inspection
- Be kept for 2 years from the date of the last entry
- Have entries written in indelible ink
- Have two members of staff sign the register, one of whom would be a witness
- Have entries in chronological order, made on the day of transaction or on the following day
- Have no cancellations or obliterations or alterations (corrections must be made in indelible ink in the margin or as a footnote and must be signed and dated).

Controlled drugs in Schedules 1 or 2 may only be destroyed in the presence of a person authorized by the Secretary of State, e.g. a police officer or Home Office inspector. Such an authorized person would be required to be present for the destruction of out-of-date stock items from Schedule 1 or 2. Details of the drug being destroyed must be entered in the controlled drugs register, including the drug name, form, strength and quantity as well as the date of destruction and the signature of the person in whose presence the drug was destroyed.

Whilst the legislation may differ in detail from country to country (and from state to state in the USA), similar laws apply to the secure storage and record keeping of this group of drugs.

The Animals (Scientific Procedures) Act 1986

The Animals (Scientific Procedures) Act 1986 governs the use and care of experimental animals for research purposes. It is specific about the use of analgesic and anaesthetic agents. Similar legislation exists in the European Community and there is Federal legislation on the subject in the USA. The Canadian Council on Animal Care issues welfare guidelines for animals used for research in Canada, including anaesthetic and analgesic use.

Duty of care

The principles of the duty of care, as defined in Halsbury's Laws of England, apply equally to veterinary surgeons as to medical practitioners, with one distinct difference, namely that the duty of care is to the client/animal owner in making a number of decisions relating to anaesthesia. These include:

- A duty of care in deciding whether anaesthesia may be performed with a reasonable degree of safety
- A duty of care deciding on the most appropriate technique of anaesthesia
- A duty of care in the administration of the anaesthetic
- A duty of care in fully consulting other veterinary surgeons dealing with the case and offering full and proper advice to the animal owner.

Negligence

The anaesthetist must bring to his/her task a reasonable degree of skill and knowledge and must exercise a reasonable degree of care. Whether this has been done is a matter that must be determined by the facts pertaining to each individual case. It is clear, however, that failure to do so, which results in injury to (or death of) an animal will give the owner the right to bring a legal action for damages. In general, a veterinary surgeon in practice anaesthetizing an animal will be judged against the standard of the good, careful and competent general practitioner. However, a veterinary surgeon of specialist or consultant status will be judged against the standard of his/her peers.

There is also the very important aspect of the responsibility of the veterinary surgeon for negligence by any person assisting him/her with the anaesthesia of an animal. In general practice, it is likely that a veterinary surgeon as an employer would be responsible for the negligence of an employee. It is likely that when assessing an action for negligence of a lay assistant, the courts would have regard to their level of training and qualifications. Hence, it is essential to ensure that any person asked to assist with anaesthesia is competent to carry out the tasks assigned to them.

In recent years there have been two high profile court cases involving dogs being returned to their owners before they were fully recovered from anaesthesia. Both animals died. The courts found the veterinary surgeons to be negligent.

There is often confusion between negligence and disgraceful professional conduct which could lead to disciplinary action by the Royal College of Veterinary Surgeons. Negligence *per se* does not necessarily amount to disgraceful professional conduct unless it is so gross and excessive that it is likely to bring the veterinary profession into disrepute. It is only then that a disciplinary action may ensue.

Consent

There is a definite difference in law between the duty to obtain consent from an owner for a particular procedure to be carried out on an animal, and the duty to inform them of the material risks. Whilst there is a considerable amount of information and case law on the subject in human medicine compared to the veterinary field, it is reasonable to assume that the courts would follow a similar course of action. Failure to obtain consent may constitute a trespass, whereas failure to warn of material risks may give rise to an obligation to compensate for damages caused by that breach of duty. It could result in a claim for compensation in respect of a complication or side effect of the treatment even if that procedure was conducted properly. Consent is a state of mind – a decision by the animal owner. The competent adult owner, over 18 years of age, has a fundamental right under common law to give or withhold consent to examination, investigation or treatment. Consent may be *implied* or *express*:

- **Consent is implied** when an owner brings an animal to a veterinary surgeon for examination and there is physical contact between the veterinary surgeon and the animal. Implied consent does not necessarily imply that the material risks of any procedure have been explained or understood
- **Express consent** should be obtained for any procedure which carries a material risk and this, of course, applies to anaesthesia. Whilst express consent may be obtained orally or in writing it is always preferable to obtain written consent wherever possible. It is not acceptable for an owner to sign a blank piece of paper; it is essential that they have given their consent for a procedure and to provide evidence that the material risks have been explained to them. In the exceptional situation that oral consent is obtained, it is essential that a record of the advice offered and that consent was given should be written in the case notes. Written consent is not necessary to defend an action although it does provide evidence that consent was obtained.

It may occasionally be necessary to provide treatment and carry out a procedure without consent, although this is rarely used except for a life-saving procedure where it is not possible to contact the animal owner. When this is done a note should be made in the case notes to explain the absence of formal consent.

Adult owners have a right to refuse to consent to a particular procedure with or without good reason. If consent is refused for an anaesthetic procedure that is considered to be the most appropriate, then reasonable attempts should be made to persuade the owner that the technique carries the least risk of adverse sequelae. However, it is not acceptable to coerce owners into accepting a specific technique. In certain situations it may be necessary to point out to owners that a failure to prevent suffering may well bring them into breach of the Protection of Animals Act 1911.

A copy of the specimen consent form recommended by the Royal College of Veterinary Surgeons is shown in Figure 1.1.

A veterinary surgeon may administer a veterinary medicine outwith the data sheet recommendations ('off-label'), a human medicine, a specially prepared medicine or an imported medicine under certain circumstances. The veterinary surgeon should explain fully what is involved and ideally obtain the owner's written consent. A sample consent form can be found on the Veterinary Defence Society website (www.veterinarydefencesociety.co.uk). It is also necessary to inform the owner and obtain their consent when drugs are being used in a clinical trial.

Personnel

The role of the veterinary nurse or veterinary technician in anaesthesia is often the subject of debate within the profession. It is well accepted that both the maintenance of anaesthetic equipment and preparation for anaesthesia can be delegated to these staff. They also play an important part in the restraint and management of animals during induction of anaesthesia. However, in the UK the induction and maintenance of anaesthesia is an act of veterinary surgery under the Veterinary Surgeons Act 1966. Veterinary nurses are often involved in the monitoring of anaesthesia but the ultimate responsibility is that of the veterinary surgeon (see negligence above).

A similar situation applies in North America, even though it appears that more responsibility is taken by veterinary technicians. In most states and provinces the law clearly states that the technician must be under the supervision of a veterinary surgeon, and most stipulate that they must be under *direct* supervision. This has come to be interpreted that the veterinary surgeon must be on the premises even if not in close proximity to the animal. This appears to be legal and acceptable. However, if there are problems, the veterinary surgeon is still ultimately responsible.

CONSENT FOR ANAESTHESIA AND SURGICAL PROCEDURES

Species and breed ....

Name ....

Colour ....

Age .... Sex M/F/NM/NF

Microchip/tattoo/brand ....

Owner/agent's name ....

Address ....

....

....

Telephone Home ....

Work ....

Mobile ....

Operation/procedure ....

I hereby give permission for the administration of an anaesthetic to the above animal and to the surgical operation/procedure detailed on this form together with any procedures which may prove necessary. The nature of these procedures and of such other procedures as might prove necessary have been explained to me and I understand that all anaesthetic techniques and surgical procedures involve some risk to the animal. I accept that the likely cost will be as detailed on the attached estimate, and that in the event of further treatment being required or of complications occurring which will give rise to additional costs, I shall be contacted as soon as practicable so that my consent to such additional costs may be obtained.

Signature ....

Owner/agent's name ....
(Block capitals)

Date ....

1.1 Specimen consent form recommended by the Royal College of Veterinary Surgeons.

2

Pre-anaesthetic assessment

Lysa P. Posner

Introduction

Benefits of evaluating veterinary patients before general anaesthesia are often underestimated. With the advancement of veterinary medicine and surgery, the veterinary surgeon nowadays will routinely anaesthetize older and sicker patients. At present, peri-anaesthetic mortality for dogs and cats is approximately 1 in 2,000 patients. By comparison, peri-anaesthetic mortality in people is approximately 1 in 10,000 patients. Thus, there is still room for veterinary surgeons to decrease peri-anaesthetic mortality rates. One approach to minimize morbidity and mortality is to identify at-risk patients and modify the anaesthetic plan accordingly.

The American Society of Anesthesiologists (ASA) has developed a scale to rate physical status (Figure 2.1). A patient is assigned a category status from 1 to 5. 1 denotes healthy, and 5 is moribund. An 'E' following the number denotes 'emergency'. This scale has been shown to be predictive of anaesthetic morbidity and mortality in veterinary patients. Animals with an ASA score of 3 or greater are almost four times more likely to suffer peri-anaesthetic complications compared to those in ASA category 1 or 2. Thus, accurately assigning an ASA score is a proven way to identify at-risk patients. In order to assign an ASA status properly, a thorough pre-anaesthetic evaluation must be performed.

ASA scale	Physical description	Veterinary patient examples
1	Normal patient with no disease	Healthy patient for ovariohysterectomy or castration
2	Patient with mild systemic disease that does not limit normal function	Controlled diabetes mellitus, mild cardiac valve insufficiency
3	Patient with severe systemic disease that limits normal function	Uncontrolled diabetes mellitus, symptomatic heart disease
4	Patient with severe systemic disease that is a constant threat to life	Sepsis, organ failure, heart failure
5	Patient that is moribund and not expected to live 24 hours without surgery	Shock, multiple-organ failure, severe trauma
E	Describes patient as an emergency	Gastric dilatation–volvulus, respiratory distress

2.1 American Society of Anesthesiologists (ASA) scale of physical status.

Patient assessment

Veterinary patients are a heterogenous group, both in physical stature and disease state. Many companion animals are also anaesthetized for procedures other than surgery. Knowledge of the procedure can help direct the focus of a pre-anaesthetic evaluation, although the veterinary surgeon must resist focusing only on the obvious problem. Fractious or feral patients may require anaesthesia to facilitate examination, and may be healthy (feral cat for castration) or severely compromised (aggressive dog hit by car). Furthermore, patients may require anaesthesia to allow imaging or diagnostics (medical imaging, endoscopy, angiography). Again, patients range from healthy (radiographic examination for hip dysplasia) to severely compromised (magnetic resonance imaging for brain tumour). However, the vast majority of patients are anaesthetized to allow surgery. Patients range from healthy (routine ovariohysterectomy) to critically ill (intestinal obstruction). It is important to understand the surgical/diagnostic plan and whether anaesthesia is elective, scheduled or urgent. Pre-anaesthetic assessment must therefore be tailored to each patient.

History

Each patient should have a complete history taken from the owner. This is an opportunity not only to gather useful information about the patient, but also to engage the owner and allow questions and concerns to be raised. Some animals cannot be handled for physical examination or diagnostic testing (wildlife or fractious animals), and the history may be the only knowledge of the patient the veterinary surgeon will have before anaesthesia is induced. The patient history should include the following details.

Signalment

Basic information should include species, breed, age, gender and whether the patient has been neutered. Knowledge of breed characteristics and certain medical conditions pertinent to the breed can provide information about additional anaesthetic concerns (see later). Age might influence whether further diagnostic tests are warranted, and influence choice of drugs and the doses used.

Chief complaint/reason for surgery

This information should include duration and severity of the presenting problem. It should include any abnormal physical signs and any treatment received. Although this will narrow the focus, the veterinary surgeon should remain cautious, so as not to have 'tunnel vision', and remember to assess the whole patient.

Complete medical history

This information should include any other pertinent medical history, including vaccination and, in relevant areas, heartworm status. It is important to ask the owner directly about each individual organ system (Figure 2.2) as many animals have concurrent diseases that could affect the way anaesthesia is managed. It is also useful to know if the animal has undergone anaesthesia before and whether there were any adverse effects. Good record keeping within a practice can provide useful information.

Body system/ other	Points of interest
Owner	Complete contact information, special considerations, e.g. consent, 'do not resuscitate' orders
Medical history	Present and previous illness, surgery and anaesthetics, current medications, vaccination status, heartworm status
Pre-anaesthetic preparedness	Fasted, clean, signed consent form
General	Attitude, activity, appetite, gain or loss of weight
Integument	Itch, hair loss, wounds, infection
Cardiovascular system	Activity, stamina, cough, fainting episodes
Respiratory system	Cough, sneeze, wheeze, dyspnoea, gagging, change of voice
Gastrointestinal system	Faeces, vomiting, regurgitation
Genitourinary system	Urination, reproductive status, pregnancy
Central nervous system	Mentation, balance, tremor, seizure, aggression

2.2 Guidelines on which areas to concentrate on while taking a patient's history.

Preparation for anaesthesia

Fasting/water deprivation

Fasting is routinely recommended before general anaesthesia to decrease the amount of food and fluid in the stomach, and decrease risk of aspiration. Fasting is considered unpleasant by many owners and can be deleterious in some patients. Young or thin animals or patients with a fast metabolism are at risk for hypoglycaemia. Patients with increased fluid requirements (fever, renal insufficiency, diabetes) can quickly become dehydrated during long periods of water deprivation. In people, allowing an abbreviated fast does not result in increased morbidity in healthy patients. Furthermore, prolonged fasting in animals has been associated with increased incidence of reflux and increased gastric acidity. Based on this information, it is probably prudent to have a moderate fasting period (6–8 hours for food and 2–4 hours for water) before the premedication stage of anaesthesia for average, reasonably healthy patients.

Owner comprehension and permission

Before anaesthesia, the owner should understand both anaesthetic and surgical risks. A frank discussion should take place about what to do in an emergency situation (e.g. 'do not resuscitate' orders). The owner should also sign a consent form (see Chapter 1).

Cleanliness

Due to the hair coat of domestic pets, many veterinary surgeons recommend that all anaesthetic/surgical patients are recently bathed and are free of fleas and ticks. The patient's coat, season, geographical location and procedure performed should dictate whether this is necessary.

Physical examination

Ideally, every patient should have a complete physical examination within the week before surgery and a further cursory examination on the day of anaesthesia. Patients presented for emergency anaesthesia should be evaluated as completely as possible. General assessment should include the following areas.

Body condition score

Patients are generally given a score from 1 to 9 (1 is cachectic and 9 is obese). Body condition can provide information about chronicity of a disease process, and can serve as an alert for potential problems during anaesthesia. In general, obese animals have diminished cardiovascular function and are at risk for hypoventilation, while cachectic animals have poor reserves and are at risk for hypothermia and hypoglycaemia.

Hydration

All patients should have hydration status evaluated. Skin turgor, moisture of mucous membranes and sunken eyes can all be used to assess hydration physically. Hydration estimation is important because dehydrated animals are likely to have decreased intravascular volume and electrolyte abnormalities. Whenever possible, rehydration and electrolyte stabilization should take place before anaesthesia (see Chapter 16).

Cardiovascular system

All patients should have mucous membrane colour and capillary refill time assessed, and the heart auscultated for rate, rhythm and murmurs. Pulses should be examined for subjective assessment of vascular tone and synchronicity with heart sounds. Murmurs and arrhythmias can be indicators of significant cardiac dysfunction and should be further evaluated before anaesthesia (e.g. radiographs, electrocardiogram (ECG)).

Pulmonary system

All patients should have breathing patterns observed at rest, colour of mucous membranes assessed and lungs auscultated for breath sounds. Additionally, the trachea should be palpated and an attempt made to elicit a cough. Inducible coughs can indicate tracheitis or collapsing trachea, both of which could increase perianaesthetic morbidity. Attention is directed to increased respiratory rates, dyspnoea, areas of diminished or wet breath sounds, crackles or wheezes. These changes can all indicate decreased pulmonary performance and the need for further assessment (e.g. radiographs, pulse oximetry, arterial blood gas measurement).

Gastrointestinal and urinary systems

Abdominal palpation should be performed to identify discomfort or structural abnormalities. The gastrointestinal system is often considered irrelevant in the pre-anaesthetic evaluation, but disease states can have an effect on anaesthetized patients. Viscus dilation, pancreatitis and abdominal cavity inflammation are painful conditions. Enlargement of abdominal organs can impede venous return and place pressure on the diaphragm causing hypoventilation. Decreased venous return can decrease cardiac output causing low blood pressure. Impaired ventilation can result in hypoxaemia and hypercapnia.

Integument

The skin should also be evaluated for infection and skin characteristics. Although this is often overlooked in a pre-anaesthetic examination, the health of the skin can affect how anaesthesia is performed. Catheters and epidural/spinal injections should not be placed through infected skin, as this increases the possibility of transferring infection to within the body. Additionally, skin characteristics can point to other concurrent disease processes (e.g. thin, friable skin to Cushing's disease; ulcerated skin to autoimmune diseases). Some breeds tend to have thicker skin, and this can make vein catheterization challenging.

Neurological system

A basic neurological examination should be performed. Since all anaesthetics affect the central nervous system (CNS), it is prudent to find any problems before anaesthesia is induced. Patients with CNS depression are sensitive to many anaesthetic drugs and an exaggerated response may be observed with even low doses of anaesthetics. Animals that may have elevated intracranial pressure should be anaesthetized cautiously as intracranial pressure can increase further with certain drugs (e.g. ketamine), intubation and with hypercapnia (common during anaesthesia) (see Chapter 26). Patients with neuromuscular disease can have weakened respiratory musculature leading to hypoventilation and hypoxaemia under anaesthesia.

Clinical diagnostics

In addition to a thorough physical examination, many patients may require additional tests before anaesthesia. Which tests are performed is based on patient age, surgical procedure, concurrent disease processes and the owner's ability to pay. Although it is tempting to simply 'run every test', it is wiser to run tests on body systems where results will alter the anaesthetic plan. As more information is obtained, the risk assessment associated with anaesthesia may change and owners should be updated with this information before the animal is anaesthetized.

Although there is controversy regarding the percentage of patients that benefit from routinely running full pre-anaesthetic blood tests, it is clear that if testing is not performed, no abnormalities can be found. Many practices compromise by running inexpensive basic bloodwork prior to anaesthesia.

Packed cell volume, total solids, blood glucose and blood urea nitrogen

Minimum bloodwork in young, otherwise healthy animals presented for elective procedures should consist of packed cell volume (PCV), total solids (TS), blood glucose and blood urea nitrogen (BUN). These four tests can detect anaemia, hypo-/hyperproteinaemia, kidney disease and hypo-/hyperglycaemia. This wealth of information can be obtained with little blood, equipment or cost. If any abnormalities are noted, then further testing or evaluation can be performed.

Complete blood count, serum chemistry and urinalysis

In older or infirm animals, more comprehensive testing should be performed to screen for occult problems. In general, complete blood count (CBC), serum chemistry and urinalysis should be completed. These three tests can be diagnostic for diseases such as diabetes (see Chapter 25), or indicate the need for further tests (e.g. bile acids to check liver function).

Tests for heartworm

Depending on the geographical location of a veterinary facility or travel history of the patient, prevalence of heartworm disease in dogs and cats can greatly vary. In endemic areas, heartworm status should be known before anaesthesia is induced, as heart failure and sudden death are possible with heartworm disease.

Tests for thyroid function

Ideally, any animal that shows physical evidence of thyroid dysfunction should be evaluated before anaesthesia. Hypothyroidism in dogs is associated with obesity and a hypometabolic state. Hyperthyroid cats are generally underweight, have high metabolic demands and often have hypertrophic cardiomyopathy. Both of these thyroid conditions and subsequent effects on other organ systems increase anaesthetic risk. When possible, hypo- or hyperthyroid animals should be treated before the anaesthetic episode (see Chapter 25).

Coagulation profile

Animals at risk for increased bleeding based on breed (e.g. Dobermann), disease (e.g. portosystemic shunt) or procedure (e.g. liver biopsy) should be screened for the presence of coagulopathies. When possible, blood coagulation tests or specific factor determination should be performed in advance of the scheduled procedure. Abnormal results can become grounds to cancel elective surgical procedures due to a high risk of uncontrollable bleeding. Non-elective procedures must often proceed, but with knowledge that excessive bleeding might occur and the need for blood products will be increased (see Chapter 16).

Radiological examination

The most used imaging modality in veterinary private practices remains radiography. Radiography can be used to assess the size and shape of many internal organs (heart, liver, kidney) and can identify abnormal organ position (e.g. gastric dilatation–volvulus (GDV)), structures (e.g. tumour) or densities (e.g. air, fluid). Radiographs can be taken for routine screening (post-trauma or geriatric patients) or when assessing a particular problem.

Electrocardiography

Routine ECG screening is recommended for older animals, patients with evidence of cardiac disease or patients with underlying disease that might lead to arrhythmias (hyperkalaemia, splenomegaly, GDV, post-traumatic myocarditis). For veterinary surgeons who do not feel comfortable evaluating ECGs, advancements in technology now allow for ECG consultation with a cardiologist through a telephone line.

Echocardiography

An echocardiographic examination should be performed in patients that have evidence of cardiac disease on physical examination, radiographical changes to the heart and/or an abnormal ECG. Echocardiography should also be performed in patients that have a disease associated with changes in cardiac function (e.g. feline hyperthyroidism). This examination will provide further information on anatomical or contractile changes. This information is useful for establishing anaesthetic risk, and to assess the ability of the cardiovascular system to cope with stress.

Computed tomography and magnetic resonance imaging

More specialized diagnostics can provide even further information, but unfortunately these imaging modalities require general anaesthesia for veterinary species and are therefore rarely useful prior to induction of anaesthesia. Management of the patient for computed tomography or magnetic resonance imaging can be found in Chapter 26.

Other anaesthetic considerations

Recent trauma

Traumatized patients can have multiple changes or injuries that increase anaesthetic risk. Recently traumatized animals often require anaesthesia for surgical repair of obvious injuries (e.g. fractured limbs). It should be remembered that these patients often have more than one injury (see Chapters 19, 21 and 26). It is commonplace for these patients to have hidden injuries that are potentially life-threatening (e.g. pneumothorax). Traumatized patients should be evaluated for presence of shock, bleeding, abdominal or thoracic injuries or cardiac abnormalities. It is imperative that the veterinary surgeon does not lose sight of the whole patient in a rush to fix the obvious problem.

Breed considerations

While it is obvious that the Great Dane, Bulldog and Yorkshire Terrier are all dogs, they can require different anaesthetic management. Below is a short list of breeds that have known risk factors associated with anaesthesia/surgery.

Dobermann

Abnormal concentrations of von Willebrand factor occur in 73% of Dobermanns. With such a high frequency, it is reasonable that all Dobermanns are screened before elective surgery. If a Dobermann is presented for emergency anaesthesia and the status is unknown, the buccal mucosal bleeding time (BMBT) should be assessed. A dog deficient in von Willebrand factor or with prolonged BMBT may require additional treatment (desmopressin acetate, cryoprecipitate or whole blood) to limit bleeding during surgery (see Chapter 16).

Miniature Schnauzer

Miniature Schnauzers, particularly bitches, are at risk for developing sick sinus syndrome. They may appear normal on physical examination, but it is possible for occult disease to be unmasked by anaesthesia. It is therefore recommended that all Miniature Schnauzers have an ECG evaluated before any anaesthetic drugs are given. If sick sinus syndrome is detected before an elective procedure, the anaesthetic should be cancelled and the heart disease evaluated (see Chapter 19).

Boxer

Certain familial lines of Boxers appear to be quite sensitive to the effects of acepromazine, and can have an exaggerated response to the sedative and hypotensive effects of the drug. There are anecdotal reports of dogs fainting from what is assumed to be hypotension. Interestingly, bradycardia has been reported to occur alongside hypotension, prompting the recommendation that an anticholinergic (e.g. glycopyrronium) is used with acepromazine in Boxers or that acepromazine is avoided in this breed altogether.

Brachycephalic breeds

The brachycephalic breeds (e.g. Bulldog, Pug) are thick-necked dogs that often have small tracheas, elongated soft palates and stenotic nares. Additionally, the laryngeal mucous membranes are prone to swelling, which can compromise an already tenuous airway. Recommendations for these breeds include gentle intubation with an appropriately sized endotracheal tube (which might be smaller than expected based on the weight of the dog), and late extubation performed with the dog in sternal recumbency. Dogs of these breeds should be monitored post extubation for a number of hours for any sign of respiratory distress. Heavy sedation should be avoided unless the patient can be closely monitored with attention to oxygenation and ventilation.

Greyhounds and sighthounds

Anaesthetic recovery from thiopental occurs through redistribution. The drug moves from brain to blood to fat and is eventually removed through hepatic metabolism. Therefore, dogs with low fat stores, either through genetics or disease, tend to have higher concentrations of intravenously administered drugs in circulating blood, and this can lead to lengthy recoveries and potential overdosing. Sighthounds tend to be lean dogs with a low fat:body mass ratio. In addition to lower fat deposits, Greyhounds are missing a liver enzyme needed for metabolism of barbiturates; therefore the effects can be prolonged (up to four times longer than in mixed breed dogs). Although barbiturates do not depress the cardiovascular system in Greyhounds or sighthounds any more than in other breeds, the prolonged recovery would suggest they not be used in these breeds, or used with care. There are better alternatives available for induction such as propofol or a ketamine/diazepam combination.

Concurrent drug use

Many veterinary patients require anaesthesia while receiving medications for other disease processes. It is imperative that the drugs are identified and a decision made whether to discontinue their administration, or to avoid certain anaesthetic drugs.

Antibiotics

Many animals will concurrently be receiving antibiotic therapy, although most do not interfere or cause a problem with anaesthesia. However, the aminoglycoside antibiotics (e.g. gentamicin) can be nephrotoxic. Patients receiving aminoglycosides should be screened for renal disease and precautions taken to limit renal damage under anaesthesia (i.e. good perfusion, good hydration). Additionally, the aminoglycosides can interfere with neuromuscular transmission and could potentiate the neuromuscular blockade from peripherally acting neuromuscular-blocking drugs (e.g. atracurium) or disease (e.g. myasthenia gravis).

Cardiac drugs

Drugs for treatment of heart failure are becoming commonly used in veterinary practice. It is imperative the veterinary surgeon knows the class of drugs used and the potential effects during anaesthesia. In general, cardiac drugs should be continued during the peri-anaesthetic period and side effects should be anticipated.

Angiotensin converting enzyme inhibitors: Angiotensin converting enzyme (ACE) inhibitors (e.g. ramipril, enalapril, benazepril) are commonly used as vasodilators to prevent and treat heart failure (decrease afterload). These drugs interfere with the renin–angiotensin–aldosterone system and can result in clinically significant hypotension under anaesthesia.

Cardiac glycosides: Cardiac glycosides (e.g. digoxin) are positive inotropes used to prevent and treat heart failure as well as to treat some arrhythmias (increase cardiac contractility and output, and slow heart rate). Although these drugs allow the heart to work more productively, there is a narrow therapeutic margin and overdoses can result in ECG and contractility abnormalities. Patients treated with cardiac glycosides are sensitive to hypomagnesaemia, hypokalaemia, hypovolaemia and hypoxaemia, and these conditions will increase ventricular arrhythmias. Patients receiving digoxin should not receive anticholinergics.

Beta blockers: Beta blockers (e.g. propranolol, esmolol) are class II anti-arrhythmics and block beta-1 and beta-2 adrenergic receptors. These drugs are primarily used to treat tachyarrhythmia and their use alongside anaesthetic drugs can result in bradycardia and decreased cardiac contractility.

Analgesics

Opioids: Opioids (e.g. morphine, methadone, hydromorphone, fentanyl) are drugs that bind to opioid receptors and provide analgesia. Aside from analgesia these drugs can cause clinically significant bradycardia, second-degree heart block, respiratory depression and vomiting, and are synergistic with other anaesthetic drugs. Care should be taken routinely to monitor the patient's heart and respiratory rate when using these drugs.

Tramadol: This is by classification a mu opioid agonist, but analgesia is also from inhibition of noradrenaline and serotonin uptake. Tramadol is gaining favour in the veterinary community because it is not controlled, has reasonable efficacy and can be administered orally. However, tramadol should be used with caution in patients taking monoamine oxidase (MAO) inhibitors or tricyclic antidepressants, which also increase circulating serotonin levels. Elevated serotonin levels can lead to 'serotonin syndrome' which can be expressed as drowsiness, restlessness, altered mentation, muscle twitching, high body temperature, shivering, diarrhoea, unconsciousness and death.

Non-steroidal anti-inflammatory drugs (NSAIDs): These are frequently used for analgesia in anaesthetized patients. These drugs are potent analgesics through interference with prostaglandin synthesis in the arachidonic acid inflammatory pathway. Although inhibition of certain prostaglandins results in analgesia, inhibition of other prostaglandins necessary for normal physiological functions can be detrimental. NSAIDs can interfere with gastric mucosal protection, renal blood flow and coagulation. Different NSAIDs have different side effects and safety profiles, particularly with different species, so the veterinary surgeon must be familiar with the particular NSAID and the species in which it is used. Patients that are dehydrated, hypovolaemic, hypotensive or who might become this way, should not be given NSAIDs. Furthermore, patients with a history of vomiting or diarrhoea, or those given corticosteroids should also not receive NSAIDs.

N-methyl-D-aspartate (NMDA) antagonists

Ketamine and amantadine: These are used to treat chronic pain states. Ketamine is routinely used as an injectable anaesthetic, but can be used at sub-anaesthetic doses to treat refractory pain. When used at low doses it is unlikely that either of these drugs would significantly interact with other anaesthetics.

Behaviour modification drugs

Selegiline (L-deprenyl): This is used to treat dogs with canine cognitive disorder ('old dog dementia') and separation anxiety. Selegiline is an MAO inhibitor which results in increased levels of dopamine as well as other monoamines, such as serotonin. Dogs receiving selegiline should not be given pethidine (meperidine) or tramadol, both of which interfere with serotonin reuptake and can lead to 'serotonin syndrome' (see earlier).

Clomipramine: This is a tricyclic antidepressant that prevents reuptake of serotonin and noradrenaline. The same precautions should be taken as for selegiline (see above).

Incontinence drugs

Phenylpropanolamine: This is a sympathomimetic which increases urethral sphincter tone due to increased noradrenaline release. The increase in noradrenaline can result in clinical hypertension and/or tachycardia. Tramadol also inhibits reuptake of noradrenaline and should be avoided in patients taking phenylpropanolamine.

Ephedrine/pseudoephedrine: These are sympathomimetics which increase urethral sphincter tone (pseudo-ephedrine is an isomer of ephedrine) by increasing noradrenaline. Clinical signs and cautions are the same as for phenylpropanolamine (see above).

Anticonvulsants

Phenobarbital: This is a barbiturate commonly used to treat epilepsy. Phenobarbital is a gamma amino butyric acid (GABA) receptor agonist. Many other anaesthetic drugs work via the GABA receptor, such as thiopental, pentobarbital, benzodiazepines (diazepam, midazolam) and inhalants (isoflurane). Therefore, patients treated with phenobarbital may have exaggerated CNS effects to these anaesthetic drugs (synergy). In general, it is best to continue phenobarbital therapy and adjust the anaesthetic drug doses accordingly.

Chemotherapy drugs

There are dozens if not hundreds of drugs used for cancer treatment. Most of these drugs can affect the bone marrow while others may be nephrotoxic, cardiotoxic or hepatotoxic. It is beyond the scope of this chapter to list all the drugs, but it is imperative that the veterinary surgeon is prepared to look for such changes in any patient undergoing chemotherapy and also requiring anaesthesia.

Nutraceuticals

Many owners administer a variety of 'natural' therapies to their pets, and often assume they are benign, and therefore do not report their use when asked if their pets receive any 'medications'. However, many of the over-the-counter remedies and nutraceuticals have chemical properties that can react with anaesthetic drugs. For example, St John's wort has been linked to serotonin syndrome in people also taking tricyclic antidepressants or MAO inhibitors. From this, it is reasonable to assume that St John's wort might have negative interactions with tramadol (see earlier). It is therefore wise to ask if the owner is giving 'anything else' and research the potential interactions of any non-medically prescribed drug with which a veterinary surgeon might not be familiar.

Concurrent disease states

Many patients requiring anaesthesia will have concurrent diseases. It is prudent to be familiar with the diseases and how they might affect the patient in the peri-anaesthetic period (see Chapters 17–28).

Assigning ASA category

After completion of a thorough physical examination and interpretation of the data from ancillary tests, an ASA physical status can be assigned. Knowing a patient's physical status will better aid the veterinary surgeon in assigning relative anaesthetic risk for that patient, and in altering the anaesthetic protocol accordingly.

References and further reading

Atkins CE, DeFrancesco TC, Coats JR *et al.* (2000) Heartworm infection in cats: 50 cases (1985–1997). *Journal of the American Veterinary Medical Association* **217**, 355–358

Brady M, Kinn S and Stuart P (2003) Preoperative fasting for adults to prevent perioperative complications. *Cochrane Database of Systematic Reviews.* www.cochrane.org

Brooks M, Dodds WJ and Raymond SL (1992) Epidemiologic features of von Willebrand's disease in Doberman pinschers, Scottish terriers, and Shetland sheepdogs: 260 cases (1984–1988). *Journal of the American Veterinary Medical Association* **200**, 1123–1127

Dyson DH, Maxie MG and Schnurr D (1998) Morbidity and mortality associated with anesthetic management in small animal veterinary practice in Ontario. *Journal of the American Animal Hospital Association* **34**, 325–335

Galatos AD and Raptopoulos D (1995) Gastro-oesophageal reflux during anaesthesia in the dog: the effect of preoperative fasting and premedication. *Veterinary Record* **137**, 479–483

Hosgood G and Scholl D (2002) Evaluation of age and American Society of Anesthesiologist (ASA) physical status as risk factors for perianesthetic morbidity and mortality in the cat. *Journal of Veterinary Emergency and Critical Care* **12**, 9–16

Kawashima Y, Takahashi S, Suzuki M *et al.* (2003) Anesthesia-related mortality and morbidity over a 5-year period in 2,363,038 patients in Japan. *Acta Anaesthesiologica Scandinavica* **47**, 809–817

Robinson EP, Sams RA and Muir WW (1986) Barbiturate anesthesia in greyhound and mixed-breed dogs: comparative cardiopulmonary effects, anesthetic effects, and recovery rates. *American Journal of Veterinary Research* **47**, 2105–2112

3

Postoperative care: general principles

Daniel Holden

Introduction

Advances in veterinary medicine, anaesthesia and surgery have increased the ability to operate on a wider range of patients. This has led to greater demands for a high level of postoperative care, which has naturally extended to the development of intensive care units, and specialist veterinary surgeons and nurses working within university teaching hospitals and larger practices. In many practices, however, the recovery area doubles as the ward or patient preparation area; this arrangement need not necessarily compromise patient care if vigilance and attention to detail are maintained.

The recovery room

In ideal circumstances, the recovery room is a separate area adjacent to the operating theatre(s), where patients are monitored and undergo stabilization for variable periods of time before returning to the ward area. Size should reflect both the number and the type of cases seen. A separate area within the room for cats and small mammals/exotics is beneficial. It should be possible to observe all patients easily and the area should be well ventilated (current Department of Health regulations for human units recommend 15 air changes per hour) to ensure effective elimination of waste anaesthetic gases; active extraction may be required if occupational exposure limits are exceeded. Ambient temperature should be kept at 23–25°C. The following equipment should be readily available:

- A fully equipped anaesthetic machine (preferably with a ventilator and scavenging)
- Oxygen flowmeters (on wall or on size E cylinder)
- Equipment for induction of anaesthesia
- Equipment for management of cardiopulmonary arrest
- Portable suction apparatus
- Equipment for patient warming/cooling
- Equipment for intravenous access and fluid therapy.

In the immediate period after surgery, close monitoring of the patient should continue in the recovery area. If this involves transfer of care to other staff, then a comprehensive exchange of information should take place as part of the handover process, including the following information:

- Patient's name, species, breed, age, sex, weight
- Relevant pre-existing disease (if any)
- Operation/procedure performed and staff involved
- Anaesthetic protocol
- Spontaneous or intermittent positive pressure ventilation
- Use of neuromuscular-blocking drugs and their reversal agents
- Pain control
- General condition during procedure
- Body position for the procedure
- Untoward events during the procedure.

Postoperative monitoring and complications

Monitoring should be performed at the same intensity and frequency as during the procedure until the patient's vital signs have normalized. The most important areas that require regular attention are:

- Airway
- Breathing and gas exchange (see also Chapters 7, 20 and 29)
- Circulation (see also Chapters 7, 19 and 29)
- Level of consciousness (see Chapter 7)
- Body temperature
- Pain management (see Chapters 8–11)
- Patient comfort.

Airway

Airway-related complications are among the most common problems in the postoperative period. Any intubated patient should never be left unattended. Extubation is usually performed once signs of return of the swallowing reflex are apparent; it may be preferable in cats (and other species prone to laryngeal spasm and oedema) to remove the tube earlier. Tube removal should be timed to coincide with expiration, so that any accumulated debris or secretions are then exhaled or expectorated. Following extubation, the patient's neck should be gently extended and the tongue drawn forward to maintain airway patency. Severely brachycephalic individuals may tolerate the presence of the tube for surprisingly long periods; this is not problematic, provided that the patient is carefully monitored and prompt extubation is performed when required.

Clinical signs of airway obstruction include stertorous (snoring) or stridorous breathing, flaring of the nostrils and asynchronous motion of the thoracic and abdominal walls. Total obstruction results in an absence of airflow at the mouth and nostrils. Common causes of postoperative airway obstruction include:

- Soft tissues, most commonly the tongue and pharynx: elevation of the chin and withdrawal of the tongue usually relieves signs
- Foreign material (e.g. blood clots, saliva, vomitus, teeth, swabs): especially common after ear, nose and throat (ENT), endoscopic or dental procedures. Removal of the offending material with forceps or suction is required
- Laryngeal spasm: reflex contraction may occur following airway irritation or following upper airway surgery. Oxygen should be given by facemask and gentle suction of the pharynx and larynx performed. Atropine may be required to prevent any reflex bradycardia that may ensue. If the problem persists or the patient does not tolerate oral suction, then re-intubation may be necessary
- Laryngeal oedema: this is usually more problematic in patients with smaller diameter airways (e.g. cats, neonates) and may result from traumatic intubation, excessively large tubes or allergy/anaphylaxis. Administration of humidified oxygen may help. Intravenous short-acting corticosteroids are often given although there is little evidence to support their use. In severe cases, nebulized or intravenous adrenaline (0.02 mg/kg) may be required.

Breathing and gas exchange

Adequate ventilation is essential, not only to maintain sufficient uptake of oxygen and elimination of carbon dioxide, but also to permit the elimination of volatile anaesthetic agents. Pulse oximetry is an invaluable tool for assessment of saturation of haemoglobin with oxygen (see Chapter 7); its efficacy may, however, be hampered by patient movement and poor probe contact. Clinical examination of the patient is often unreliable at detecting even severe hypoxaemia (S_pO_2 <80%).

Hypoxaemia in the postoperative period may be due to the following factors:

- Decreased inspired oxygen: supplemental oxygen may be required, particularly if nitrous oxide was a component of the inspired gas mixture during the procedure, as this may lead to diffusion hypoxia (see Chapter 14)
- Hypoventilation. Potential causes include:
  - Impaired control of respiration
  - Drugs (injectable and volatile agents, opioids, benzodiazepines, alpha-2 agonists)
  - Hyperventilation during surgery
  - Central nervous system (CNS) disease or injury
  - Hypothermia
  - Endocrinopathies (e.g. hypothyroidism, hyperadrenocorticism).

Therapy for the above causes of hypoventilation consists of oxygen administration and reversing the effects of implicated drugs using specific antagonists. Intubation and positive pressure ventilation may be necessary. The use of doxapram may be helpful, but it is a general CNS stimulant and excessive use may precipitate hypertension, tachycardia and seizures.

- Impaired respiratory mechanics:
  - Airway obstruction
  - Respiratory muscular weakness (epidural/spinal anaesthesia, residual neuromuscular blockade, neuromuscular disease, electrolyte disturbances)
  - 'Splinting' of the abdomen and/or diaphragm (obesity, pain, tight dressings, abdominal distension)
  - Bronchospasm (anaphylaxis, drugs, asthma/bronchitis)
  - Chest wall disease or injury.

Patients in this group also require oxygen, and therapy of the underlying cause wherever possible. Opioids should not be excluded for analgesia in these cases, as they may actually facilitate improved respiratory mechanics. Patients with chest wall pain may benefit from intercostal or interpleural analgesic techniques (see Chapter 10).

- Venous admixture: dependent lung parenchyma becomes atelectatic due to a fall in functional residual capacity (FRC) of the lung (resulting from reduced respiratory muscle tone). This results in alveoli that cause mismatching of ventilation and perfusion. In humans, this effect is enhanced by pain, age, obesity and pulmonary parenchymal disease (e.g. oedema, pneumonia, contusions). Careful auscultation to detect pulmonary crackles and/or areas of decreased resonance is essential; radiography may be necessary to detect more subtle pulmonary changes. Therapy consists of oxygen therapy and vigorous management of the underlying cause (e.g. analgesia, diuretics).

Oxygen therapy

Oxygen therapy is vital in the management of many postoperative complications, but care should be taken to ensure that the stress created in the patient by the method of administration does not offset the benefit of oxygen therapy. A wide variety of techniques exists (although no single one is perfect).

Enclosed techniques: In these systems, oxygen flows into a contained area over the head or muzzle of the animal. Most oxygen masks are made of transparent plastic, through which the animal can be observed. Several methods have been described by which increased inspired concentrations of oxygen can be achieved, including placement of a plastic bag over the head, into which oxygen is pumped, and the use of an Elizabethan collar with plastic wrap covering the front (Figure 3.1). One must remember to leave a hole for carbon dioxide to escape and placement of the hole should allow oxygen (heavier than air) to accumulate near the patient.

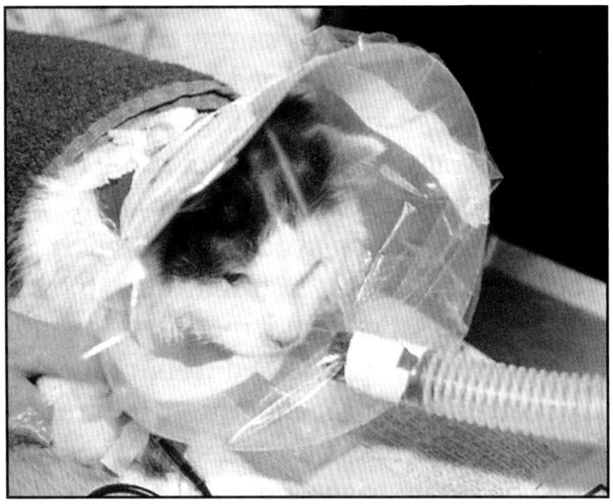

3.1 Cat with head tent for delivery of oxygen using Bain breathing system.

Advantages of these methods include a relative ease of use and rapid placement in emergency situations. Depending on flow rates and tightness of fit, very high oxygen concentrations can be achieved and access to the rest of the patient is still possible. Disadvantages are usually ones of tolerance; severely dyspnoeic or very mobile patients may not tolerate these systems, and build-up of excessive heat and carbon dioxide can limit their usefulness or even lead to respiratory acidosis.

Nasal administration: A urinary catheter or soft polythene nasal feeding tube is commonly used. Catheters may vary in size from 5 to 10 French (Fr) depending on the size of the animal. The catheter is measured from the nares to the medial canthus of the eye, and marked. Following desensitization of the nostril, the lubricated catheter is inserted gently into the nostril in a ventromedial direction (Figure 3.2a) and advanced to the mark. Once the catheter is in place, it is contoured around the alar fold, and sutured or glued in place on the side of the face (Figure 3.2b). For the most secure placement, a suture should be placed as close to the nasal-cutaneous junction as possible. The nasal catheter is attached to an oxygen delivery system with flow rates of 100–200 ml/kg/minute. In very hypoxic animals, bilateral nasal oxygen lines can be used. If the nasal catheter is guided further into the nasopharynx under sedation, inspired oxygen concentrations (F_iO_2) of up to 80% may be achieved in some animals. Knowing the F_iO_2 makes interpretation of arterial blood gases more informative.

Some animals can be best managed using human bilateral nasal 'prongs' that only penetrate 1 cm or less into the nasal cavity (Figure 3.3). Inspired oxygen concentrations of 30–50% can easily be achieved using this type of system, although panting probably limits the effectiveness of prongs.

Some animals will not tolerate nasal catheters or prongs and inspired oxygen concentrations may not be high enough for very hypoxic animals, particularly if they are mouth breathing. This is not a useful technique in brachycephalic animals or patients with facial disease or pain.

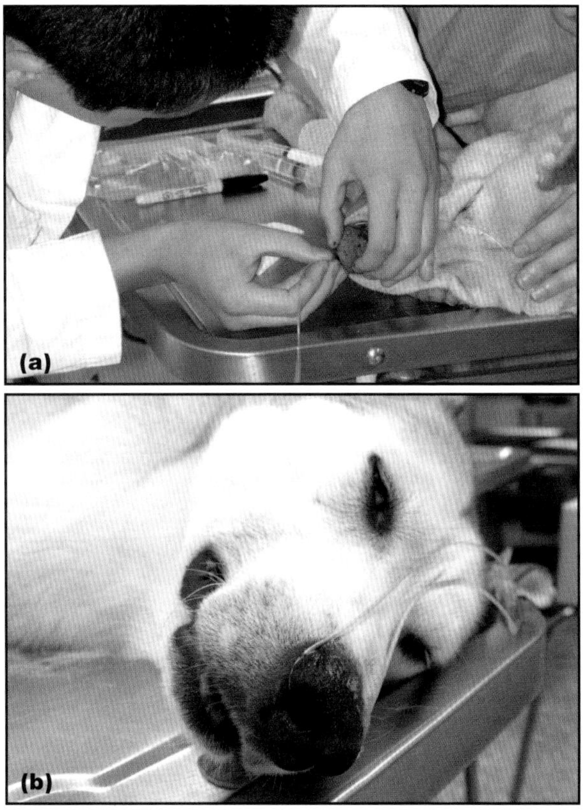

3.2 **(a)** Placing nasal oxygen catheters. **(b)** Dog with two nasal oxygen catheters in place.

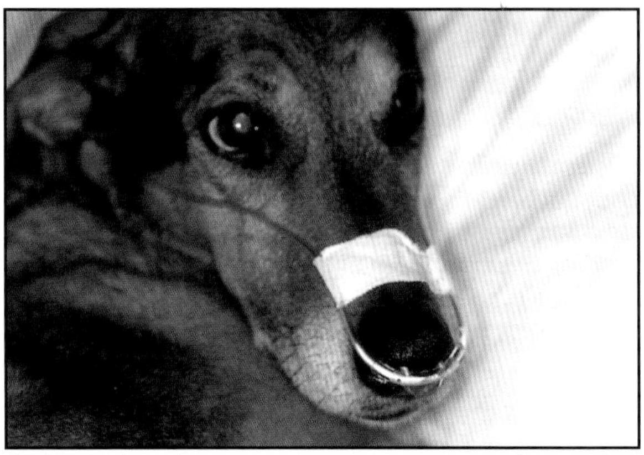

3.3 Nasal oxygen prongs that are manufactured for human patients can be used in many canine patients to provide oxygen supplementation.

Oxygen cages: These are now widely available to the veterinary market. As well as providing a higher concentration of inspired oxygen, a good oxygen cage should also allow control of internal cage temperature and humidity. A good oxygen cage should be capable of reaching oxygen concentrations in excess of 80%, for use with severely hypoxic animals (Figure 3.4). However, the time needed to achieve these concentrations may be prohibitively long. Poor-quality cages will only reach oxygen concentrations of about 50–60%. Oxygen cages and incubators can be invaluable for severely hypoxic cats, where the ability to administer a high oxygen concentration non-invasively is essential. Oxygen cages can be expensive to purchase and potentially wasteful of oxygen, since each time the door is opened much of the oxygen inside is lost.

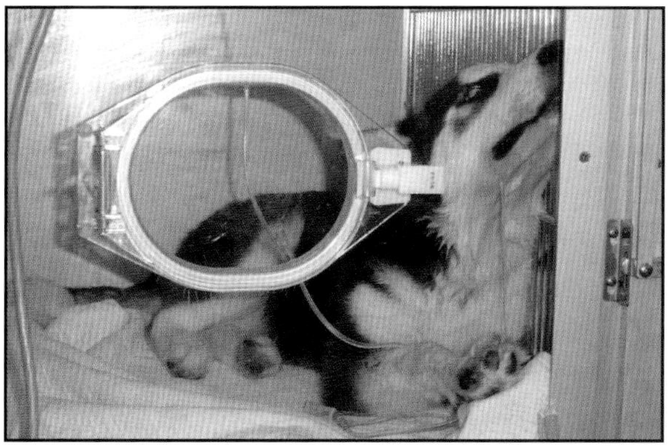

3.4 Cyanotic dog in an oxygen cage showing signs of dyspnoea. Note the extended neck to keep the airway open and nausea (drooling). (Courtesy of Dr SL Cantwell, University of Florida)

Circulation

Following simple routine procedures in fit, healthy patients, all that may be required is frequent monitoring of vital signs (heart and pulse rate, pulse quality, mucous membrane colour, capillary refill time, extremity temperature) to ensure a smooth recovery. Arterial blood pressure monitoring is essential in patients with unstable haemodynamics, or in those that have undergone more invasive or prolonged procedures. Central venous pressure may also be helpful in managing postoperative hypovolaemia, or in patients that are preload sensitive (e.g. myocardial disease).

The most common potential circulatory problems in the postoperative period include hypotension, hypertension and arrhythmias.

Hypotension

This is arguably the commonest cardiovascular complication and may be multifactorial. Potential causes can be grouped as follows:

- Decreased preload:
  - Blood loss:
    - Ongoing
    - Inadequately replaced
    - Coagulopathy
  - Reduced venous return:
    - Aggressive rewarming
    - Drugs (anaesthetic agents, spinal anaesthesia, vasodilators)
    - Massive pulmonary embolism
    - Sepsis
    - Increased intrathoracic pressure (pneumothorax, intermittent positive pressure ventilation)
- Decreased contractility:
  - Drugs
  - Pre-existing myocardial disease
  - Hypoxia/ischaemia
  - Acid–base and electrolyte disturbances
- Decreased afterload:
  - Regional anaesthesia-induced sympathetic blockade
  - Sepsis
  - Other vasodilator drugs
  - Over-aggressive rewarming of a hypothermic patient.

In all cases, fluid support should be given to provide volume and minimize further acid–base and electrolyte changes while the underlying cause is identified. Inotropes should be considered if myocardial dysfunction is suspected. Vasopressors (ephedrine, noradrenaline) may be appropriate in sepsis or other causes of inappropriate vasodilation.

Hypertension

This is most commonly caused by:

- Pain (wound/other trauma, full urinary bladder)
- Hypoxia
- Hypercapnia
- Pre-existing hypertensive disease:
  - Hyperadrenocorticism
  - Hyperthyroidism
  - Chronic renal failure
  - Diabetes mellitus
  - Phaeochromocytoma
  - Hyperaldosteronism
- Iatrogenic causes (eg vasopressors).

Patients should be given oxygen (and intubated and ventilated if severely hypercapnic) and analgesia while the underlying cause is determined and treated. Specific antihypertensive therapy is rarely necessary.

Arrhythmias

Arrhythmias are, in many cases, of little or no haemodynamic significance. Their effect on tissue perfusion should be assessed (if only by way of physical examination) and if signs of low cardiac output are evident, the underlying cause should be addressed while specific anti-arrhythmic therapy is provided. Causes of arrhythmias include:

- Residual effects of anaesthetic drugs
- Pre-existing cardiac disease
- Acid–base and electrolyte imbalance
- Hypoxaemia/hypercapnia
- Pain
- Excessive vagal tone
- Hypothermia.

Level of consciousness

The duration of the unconscious state depends on a number of factors. These include:

- Drugs used perioperatively: agents that have active metabolites (e.g. ketamine) or drugs with a long duration of action may delay return to consciousness
- Duration of anaesthesia and surgery: a greater risk of drug accumulation and increased risk of other factors influencing recovery, e.g. hypothermia, hypoglycaemia, hypoxaemia
- Intercurrent disease: hepatic, renal or thyroid dysfunction may all delay metabolism and/or clearance of any anaesthetic drugs used
- Adverse intraoperative events: hypoglycaemia, hypoxaemia, hypercapnia, hypotension and haemorrhage all prolong recovery.

Level of consciousness should be carefully and regularly assessed at the same frequency as was employed intraoperatively. Ocular and cough reflexes, jaw tone and response to gentle manipulation or other physical or verbal stimulation can all be used to assess the return of consciousness. Care should be taken to ensure that animals that have received neuromuscular-blocking drugs as part of their anaesthetic protocol have had the blockade adequately reversed, as assessment of return to consciousness may be hampered by residual paralysis. Patients undergoing diagnostic or surgical procedures involving the CNS may require other specific assessments or might warrant deliberate prolongation of sedation or anaesthesia as part of the recovery process (see Chapter 26).

Emergence delirium is a term used to describe a state during recovery from anaesthesia characterized by vocalization, abnormal repetitive movement and unresponsiveness to verbal reassurance or commands. The aetiology of this condition is uncertain, but in humans it appears more common in children, the elderly, patients who are anxious or agitated prior to anaesthesia and patients with psychological disturbances. It has been poorly studied in animals, but appears more common in unpremedicated patients and those who experience rapid recovery (use of sevoflurane and desflurane has been implicated). Adequate analgesia should obviously be ensured and further sedation (acepromazine 0.01–0.03 mg/kg or medetomidine 1–5 μg/kg) may be necessary to minimize the risk of trauma to the patient and surgical site.

Body temperature

Despite widespread awareness of the risk, hypothermia is still a common occurrence in anaesthetized dogs and cats. The causes are many and varied:

- Lack of endogenous heat production:
  - Intercurrent disease (hepatic, metabolic, thyroid)
  - Starvation/cachexia
  - Trauma
  - Extremes of age
- Impaired thermoregulation leading to increased heat loss:
  - Intercurrent disease
  - Drugs (e.g. acepromazine)
  - Trauma
- Exposure to cold surfaces and environment during premedication, anaesthesia and surgery
- Radiant and evaporative losses during clipping, surgical preparation and tissue or organ exposure (especially during body cavity surgery)
- Delivery of cold, dry anaesthetic gases to the lungs
- Further radiant losses during the recovery period.

The effects of hypothermia are complex and may result in hypoventilation, arrhythmias, delayed drug metabolism, hypoxaemia and CNS dysfunction. Therapy should be directed at elevating core temperature as well as the ambient temperature of the patient's immediate environment. This may require measures such as urinary bladder lavage with warmed 0.9% saline and the use of waterbeds, heatpads or more sophisticated methods such as warm air devices like the Bair Hugger® (Figure 3.5) or Warmtouch®. Oxygen supplementation is essential as postoperative shivering can raise oxygen consumption by 300–400%.

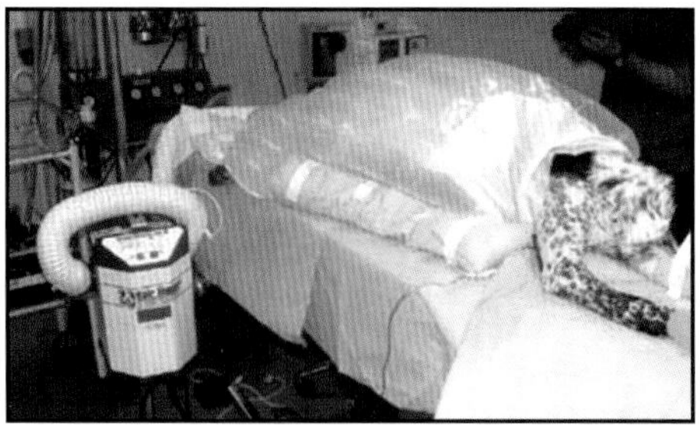

3.5 Bair Hugger® warming system.

An elevated core body temperature in the immediate postoperative period is uncommon, but may represent pyrexia due to infection, a febrile transfusion reaction or sepsis. True hyperthermia may occasionally occur in larger dogs undergoing low-flow anaesthesia using absorber systems (see Chapter 5), or may represent true malignant hyperthermia. Patients in this latter category are extremely rare, but if this is suspected any volatile agents should be discontinued and dantrolene (if available) should be administered immediately at a dose of 2.5–5 mg/kg.

Pain management

Pain assessment and management are discussed in further detail in Chapters 8–11. Difficulties in accurate detection and quantification of postoperative pain should not prevent the veterinary surgeon from administering effective analgesia. The use of pre-emptive analgesia in dogs and cats is now becoming commonplace, and both opioids and non-steroidal anti-inflammatory drugs (NSAIDs) are widely used perioperatively. Assessment of postoperative pain should be performed by careful observation of the patient's attitude and behaviour, degree of vocalization (often more in dogs than in cats) and assessment of responses to stroking, gentle manipulation and very gentle examination of the wound and its immediate area. The patient's willingness to eat, drink, move and interact with personnel are all useful parameters to assess. Previous drug administration and other history should be checked before other analgesics are given.

Patient comfort

It is axiomatic that all patients should be kept as comfortable as possible at all times during the immediate recovery period. All dressings, points of intravenous access or drains should be checked to ensure that excessive tightness or traction is avoided. Recumbent patients should be turned regularly (every 1–2 hours) and care should be taken to avoid limb compression or compromise of venous drainage. Bedding should be kept warm and dry and should be of sufficient texture and depth to prevent decubital sores or other injuries. Prompt, calm and kind interaction with staff to provide reassurance and 'TLC' is also important to allay anxiety or agitation during the recovery process.

Prolonged recovery from anaesthesia

Common causes of prolonged recovery from anaesthesia include the following:

- Hypothermia due to intercurrent disease, prolonged surgery and anaesthesia, patient debilitation, cold environment
- Drugs with active metabolites with a long duration of action may delay return to consciousness
- Prolonged anaesthesia and surgery not only carry a greater risk of drug accumulation but also incur an increased risk of other factors influencing recovery, e.g. hypothermia, hypoglycaemia, hypoxaemia
- Intercurrent disease: hepatic, renal or thyroid dysfunction may all delay metabolism and/or clearance of any anaesthetic drugs used
- Adverse intraoperative events: hypoglycaemia, hypoxaemia, hypercapnia, hypotension and haemorrhage all prolong recovery.

The following basic steps are suggested as a guide to the management of patients that do not recover from anaesthesia within the expected timeframe:

1. Check the patient's airway – if respiration is stertorous or stridorous, or if there are any doubts as to the patient's ability to maintain an airway, then re-intubate.
2. Check respiratory function – ensure that both oxygen saturation and ventilation are adequate:
   - Provide supplemental oxygen to all patients in prolonged recovery
   - Patients with severe hypoxia (S_pO_2 <85%) and/or hypercapnia (end-tidal carbon dioxide >55 mmHg) may need intubation and ventilatory support
   - Ensure adequate reversal of any respiratory depressant agent using specific antagonists.
3. Check circulatory status: heart rate, pulse rate and volume, mucous membranes and capillary refill, urine output and core/peripheral body temperature. Ensure intravenous access and look for signs of continued operative haemorrhage or bleeding from other sites. Provide intravenous fluid support if signs of hypotension are present.
4. Check body temperature – if core body temperature is reduced then institute warming mechanisms:
   - Raise the environmental temperature
   - Provide passive insulation to prevent further heat loss
   - Warm intravenous fluids
   - Consider active external warming techniques (warm air blowers, heat pads, waterbeds)
   - Consider colonic or urinary bladder lavage with warmed sterile saline.
5. Check for signs of pain and provide analgesia if necessary – cranial abdominal or thoracic pain may produce hypoventilation leading to reduced elimination of volatile agents.
6. Collect blood and evaluate packed cell volume, total solids, glucose, urea and electrolytes for signs of disturbance. Arterial blood gas analysis (if available) is invaluable in determining pulmonary functional status.
7. Consider systemic disease (hepatic, renal, endocrine) or intraoperative neurological insult.
8. Continue to provide respiratory, cardiovascular and thermal support and monitor vital signs at frequent regular intervals until signs of improvement are observed.

References and further reading

Fitzpatrick RK and Crowe DT (1986) Nasal oxygen administration in dogs and cats: experimental and clinical investigations. *Journal of the American Animal Hospital Association* **22**, 493–503

McGaffin PA and Cristoph AB (1994) Assessment and monitoring of the post anaesthesia patient. In: *The Post Anaesthesia Care Unit, 3rd edn*, ed. CB Dran, pp. 261–288. WB Saunders, Philadelphia

Tuckey J (2000) Care of the postoperative unconscious patient. *Anaesthesia and Intensive Care Medicine* **1(1)**, 3–6

Wingfield WE and Raffe MR (eds) (2001) *The Veterinary ICU Book*. Teton New Media, Jackson, Wyoming

4

The anaesthetic machine and vaporizers

Hatim Alibhai

Introduction

Accurate and continuous delivery of gas and vapour mixtures of desired compositions is possible by the use of an anaesthetic machine and vaporizer. Several manufacturers produce anaesthetic machines for human or veterinary use and, although the equipment is varied, the basic design remains the same and a working knowledge of the basic components will enable familiarity with newer designs.

A standard machine consists of a rigid steel or aluminium framework on rubber antistatic wheels with brakes. Antistatic measures improve flowmeter performance.

Anaesthetic machines are designed to suit a wide variety of environments. Compact (portable) or wall-rail mounted machines (Figure 4.1) may be suitable in areas where space is restricted and they may have single or twin positions for vaporizers on the back bar (Figure 4.2). Ceiling- or trolley-mounted machines are large and heavy with many components, including an integrated array of monitors. Machines intended for use in magnetic environments are made from non-ferrous metals. Modern machines have very easy-to-clean surfaces, and drawers, shelves and rails to accommodate specialist accessories. Modern machines are mains powered and have a rechargeable battery.

The basic anaesthetic machine consists of:

- A gas supply
- Pressure gauges
- Pressure-reducing valves
- Flowmeters
- Vaporizers
- A common gas outlet
- A breathing system (see Chapter 5)
- A ventilator (on modern machines).

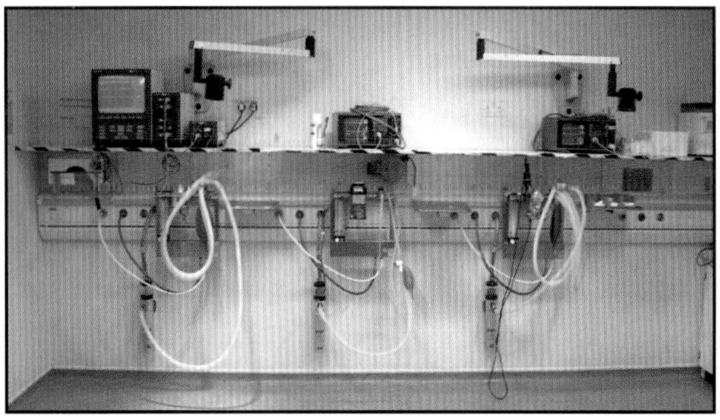

4.1 Three wall-mounted anaesthetic machines in a busy preparation room.

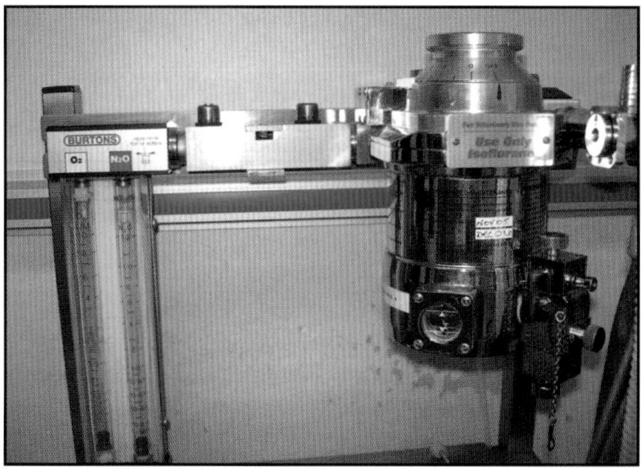

4.2 A wall-mounted machine with twin positions for vaporizers on the back bar.

Gas supplies

The supply of medical gases in any veterinary clinic or hospital takes the form of cylinders or piped gases.

Cylinders

Historically, these were made from low-carbon steel, but modern standard cylinders in the UK are now constructed from molybdenum steel. Cylinders designed for the home or use in magnetic resonance imaging (MRI) facilities are made from aluminium alloy. Extremely portable cylinders are made from lightweight steel or aluminium and have a wrapping of fibreglass in epoxy resin matrix. Impact, pressure and tensile tests are carried out regularly by manufacturers; colour-coded plastic discs around the neck of the cylinder indicate when the next tests are due (Figure 4.3).

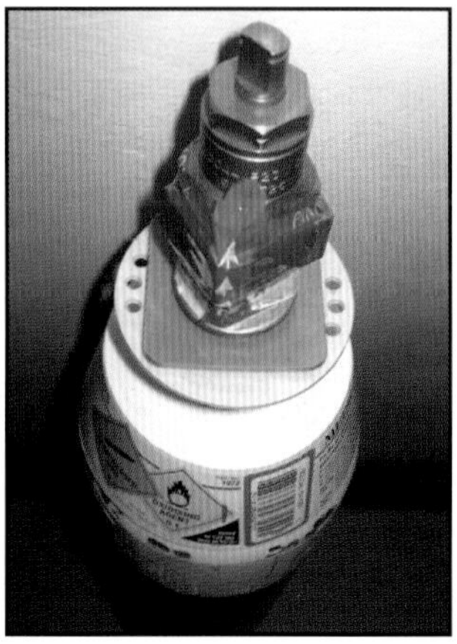

4.3 A size E oxygen cylinder with colour-coded plastic discs showing when cylinder testing is next due.

Oxygen and medical air are stored in cylinders as compressed gas; oxygen is stored at a pressure of 13,700 kPa. Nitrous oxide and carbon dioxide liquefy at the pressures used to fill the cylinders and in fact most of the gas content is in liquid form. Nitrous oxide is stored in the liquid phase, in equilibrium with its vapour at the top of the cylinder, at a pressure of 4400 kPa. Cylinders containing liquefied gas are filled to a *filling ratio* (the weight of liquid in the cylinder divided by the weight of water that it could hold); the filling ratio for nitrous oxide is 0.75. This ratio is very important because if the cylinder were completely filled, a small rise in temperature would cause a large rise in pressure and possibly cause the cylinder to rupture. Cylinders with liquefied gas must always be used vertically with the valve uppermost, otherwise liquid will be discharged when the valve is opened.

Cylinders are available in sizes A to J: Figure 4.4 shows the capacity of the commonly used ones.

Cylinder identification

Identification information on what a cylinder contains is provided on a label (Figure 4.5), with further information engraved on the side of the valve block. This engraving indicates tare weight, chemical formula of contents, test pressure and dates when tests were carried out.

Cylinders also conform to a colour code in order to prevent accidental misuse of gas or vapour, and are painted so that their contents are known. In the UK, oxygen cylinders are painted black with a white shoulder; nitrous oxide, blue; carbon dioxide, grey. In North America, the cylinder colours are the same except that oxygen is stored in green, or green and white cylinders.

Cylinder storage

Medical gas cylinders should be stored as described in Figure 4.6. They must not be subjected to extremes of heat or cold, and should not be stored near flammable materials such as oil or grease, nor near any source of heat. They should be kept dry and away from corrosive chemicals. Full and empty cylinders should be stored separately. E-sized and smaller cylinders should be stored horizontally, or vertically in a specially designed trolley, whereas F-sized and larger cylinders should be stored vertically. Smoking and naked flames should be prohibited in the vicinity of a cylinder or in confined spaces where cylinders are stored; warning notices to this effect should be posted and clearly visible. Large clear signs should indicate the cylinder storage location and the nature of gases kept there. Cylinders are filled to high pressures and explosions are possible if they are dropped or exposed

	UK				USA		
	E	F	G	J	E	F	G
Dimensions	34 x 4	36 x $35\frac{1}{2}$	54 x 7	$56\frac{1}{2}$ x 9	26 x $4\frac{1}{2}$	51 x $5\frac{1}{2}$	51 x $8\frac{1}{2}$
Oxygen	680	1360	3400	6800	650	2062	5300
Nitrous oxide	1820	3640	9100	18200	1590	5260	13800

4.4 Dimensions (height x outer diameter in inches) and approximate capacity (in litres measured at room temperature and pressure) for various commonly used gas cylinders. (Adapted from Ward (1975) and Dorsch and Dorsch (1999).)

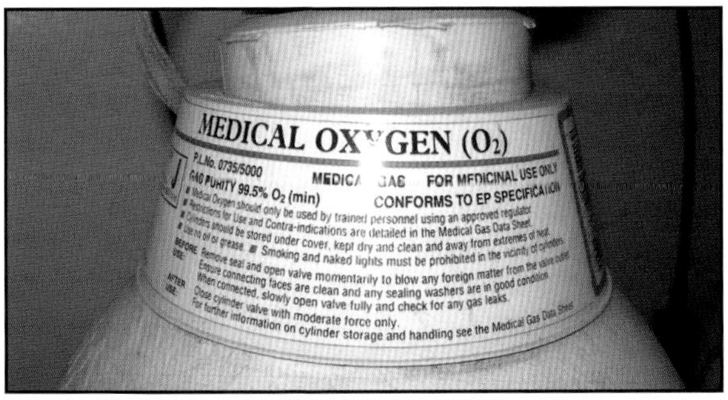

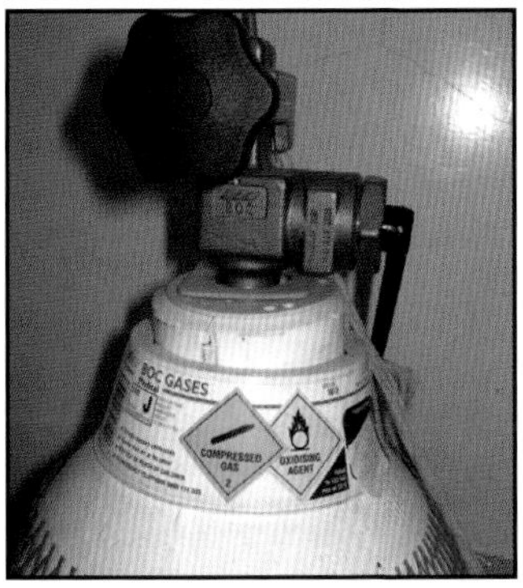

4.5 Plastic label attached to a size F oxygen cylinder showing contents and other information.

- Cylinders should be stored:
  - Under cover
  - Not subjected to extremes of heat or cold
  - In dry clean well ventilated storage areas
  - Separately from industrial and non-medical gases
- Cylinders should not be stored:
  - Near stocks of combustible material
  - Near sources of heat
- Full and empty cylinders should be stored separately
- Full cylinders should be used in strict rotation (the earliest date cylinder should be used first)
- F-sized and larger cylinders should be stored vertically in concrete-floored pens
- E-sized and smaller cylinders should be stored horizontally
- Emergency services should be advised of the cylinder store location and the nature of gases kept there
- Warning notices prohibiting smoking and naked lights should be posted clearly on the storage compound

4.6 Storage of medical gas cylinders.

to high temperatures. Further information on the safe storage and handling of cylinders may be found on the BOC website (www.bocmedical.co.uk).

Cylinder valves

Cylinder valves seal and secure the contents within the cylinder. All cylinders come with a plastic wrapping around the valve to prevent dust gathering and blocking the exit port (Figure 4.7). The cylinder valve is turned on or off with a spindle; only sufficient force should be used to close a valve. ***Valves must not be lubricated and must be kept free from carbon-based oils and greases; failure to observe this can result in explosion.***

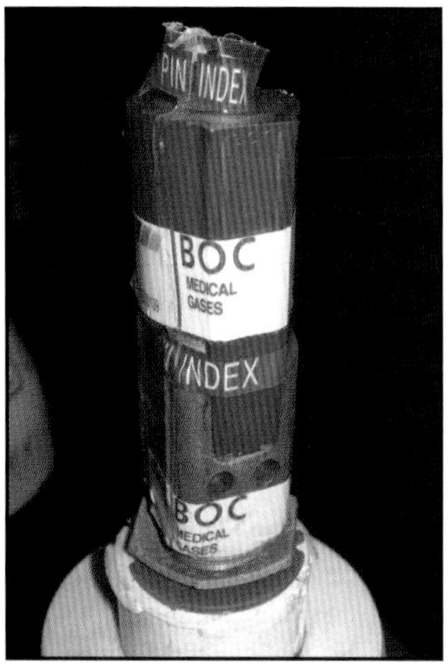

4.7 Size E oxygen cylinder with protective plastic wrapping around the valve block.

Pin index system

Pin index system valves are fitted to the small cylinders that are commonly connected to anaesthetic machines. This prevents the fitting of a cylinder of the wrong gas to a yoke on the anaesthetic machine. The cylinder valve block bears a specific configuration of holes for each medical gas, which fit on a matching configuration of pins protruding from the yoke on the anaesthetic machine (Figures 4.8 and Figure 4.9). This allows only the correct gas cylinder to be fitted to that yoke. The exit port for the gas will not fit and seal against the Bodok seal (Figure 4.10) on the yoke unless the holes and the pins are aligned. The Bodok seal should be inspected for damage prior to use, and spare seals should always be available.

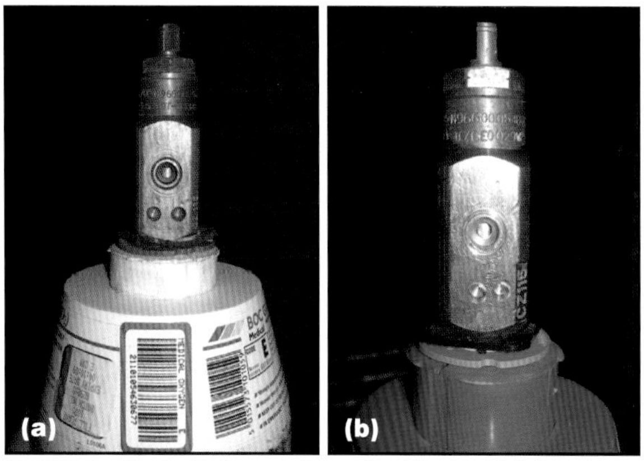

4.8 Pin indexing on the valve blocks of **(a)** a size E oxygen cylinder and **(b)** a size E nitrous oxide cylinder.

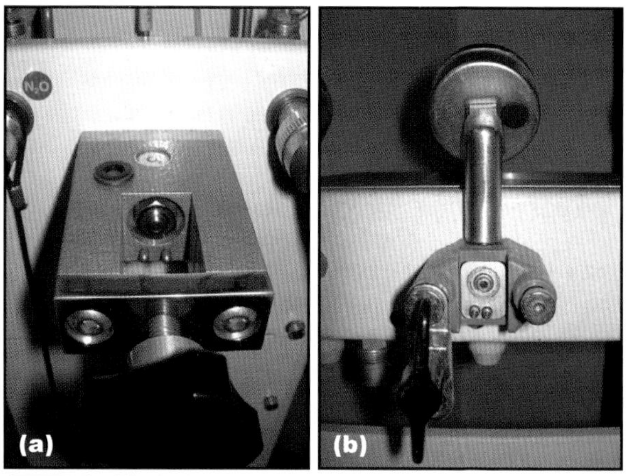

4.9 Pin-indexed yokes for **(a)** a size E oxygen cylinder and **(b)** a size E nitrous oxide cylinder.

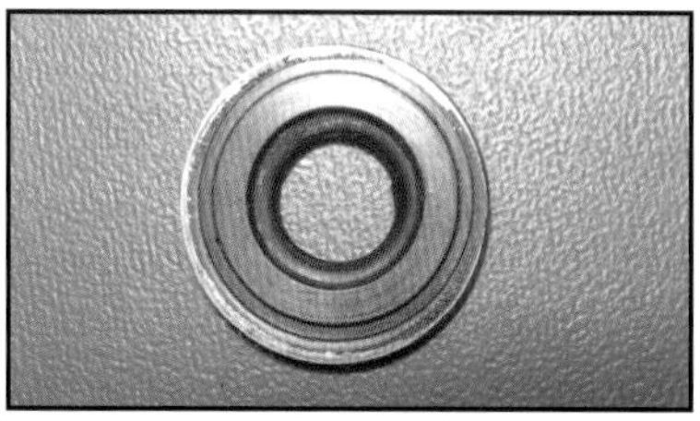

4.10 A Bodok seal.

Cylinder yokes may also be fitted with one-way, spring-loaded check valves. These prevent retrograde gas flow through the inlet nipple of vacant hanger yokes when a pipeline gas source is in use. They also allow changing of empty cylinders, by preventing gas transfer from a high-pressure (fresh) cylinder to a low-pressure (used) cylinder. Check valves are difficult to locate within the yokes: their presence is confirmed by removing a cylinder from the yoke under test and allowing an alternative source of the same gas to be turned on. A hiss at the yoke will indicate a malfunctioning or absent check valve. If the check valve function is unknown then it is safer to close the cylinder that is empty before opening a new one.

Pipeline supply

The source of pipeline gas supply can be a cylinder manifold, liquid oxygen storage tank or oxygen concentrators.

Cylinder manifold

Many large veterinary hospitals have cylinder manifolds that supply oxygen and nitrous oxide. An average cylinder manifold configuration has two banks of gas cylinders with a centrally located panel (Figure 4.11), which provides a nominal output of 400 kPa (4 bar). The changeover from 'duty' to 'standby' bank should ideally be automatic, achieved through a pressure-sensitive device that detects when the cylinders are nearly empty. This changeover also alerts staff to change the cylinders. The arrangement should also contain a manually operated emergency bank with two cylinders. The total capacity of the bank should be based on 1 week's supply of gas, with a minimum of 2 days' supply on each bank and a supply for 3 days on the spare cylinders held in the manifold room. Nitrous oxide manifolds have heaters fitted to the supply line to prevent freezing during periods of high demand.

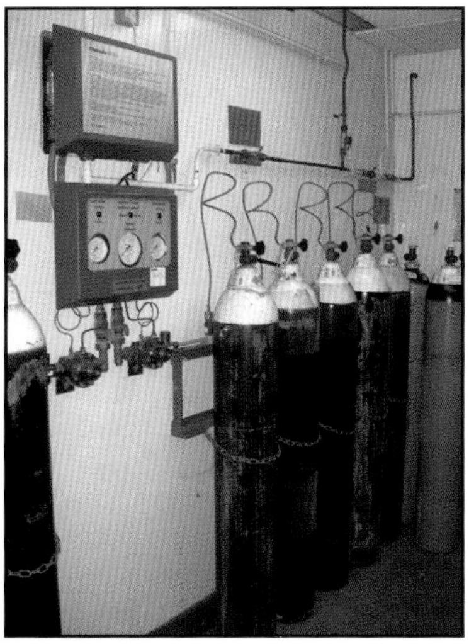

4.11 An oxygen cylinder manifold.

The manifold room should be:

- Constructed from sturdy material which is fireproof
- Well ventilated
- Ideally located to allow delivery and distribution in the hospital
- Well lit
- Temperature regulated
- Contain only cylinders used for pipeline supply
- Not used as a general store
- Fitted with warning signs on the outside and inside of the building.

Only suitably trained persons should be allowed to change cylinders and a logbook must be completed when they are changed.

Liquid oxygen storage

When the annual consumption of a veterinary hospital is considered too great for a cylinder manifold, a vacuum-insulated evaporator (VIE) for liquid oxygen is the most economical way to store and supply oxygen (Figure 4.12). This has significant advantages:

- It is a semi-permanent installation and is filled from a remote point, which removes the need for manually handling and connecting large cylinders

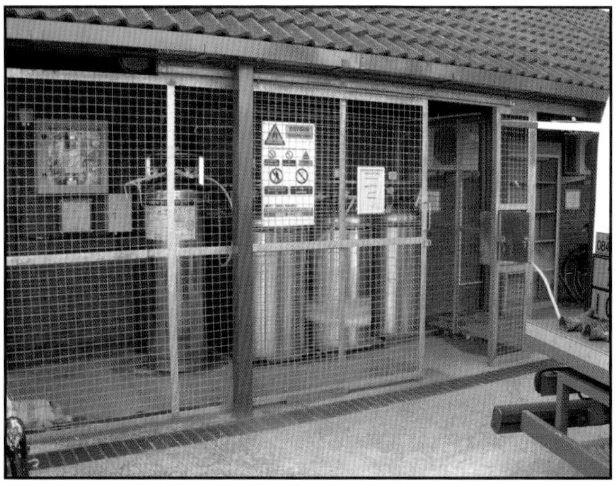

4.12 Vacuum-insulated evaporators (VIE) for liquid oxygen.

- The VIE has a pressure regulator that allows oxygen to enter the pipelines and maintains the pressure throughout the pipelines at 400 kPa
- A safety valve, which functions at 1700 kPa, allows gas to escape during periods of low demand. During periods of high demand, a control valve opens, allowing liquid oxygen to evaporate by passing through superheaters.

Oxygen liquefies at –150°C to –170°C, and is stored at pressures of up to 500–1000 kPa. The storage vessel rests on a weighing balance to measure the mass of liquid. When required, fresh supplies of liquid oxygen are pumped from a tanker into the vessel. At atmospheric pressure and temperatures of 15°C, liquid oxygen can give 842 times its volume in gas.

Oxygen concentrators

These devices separate oxygen from air by chemical means, and all the currently available models are electrically powered. Low-pressure generators will supply one anaesthetic machine (Figure 4.13), whereas high-pressure models can be connected to the manifold of an existing pipeline system.

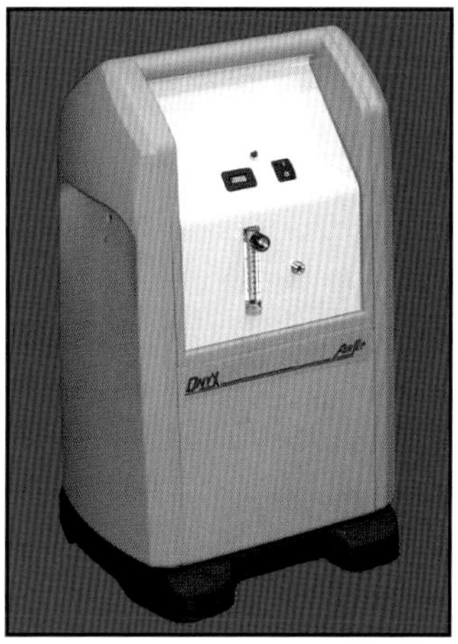

4.13 The Krutech Onyx 8 low-pressure oxygen generator. This unit delivers up to 8 l/minute of dry oxygen with a 94% purity at a pressure of 130 kPa.

Distribution systems

Medical gases are distributed throughout the hospital at a pressure of 400 kPa, through pipelines designed to achieve a minimum pressure drop from the source to the point of use. Oxygen, nitrous oxide and medical air are the most common gases normally distributed by pipeline in veterinary hospitals within the UK. Newly installed gas pipelines should be inspected and purged according to the laws of the country in which the hospital is located. The gases are fed into a labelled and colour-coded pipeline distribution network, which terminates in self-sealing (Schrader) sockets either in the wall (Figure 4.14) or on a ceiling mount. A European standard governs the dimensioning and construction of the terminal unit and its associated probe. A flexible pipeline connects the terminal outlet to the anaesthetic machine or other medical equipment. Each flexible pipeline has three components:

- The Schrader probe (Figure 4.15). To prevent misconnection to the wrong gas service, the probe for each gas supply has a protruding indexing collar with unique diameter, which only fits the Schrader assembly for the same gas

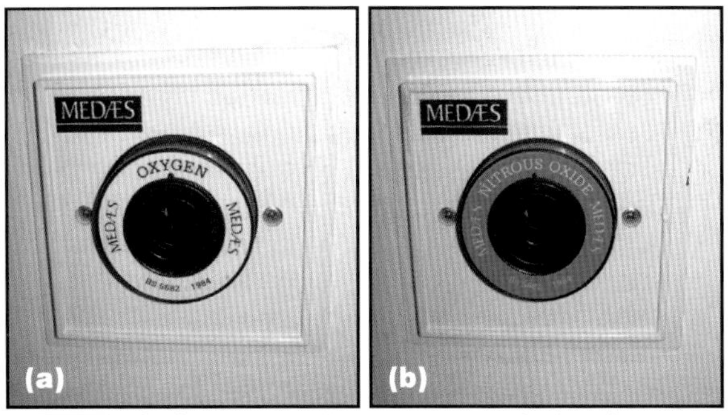

4.14 Self-sealing wall mounted terminal outlets ('Schrader sockets') for **(a)** oxygen and **(b)** nitrous oxide.

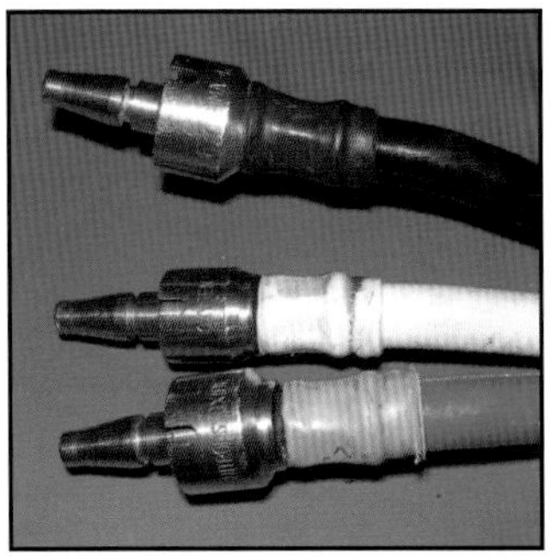

4.15 Schrader probes and hoses for the terminal outlets. From top to bottom: medical air; oxygen; nitrous oxide.

- Flexible hose. Modern hoses are colour-coded for each gas: oxygen is white; nitrous oxide is French blue; medical air is black and white
- Non-interchangeable screw thread (NIST) for connection to the anaesthetic machine (Figure 4.16). This ensures a hose connection specific to each gas service. It comprises a nut and probe: the probe has a unique profile for each gas, which fits only the union on the machine for that gas. The nut has the same diameter and thread for all services, but can only be attached to the machine when the probe is engaged. The term NIST is therefore misleading, because the screw thread does not determine the unique fit. A one-way valve ensures unidirectional flow.

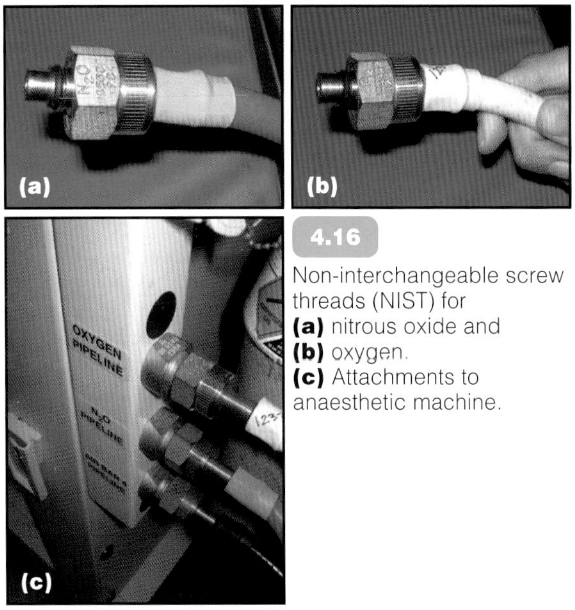

4.16 Non-interchangeable screw threads (NIST) for **(a)** nitrous oxide and **(b)** oxygen. **(c)** Attachments to anaesthetic machine.

Alarms

There are several different types of alarm used within the hospital medical gas system: the main plant alarms and the local alarms. The main alarm is to provide an indication of the plant status and to provide advance warnings that something might be in process of failure. In addition to the indicators on the main plant panel, a visual indicator will appear on each manifold providing more detailed information on the nature of the fault. The local alarm is more an indication that the problem has already occurred at the point of use. Each local area is monitored by a pressure switch that detects high or low pressure within the pipeline, near an area valved service unit in the local zone. Alarms are both visual and audible; the audible alarm can be muted for 15 minutes. If the fault has not been rectified, the alarm will reset itself until the problem has been cured.

The anaesthetic machine

Most anaesthetic machines should have the following features to ensure the safe delivery of anaesthetic gases and vapours:

- Pressure gauges (colour coded for each gas)
- Pressure-reducing valves (pressure regulators)
- Flowmeters that are colour-coded for oxygen, nitrous oxide and medical air
- Baffling the oxygen flowmeter so that it is the last gas to be mixed with the other gases (to prevent delivery of a hypoxic mixture to the patient in the event of a cracked flowmeter tube)
- Oxygen low pressure provides the cut-off for nitrous oxide
- Pin index system for cylinders and a NIST for pipelines
- An oxygen failure alarm
- At least one reserve oxygen cylinder on machines that use pipeline supply, and two oxygen cylinders on machines that do not use a pipeline supply.

Pressure gauges

These measure the pressure of the gas in the pipeline and cylinders, using Bourdon gauges. The pressure gauges in older machines are mounted above the cylinder yoke, while in modern machines they are mounted on the front panel (Figure 4.17).

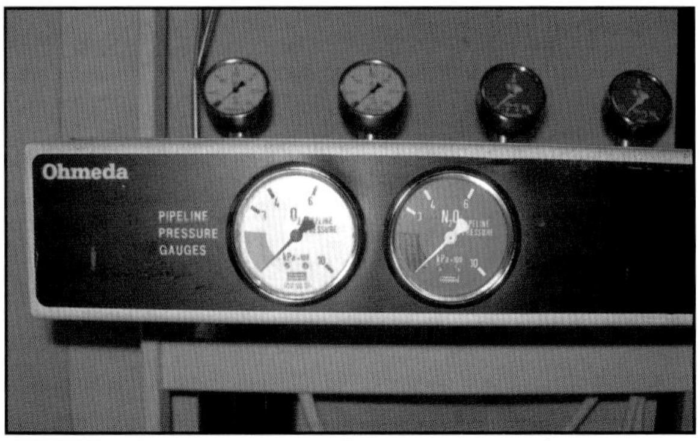

4.17 Pressure gauges for oxygen and nitrous oxide on the front panel of a modern anaesthetic machine.

The gauges are labelled, colour-coded and calibrated for each gas or vapour. The pressure gauge for oxygen indicates the gas volume in the cylinder, calculated using Boyle's law (PV=K). For example, an E-sized cylinder contains 680 litres of gas when filled to 13,700 kPa at 20°C. At the same temperature, a pressure gauge registering 4500 kPa indicates that only 230 litres remain.

The nitrous oxide pressure gauge does not act as the contents gauge; it measures the saturated vapour pressure of gaseous nitrous oxide in equilibrium with its liquid phase. This remains constant until all the liquid evaporates, after which the pressure falls rapidly. Gas volume in a nitrous oxide cylinder is determined by weighing the cylinder and applying the formula:

Gas present (litres) = (net-tare) weight (in grams) x 22.4/44

(The tare weight of a nitrous oxide 'E' cylinder is about 5800–6400 g)

Pressure-reducing valves (pressure regulators)

Pressure-reducing valves (Figure 4.18) are used:

- To *reduce* the high pressure delivered from a cylinder, so that sudden surges of pressure cannot be delivered to the patient
- To *maintain* a constant reduced pressure (generally 400 kPa) as the contents of the cylinder are exhausted.

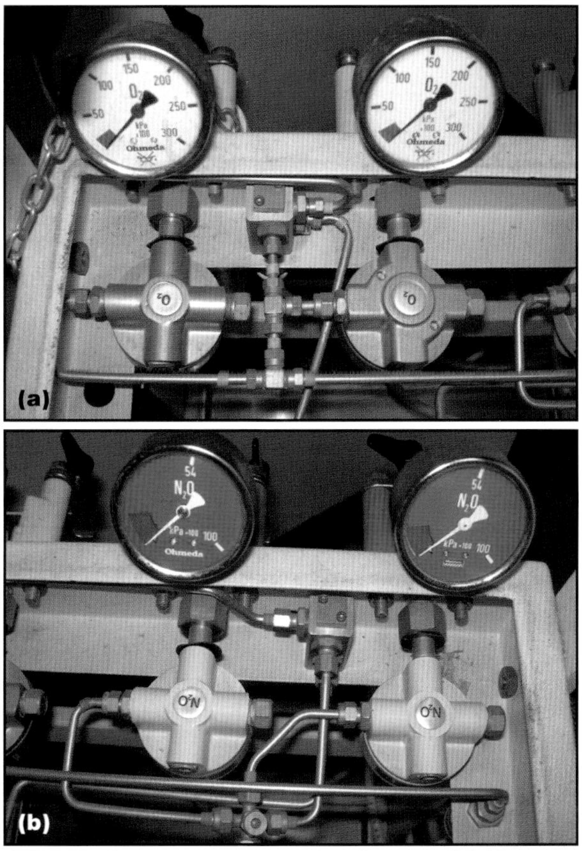

4.18 Pressure regulators. **(a)** Oxygen. **(b)** Nitrous oxide.

Machines holding more than two cylinders have one regulator per cylinder. Piped gases are regulated at their source. Complex pressure regulators incorporating pressure gauges, regulators, flowmeters and a 'bull-nosed' connector are available for the attachment of pipelines to larger cylinders.

Pressure relief valves (opening at a pressure of 570–700 kPa) are fitted downstream on the anaesthetic machine to allow the escape of gas should the regulators fail; these valves may be spring-loaded so that they open at high pressure and close when the pressure falls. Some may rupture and need to be replaced by a qualified engineer. Modern anaesthetic machines have primary and secondary pressure regulators. Primary regulators are used to reduce high cylinder pressures and thus lower the machine working pressure. Some machines allow cylinder reducing valves to work below 420 kPa (60 psi) thus giving the pipeline preference and allowing pipeline gas to be used instead of cylinder gas. It is preferable to leave the reserve cylinder on, but some cylinders may leak and empty their contents slowly if accidentally turned on.

Using oxygen from an auxiliary port to drive a ventilator (or during peak usage of pipeline gases) may cause a fluctuation in the working pressure of the anaesthetic machine. A secondary reducing valve set below the anticipated pressure drop smoothes out the supply, minimizing fluctuations.

All regulators are tested before being installed to withstand pressures of 30 MPa with no disruption and with no variation of their output over a wide flow range.

Gas flow measurement and control valves

Control (needle) valves control the gas flow into the flowmeters by manual adjustment. These valves provide the final stage of pressure reduction, and pressures beyond the flowmeters in the back bar range from 1–8 kPa. The flowmeter (also called a rotameter) is a tube made of transparent tapered (wider at the top of the flowmeter) glass or plastic, with a lightweight ball or bobbin (e.g. non-rotating H-float, skirted bobbin and non-skirted bobbin) floating on the gas flow (Figure 4.19). The bobbin (or ball) is held in the tube by gas flow passing around it, and the higher the flow rate, the higher the bobbin rises in the tube. The flows within the tube are both laminar (low flows) and turbulent (higher flows), thus making both viscosity and density of the gas significant in calibration. The flow

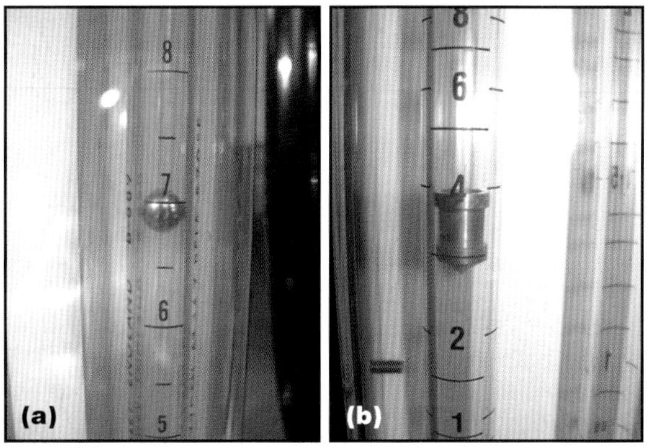

4.19 Flowmeter. **(a)** Ball. **(b)** Bobbin.

rate is etched on to the tube (in litres/minute for flows above one litre, and 100 ml/minute for flows below one litre). Gas flow is read from the top of the bobbin; when a ball is used the reading is taken from the centre of the ball. Neoprene washers at either end make them leak proof. Flowmeters are designed to be read in a vertical position. Calibration is done at room temperature and sea level and the error margin is ±2%. The commonest causes of inaccurate flow measurements are dirt and static electricity. This could be a problem at low flow rates, when there is a narrow clearance between bobbin and flowmeter wall. Static electricity builds up over time and can cause the bobbin to stick to the sides of the flowmeter tubing; using an antistatic material coating on the inside and outside of flowmeters will prevent this. An application of antistatic spray will generally solve the problem of a sticky bobbin.

The needle valve control knobs are colour- and touch-coded and bear the name of the gas: the oxygen knob is large and white in colour and has larger ridges than the other knobs. In the UK, flowmeters are arranged in a block, with the oxygen flowmeter to the left and nitrous oxide on the right, and those for medical air and carbon dioxide in between these where fitted (Figure 4.20). The flowmeters are arranged vertically and adjacent to each other so that their upper ends discharge into the manifold. In older flowmeter blocks, this resulted in oxygen (instead of nitrous oxide) leaking out if the central flowmeter tube was damaged, resulting in a hypoxic mixture being delivered to the patient. Later designs of the flowmeter block ensure that oxygen is the last gas to be delivered to the back bar (by baffling the oxygen tube). In the USA and Canada, this problem is solved by placing the oxygen flowmeter to the right of the block and nitrous oxide to the left.

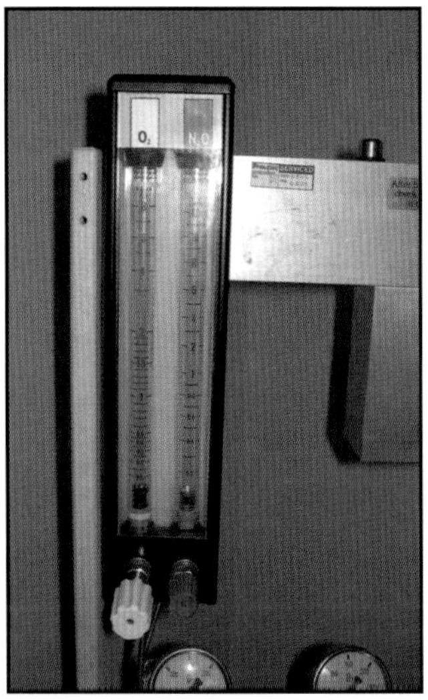

4.20 A flowmeter block. Note protrusion of oxygen flow control.

On some modern machines, it is impossible to deliver nitrous oxide without the addition of a fixed percentage of oxygen; the interactive nitrous oxide and oxygen controls prevent hypoxic mixtures being delivered to the patient. Figure 4.21 shows the Quantiflex MDM, which was one of the earlier machines designed to prevent delivery of hypoxic mixtures.

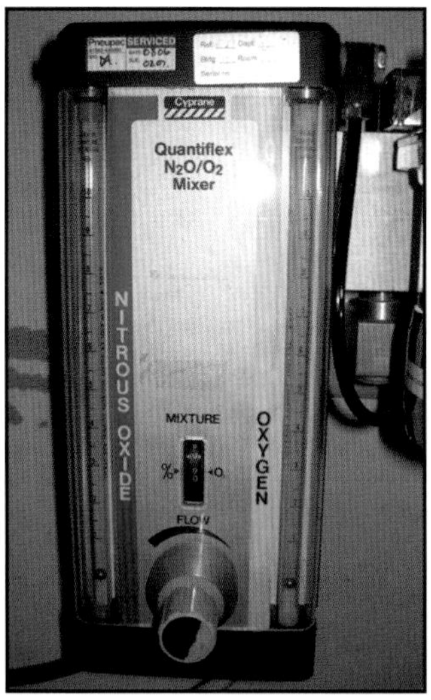

4.21 The Quantiflex MDM. Note that the oxygen flowmeter is on the right, and that for nitrous oxide on the left.

Low-flow anaesthesia (see Chapter 5) requires flowmeters that measure flows accurately below 1 l/minute; to achieve this, an arrangement of two flowmeters in series is used (Figure 4.22). One flowmeter reads to a maximum of 1 l/minute, allowing fine adjustment of flow. One flow control valve per gas is needed for both the flowmeters.

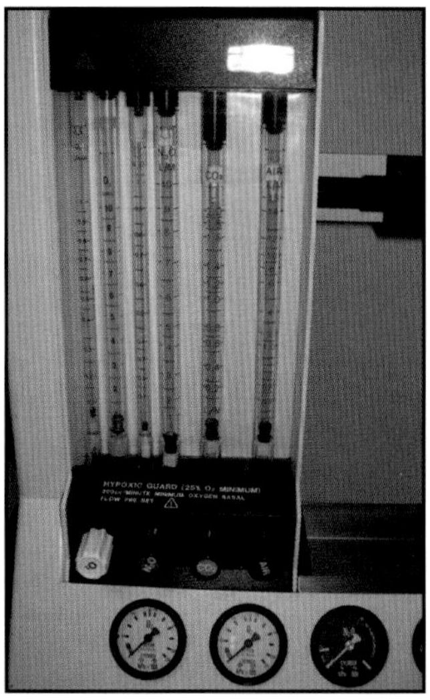

4.22 'Cascade' flowmeters: these allow accurate measurement of gas flows less than 1 l/minute.

In modern anaesthetic machines designed for human use, highly accurate microprocessors are used to control the flow of gas.

Back bar

The back bar supports the flowmeter block, vaporizers and some other components (Figure 4.23). The back bar on older anaesthetic machines has the vaporizer (alone or in series) mounted downstream from the flowmeter block and bolted to the bar with tapered cagemount connector fittings; this makes servicing individual components very difficult. Modern back bars allow greater flexibility in allowing vaporizers to be removed and exchanged with ease for servicing and refilling. The Ohmeda 'Selectatec' fitting is the most popular in the UK (Figure 4.24a). The vaporizer assembly has two female ports with a locking mechanism (Figure 4.24bc), which fit on to two vertically

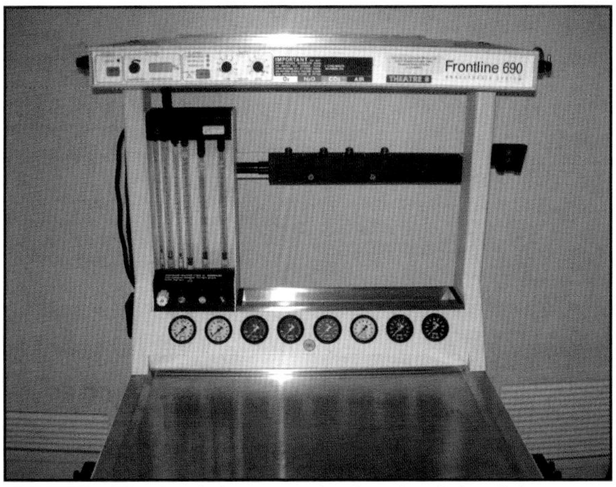

4.23 The back bar, attached to the right of the flowmeter block.

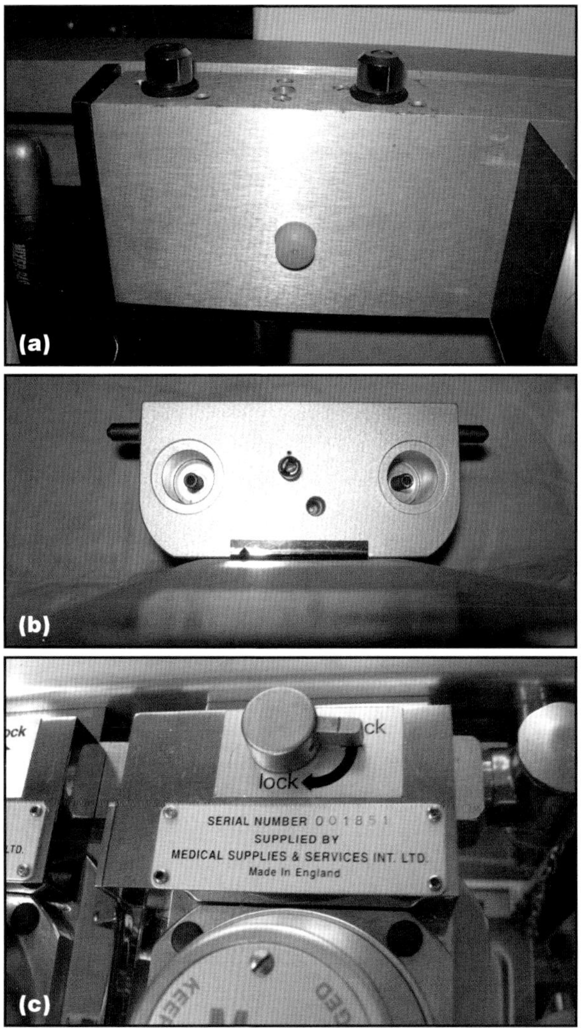

4.24 **(a)** A 'Selectatec' station for vaporizer attachment to the back bar. **(b)** Matching vaporizer assembly showing two female ports, accessory pin and locking recess. **(c)** Locking mechanism on a TEC3 vaporizer.

mounted male ports on the 'Selectatec' fitting; between the inlet and the outlet ports is an accessory pin and locking recess. The vaporizers have to be locked on to the bar by turning a knob. This system prevents the use of older vaporizers on the modern back bar.

In order to ensure an airtight seal, O-rings are placed on the male ports on the back bar. Modern TEC vaporizers (4–7) also incorporate an extension rod, which protrudes sideways from the vaporizer when it is turned on: this displaces an equivalent rod in the vaporizer adjacent to it and prevents that one from being turned on as well (Figure 4.25).

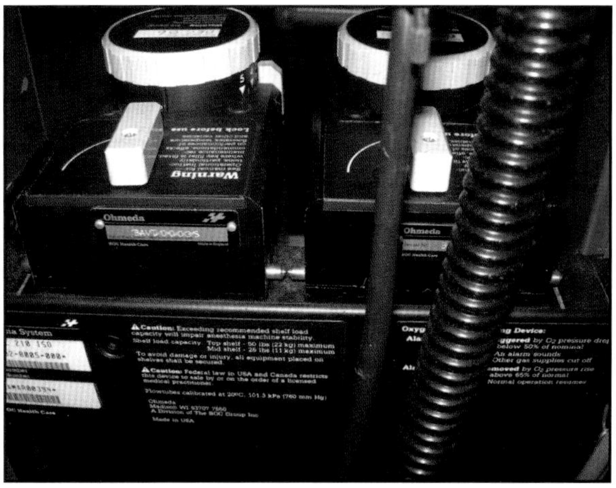

4.25 Safety interlock, showing an extension rod protruding from each vaporizer; the rod extends sideways from one vaporizer as it is turned on, and immobilizes the equivalent pin on the adjacent vaporizer.

In modern back bars, back pressure from minute volume divider ventilators can damage flowmeters and a pressure-relief valve (often set at 30–40 kPa) is fitted in the same housing as a non-return valve at the right hand side of the back bar (see below).

Common gas outlet

The common gas outlet (Figure 4.26) connects the anaesthetic machine to breathing systems, ventilators or oxygen supply devices (e.g. masks). The outlet has a 22 mm male/15 mm female outlet. The common gas outlet is either fixed or swivelled; the latter is useful because it reduces the need for the machine to be moved and facilitates breathing system positioning, with reduced risk of hoses kinking.

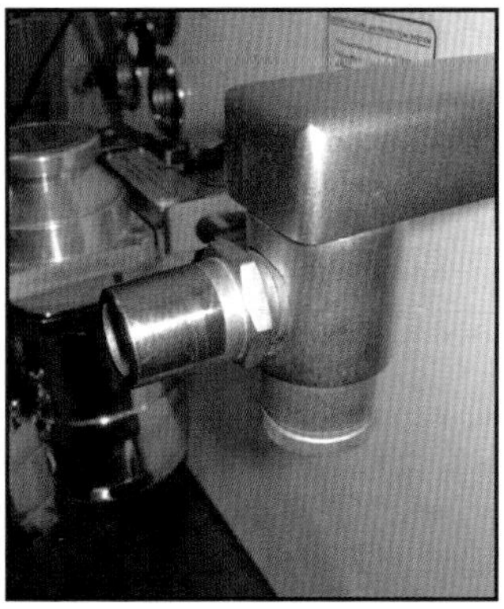

4.26 Common gas outlet.

Auxiliary gas sockets

One or more mini-Schrader gas sockets are fitted to modern machines to deliver air or oxygen to power ventilators (Figure 4.27) and suction units. The working pressure for these sockets is 400 kPa.

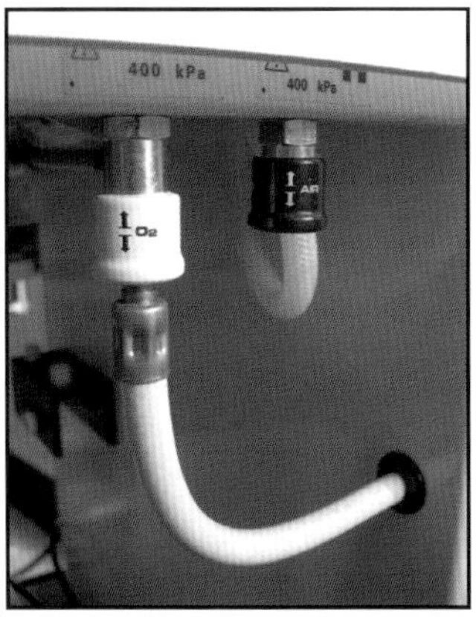

4.27 Auxiliary gas sockets for oxygen and medical air.

Non-return and pressure-relief safety valve

This is situated either on the back bar or near the common gas outlet (Figure 4.28). It opens when back pressure exceeds 35 kPa, usually from the use of minute volume divider ventilators. This prevents damage to flowmeters and vaporizers.

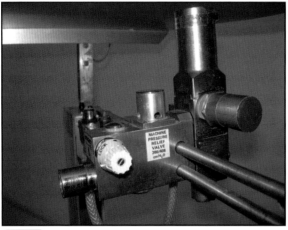

4.28 Pressure-relief valve.

Emergency oxygen flush

The oxygen flush receives oxygen directly from the pipeline or cylinder, thus bypassing the vaporizer (Figure 4.29). When activated by a button, oxygen is delivered at a high flow of 30–70 l/minute at a pressure of 400 kPa. Care should be exercised when using this with patients attached to breathing systems: it exposes them to risk of barotrauma.

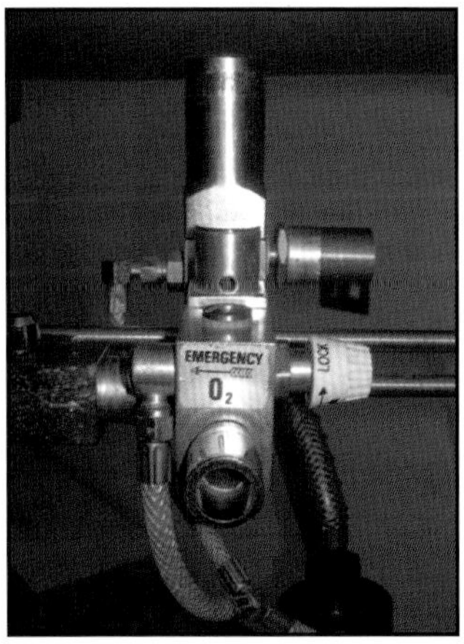

4.29 Emergency oxygen flush: this supplies oxygen directly to the breathing system at a rate of 30–70 l/minute. Note that in modern machines, the valve does not have a locking facility (to prevent barotrauma).

Emergency air-intake valve

This valve opens with a loud beep when the gas flow from the anaesthetic machine ceases, allowing the patient to breathe room air until flow is restored.

Overpressure valve

This allows release of excessive pressure downstream from the common gas outlet; as the valve opens it may also sound an alarm. The device is useful in testing breathing systems for leaks.

Oxygen failure alarm

Oxygen failure devices are very important on anaesthetic machines. Ideally, falling oxygen supply should curtail nitrous oxide flow and simultaneously sound an alarm, which should be gas driven and depend on the pressure of oxygen alone. It should not require batteries or mains electrical supply. The British Standard states that the alarm should be activated when the oxygen pressure falls to approximately 200 kPa.

Vaporizers

A vaporizer is a device that delivers clinically safe and effective concentrations of anaesthetic vapour. Most inhaled anaesthetics are liquids at room temperature and pressure, and therefore need to be vaporized before being delivered to the patient.

The saturated vapour pressure (SVP) of most volatile anaesthetics is much greater than that needed to produce anaesthesia (see Chapter 14). For example, the SVP of isoflurane at 20°C is approximately 240 mmHg, which yields a maximum concentration of 32%; breathing this concentration of isoflurane would be rapidly fatal and thus vaporizers are used to dilute the saturated vapour of volatile anaesthetics and yield a range of safe and useful concentrations. This dilution is achieved by splitting the flow of gas to the vaporizer into two streams. One passes through the vaporizer chamber (which contains saturated vapour), whilst the other stream bypasses the chamber. The ratio between these two flows (the splitting ratio) is what the control dial of the vaporizer dictates.

Gas can be made to flow through a vaporizer in one of two ways:

- Under positive pressure of gas delivered from flowmeters proximal ('upstream') to the vaporizer. This type is called a *plenum vaporizer* (plenum is a term which describes a pressurized chamber). This is the most familiar type, fitted to the back bar of the anaesthetic machine. Resistance to gas flow is relatively high
- Under negative pressure developed distal ('downstream') to the vaporizer. This is known as a *draw-over vaporizer* and the negative pressure is generated by the patient's inspiratory effort. Such vaporizers have a low resistance to gas flow and are normally used 'in-circuit' in the Komesaroff and Stephens' anaesthetic machines (see below).

Vaporizer performance

The amount of volatile liquid anaesthetic vaporized depends on:

- The SVP of the agent
- Temperature
- Gas flow through the vaporizer
- The amount of contact between the liquid and the gases
- The dimensions of the vaporizing chamber
- Movement and tilting of vaporizers: always keep upright. If tilted, liquid anaesthetic may contaminate the bypass and expose the next patient to very high vapour concentrations
- Back pressure, e.g. from minute volume divider ventilators (Chapter 6).

In simple vaporizers (such as the Boyle's bottle), liquid anaesthetic evaporates so that its temperature and hence SVP fall. Also, the degree of saturation of gas leaving the vaporizing chamber is very dependent on gas flow (with higher concentrations achieved at lower flows). This problem of flow and temperature dependence is overcome in the design of modern vaporizers.

Plenum vaporizers

Temperature-compensated (TEC) vaporizers

Examples include the Ohmeda TEC3, TEC4 and TEC5, the Dräger Vapor and the Penlon Sigma Delta (Figure 4.30). Temperature compensation prevents the fall in output that would otherwise occur as the liquid anaesthetic evaporates and cools. This is achieved by altering the splitting ratio with temperature, so that more gas flows through the vaporization chamber as the temperature falls. TEC vaporizers contain a temperature-controlled valve, which adjusts the splitting ratio; this may involve the use of either a bimetallic strip or an aneroid bellows.

When purchased, performance data are provided with the vaporizer (in graphical form) indicating actual output (compared with control dial setting) over a range of temperatures and gas flows and it is important to consult these before use. For example, at flows less than 1 l/minute, the splitting ratio may alter and affect vaporizer output.

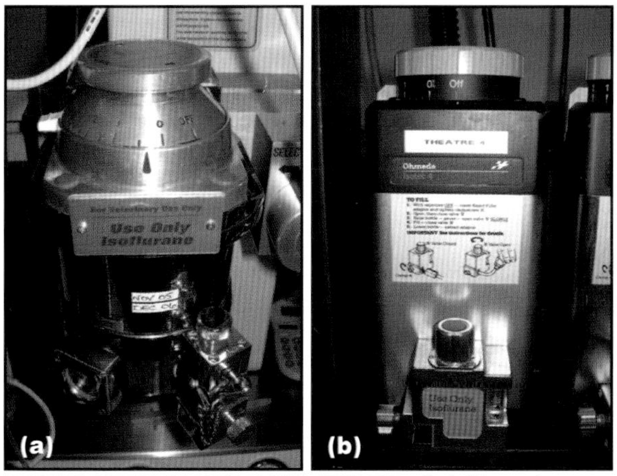

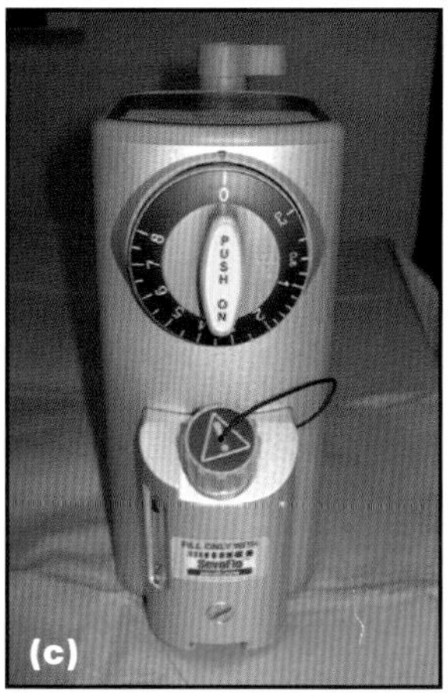

4.30 **(a)** Ohmeda TEC3 and **(b)** TEC4 vaporizers for isoflurane. **(c)** Penlon Sigma Delta vaporizer for sevoflurane.

Measured flow vaporizers

Examples include the 'copper kettle' (not used in the UK) and the TEC6 for use with desflurane (Figure 4.31). Desflurane has a very low boiling point (23°C), so that it would not stay in liquid form in the reservoir of a conventional vaporizer. Consequently, the liquid anaesthetic is contained within an electrically heated chamber that raises the temperature of the desflurane to 39°C, at which the SVP is 1500 mmHg. Pure vapour under pressure is then released into the carrier gas as required, dependent on the control dial setting.

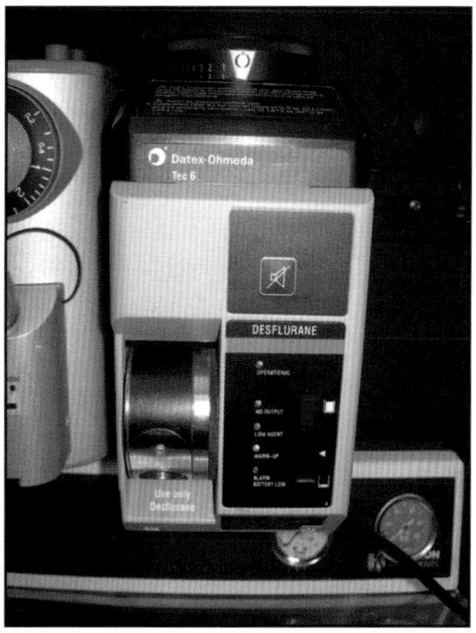

4.31 TEC6 vaporizer for desflurane.

Filling of plenum vaporizers

In older designs, a screw-threaded stopper in the filling port is unscrewed and liquid anaesthetic poured in. This allows the possibility of filling the vaporizer with the wrong agent and thus agent-specific filling devices have been developed:

- Key-indexed filling systems: the proximal end of the 'key' will only fit on to the neck of the bottle of a specific agent, whilst the distal end will only fit into a vaporizer calibrated for that agent (Figure 4.32)
- Sevoflurane and desflurane are sold in sealed bottles and will only fit into the filler ports on the correct vaporizer (Figure 4.33).

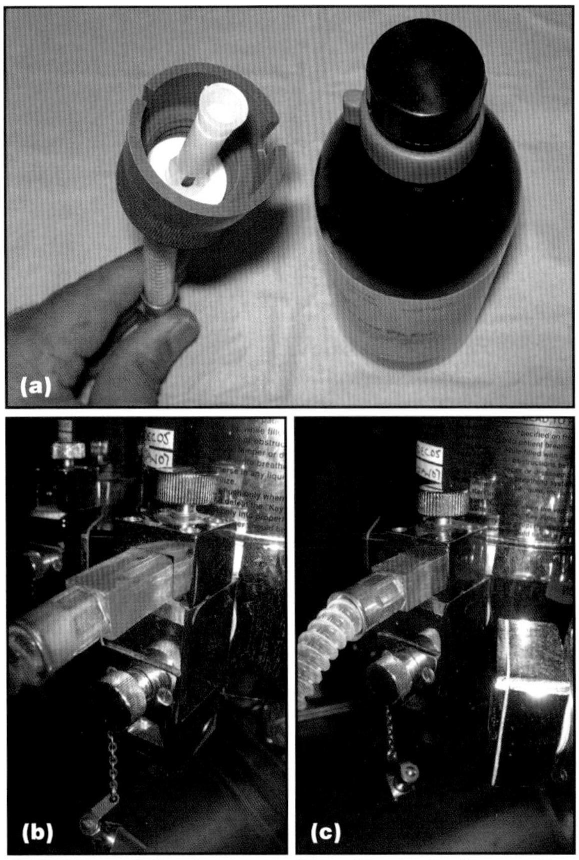

4.32 **(a)** Proximal end of key-filler for isoflurane: the grooves on the screw top will only fit on to the collar of an isoflurane bottle. **(b)** and **(c)** Distal ends of key-fillers for isoflurane (purple) and halothane (red): these 'keys' will only fit into the filling ports of matching vaporizers.

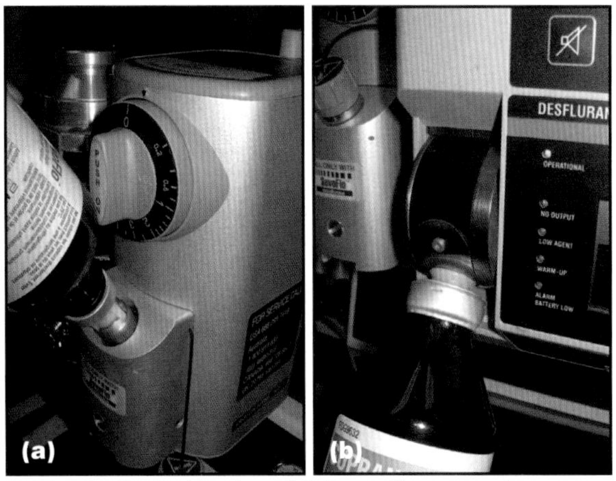

4.33 Sealed bottles of **(a)** sevoflurane and **(b)** desflurane fitting into the filling ports of their specific vaporizers.

Checking plenum vaporizers before use

Before the gas flow is turned on, vaporizers should be checked to ensure that:

- They contain enough liquid anaesthetic (and are not overfilled)
- The filling port is tightly closed
- The control dial turns smoothly. 'Sticking' of the dial can be a problem with halothane vaporizers, where thymol (added to halothane as a preservative) can accumulate and make the dial difficult to turn. To avoid this, it is recommended that halothane vaporizers are drained and refilled at regular intervals (usually weekly).

Position of vaporizers on the back bar

If two or more vaporizers are fitted to the back bar, their relative position is important. In simple terms, the vaporizer for the more volatile agent should be mounted upstream (i.e. closer to the flowmeters). More correctly, vaporizer position depends on the ratio between the SVP and the minimum alveolar concentration (MAC; see Chapter 14). The vaporizer for the agent with the lowest ratio should be placed upstream and that with the highest ratio downstream (Figure 4.34). The arrangement of sevoflurane–isoflurane–halothane (from upstream to downstream) minimizes the potential for vaporizer contamination from considerations of SVP and potency (MAC).

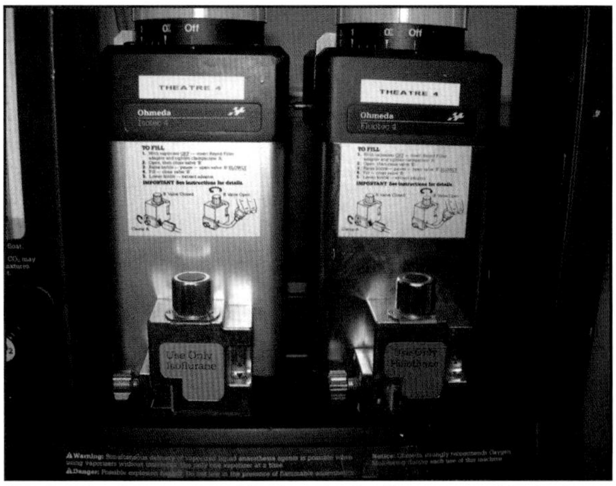

4.34 Correct positioning for isoflurane and halothane vaporizers on the back bar, based on the ratio of SVP/minimum alveolar concentration.

'Vaporizer in circuit' anaesthetic machines

Examples of these include the Komesaroff and Stephens' machines. These are basically circle breathing systems (see Chapter 5) with one or more draw-over (low-resistance) vaporizers positioned within the circle.

The basic design of the Komesaroff machine consists of an oxygen supply, pressure-reducing valve and flowmeter attached to a circle breathing system, which incorporates one or two in-circuit vaporizers (Figure 4.35). The Stephens' machine is similar in design but incorporates a single in-circuit vaporizer and does not have an integral oxygen supply (Figure 4.36).

These machines are economical to use because of the very low fresh gas flows required, but do need some practice to operate. Disadvantages include the possibility of anaesthetic overdosage, especially if intermittent positive pressure ventilation is used. Also, performance of the draw-over vaporizers may be affected by contamination with water vapour.

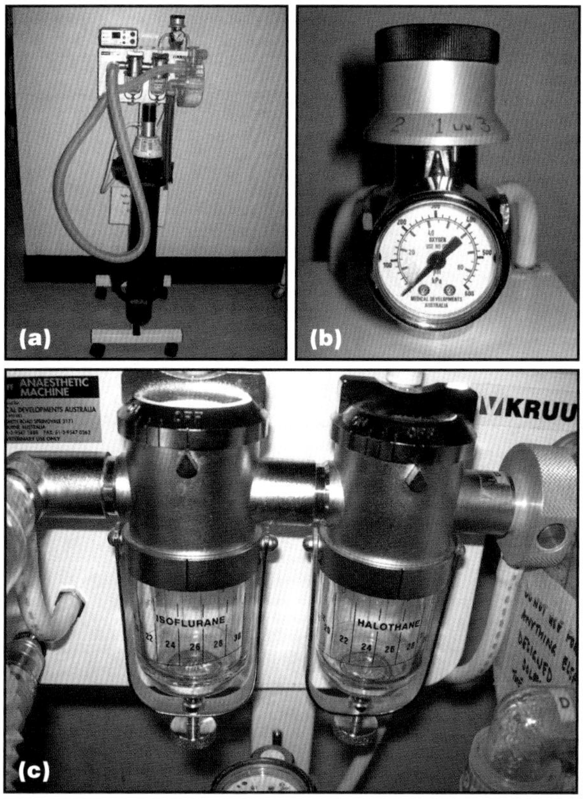

4.35 The Komesaroff anaesthetic machine. **(a)** Complete unit. **(b)** Flowmeter on the Komesaroff machine, designed for delivering very low flows. **(c)** Low-resistance draw-over vaporizers for isoflurane and halothane.

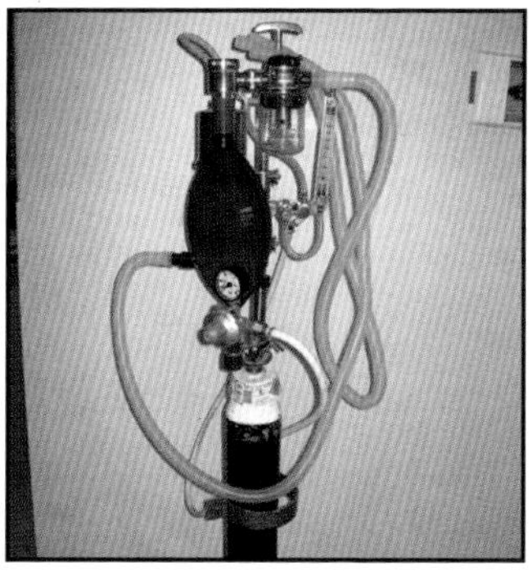

4.36 The Stephens' anaesthetic machine.

Checking the anaesthetic machine before use

The anaesthetic machine should always be checked before use (Figure 4.37).

1. Ensure flow control valves are turned off.
2. Ensure cylinders are turned off and fitted securely on the hanger yoke.
3. Press the oxygen flush valve until no gas flows from the common gas outlet.
4. Check that flowmeters and pressure gauges are at zero.
5. Open the oxygen cylinder valve (slowly, anticlockwise) and observe the registered pressure. Open then close the oxygen flowmeter control valve to ensure smooth function. Press the oxygen flush valve. (On machines that carry a second oxygen cylinder, the tested cylinder should be closed first and the test repeated on the second cylinder.)
6. Label the cylinders either 'In Use' or 'Full' depending on the registered pressure.
7. Replace cylinders with little remaining gas.
8. Open the oxygen cylinder that is 'In Use' and set the oxygen flow to 2 l/minute. Examine the status of the nitrous oxide cylinders as in Step 5. Label the nitrous oxide cylinders.
9. Set the nitrous oxide flow to 4 l/minute then turn off the oxygen supply; ensure low oxygen warning device operates.
10. Check the vaporizer (see text).
11. Check overpressure and emergency air intake valves.

4.37 Checking the anaesthetic machine before use.

References and further reading

Al-Shaikh B and Stacey S (2001) *Essentials of Anaesthetic Equipment, 2nd edn.* Churchill Livingstone, New York

Davey AJ and Diba A (2005) *Ward's Anaesthetic Equipment, 5th edn.* Elsevier Saunders, Philadelphia

Dorsch JA and Dorsch SE (1999) *Understanding Anesthesia Equipment, 4th edn.* Lippincott Williams & Wilkins, Pennsylvania

Laredo FG, Sanchez-Valverde MA, Cantalapiedra AG *et al.* (1998) Efficacy of the Komesaroff anaesthetic machine for delivering isoflurane to dogs. *Veterinary Record* **143,** 437–440

Ward CS (1975) Anaesthetic equipment: physical principles and maintenance. Baillière Tindall, London

5

Breathing systems and ancillary equipment

Lynne Hughes

Definition and function of breathing systems

Breathing systems are interposed between an anaesthetic machine and a patient, i.e. between the common gas outlet and an endotracheal tube or a facemask.

They serve to:

- Deliver oxygen and anaesthetic agents from the anaesthetic machine to the patient
- Remove carbon dioxide exhaled by the patient
- Provide a means of ventilating the lungs, by applying pressure on the reservoir bag.

Ancillary functions include delivery of waste anaesthetic gases to a scavenging system, measurement of airway pressure, gas sampling and volume measurements.

Other definitions relating to breathing systems

- Rebreathing: to inhale previously respired gases, from which carbon dioxide may have been removed. In some cases this may lead to accumulation of carbon dioxide; however, in the context of anaesthetic breathing systems it is possible for patients to rebreathe either partially or fully without an increase in arterial carbon dioxide tension (hypercapnia). The amount of rebreathing will depend on the gas flow, the apparatus deadspace and the design of the breathing system.
- Apparatus deadspace: the volume of the breathing system occupied by gases that are rebreathed without any change in composition.
- Minute volume: the sum of all gas volumes exhaled in 1 minute. It is calculated as a multiple of tidal volume and respiratory rate. An approximate value is 200 ml/kg.
- Tidal volume: the volume of gas exhaled in one breath. An approximate value is 10–20 ml/kg.

Basic components of breathing systems and their function

These features are summarized in Figure 5.1.

Components of breathing systems (and their synonyms)	Functions	Notes
Breathing tubes (limbs)	To convey gases to and from patient To allow flexibility in positioning of breathing system To act as a reservoir	May be rubber or plastic Smooth internal bore causes less turbulence Corrugated tubing is capable of expansion
Reservoir bag (breathing bag, rebreathing bag)	To allow accumulation of gas during exhalation To act as a reservoir for inhalation To visualize breathing To provide a method of assisting ventilation To protect the patient from excessive pressure	Should contain at least twice tidal volume of patient Sizes from 0.5–4 litres Ellipsoid shape Open-ended or closed Compliance accommodates rise in pressure
Carbon dioxide absorbent (Waters' canister, soda lime, baralyme)	To absorb carbon dioxide. This allows complete rebreathing of exhaled gases	See section on Breathing systems with carbon dioxide absorption
One-way valves (unidirectional valves)	To ensure that gases flow towards the patient in one breathing tube and away from the patient in the other To prevent mixing of fresh gas with carbon dioxide-rich gas	Present in the circle system Valve leaflet/disc may sit horizontally (turret or dome type) or vertically. Horizontal is preferable
Pressure relief valve (pop-off valve, scavenging valve, spill valve, expiratory valve, APL valve, etc.)	To limit the build up of pressure within the system To release waste gases To allow safe connection to a scavenging system	Most have a lightweight disc on a narrow seating held in place by a spring APL valve limits the maximum pressure in the breathing system
Fresh gas inlet	To connect the breathing system to the common gas outlet on the anaesthetic machine	Attach with 'push and twist' action for maximum security

5.1 Basic components of breathing systems and their function.

Names and classification of breathing systems

The classification of breathing systems is confusing and terminology is complicated. They have been classified in various ways:

- According to their function (open, semi-open, semi-closed, closed)
- Whether they allow rebreathing
- Whether they contain absorbent to remove carbon dioxide
- The systems without carbon dioxide absorption were classified by Mapleson in 1954 (A to F).

For the purposes of this chapter, the most common name for the breathing system will be used and reference will be made to alternative names and classifications. Descriptions of the passage of gas in each system are included in relation to the spontaneously breathing patient only. For further details on classification systems, the mechanical aspects of individual systems and their detailed use during intermittent positive pressure ventilation (IPPV), the reader is directed to a standard textbook on anaesthesia equipment.

In veterinary anaesthesia, the simplest method of describing breathing systems is by grouping them into systems with similarities in their mode of use.

Breathing systems without carbon dioxide absorption

Some general points when using breathing systems *without* carbon dioxide absorption:

- There are no unidirectional valves in any of these systems and so clearance of carbon dioxide is dependent on using an adequate flow of fresh gas
- The fresh gas flow should not be altered during anaesthesia, unless there is a change in the patient's minute volume
- In order to prevent rebreathing of alveolar gas, all fresh gas flows are based on a multiple of minute volume. Their proper function also depends on an end-expiratory pause. If the respiratory pattern alters, and especially if respiratory rate increases during anaesthesia, the fresh gas flow should be recalculated and increased
- When the vaporizer setting is altered, the patient receives the new percentage of anaesthetic agent at the next breath. This makes it possible to alter depth of anaesthesia rapidly
- Inspired gas is cold and dry and will contribute to the development of hypothermia, especially in small patients
- High fresh gas flow increases the cost of anaesthesia and also the amount of atmospheric pollution
- To increase the efficiency of these systems, a capnograph may be used to monitor levels of inspired carbon dioxide and the gas flow reduced until rebreathing is detected (see Chapter 7)
- If nitrous oxide is used, the total fresh gas flow may be divided between oxygen and nitrous oxide; the usual oxygen:nitrous oxide ratio is 1:2.

The *T-piece* and the *Bain* systems are functionally similar and require fresh gas flows of at least twice the minute volume to prevent carbon dioxide accumulation. Both may be used for the spontaneously breathing patient, but are most economical when used for IPPV. The T-piece is most often used for cats and small dogs, while the Bain is suitable for larger dogs. However, in North America the Bain is commonly used for patients less than 10 kg bodyweight and the T-piece is rarely used.

The *Magill* and *Lack* systems allow partial rebreathing of gas from the patient's anatomical deadspace. Thus, a fresh gas flow equal to alveolar ventilation should prevent accumulation of carbon dioxide. However, if these systems are used to provide IPPV, this advantage is lost and gas flows in the order of two to three times the minute volume are required. Both systems are suitable for small to medium dogs. These breathing systems are not commonly used in North America.

The T-piece

This section includes various modifications of the T-piece, with and without bags, e.g. Ayre's T-piece, Jackson-Rees modified T-piece (Mapleson D, E and F) (Figure 5.2).

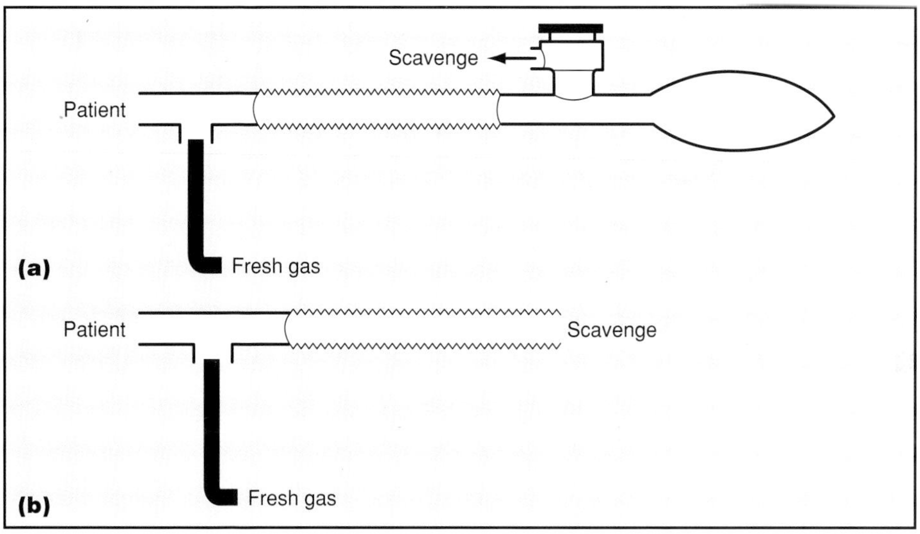

5.2 T-pieces. **(a)** Paediatric T-piece with APL valve (Mapleson D). **(b)** Ayre's T-piece (Mapleson E). (continues) ▶

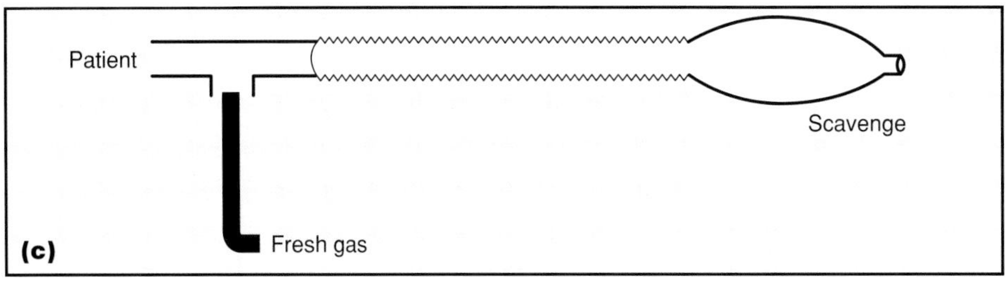

5.2 (continued) T-pieces. **(c)** Jackson-Rees modified T-piece (Mapleson F).

Fresh gas enters the system close to the patient (at a T-junction) and fills the breathing tubing, from where it is inhaled. After a short pause, exhaled gas passes into the breathing tubing and is driven by the continuous flow of fresh gas to the exterior through the tubing itself, or an open-ended reservoir bag, or an expiratory valve. The tubing thus refills with fresh gas during the expiratory pause. A high fresh gas flow of two and a half to three times the minute volume (or approximately 600 ml/kg/minute) is required to prevent rebreathing of alveolar gas (Figure 5.3). Additional points of interest include:

- There are no one-way valves or absorbent canisters in this system. Thus, resistance to breathing is low and the system is suitable for small patients. The resistance from the adjustable pressure limiting (APL) valve on the paediatric Mapleson D is small (2–3 cmH_2O) when the valve is fully open
- The requirement for high fresh gas flows makes this system uneconomical in patients greater than 10–12 kg
- It must be possible to contain the patient's tidal volume within the breathing tubing and the reservoir bag, otherwise waste gas (or air) will be entrained during inspiration
- The narrow breathing tubing may cause resistance during peak expiratory gas flow. This is of importance in larger dogs
- In the Jackson-Rees modification, waste gas is scavenged through a tail on an open-ended reservoir bag. Extreme care must be taken to ensure that the tail does not become twisted and obstruct the outflow of gas: the high pressures generated can cause a reduction in venous return, pneumomediastinum and/or pneumothorax, resulting in disaster
- IPPV is possible by partially or intermittently blocking an open-ended reservoir bag, or by partially closing the APL valve on other (Mapleson D) versions.

Disposable paediatric versions of this system are in common use in veterinary practice. Models should be chosen with an APL valve (Mapleson D). This ensures that, during routine use, pressure in excess of the limit cannot be transmitted to the patient: a suitable pressure limit is 35 cmH_2O. This is the maximum pressure that can be generated before the valve opens. In addition, easy and safe scavenging is possible via a standard scavenging shroud. Disposable systems must be discarded on a regular basis.

The Bain system (Mapleson D)

Two versions of the Bain system are available: in the co-axial version, tubing carrying fresh gas is situated inside the expiratory tubing (Figure 5.4); in the parallel version, the two lengths of tubing run side by side. This system is functionally similar to the T-piece in its mode of action. Prior to inspiration, fresh gas is delivered in close proximity to the patient and fills a length of breathing tubing, from where it is inhaled. Exhaled gas passes through the expiratory limb of the breathing system to a reservoir bag, a pressure relief valve and then to the exterior. Some mixing of fresh gas and exhaled gas occurs in the tubing but, provided fresh gas flow is adequate, no significant rebreathing of carbon dioxide-rich alveolar gas should occur. Fresh gas flows of two to four times the minute volume are recommended for spontaneously breathing animals: in practice, once to twice the minute volume is usually adequate (200–400 ml/kg/minute; see Figure 5.3). This may be lowered further if a capnograph is used to detect rebreathing. As the reservoir for fresh gas (the breathing tubing and the breathing bag) is more capacious than the Ayre's T-piece, the system is suitable for larger patients.

Breathing system	Multiple of minute volume	Fresh gas flow (ml/kg/minute)	Size of animal	Suitable for IPPV?
T-piece	2.5–3	500–600	Uneconomical if >10 kg	Yes
Bain	1–2	200–400	Uneconomical if >15–20 kg	Yes
Magill	0.8–1	160–200	Uneconomical if >25–30 kg	Best not unless gas flow increased
Lack	0.8–1	160–200	Uneconomical if >25–30 kg	Best not unless gas flow increased
Mini-Lack	1	200	Up to 10 kg	Yes, if gas flow increased to 600 ml/kg/minute
Humphrey ADE, A mode	0.5–0.75	100–150	Up to 10–20 kg	Yes (manual)

5.3 Gas flows and suggested patient size for breathing systems without carbon dioxide absorption. Provided inspired carbon dioxide levels are monitored, gas flows may be reduced further than those stated above. In the Lack system fresh gas flows of 120 ml/kg/minute have not caused rebreathing in dogs greater than 15 kg. Note that comments on economy are based on an arbitrary fresh gas flow less than 6 l/minute.

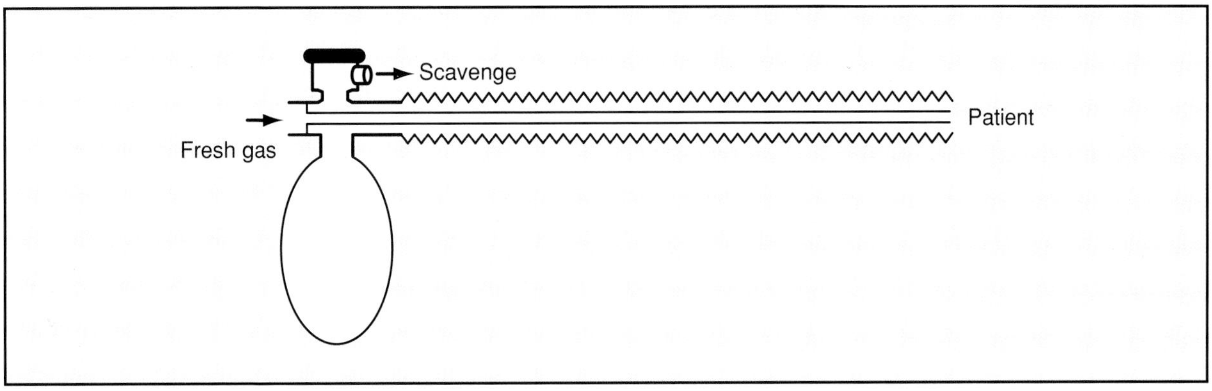

5.4 The Bain system (Mapleson D).

When used for IPPV, the pressure relief valve may be closed during lung inflation only and opened immediately following compression of the bag. Extreme care should be taken when using the Bain for IPPV, as pressures within the system may build up rapidly if high gas flows are used. High gas flows during IPPV may lead to hypocapnia and are seldom required.

The Magill system (Mapleson A)

The Magill system consists of a reservoir bag (situated beside the fresh gas inlet), wide-bore breathing tubing and a pressure relief valve (Figure 5.5). Fresh gas fills the reservoir bag and the breathing tubing before reaching the patient, so that, when the patient inhales, the bag empties. The initial portion of exhaled breath (deadspace gas) passes along the breathing tubing to the partially empty bag, until the pressure increases sufficiently to open the pressure relief valve. Since the pressure relief valve is situated close to the patient, alveolar gas is preferentially vented and deadspace gas is retained for rebreathing. In the spontaneously breathing patient, the only requirement for fresh gas is to replace alveolar gas: approximately 0.8 times the minute volume (160 ml/kg/minute; see Figure 5.3).

The Lack system (Mapleson A)

The Lack system also allows rebreathing of deadspace gas and requires a similar fresh gas flow to the Magill (160 ml/kg/minute). This system has two lengths of breathing tubing, one which transports fresh gas to the patient and the other which brings exhaled gas to the scavenging system. The bag is situated between the common gas outlet and the inspiratory tubing. As in the Magill system, when the patient inhales the bag will empty, allowing the first portion of exhaled gas to pass into the inspiratory tubing. This, combined with continuous fresh gas flow, will increase the pressure in the system and drive the second portion of the exhaled breath (alveolar gas) into the expiratory tubing where it exits through the pressure relief valve. There are no unidirectional valves to prevent the patient inhaling from both the inspiratory and expiratory tubes. Like the Bain system, the Lack is available in parallel and co-axial versions (Figure 5.6ab).

The mini parallel Lack (Figure 5.6c) was designed as an alternative to the T-piece for patients under 10 kg; the tubing connectors are too narrow for larger patients. The recommended gas flow is 200 ml/kg/minute (see Figure 5.3), although it has been used successfully in cats at lower gas flows (Walsh and Taylor, 2004).

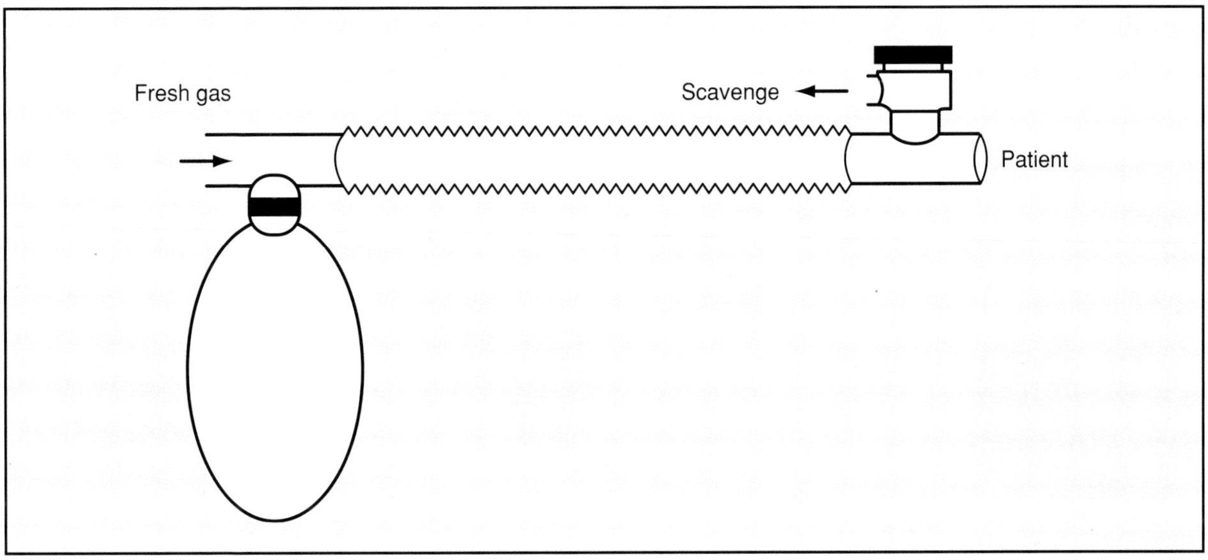

5.5 The Magill system (Mapleson A).

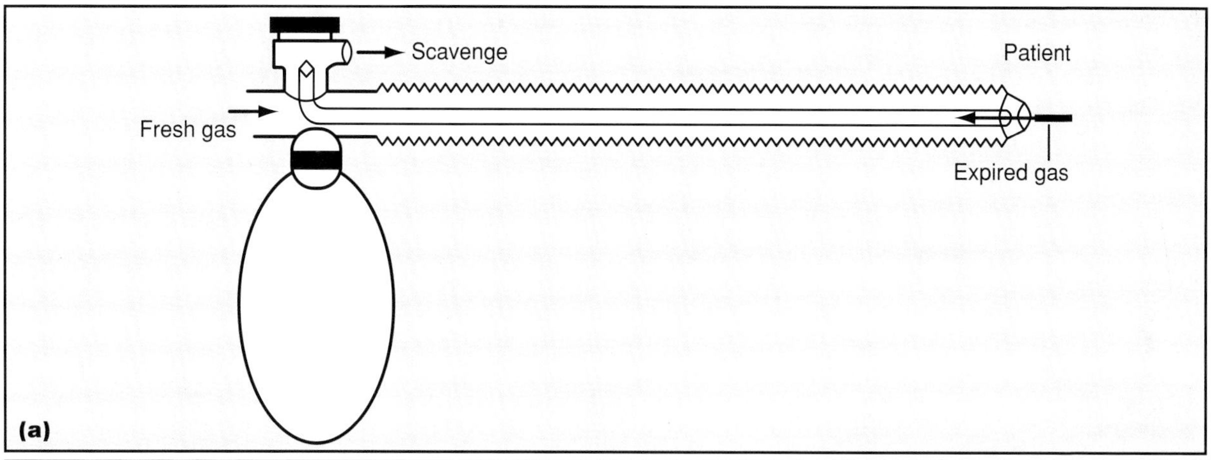

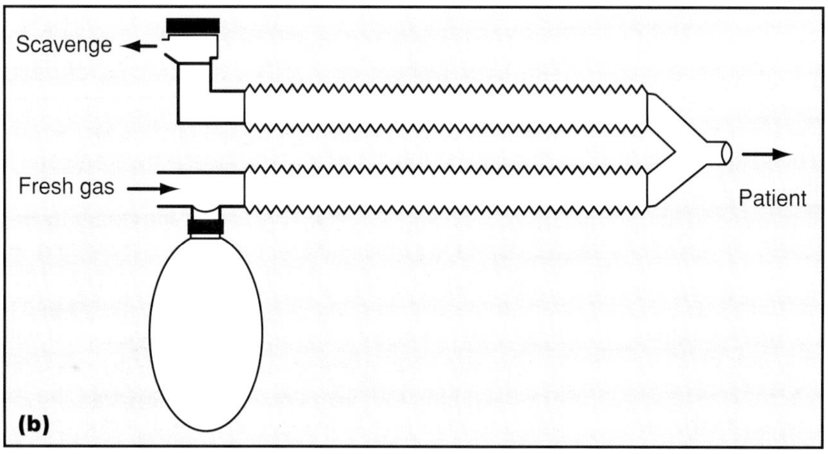

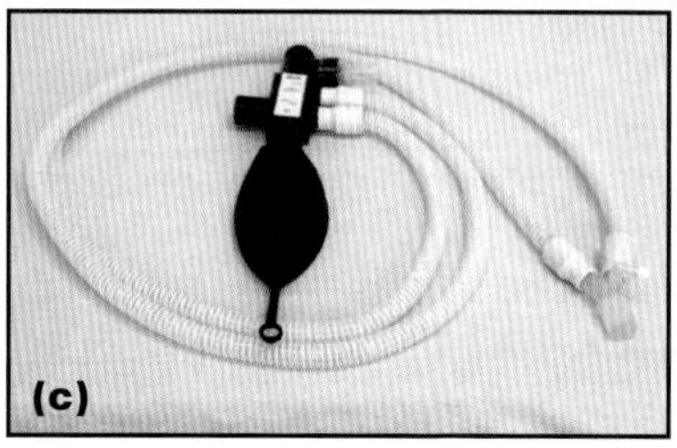

5.6 **(a)** The Lack system (Mapleson A). **(b)** The parallel Lack (Mapleson A). **(c)** The mini-Lack.

The Humphrey ADE system

The Humphrey ADE is a versatile breathing system, which may be used in three different modes by altering a lever switch (Figure 5.7). As there are a number of versions on the market, the reader is directed to the manufacturer's instructions (Arnolds Veterinary Products Ltd.) for detailed descriptions of the use of each system. The notes below are intended to give a summary of the modes of use only.

The main component of the system is the Humphrey block, which attaches to the common gas outlet on an anaesthetic machine. The constituents are:

- A lever which can be moved to the upright (A mode) or downward (E mode) positions. The lever rotates a metal cylinder with openings which allow the passage of gas into other components
- An APL valve with a red spindle (to indicate performance) and a scavenging shroud. The APL valve offers a small amount of positive end-expiratory pressure (PEEP) of about 1 cmH_2O, which may assist in preventing alveolar collapse
- An over-pressure relief valve which opens at pressures in excess of 60 cmH_2O
- A closed reservoir bag
- A port for connection to a ventilator
- Two connection ports for lengths of 15 mm smooth-bore breathing tubing. The breathing tubes are connected at a Y-connection leading to the patient.

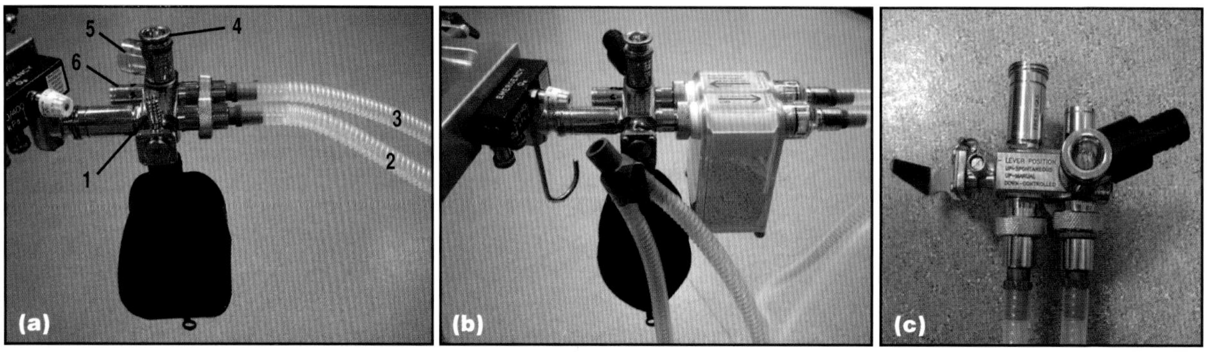

5.7 The Humphrey ADE system. **(a)** Without canister, with parallel breathing tubing and reservoir bag. The ventilator port is not visible. 1 = Lever to select spontaneous or controlled ventilation. The lever is in the 'up' or Mapleson A position for spontaneous ventilation; 2 = Inspiratory tubing; 3 = Expiratory tubing; 4 = APL valve with visible indicator; 5 = Scavenging shroud; 6 = Safety pressure relief valve. **(b)** With soda lime canister attached. **(c)** Top view.

When the patient is breathing spontaneously and the lever is in the upright position, the Humphrey ADE may be used in a mode similar to the Lack (Mapleson A). The A mode is more economical than the Lack and gas flows of 100–150 ml/kg/minute will prevent rebreathing of alveolar gas. This system has also proved suitable for manual ventilation, without altering the gas flow. When the position of the lever switch is facing downwards and respiration is controlled by a ventilator, the system may be used in a similar mode to the T-piece (Mapleson E). It is also possible to use the system in a fashion analogous to the Bain (Mapleson D), but this is now considered unnecessary as the A mode is more economical. A recent modification of the Humphrey ADE is the inclusion of a removable absorbent canister so that the system may be used in circle mode (see below). This further increases efficiency, and its use is recommended by the manufacturer in dogs greater than 10–20 kg.

The Humphrey ADE is suitable for use in cats and dogs. The 15 mm smooth-bore tubing has a low internal volume, reduces turbulence, encourages laminar gas flow and does not increase resistance to breathing when compared to standard 22 mm corrugated tubing. A smaller reservoir bag (500 ml or 1 l) should be used in cats and small dogs.

Breathing systems with carbon dioxide absorption

The *circle* and *to-and-fro* systems allow rebreathing of exhaled gases, from which carbon dioxide has been removed by an absorbent. Fresh gas flow must include oxygen at a rate at least equal to that required by the body for cellular metabolism. These systems are most economical when used for 'low-flow' anaesthesia (see below). Both systems may be used in the spontaneously breathing patient, or may be used to provide IPPV. Unless specifically stated, most systems manufactured for the veterinary market are not suitable for spontaneously breathing patients weighing less than 12–15 kg. The advantages and disadvantages of using these systems are summarized in Figure 5.8.

The circle system

The arrangement of the components of the circle system ensures that gases move in one direction only, in a circular fashion (Figure 5.9a). Inspired gas is a mixture of fresh gas and previously exhaled gas, from which carbon dioxide has been removed. The system contains two unidirectional valves: one allows the patient to inhale only through an inspiratory breathing tube (limb), which connects to the patient at a Y-piece; another prevents exhaled gas from entering the inspiratory limb, instead it enters the expiratory breathing tube (limb), which is also connected to the Y-piece. The other basic components of the system are an absorbent canister, a closed reservoir bag and a pressure relief valve. The exact arrangement varies from manufacturer to manufacturer. Some systems include a pressure manometer, which is useful when carrying out IPPV.

Specific advantages of the circle system include:

- The apparatus deadspace is small provided the unidirectional valves are functioning correctly: it is only in the Y-piece that mixing of inspiratory and expiratory gases may occur
- Removal of carbon dioxide is efficient because the passage of gas in a circle ensures that all exhaled gas must pass through the canister
- The pressure relief valve is situated remotely from the patient, allowing ease of access
- Dust from the absorbent should not reach the patient as it will settle in the breathing tube
- The risk from hyperthermia is reduced, as heat generated by the absorption of carbon dioxide may be dissipated by the breathing tubes.

The to-and-fro system

In the to-and-fro system, fresh gas enters the system near the patient. The patient exhales through a Waters' canister, for absorption of carbon dioxide, into a closed reservoir bag and gas returns to the patient by the same route (Figure 5.9b). Excess gas is vented through a pressure relief valve situated close to the patient connector. This system has several disadvantages when compared with the circle:

Advantages
Absorbs carbon dioxide
Allows rebreathing of exhaled gas, therefore allowing low fresh gas flows to be employed – this results in greater economy
Warms inspired gas
Moistens inspired gas
Low-flow systems result in less environmental pollution
Disadvantages
Channelling or tracking of gases may occur if the canister is not packed correctly or if the granules fragment (particular problem in the to-and-fro system)
Absorbent presents resistance to breathing
May generate excessive heat when used for large breed dogs
Water may collect in the breathing tubes (particular problem in the circle)
Absorbents may react with some anaesthetic agents to form toxic byproducts (see Figure 5.10)
Absorbents may generate caustic dust, which may reach the respiratory tract (particular problem in the to-and-fro system)
Deadspace may increase with the duration of the anaesthetic (particular problem in the to-and-fro system)
May cause 'drag' on the endotracheal tube (particular problem in the to-and-fro system)
Canister may be switched out of the system in some designs (particular problem in the circle)
Canister may be difficult to clean
Canister is prone to leakage

5.8 Advantages and disadvantages of using an absorbent canister.

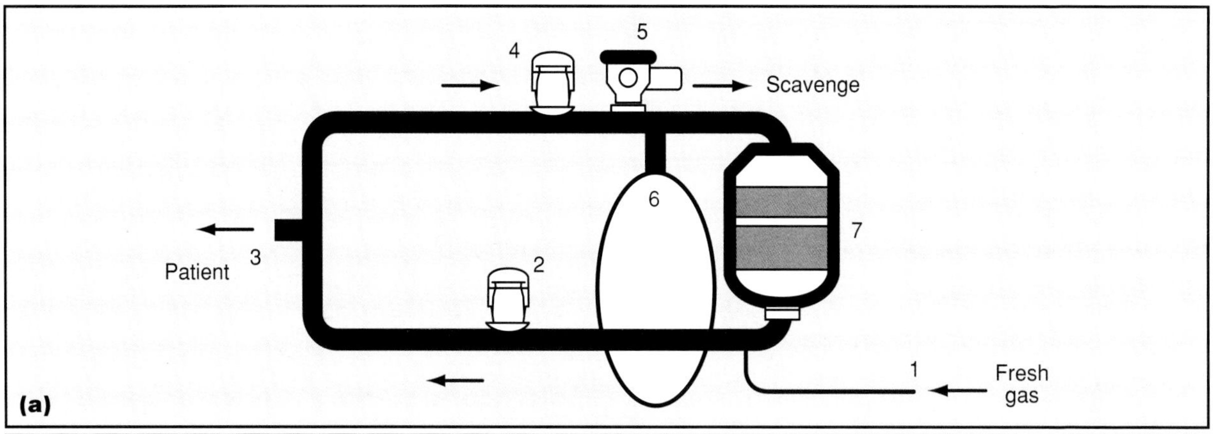

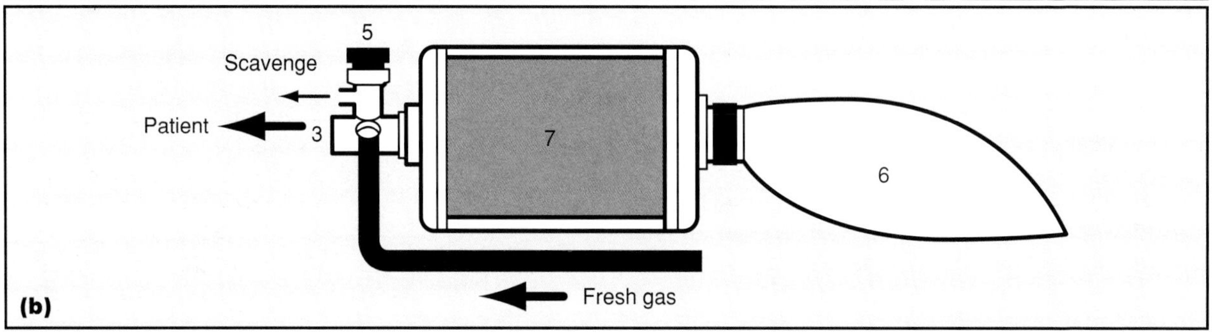

5.9 **(a)** The circle system. **(b)** The to-and-fro system. 1 = Fresh gas inflow; 2 and 4 = Inspiratory and expiratory unidirectional valves; 3 = Patient connector; 5 = Pressure relief valve; 6 = Reservoir bag; 7 = Absorbent canister.

- The canister is usually positioned horizontally and, as the absorbent settles and granules disintegrate, spaces will appear above the absorbent. This allows channelling of gases through areas with no absorbent, with resultant reduction in absorption of carbon dioxide
- The canister is situated in close proximity to the patient, increasing the possibility of caustic dust reaching the respiratory tract, especially during IPPV
- The system is bulky and heavy, and exerts considerable drag on the endotracheal tube
- The pressure relief valve is situated close to the patient, which may be inconvenient during surgery
- As anaesthesia progresses, the absorbent becomes increasingly exhausted from the surface closest to the patient; over time this results in an enlargement in apparatus deadspace
- When used for small patients (less than 10 kg) a significant portion of alveolar gas may never reach working absorbent, resulting in rebreathing of carbon dioxide-rich gas.

Substances used to absorb carbon dioxide

In the anaesthetized patient, if carbon dioxide is removed from the exhaled breath, then the remainder of the respiratory gases may be recycled and inhaled. The advantages of a breathing system containing absorption of carbon dioxide include:

- Decreased fresh gas requirement (oxygen ± nitrous oxide)
- Decreased expense of volatile agent
- Decreased environmental pollution
- Decreased loss of heat and moisture from the patient.

The most common substances used to absorb carbon dioxide are calcium hydroxide and sodium hydroxide. Barium hydroxide was removed from the market in Europe in 2004. Various advances in manufacturing have resulted in the addition of other compounds to increase the effectiveness of the absorbent and reduce the production of toxic byproducts (Figure 5.10).

Compound	Properties	Possible problems
Calcium hydroxide	Main component of soda lime	Very soft unless mixed with other substances
Sodium hydroxide	Enhances reactivity and ability to bind water. Usually present in soda lime.	If dry, causes degradation of isoflurane, enflurane and desflurane to carbon monoxide, and degradation of sevoflurane to compound A, formaldehyde and methanol
Potassium hydroxide	As sodium hydroxide	As sodium hydroxide. Now discontinued
Barium	Contains water of crystallization. Does not require hardeners	Produces more carbon monoxide and compound A than soda lime. Removed from market

5.10 Main constituents of carbon dioxide absorbents and their properties. (continues) ▶

Compound	Properties	Possible problems
Water	14–19% essential for chain reaction to occur	If there is inadequate water, absorbents will exhaust quickly, can produce toxic compounds and may absorb anaesthetic agents. Excess water will increase resistance and stickiness
Indicators	Acid or base whose colour depends on the pH. Used to reveal when the absorbent is exhausted	It is important to be familiar with the expected colour change Ethyl violet may be deactivated in light
Zeolite	Increases porosity, hardness and water content	May absorb anaesthetic agent if absorbent is very dry
Silica	To overcome softness of calcium hydroxide	
Calcium chloride and calcium sulphate	Enhance reactivity, ability to bind water and improve the hardness	Colour may change if dried out

5.10 (continued) Main constituents of carbon dioxide absorbents and their properties.

Carbon dioxide is removed from exhaled gases by a chemical reaction. The reaction both requires and generates water – on balance more water is generated than is required. The reaction also generates heat and a pH change. Several steps are involved but they may be summarized as follows:

1. $H_2O + CO_2 \rightarrow H_2CO_3$
2. $2H_2CO_3 + 2NaOH + Ca(OH)_2 \rightarrow$ $CaCO_3 + Na_2CO_3 + 4H_2O + \text{heat}$

Absorbent materials are granular. The following details are important:

- The size of the granules. A combination of small and large granules is preferable as this minimizes resistance to breathing, increases the surface area for contact and absorption, and decreases caking and channelling
- Granules may fragment, producing dust. If excessive, dust may:
  - Result in increased resistance to breathing
  - Cause caking of granules and channelling of gases through the spaces which are formed
  - Reach the patient, where it will cause caustic burns of the respiratory tract
  - Settle on valves and other moving parts, causing them to malfunction
  - Migrate on to gaskets and rubber seals, causing them to leak.

Modern manufacturing techniques help reduce the quantity of dust produced by absorbents.

Signs of exhaustion of the carbon dioxide absorbent include:

- Colour change – the colour varies with the pH indicator used
- A canister that is cold to the touch when in use
- Increased inspired carbon dioxide detected by a capnograph
- Signs of hypercapnia, i.e. increased respiratory rate, heart rate and blood pressure, in association with a bounding pulse and wound oozing
- Granules that are hard, not crumbly (gloves should be worn when carrying out this test).

Depleted absorbents may appear to regenerate as the granules dry out when not in use. However, the additional capacity to absorb carbon dioxide is minimal and the indicator usually reverts to the exhausted colour after only a few breaths. Absorbent should be replaced as soon as the indicator change is noticed.

Absorbent canisters are manufactured in many shapes and sizes. The desirable features of a canister are:

- Transparent walls, so that the colour change can be visualized: this is the norm for modern canisters
- Large cross-sectional area, to decrease resistance and dust migration: this is a feature of most circle absorbers, but not of the to-and-fro
- Large enough to contain the tidal volume of the patient in the intergranular space: there is variation between manufacturers in the sizes of canisters
- Situated in the vertical position, to prevent gas channelling through unfilled portions: this is usual in the circle, but not in the to-and-fro.

Practices that avoid the production of toxic byproducts from absorbents include:

- Not allowing the absorbent to dry out, i.e. turning off the anaesthetic machine and/or disconnecting the oxygen supply when not in use, so that there is no possibility of prolonged gas flow through the absorbent
- Turning off the vaporizer when not in use
- Checking the absorber for excessive heat; heat increases the production of toxic byproducts.

Precautions for the care and handling of soda lime include:

- Wet soda lime is caustic – avoid touching it (wear gloves), inhaling it (wear a mask) or allowing it to enter the eyes
- Handle the absorbent gently to avoid fragmentation of granules and dust production
- Reseal the package after opening to prevent the absorbent reacting with air, deactivation of the indicator by light and loss of moisture
- Store at temperatures above freezing to prevent granules expanding and disintegrating.

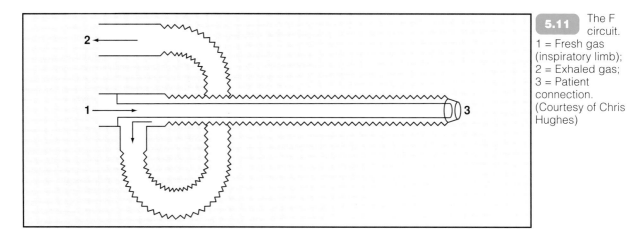

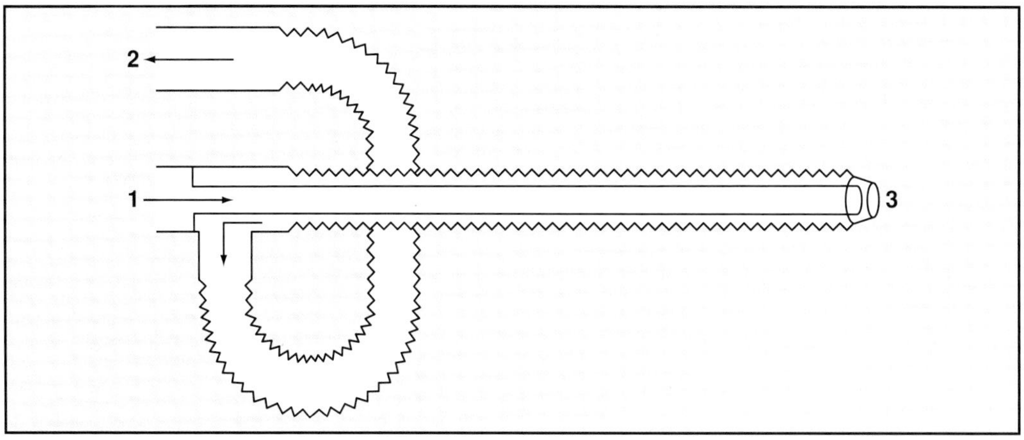

5.11 The F circuit. 1 = Fresh gas (inspiratory limb); 2 = Exhaled gas; 3 = Patient connection. (Courtesy of Chris Hughes)

F circuit

The universal F circuit (Figure 5.11) is not a complete breathing system in itself: it is a co-axial (tube-within-a-tube) system of breathing tubing in which the inner and outer tubes diverge at one end. The patient is attached at the co-axial end, while the other ends can be connected to the inspiratory and expiratory side of a breathing system.

It is most commonly used as part of a circle breathing system when the diverging ends are attached in the same manner as the traditional lengths of tubing. It is usual for the inner tubing to be the inspiratory limb and the outer tubing the expiratory. Characteristics include:

- One length of tubing instead of two attached to the patient. This streamlined version is less bulky and may cause less drag
- It is thermally efficient, as heat from the exhaled breath warms the inspired gases
- Water vapour condensing in the outer expiratory tube is more likely to cause an obstruction than in the two tube system.

The F circuit is manufactured in various lengths which are useful for special anaesthetic procedures such as magnetic resonance imaging (MRI).

Low-flow anaesthesia

The circle and to-and-fro systems may be utilized with low flows in veterinary anaesthesia. When considering the minimum fresh gas flow, only the oxygen required for cellular metabolism need be supplied, as exhaled gas is rebreathed. Any additional gas must be vented through the pressure relief valve. These systems are thus economical to run and result in less atmospheric pollution. Estimates of oxygen requirements in dogs and cats under general anaesthesia vary from 2–7 ml/kg/minute. As this figure is dependent on metabolic rate, age, temperature, etc., a safe estimate that also affords ease of calculation is 10 ml/kg/minute.

True 'low-flow' anaesthesia involves provision of just enough fresh gas for metabolism, for the entire duration of anaesthesia. The breathing system is used in the 'closed' mode with the pressure relief valve remaining shut. This method requires considerable skill to maintain and alter depth of anaesthesia and for this reason a simpler and more reliable method is detailed below.

Using low-flow anaesthesia in veterinary practice

- Following induction of anaesthesia and endotracheal intubation, a fresh gas flow of 100 ml/kg/minute should be provided for 5–10 minutes. The pressure relief valve should be fully open during this period. The advantages of an initial high flow include purging the system of air (nitrogen) and filling it with fresh gas (oxygen and anaesthetic agent) and also providing sufficient inhaled anaesthetic agent for rapid stabilization of anaesthetic depth.
- Once anaesthetic depth is stabilized, the fresh gas flow may be reduced to approximately 10 ml/kg/minute. Alternatively, 0.5–1 l/minute is adequate for all dogs weighing less than 50 kg. Moreover, many vaporizers require a fresh gas flow of at least 0.5 l/minute to ensure accuracy. At this stage, the pressure relief valve should be partially closed so that the reservoir bag contains adequate gas, but without any detectable increase in pressure within the system; the valve may require occasional adjustment during anaesthesia.

Some general points should be considered when using low-flow anaesthesia:

- The contribution of fresh gas to the overall volume of the breathing system is small when using low-flow anaesthesia; many circle breathing systems in use in veterinary practice have a volume in excess of 4 litres. Moreover, exhaled breath usually contains less volatile agent than was inspired by the patient, especially at the beginning of an anaesthetic. The net result is that the exhaled breath 'dilutes' the effect of the fresh gas, and the patient inhales considerably less volatile agent than the vaporizer setting would suggest. The lower the fresh gas flow used and the larger the patient, the greater the discrepancy between the vaporizer setting and the inspired breath. In addition, this is more noticeable with halothane,

because it takes longer to equilibrate in the body than do isoflurane or sevoflurane. The example below illustrates this:
The minute volume of a 15 kg dog is approximately 3 l/minute (200 ml/kg/minute). If the fresh gas flow during the initial high-flow period is 1.5 l/minute (100 ml/kg/minute), then the diluting effect of the patient's breath is 2:1. However, if the fresh gas flow during the low-flow period is 150 ml/minute (10 ml/kg/minute), then the fresh gas containing volatile agent is diluted 20:1 by the patient's exhaled breath. This explains why it is difficult to stabilize (or change) depth of anaesthesia rapidly using volatile agents and a low-flow system. Over time, the patient exhales increasing amounts of volatile agent and the concentration difference between the vaporizer and inspired percentage of that agent reduces

- The initial vaporizer setting should be maintained until depth of anaesthesia is well stabilized. When the gas flow is reduced, a higher vaporizer setting is usually required, for the reason stated above
- During the course of an uneventful anaesthetic, the vaporizer setting may be increased or decreased by small increments (0.5–1.0%), without varying the gas flow
- If it is necessary to alter the depth of anaesthesia rapidly:
  - The vaporizer setting should be adjusted
  - The gas flow should be increased to 100 ml/kg/minute for several minutes and the pressure relief valve opened fully
  - The contents of the reservoir bag may be 'dumped' into the scavenging system although this is not essential
  - This allows the new vapour setting to wash into the system rapidly. When the required depth of anaesthesia has been achieved, the lower gas flow should again be used
- During the low-flow period, the pressure relief valve may be partially closed, but some gas will be vented to the scavenging system
- If nitrous oxide is used in a rebreathing system, care should be taken to provide adequate inspired oxygen. Because oxygen is continuously consumed by the patient, and nitrous oxide is not, the proportion of oxygen in the system will decrease over time. In the absence of an inspired oxygen analyser, a 1:1 mixture of oxygen:nitrous oxide should be used, and oxygen flow should be set at a minimum of 20 ml/kg/minute
- If the reservoir bag empties, it should be refilled by increasing the gas flow at the flowmeter. Using the oxygen flush mechanism will result in dilution of the volatile anaesthetic agent
- At the conclusion of anaesthesia, gas flow should again be increased and/or the contents of the reservoir bag 'dumped' to flush out exhaled anaesthetic agent, which would otherwise recirculate and prevent the patient from awakening.

Checking and leak testing of breathing systems

Prior to use, all breathing systems should receive a thorough check-over. This is especially important when a system is used for the first time or following reassembly after cleaning.

1. Inspect the system checking that:
   - All components are present and assembled correctly
   - There are no obvious holes, obstructions or foreign bodies in tubing
   - The inner tube of co-axial systems is attached at both ends.
2. Attach to the common gas outlet with a 'push and twist' action and ensure the connection is secure.
3. Test the system for leaks:
   - Close the pressure relief valve, or the tail on an open-ended bag
   - Close the patient connector with a finger or suitable plug
   - Fill the system with oxygen to a pressure of 30–40 cmH_2O
   - Turn off the oxygen flow and ensure that the system maintains the set pressure for at least 10 seconds. In the absence of a pressure gauge the bag should be filled until it appears under pressure and it should be observed for signs of deflation
   - Open the pressure relief valve and ensure that the pressure is immediately relieved
   - Remove the plug from the patient connector.
4. Check the function of the unidirectional valves on the circle.
5. Specific tests are required to check the integrity of the inner tube of co-axial systems (Bain and Lack). Note that these tests must be carried out with care as they can result in disconnection of the inner limb at one or other end:
   - Bain: with an oxygen flow of 2 l/minute, *briefly* occlude the inner limb (with a pencil or plunger from small syringe) and note that the reservoir bag remains deflated. As this generates considerable back pressure in the anaesthetic machine the following may also happen: the flowmeter bobbin will drop, if the machine is fitted with a high-pressure safety valve, it will alarm (if not, the breathing system may be propelled from the common gas outlet)
   - Lack: using a suitably sized endotracheal tube, cover the inner tubing at the patient end. Blow down the endotracheal tube and if any movement is observed in the reservoir bag then there is leakage from the inner limb. (Alternative method: with the pressure relief valve closed, occlude the inner limb and ensure that the reservoir bag distends).

Common hazards caused by breathing systems

The medical literature contains numerous descriptions of hazards caused by faulty breathing systems, or errors in their use. This section covers the most common errors encountered in veterinary practice, their consequences and main causes:

- Disconnection of the breathing system (and resultant hypoxia) caused by:
  - Failure to secure breathing systems using a 'push and twist' action when attaching components. The most common site of disconnection is between the breathing system and the endotracheal tube. This is particularly hazardous during surgery of the head and neck, when the area is covered by drapes
  - Attaching components that are manufactured from different materials. In this case the friction generated will not be as strong as if the two components are made of the same material
- Increased deadspace (and resultant hypercapnia) caused by:
  - Exhausted absorbent in the circle or to-and-fro systems. This may not be noticed if the centre of the canister is fully exhausted while the absorbent around the outside has not changed colour
  - Channelling of gases along the top of an inadequately packed Waters' canister in the to-and-fro
  - Non-functioning unidirectional valves in a circle, which allow mixing of fresh gas with exhaled gas
  - Inadequate fresh gas flow when using systems without carbon dioxide absorption
  - Use of overlong elbow (or other) connectors between the endotracheal tube and the breathing system
  - Disconnection of the inner tubing in a co-axial Bain system
  - Inadvertent switching of the absorbent out of use; this is possible in some older circles
- Excessive pressure at exhalation (and resultant prevention of adequate venous return, barotrauma to the lungs, pneumomediastinum or pneumothorax) caused by:
  - Failure to open the pressure relief valve following leak testing of the breathing system
  - Obstructions of the scavenging outlet, as described above in the open-ended bag of the Jackson-Rees modified T-piece
  - A faulty pressure relief valve which fails to open. This is most likely if disposable breathing systems are re-used indefinitely or if the valves of re-usable systems are over-tightened
  - Obstruction of the pressure relief valve with soda lime granules
  - Obstruction or kinking of the breathing tubing or the neck of the bag by other equipment (often a table)
  - The presence of foreign bodies in the breathing system. This has been reported as a manufacturing or packaging fault
  - The presence of large quantities of water in the expiratory limb of a circle breathing system, particularly if the limb hangs off the table in a loop
- Generation of negative pressure at inspiration (and resultant pulmonary oedema) caused by:
  - Inadequate fresh gas flow resulting in an empty bag when the patient inhales. Some breathing systems incorporate a valve, which allows entrainment of air to combat this
  - Excess 'pull' from an active scavenging system, which empties the bag
  - Failure of the inspiratory valve on the circle system to open
- Hyperthermia (and resultant tachycardia and arrhythmias) caused by heat generated during low-flow anaesthesia when using breathing systems with an absorbent. The incidence is increased in giant-breed dogs and in warm weather.

Disposable breathing systems are in common use in medical anaesthesia, where they are discarded on a routine basis: approximately once a week. As the systems are not designed for prolonged use, faults will develop over time. It is vital that these systems are checked prior to every use and that the veterinary practice develops a routine of discarding them. The most common faults include:

- Unidirectional valves which fail to operate – this may be difficult to detect without a capnograph
- Pressure relief valves which fail to open
- Cracking, splitting or distortion of the attachment for the common gas outlet
- Holes in the breathing tubing or bag
- Disconnection of the inner limb of co-axial systems.

Care and maintenance of breathing systems

For the purposes of this section, breathing systems may be divided into disposable and re-usable. As a general principle, the closer the equipment is to the patient, the greater the need to sterilize or discard it.

Disposable systems (single or limited use)

- Should be chosen if it is suspected that a patient has an infectious disease. The system should be discarded after use.
- Should be fully checked prior to every use.
- If re-used for a limited period, should be discarded on a routine basis (e.g. after a certain number of cases or on a certain date).

Re-usable systems

It is important to adhere to a set routine of thorough cleaning and rinsing, followed by disinfection or sterilizing. It is preferable to fully sterilize re-usable breathing systems periodically, using heat or chemical methods appropriate to the material from which they are manufactured. In the intervening periods they should be dismantled, washed in hot soapy water and soaked in a suitable disinfectant solution on a routine (weekly) basis. In addition, moisture collecting in the breathing tubing from the circle system should be drained daily and the contents of absorbent canisters should be replaced when the colour change is noticed – not left till the following morning.

All re-usable systems must be checked fully when reassembled.

The medical literature contains several case reports documenting cross-infection of patients by anaesthetic-related equipment. Although this evidence is scant in the veterinary field, the potential for transmission of infections via this route should not be ignored and procedures should be put in place to minimize the risk.

Endotracheal tubes

Endotracheal tubes may be manufactured from red rubber, PVC or silicone (Figures 5.12 and 5.13). There is generally a pilot balloon, which is used as an indicator that the cuff is inflated. The Murphy eye is an oval hole opposite the bevel. This allows gas to flow through the tube should the bevel become obstructed or be positioned against the wall of the trachea.

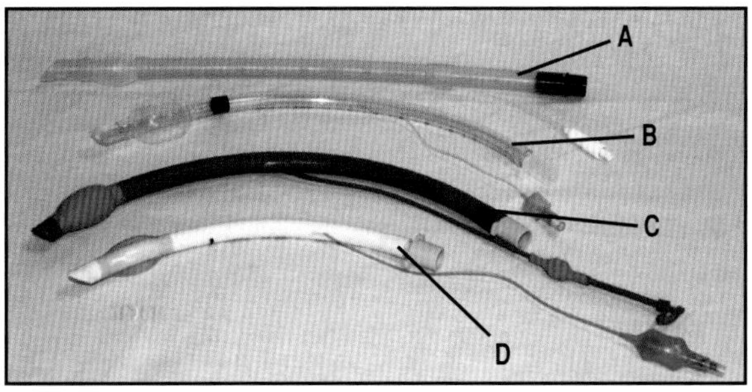

5.12 Endotracheal tubes manufactured from different materials. A = Silicone; B = PVC low-pressure, high-volume cuff; C = Red rubber; D = PVC high-pressure, low-volume cuff.

Armoured tubes are thick-walled tubes with a spiral wire coil embedded in the wall (Figure 5.14). They are used to prevent kinking during maximal neck flexion. Several problems have been associated with their use: they are difficult to insert and require an introducer, and if the animal bites down on them they may become permanently obstructed.

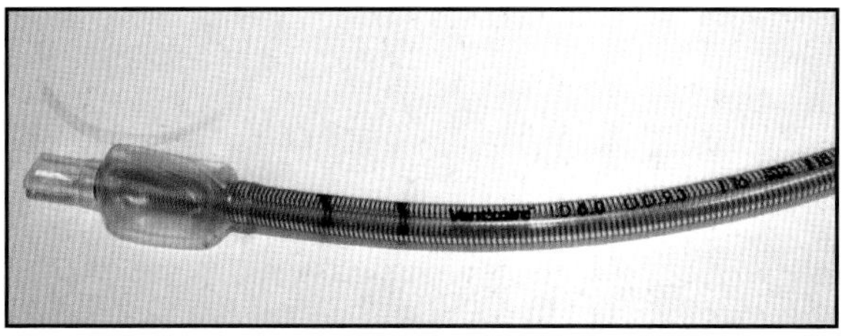

5.14 An armoured endotracheal tube. (Courtesy of Elizabeth Leece)

There are different cuff types:

- High-pressure, low-volume. These provide superior protection of the airway, although the narrow area of high pressure generated by the profile of the cuff may damage the tracheal mucosa
- Low-pressure, high-volume. Because the region of pressure is spread over a wider area, there is less risk to the tracheal mucosa. However, liquid may pass the cuff due to the small folds that may develop in the cuff.

Feature	Red rubber	PVC	Silicone
Durability	May be re-used but will perish over time, especially in sunlight	Disposable	May be re-used
Repair	Cannot be repaired	Cannot be repaired	May be repaired
Available sizes	2–16 mm ID	2–11 mm ID	2–16 mm ID
Withstands autoclave	Yes	No	Yes
Mould to shape when warmed	No	Yes	Yes
Withstands kinking	No, especially when old	Better than red rubber	Better than red rubber
Irritant	Yes	No	No
Expense	Moderate	Inexpensive	Most expensive
Blockages visible	No	Yes	Perhaps
Pre-formed curve	Yes	Yes	No
Ease of insertion	Easy to insert	Easy to insert	May require stylet to form curve
Self-sealing pilot balloon for cuff inflation	No	Yes	Yes
Types of cuff available	Low-volume, high-pressure	• Low-volume, high-pressure • High-volume, low-pressure	Low-volume, high-pressure

5.13 Comparison of manufacturing materials of endotracheal tubes. ID = Internal diameter.

When selecting endotracheal tubes:

- Choose the widest diameter that will pass easily through the narrowest part of the airway. However, care must be taken not to damage the larynx or trachea by placing a tube that is too big, and if in doubt a slightly smaller tube should be chosen. Narrow tubes increase resistance to gas flow and so increase the work of breathing. It is best to have two or three possible sizes of tube available for every animal. A guide to sizes is shown in Figure 5.15
- Choose the shortest tube that can be adequately secured (see section below). This also decreases the work of breathing, decreases the possibility of intubating a main bronchus and decreases apparatus deadspace. Tubes may be cut to the correct length
- Choose a tube with a cuff, as this is preferable in most situations; the cuff will result in superior protection of the airway. Opinions vary on whether cuffs are desirable when intubating cats. The cuffs of modern disposable tubes are manufactured from very thin material which may not restrict the diameter of the airway to the same extent as red rubber tubes. A cuff is especially important if:
  - The animal is not fasted: it is more likely to regurgitate
  - The procedure involves the gastrointestinal tract, upper abdomen or mouth
  - A smaller tube than expected is used.

Sizes (internal diameter) (mm)	Cuffed and/or uncuffed	Approximate lean bodyweight (kg)
2.0, 2.5, 3.0	Cuffed and uncuffed	1–2.5
3.5, 4.0, 4.5	Cuffed and uncuffed	2.5–5
5, 6	Cuffed and uncuffed (size 5)	4–9
7, 8	Cuffed	7–15
9, 10	Cuffed	15–25
11, 12	Cuffed	25–45
14, 16	Cuffed	>40

5.15 Suggested sizes of endotracheal tubes suitable for small animal practice. Note that there is large individual variation in tracheal diameter in dogs and this table is intended as a guideline only. The Bulldog breed has a high incidence of hypoplastic (narrow) trachea.

Technique for intubating dogs and cats

Prior to inserting an endotracheal tube, the procedure is as follows:

- Pre-measure the tube against the patient. It should reach from the incisors to the thoracic inlet, when the neck is flexed
- Ensure the tube is clean and the lumen is patent
- Inflate the cuff and leave it for 10 minutes to check for leaks (or test under water)
- Ensure there is a male 15 mm connector in place, for attachment to the breathing system
- Lubricate the tube with a water-soluble lubricant (e.g. KY Jelly), but do not occlude the bevel or the Murphy eye.

Small animals may be intubated while in lateral or sternal (or rarely dorsal) recumbency. Occasionally pathology dictates which position is best, but most often the choice is personal preference. A trained assistant is of immense benefit when intubating small animals. Dogs and cats are intubated using the following technique (Figure 5.16):

1. The assistant grasps the upper jaw, taking care not to place fingers in the mouth, and extends the head and neck towards the operator, keeping them straight and in alignment with the spine. Their other hand may be used to help extend the head; it should not be placed under the neck as this will block visualization of the larynx.
2. The operator then grasps the lower jaw, draws out the tongue gently and opens the mouth widely, facilitated by the resistance of their assistant.
3. The laryngoscope (see below) and the tongue should be held in the non-dominant hand and the tip of the laryngoscope placed on the base of the tongue, rostral to the epiglottis.
4. The laryngoscope should be used to depress the tongue and visualize the larynx. It should not be used directly on the epiglottis as the pressure may cause swelling of the epiglottis.
5. As cats are prone to laryngospasm, the larynx may be sprayed with lidocaine at this stage. Wait 30–60 seconds for the spray to desensitize the larynx, and then continue.
6. The endotracheal tube should be advanced over the epiglottis, keeping to the ventral aspect and depressing the epiglottis. It should then pass through the arytenoid cartilages and vocal folds, into the trachea.
7. In cats, if the larynx is closed when first visualized, it is preferable to wait for inhalation to occur before inserting the tube.
8. Always confirm placement of the tube in the trachea following intubation using one or two of the following methods:
   - A capnograph, which will detect exhaled carbon dioxide
   - A small piece of cotton wool or tissue paper held over the end of the endotracheal tube – this will move when the patient exhales
   - Visualization of simultaneous movement of the animal's thorax and the reservoir bag on the breathing system
   - Direct visualization of the tube in the larynx using a laryngoscope
   - Detection of water vapour on a mirror or base of the laryngoscope handle
   - Palpation of the neck to ensure the presence of only one rigid structure.

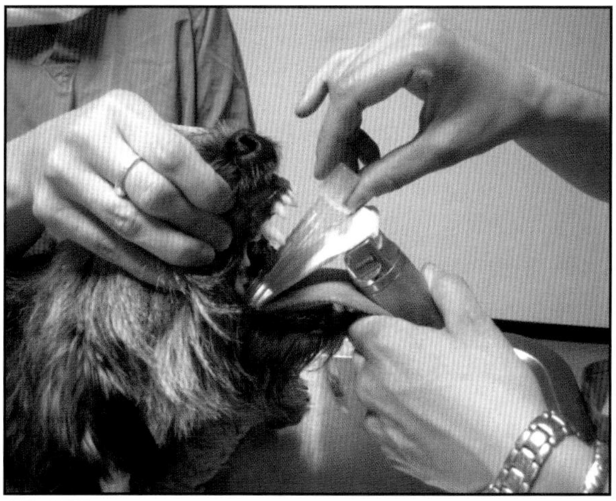

5.16 Technique for intubating dogs and cats.

Following insertion of the endotracheal tube:

1. Secure the tube in place by tying it with a bandage (e.g. white open-weave) to the top or bottom jaw, or behind the ears. The bandage needs to be tied tightly, but must not occlude the lumen of the tube. Ideally the knot should be around the connector and not the tube.
2. Position the endotracheal tube connector external to the incisors. This will ensure that the handler is not bitten when disconnecting or re-connecting the tube.
3. Turn on the oxygen flow.
4. Connect the endotracheal tube to the breathing system, using a 'push and twist' action to prevent accidental disconnection.
5. Check for gas leakage and inflate the cuff. Avoid excessive pressure in the cuff (maximum 35 mmHg/20 cmH_2O) as this will occlude the blood supply to the tracheal mucosa. To check for leaks:
   - Fill the breathing system with oxygen and briefly close the pressure relief valve
   - Inflate the cuff while squeezing the breathing bag and listening for gas leaks from the mouth – this requires an assistant
   - Stop inflating the cuff immediately when no more leaks are heard
   - Quickly open the pressure relief valve on the breathing system
   - Check the cuff inflation pressure from time to time during the anaesthetic. Most commonly it will deflate. However, nitrous oxide may diffuse into the cuff and cause it to expand.
6. Always disconnect and reconnect the breathing system from the endotracheal tube when turning the patient. Cats, especially, have suffered tracheal rupture from twisting of the endotracheal tube within the trachea.

The advantages and complications of using endotracheal tubes, in comparison with facemasks, are shown in Figure 5.17.

Advantages of endotracheal tubes when compared with facemasks

Endotracheal tubes (with an inflated cuff):
- Provide a method of inflating the lungs; facemasks result in inflation of the stomach with gas
- Prevent aspiration of foreign material (saliva, stomach contents, blood, dental debris, etc.) into the lungs
- Result in better maintenance of gas volumes in the breathing system than facemasks. This is particularly important when using a ventilator
- Result in less atmospheric pollution than facemasks
- May be secured with ties: facemasks are difficult to secure

Possible complications of endotracheal intubation

Endotracheal tubes may:
- Be inserted into the oesophagus
- Be inserted into one main bronchus
- Kink or become obstructed
- Become disconnected
- Be bitten by the patient and inhaled
- Damage the trachea or larynx or initiate laryngeal spasm
- Cause tracheal rupture if not disconnected when turning the patient

The cuff may:
- Herniate over the bevel and cause an obstruction
- Deflate during anaesthesia
- Increase in size when nitrous oxide is used
- Cause tracheal necrosis if over-inflated

5.17 Advantages and possible complications of cuffed endotracheal tubes, when compared with facemasks.

Laryngeal masks

Laryngeal mask airways (LMAs) were developed in medical anaesthesia to overcome the high incidence of haemodynamic changes and laryngeal spasm caused by intubation of the trachea in people. Their use coincided with the introduction of propofol, a drug which results in reduced laryngeal sensitivity when compared with thiopental. Although LMAs have achieved great popularity for short, uncomplicated procedures, the endotracheal tube remains the 'gold standard' for assured protection of the airway. While the use of LMAs has been reported in dogs, cats and rabbits, their full benefit in veterinary practice remains to be quantified. Intubation of dogs and cats does not present the same degree of difficulty or complexity as that exhibited in humans and laryngeal spasm in the cat is easily prevented with topical lidocaine spray. Intubation of rabbits is technically more challenging and LMAs may prove useful in this species (Bateman *et al.*, 2005). The LMA must not be used in unfasted animals or in those with a high risk of vomition or regurgitation.

Components of an LMA include (Figure 5.18):

- A transparent tube, which protrudes from the mouth in a similar manner to an endotracheal tube
- The tube is attached to an elliptical latex mask, which is positioned so that it covers the epiglottis and laryngeal opening
- Slits at the junction between the cuff and the tube prevent the epiglottis from obstructing the airway

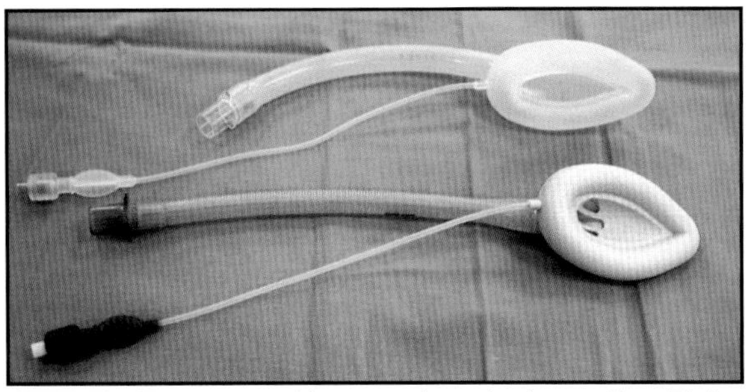

5.18 Two types of laryngeal mask airway. Top: Plain. Bottom: Reinforced (the tube is made thinner and longer, and is reinforced with a spiral of steel wire to provide added flexibility without the risk of kinking).

- A pilot balloon is used to inflate a cuff that runs around the perimeter of the mask
- Six sizes are manufactured for use in humans.

Insertion of the LMA is as follows:

1. The LMA should be lubricated prior to use and the cuff deflated.
2. With the head extended and the tongue pulled out, the LMA is inserted blindly into the mouth, keeping to the centre of the mouth and parallel to the hard palate.
3. It is advanced towards the larynx until resistance is felt; once clear breath sounds are detected the cuff should be inflated and the tube secured in place.

Facemasks

Veterinary facemasks are available in a wide range of shapes and sizes, to correspond with the diversity in the contours of our patients' faces (Figure 5.19). They should cover the nose and mouth, resulting in an airtight seal. The following points are of interest:

- Masks are valuable for preoxygenation and provision of supplemental oxygen to sick patients
- They may be used for induction of anaesthesia, although if the seal is inadequate they result in atmospheric pollution
- Masks manufactured from transparent materials are preferable, so that the patient's tongue and mucous membranes can be visualized
- Masks with a detachable rubber diaphragm provide a good seal around the face but may be poorly tolerated by conscious patients
- Care should be taken not to exert excess pressure when applying a mask as reduction in venous return from the face will cause oedema of the muzzle
- Deadspace should be minimized by using a mask with an appropriate shape, e.g. avoid the use of a conical mask in the cat
- Masks are usually well tolerated. However, if previously used, they should be washed well and flushed with oxygen as they may smell of anaesthetic agent and the patient may resist their application
- Masks do not protect the airway from aspiration of foreign material.

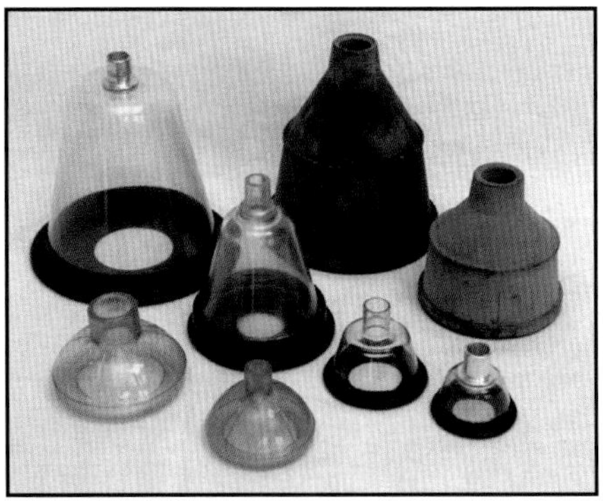

5.19 A selection of facemasks.

Laryngoscopes

The main functions of a laryngoscope are to retract the tissues of the pharynx, providing an uninterrupted view of the larynx and facilitating intubation (see section on endotracheal tubes for technique of use). Note that the blade should not be used to depress the epiglottis. A comparison of the different aids available for endotracheal intubation in small animals is shown in Figure 5.20. Laryngoscope blades should always be cleaned and disinfected after each use.

Laryngoscope (or bright light and tongue depressor)	Endoscope	Bright light and no aids
May be used to depress the tongue	No tongue depression	No tongue depression
The laryngoscope provides better visualization of the larynx and related structures	The light provides excellent visualization of the larynx and related structures	Poor visualization of larynx
Laryngoscope useful for demonstrating normal anatomy	Most useful if the larynx is not visible, e.g. pathology of temporomandibular joint	Should only be used by experienced persons
Very useful in brachycephalic and Chow-Chow dogs		Most reliable in dolichocephalic dogs only
Essential to use an aid when the patient is suffering from laryngeal pathology (paralysis, collapse, neoplasia, etc.)		No visualization of laryngeal pathology
Handling of the laryngoscope, tongue and endotracheal tube may require a period of training	Most useful if the endoscope will fit through the endotracheal tube to allow passage of the tube over the scope (railroading)	No additional equipment to handle
Many laryngoscope blades are awkward for right-handed persons	Requires expensive equipment	
A variety of sizes and shapes of laryngoscope blades are available		

5.20 Comparison of aids for intubation in small animals.

Features of laryngoscopes include:

- Detachable blades are made in several lengths; the most readily available are sizes 0, 1, 2, and 3
- The array of blade patterns available for medical anaesthesia is bewildering. However, only three are commonly used in veterinary patients: the Miller or Wisconsin (straight) and the Macintosh (curved) (Figure 5.21). Personal preference dictates which is chosen
- The light source is situated within the handle, usually battery powered. It should always be checked prior to use
- Light projections may be via a tungsten bulb in the blade, or more commonly a fibreoptic bundle from a bulb in the handle. The intensity of fibreoptic light is superior, although the bundle may degrade over time
- Blades may be plastic or metal. Metal blades are more expensive, but also more robust
- The high ridge on the right-hand side of some blades will impede the view of a right-handed person passing an endotracheal tube into the trachea with their right hand. This problem arises because blades are designed for medical use where supine humans are intubated from behind (the ridge is then on the left)
- Boxed sets are available which contain one handle and up to eight blades.

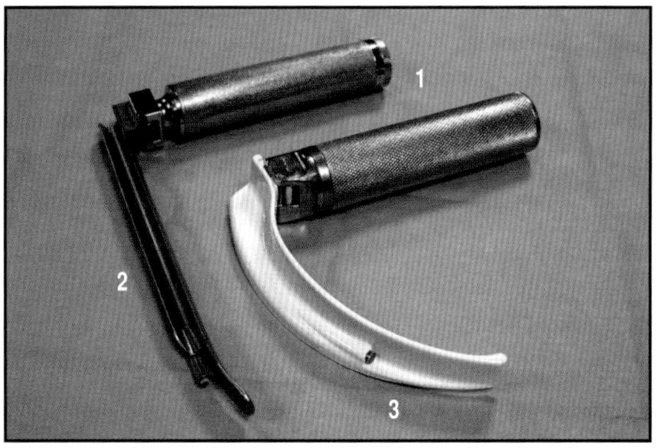

5.21 Types of laryngoscope blade. 1 = Handle containing batteries, 2 = Stainless steel Miller blade with bulb light source; 3 = Disposable Macintosh blade with fibreoptic light source.

Induction chambers

Induction chambers are usually rectangular boxes, constructed of a clear plastic material (Figure 5.22); this allows visualization of the patient in the chamber. Chambers should:

- Have a hinged lid which can be closed tightly and seal the chamber so it is leak proof
- Have a removable clear partition, allowing the use of a smaller compartment for smaller animals
- Be large enough to allow the patient to lie in lateral recumbency without flexing its neck

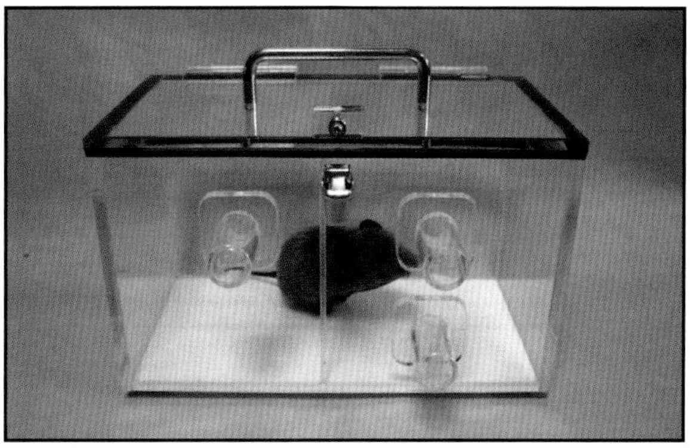

5.22 An anaesthetic induction chamber.

- Have at least two ports – one for delivery of volatile anaesthetic agents and oxygen (at the bottom) and the other for scavenging of waste gases (at the top).

Induction chambers may be used as an oxygen cage for small creatures and neonates, although they are most commonly used for gaseous induction of anaesthesia as follows:

1. Fill the chamber with 100% oxygen for 3–5 minutes prior to turning on the vaporizer.
2. Use a relatively high gas flow to increase speed of induction of anaesthesia (see Chapter 14).
3. Watch the patient continuously and remove it from the chamber as soon as it becomes unconscious.

The chamber may be used to induce anaesthesia in wild animals, e.g. fractious or feral cats, or in tiny animals, where venous access is difficult or intramuscular mass is limited, e.g. small mammals, birds or exotic pets. It may also be used as an oxygen cage or incubator for small creatures and neonates. While practical in the above patients, these boxes are not without their disadvantages:

- Pungent anaesthetic gases may cause the patient to struggle and breath-hold. This results in increased circulating catecholamines and carbon dioxide concentrations in the blood, with the associated risk of cardiac arrhythmias
- They constitute a considerable health hazard as they result in substantial atmospheric pollution when the lid is opened. A double-box system has been designed for laboratory animal work, which evacuates all waste anaesthetic gases before the box is opened.

Waste gas scavenging systems

Waste volatile and gaseous anaesthetic agents pose a threat to human health if not removed by an effective scavenging system (see Chapter 14). In addition, legislation in most countries limits the permitted exposure to airborne contaminants, including anaesthetic agents. For these reasons it is essential to install a scavenging system in all veterinary practices.

Waste anaesthetic gases leave most breathing systems via the pressure relief valve; there is a standard scavenging shroud on modern breathing systems (male 30 mm in the UK). This should be connected to 22 mm tubing, which carries the waste gas away from the patient. By convention, the scavenging tubing should be a different colour to that of the breathing system, i.e. blue or red. Scavenging from the open-ended bag of the Jackson-Rees modified T-piece is potentially hazardous and has been discussed previously.

Types of scavenging systems

Active scavenging system

This is the most effective type of scavenging and it is probable that it will be required by law in many countries in the near future. The components include (Figure 5.23):

- An extractor fan or pump which generates negative pressure; this is often capable of scavenging gas from several anaesthetic machines at once. It is usually situated above a false ceiling, where the noise nuisance is reduced. It has an outlet to the exterior (i.e. through a wall) and care should be taken in situating this outlet so that it does not in itself pose a health hazard
- A length of non-collapsible tubing connecting the extractor fan to the airbreak
- An airbreak receiver (Figure 5.24):
  - Is interposed between the extractor fan and the pressure relief valve
  - Has a visible flow indicator which is activated at flows >80 l/minute
  - Prevents transmission of sub-atmospheric (negative) pressure from the extractor fan to the patient by allowing entrainment of air
  - Prevents build up of pressure if the evacuation system fails
  - Has a filter to prevent foreign material blocking the tubing or damaging the fan
- Coloured, flexible 22 mm tubing leading from the airbreak to the shroud on the pressure relief valve on the breathing system.

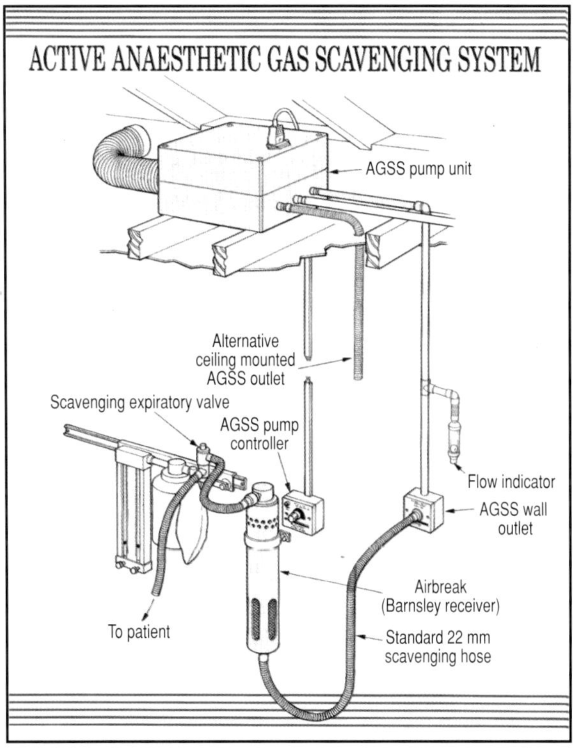

5.23 An active scavenging system. (Courtesy of Coltronics Systems)

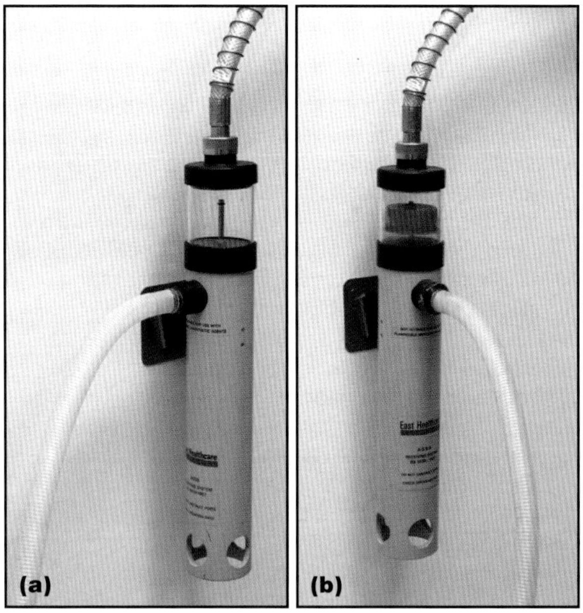

5.24 Detail of an airbreak receiver. **(a)** Airbreak off. **(b)** Airbreak on.

Active–passive scavenging system

In this system, 22 mm tubing carries waste gas from the expiratory valve on the breathing system to the grille of a ventilation system. The ventilation system must be capable of extracting gas from the room, and must be turned on. Ventilated gases must not be recirculated within the building, and care must be taken with the position of the extracted gases, as in the active system.

Passive scavenging system with adsorber

In this system, the scavenging tubing is connected to an activated charcoal container, e.g. Cardiff 'Aldasorber' (Figure 5.25). The container must be situated below the pressure relief valve, and should not be positioned near a source of heat as vapours may

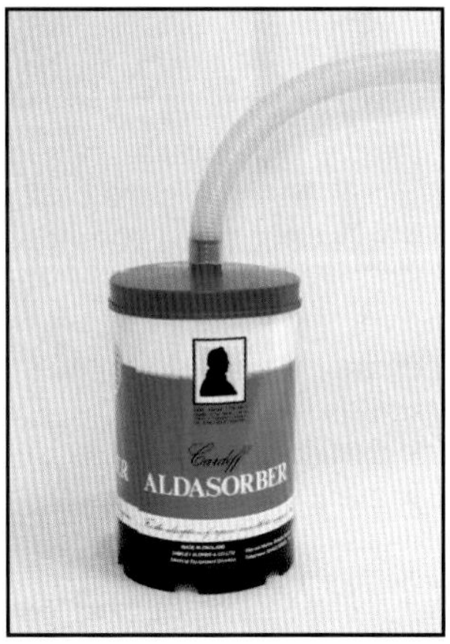

5.25 A Cardiff 'Aldasorber' with scavenging tubing attached.

be liberated. The adsorber adsorbs volatile agents only (halothane, isoflurane, sevoflurane), and does *not* adsorb nitrous oxide. There is no 'full' indicator, so the container must be weighed daily to ensure it has not exceeded the maximum weight. This requires an accurate weighing scale (±0.1 kg). Correct disposal of the container is essential.

Passive scavenging system

The scavenging tubing takes the waste gas to an outlet in a wall or leads out through a window. This system has many drawbacks. The total length of the tubing should not be excessive and there should be no constrictions or bends which may increase the resistance to expiration. The wall outlet or window opening must be lower than the expiratory valve. The outlet is subject to prevailing wind conditions; excess negative pressure may be generated or waste gas may be blown back into the building. Care must be taken with the position of the outlet, as in the active system.

Minimizing exposure to waste anaesthetic gases

In addition to installing and using an efficient active scavenging system, there are many anaesthetic practices, which, if practised *daily*, help to reduce the exposure of personnel to waste anaesthetic gases:

- Leak test all anaesthetic equipment
- Intubate all patients with a cuffed endotracheal tube and inflate the cuff where appropriate
- Avoid the use of facemasks and induction boxes
- Connect the breathing system to the patient and leak test the endotracheal tube before turning on vaporizers
- Use low-flow anaesthesia where appropriate
- Flush the breathing system with oxygen for several minutes before disconnection of the patient
- Cap the breathing system after use (this is more applicable in large animals)
- Ventilate the recovery area with a minimum of 15–20 air changes per hour, using a system that does not recirculate air
- Fill vaporizers at the end of the day in a well ventilated area, using a key (agent-specific) filler
- Vary the rostering of personnel who fill the vaporizers
- Carry out regular maintenance of anaesthetic equipment
- Monitor waste anaesthetic gases in the premises every 6 months.

Humidifiers

Humidification of inspired gases is desirable whenever there is prolonged administration of cold gases at high flows, and particularly if they bypass the turbinate system in the nares. Without humidification, respiratory secretions become thicker, mucociliary function is reduced and atelectasis may occur in the lung. In addition, losses through evaporation are increased, leading to hypothermia.

Humidifiers may be of two types:

- Heat and moisture exchangers (HMEs; Figure 5.26) are placed between the endotracheal tube and the breathing system. Their function is to conserve the heat of the exhaled breath and use it to warm the inhaled gases. Porous material absorbs heat from the exhaled gas, allowing water to condense out and be stored in or adjacent to the porous material. When the patient inhales, the heat is returned to the inhaled gas and the condensate evaporates. They are most useful when high fresh gas flows are used in systems without carbon dioxide absorption. They are designed for medical use in adult or paediatric patients; they increase deadspace and resistance to breathing and should be used with caution in small patients. It is important to follow the manufacturer's directions with regard to patient size.They should be observed frequently for plugging with secretions and they must be discarded after use
- Bubble-through humidifiers are used in conjunction with supplemental oxygen delivery systems, often in the intensive care setting. A stream of oxygen is passed through a bottle, containing sterile water, before reaching the patient. Those in common usage do not heat the gas and most will produce large water droplets, which tend to condense in the delivery system. For maximum efficiency, low gas flows should be used and the gas should be driven below the surface of the water to increase the area available for evaporation.

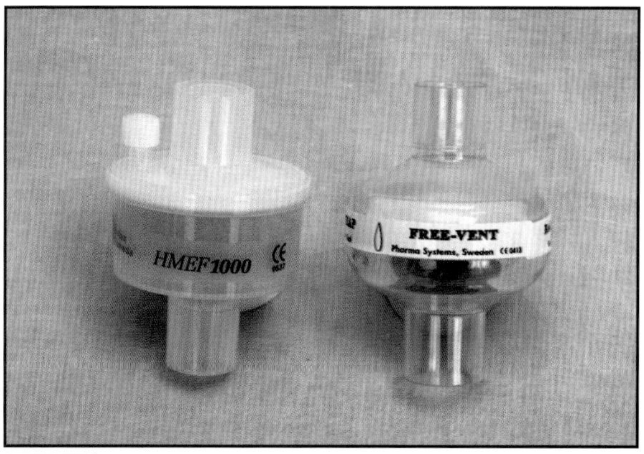

5.26 Heat and moisture exchangers (HMEs).

Magnetic resonance imaging-compatible equipment

The MRI unit contains a powerful magnet which presents unique challenges to the anaesthetist, often necessitating remote monitoring of physiological variables and anaesthetic depth, and restricted access to the patient. For this reason anaesthetic and monitoring equipment used within the *inner controlled area* (limits of the magnetic field) must not contain any iron; aluminium and plastics are suitable alternatives. While non-ferrous equipment is available, it is considerably more expensive than standard equipment. In many cases it is possible (and desirable) to position the anaesthetic machine, monitoring equipment and ventilator in the console area of the unit so they remain outside the limits of the magnet. In this case extended tubing and hosing is required to reach the patient. The personnel safety issues associated with MRIs are outside the scope of this text.

MRI-compatible equipment may be defined as equipment that, within the MRI environment, presents no safety hazard to patients or personnel, functions normally and does not interfere with the correct operation of the MRI equipment, providing instructions concerning its proper use are correctly followed.

Reasons for using MRI-compatible equipment include:

- Avoiding a projectile effect – the magnet will rapidly attract all ferrous material to it, often with disastrous results, e.g. gas cylinders, anaesthetic machines and sharp objects such as scissors
- Avoiding patient burns, which can occur from electric currents generated by the magnetic field in probes and cables
- Avoiding equipment malfunction, e.g. syringe drivers which deliver incorrect volumes of drugs
- Avoiding degradation of MRI image quality.

Equipment required for anaesthesia which is MRI-compatible includes:

- Gas cylinders: non-ferrous cylinders are available. An alternative is to store gas cylinders outside the controlled area and use an extended hose to deliver the gas to the anaesthetic machine. Under no circumstances should standard cylinders be brought into the inner controlled area
- Anaesthetic machines: non-ferrous machines are available but standard versions may be positioned outside the limits of the magnet and used with an extended breathing system (see below). Under no circumstances should standard anaesthetic machines be located within the inner controlled area
- Breathing systems: all plastic breathing systems are suitable. Several companies manufacture extra-long universal F circuits or Bain breathing systems which will reach from the console area into the MRI chamber. Ideally, these long systems should be used in conjunction with a ventilator (also positioned outside the controlled area). Expiratory valves contain metal parts which are not MRI-compatible
- Endotracheal tubes: standard rubber, PVC and silicone tubes are suitable for use in MRI units. Ferromagnetic coils within armoured tubes and in some cuff inflator balloons must be avoided (Figure 5.27), as they can cause image artefact
- Pulse oximetry: MRI-compatible probes, with fibreoptic cabling, are available from some manufacturers. Normal probes result in patient burns
- ECG: normal electrodes and cables may result in patient burns, and the cables may act as antennae. Special MRI-compatible versions are available, but extreme care must be taken with their positioning, and the trace is prone to significant artefact which makes diagnosis of abnormalities difficult
- Blood pressure monitors: the cuffs and hosing used in most oscillometric blood pressure monitors are suitable for use in the MRI unit. Extended hosing may be specially manufactured
- Capnography: plastic sampling tubing does not pose problems with MRI compatibility; however, there may be a considerable delay (20–30 seconds) in obtaining the signal due to the length of the sampling tubing
- Waste gas scavenging: use of extended plastic scavenging tubing to duct waste gases away from the patient does not pose any problems with MRI compatibility. This may be attached to a Cardiff adsorber (see above) or an active system positioned outside the controlled area.

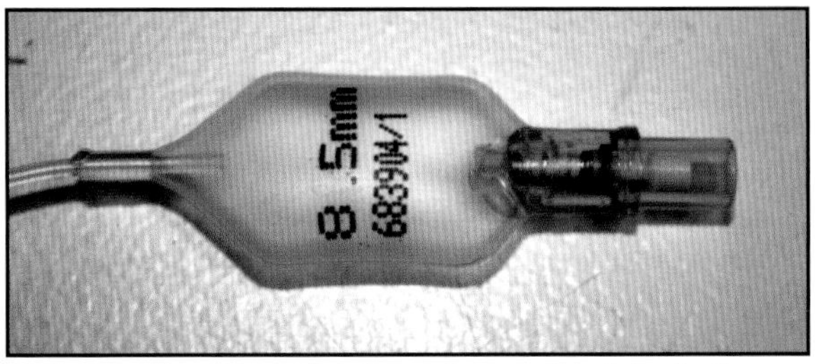

5.27 Small metal coils in some cuff inflator balloons can cause image artefacts with MRI. (Courtesy of Elizabeth Leece)

References and further reading

Al-Shaikh B and Stacey S (2001) *Essentials of Anaesthetic Equipment, 2nd edn.* Churchill Livingstone, New York

Bateman L, Ludders JW, Gleed RD *et al.* (2005) Comparison between facemask and laryngeal mask airway in rabbits during isoflurane anesthesia. *Veterinary Anaesthesia and Analgesia* **32,** 280–288

Davey AJ & Diba A (2005) *Ward's Anaesthetic Equipment, 5th edn.* Elsevier Saunders, Philadelphia

Dorsch JA & Dorsch SE (1999) *Understanding Anesthesia Equipment, 4th edn.* Lippincott Williams & Wilkins, Pennsylvania

Mitchell SL, McCarthy R, Rudloff E and Pernell RT (2000) Tracheal rupture associated with intubation in cats: 20 cases (1996–1998). *Journal of the American Veterinary Medical Association* **216(10),** 1592–1595

Walsh CM and Taylor PM (2004) A clinical evaluation of the 'mini parallel Lack' breathing system in cats and comparison with a modified Ayre's T-piece. *Veterinary Anaesthesia and Analgesia* **31,** 207–212

6

Automatic ventilators

Richard Hammond

The role of automatic ventilators

Automatic ventilators allow provision of intermittent positive pressure ventilation (IPPV) in anaesthetized or heavily sedated patients. By virtue of providing repeated, controllable breathing, automatic ventilators are an invaluable tool to allow a more effective resource allocation of the veterinary surgeon or nurse/technician to other aspects of patient monitoring and support.

There is a wide range of complex and, in many cases, technically challenging ventilators available; entire texts are dedicated to their use. In the small animal operating theatre, however, ventilation is performed for limited periods in anaesthetized patients and predominantly in those with normal lung physiology. The ventilators suitable for this purpose are therefore relatively basic in design, simple to use and can be sourced easily and inexpensively for general practice use. This chapter describes key aspects of ventilator design and respiratory physiology, as well as providing practical guidelines for assisted ventilation in the clinical situation.

Indications for IPPV

Assisted ventilation may be used to support any patient with respiratory failure. There is a marked difference between the role of the ventilator in the intensive care setting for support of a patient with pulmonary pathology and its role in the anaesthetized surgical patient.

In critically ill patients, those defined as being in respiratory failure and requiring IPPV are likely to be those with a decreased pulmonary oxygen uptake and subsequent reduced tissue oxygen delivery. In severe or multifactorial disease these patients may demonstrate concurrent failure of carbon dioxide elimination and consequent hypercapnia. More usually, due to the highly soluble nature of carbon dioxide, patients may demonstrate normal or even low arterial carbon dioxide tension in the face of hypoxaemia; this is a result of compensatory hyperventilation. In such patients, the goal of ventilatory support is complex and may include altering specific parameters of the ventilatory process (e.g. positive end expiratory pressures with high inspired concentrations of oxygen (F_iO_2)) in an attempt to reverse the hypoxaemia. Where this cannot be achieved without an associated increase in minute volume, carbon dioxide may even be added to the inspired gases to prevent further hypocapnia, metabolic alkalosis and cerebral vasoconstriction.

In contrast, in anaesthetized patients with normal lung physiology and a high F_iO_2, respiratory failure is more usually due to mild to moderate hypoventilation. This will normally result in hypercapnia without a concomitant hypoxaemia. The role of ventilation during anaesthesia is normally, therefore, to correct hypoventilation (for causes see Figure 6.1) and return arterial carbon dioxide tension to within the normal range. Minute ventilation (respiratory rate x tidal volume) defines the total volume of gas passing through the lungs per minute. This, in turn, determines the amount of carbon dioxide eliminated from the lungs (assuming inspired gases contain no carbon dioxide and also that right-sided cardiac output remains constant). Automatic ventilator set-up in these circumstances should aim to provide a correct minute volume, whilst minimizing the unwanted effects of IPPV on the animal (see below).

Inability to ventilate
The open thorax – thoracotomy, thoracoscopy and chest wall trauma
Neuromuscular blockade
Phrenic nerve paralysis
Pneumothorax
Myaesthenia gravis
Clostridium botulinum intoxication
Clostridium tetani intoxication
Spinal cord injury/oedema
Decreased lung, pleural or chest wall compliance
Decreased ventilatory drive
Anaesthetic agents (injectable and volatile)
Increased intracranial pressure
Other central nervous system (CNS) disease – infarct, encephalopathy, etc.
Hypothermia
Severe hypoxia

6.1 Causes of hypoventilation.

When to initiate IPPV

Absolute indications for IPPV during anaesthesia are those where the animal is unable to ventilate (see Figure 6.1). Relative indications and the degree of hypercapnia at which to initiate IPPV in most species remain controversial. The normal range for arterial carbon dioxide tension (P_aCO_2) is considered to be 35–50 mmHg

(4.6–6.6 kPa) and many veterinary surgeons would advocate initiation of IPPV at levels above that range. Most anaesthetic agents are non-selective central nervous system (CNS) depressants and therefore most anaesthetized patients hypoventilate. Although usually well tolerated in the healthy patient, even mild hypercapnia during anaesthesia may result in acidaemia, hyperkalaemia and reduced myocardial contractility. Further, hypercapnia and acidaemia contribute to the development of ventricular tachyarrhythmias during inhalant anaesthesia with halogenated agents. The full cardiovascular effects of hypercapnia are complex. Direct, local effects of hypercapnia include myocardial depression and peripheral arteriolar dilation. To some extent these effects are balanced by indirect effects, primarily mediated via activation of the sympathetic nervous system. This stimulation may result in tachycardia, hypertension and increased myocardial contractility, although the extent may be decreased by use of volatile agents. Higher levels of hypercapnia tend to increase vagal nervous tone and can therefore induce bradycardia, which in combination with other factors may precipitate sinus arrest. High levels of hypercapnia also result in CNS depression and narcosis, although these are unlikely to be seen at levels below 95 mmHg (12.5 kPa).

The need for IPPV should therefore be based on a multisystem evaluation, rather than on the level of hypercapnia; one should recognize that detrimental effects of IPPV may include reduction of cardiac output and further reduction of mean arterial pressure (Figure 6.2).

Advantages
More accurate control of respiratory variables
Constant arterial gas tensions create stable plasma pH and potassium concentration
Regular rhythm depresses ventilation, augments narcosis and improves operating conditions
Constant tidal volume (volume controlled) allows compliance measurement
Mechanical ventilator frees anaesthetist for other duties
Special ventilatory modes may be imposed
Disadvantages
May reduce venous return and mean arterial pressure
Pulmonary stretch may produce bradycardia
Unnoticed disconnection/cuff deflation fatal in 'paralysed' cases
Mechanical failure possible
Lung trauma more likely if inappropriate variables are set
Purchase and maintenance costs may be high
Some mechanical ventilators may be unsuitable for all patient sizes
Ventilators may become fomites and harbour transmissible respiratory pathogens

6.2 Advantages and potential disadvantages of controlled ventilation during general anaesthesia in animals.

In summary:

- Mild hypercapnia is normal during anaesthesia, usually well tolerated and often supports blood pressure – in this situation IPPV is not normally indicated
- Where ventricular arrhythmias are seen to be associated with even mild hypercapnia – initiate IPPV
- Higher levels (>60 mmHg; >8 kPa) may induce more detrimental effects including bradycardia and myocardial depression – initiate IPPV.

Classification of ventilators

There are numerous and varied systems for the classification of automatic ventilators. The following refers to only those elements of classification which enable a better understanding of their safe and effective use and pertain to those machines in common use in general small animal practice.

Control and cycling

Ventilators are described by how the flow of gas is delivered to the patient, and are either *volume* controlled (constant flow delivered) or *pressure* controlled (constant pressure delivered). In addition, volume-controlled ventilators may be time cycled, volume cycled or pressure cycled. This describes the method of transition from the inspiratory to expiratory phases. Understanding the advantages and disadvantages of each cycling method is key to enabling appropriate ventilator selection and set-up for an individual patient. Most ventilators in veterinary use are volume controlled and volume cycled, i.e. the flow delivered is constant, the tidal volume is targeted and the pressure delivered is variable and dependent upon lung compliance.

Volume-controlled ventilation with time cycling

The delivered *flow* remains constant over the period of inspiration. Inspiration is terminated once either a targeted tidal volume is delivered, or a fixed inspiratory phase time has elapsed. The inspiratory pressure does not normally affect the duration of inspiration. The pressure of the gas being delivered is variable and delivered relative to the compliance of the lung. Inspiratory pressure therefore increases over the period of inspiration to maintain a constant flow; the operator adjusts the inspiratory flow. In machines where tidal volume is fixed separately and causes cycling (see below), increasing flow will shorten the inspiratory phase time as the preset tidal volume is reached more quickly. Increased flows will also mean an increased peak airway pressure. In other machines, where the inspiratory phase time is fixed and determines cycling, increasing inspiratory flow will increase the total delivered tidal volume. Rarely, machines may allow setting of all three variables (inspiratory phase time, flow and tidal volume). In such a device, if the flow is high enough such that tidal volume is reached before the end of the set inspiratory phase, then an inspiratory pause will ensue with no inspiratory flow.

Advantages of these ventilators include:

- They are generally simple to operate and set up. The operator sets the appropriate tidal volume for the animal either directly, or indirectly by setting the flow and inspiratory phase time

- The predetermined tidal volume is delivered regardless of the changes in resistance and compliance that may occur during anaesthesia (e.g. animal is heavily draped, reducing compliance; mucus in the endotracheal tube reduces internal diameter and therefore increases resistance). The ventilator 'compensates' for such changes by increasing airway pressure during inspiration to maintain the fixed flow.

Disadvantages of these ventilators include:

- In animals weighing less than 5 kg, it may be difficult to set the appropriate tidal volume accurately. At the lower end of the control settings, even small changes in the setting for flow may markedly change the delivered tidal volume, therefore introducing the potential for significant under- or over-inflation and consequent volutrauma
- If delivery of an inappropriately high tidal volume is attempted, either by having a long inspiratory phase time or high flow, the rise in airway pressure in an attempt to deliver that volume may be potentially harmful. Some volume-controlled ventilators have an additional adjustable safety relief valve to avoid high peak airway pressures.

Most basic volume-controlled machines may not have a pressure-limiting adjustment, and rely on a high-pressure relief valve with audible warning sound for prevention of airway trauma. These are fixed and preset to between 65 and 80 cmH_2O. Some patients with high airway resistance or low compliance may require peak airway pressures in excess of 60 cmH_2O. Conversely, even one or two attempted ventilations at these airway pressures may result in volutrauma in very young animals and other patients with highly compliant lungs. A high compliance (high elasticity) may result in a more rapid rate of lung expansion for a given flow and a greater volume of lung for a given peak inspiratory pressure.

In summary:

- Volume-controlled ventilators with time cycling are more commonly encountered and generally more simple to set up and use effectively
- They deliver the preset tidal volume irrespective of changes in the animal and need less readjustment during use
- Their potential for producing volutrauma should be recognized and care taken in animals with a low tidal volume and in young animals due to high lung compliance.

Volume-controlled ventilation with pressure cycling (pressure-limited)

The delivered *flow* remains constant over the period of inspiration. Inspiration is terminated once a targeted airway *pressure* is achieved. The peak inspiratory pressure determines the duration of inspiration. The pressure of the gas being delivered is variable and delivered relative to the compliance of the lung. Inspiratory pressure therefore increases over the period of inspiration to maintain a constant flow. The rate of rise of airway pressure depends on multiple factors including gas flow, airway resistance, compliance of both lungs and chest wall, and even the nature of the gases delivered (density or viscosity depending on flow). The operator may adjust the inspiratory flow and the peak airway pressure (cycling pressure) but cannot set the tidal volume. High gas flows (especially those above which flow is expected to be laminar) will shorten the inspiratory phase time as resistance increases and therefore reduce tidal volume.

Advantages of these ventilators include:

- Tidal volume does not have to be calculated. In animals with normal airways, setting the cycling pressure to 15–20 cmH_2O, and adjusting inspiratory flow such that the inspiratory phase time appears to be 'normal' for that patient, should provide the correct tidal volume for that patient
- There is no lower limit to the size of animal that can be put on the ventilator. Setting 10–15 cmH_2O inflation pressure should provide the correct tidal volume. This setting will be within the useable range of the ventilator controls and therefore can be set as accurately for a kitten as for a St. Bernard. Limitations to animal size will be based on the ability to have a low enough flow. This is not normally a problem
- Volutrauma is less likely because the peak airway pressure is the primary setting and therefore cycling occurs before alveolar over-inflation can occur
- In patients with high resistance or low compliance due to disease, accurate setting of a higher airway cycling pressure may be needed and can be easily set
- If the effective tidal volume of a patient is reduced during a procedure (e.g. lung lobe removal, lung areas packed off for surgical access or one lung ventilation), no ventilator adjustment is needed. The ventilator still cycles at the same airway pressure irrespective of changes in tidal volume. This avoids potential over-inflation of a lower effective lung space.

Disadvantages of these ventilators include:

- Tidal volume is unpredictable and may be incorrect where normal cycling pressures are set in animals with abnormal airways
- Changes in resistance or compliance during a procedure (see above) may reduce the delivered volume of gas. Nothing on the ventilator (in most machines) will warn of such an occurrence.

Pressure-controlled ventilation with time cycling

Such machines are currently rare in veterinary anaesthesia.

The delivered *pressure* remains constant over the period of inspiration. A fixed pressure is rapidly achieved throughout the breath by delivering a decelerating inspiratory flow pattern. Once peak inspiratory pressure is reached, flow continues at a gradually reducing rate until the end of the inspiratory phase.

Inspiration is terminated by adjustment of the inspiratory phase time. The total volume of gas delivered in each breath still depends on the product of inspiratory phase time (fixed by operator) and the flow. In a volume-controlled, pressure-limited machine, flow ceases irrespective of inspiratory phase time (once the preset pressure is reached). With a pressure-controlled machine, flow continues once the preset pressure is reached. Tidal volume may be reduced but can be restored by increasing inspiratory phase time rather than peak airway pressure.

Triggering

Triggering describes how the inspiratory phase is initiated.

Time triggering

The expiratory phase time is set by the user, either directly or indirectly by means of adjusting either the inspiratory to expiratory (I:E) ratio or the respiratory rate. This is the more usual method employed during anaesthesia where management of hypoventilation is normally the primary objective. There is no allowance for spontaneous breathing. This is described as controlled mandatory ventilation (CMV).

Pressure triggering

The inspiratory effort of the patient initiates a ventilation by creating a decrease in baseline pressure. The ventilatory frequency is set by the animal, although in some machines an 'escape rate' may be additionally set in the event of a period of apnoea. Pressure triggering is used in intensive care situations where there may be respiratory muscle paresis, inadequate tidal volume and associated peripheral alveolar collapse. It is also used in those situations where the role of the ventilator is not purely to correct hypoventilation, e.g. provision of positive end expiratory pressure (PEEP). An advance on pressure triggering is flow triggering, whereby a constant flow is maintained in the breathing circuit. Changes in flow, in response to spontaneous ventilation attempts, initiate an assisted ventilation. This form of triggering reduces the work of breathing compared to pressure cycling and is found on sophisticated intensive care unit (ICU) ventilators.

Practical use of ventilators

Choosing an automatic ventilator for general veterinary practice

The requirements of a ventilator for use with anaesthesia are more basic than those needed in the ICU. It is possible to source second-hand human ICU ventilators as the technology struggles to keep up with changing clinical theory. The temptation to purchase one of these machines as an anaesthetic ventilator which will 'also do if we have the odd ICU case' is best avoided. These machines are usually highly complex, expensive to service and maintain (even sitting in storage), of gargantuan proportions and require in-depth knowledge of respiratory fluid dynamics to operate (Figure 6.3). In contrast, a ventilator designed for veterinary use (and therefore for use in animals down to 1 kg or less) or a second-hand, basic human anaesthetic ventilator is a more effective option. These are simpler to understand and use and are therefore safer from a practical viewpoint. Even a simple ventilator is suitable for postoperative support, in ICU patients for short-term use (up to 24 hours), or for resuscitation and postresuscitation situations.

6.3 Ventilators designed for ICU use are complex and multifunctional. They are rarely relevant for use in anaesthetized surgical patients.

The ideal properties of a veterinary ventilator are summarized in Figure 6.4. Although no veterinary ventilator fulfils all such requirements, many encompass the key components of the requirements for use (highlighted in italics). The following section describes

General
Compact, portable, robust and easy to operate
Economical to purchase, use and maintain
Use
Maximum inspiratory flow rates of 80 l/minute allowing: • *Variable inspiratory times of 0.5–3.9 seconds* • *Frequencies of 5–50 breaths/minute* • *A tidal volume range of 50–1500 ml* • *A variable I:E ratio (1:1–1:3.5)* • *The capability to control all the above simultaneously (altering one variable should not affect others)*
Capable of use with non-rebreathing or rebreathing anaesthetic breathing systems
Capable of rapid conversion for paediatric use
Capable of use with air, oxygen mixtures and all anaesthetics
Capable of humidifying inspired gas
Should allow 'sigh' breaths and the ability to inflate and hold by the user
Allow continuous monitoring of airway pressure and of expired volume
Safety
Electrically safe, isolated, suppressed and explosion proof
Have the ability to maintain output even when leaks develop
Capable of rapid disassembly for easy sterilization
Capable of using disposable hoses
Fitted with bacterial filters
Equipped with a pressure relief valve
Fitted with alarms for low pressure and/or circuit disconnection and high pressure and/or pressure overload
Indicate low expired minute volume and low F_iO_2

6.4 Properties of the ideal veterinary ventilator.

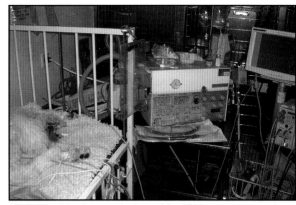

the commonly available automatic ventilators in use in the UK, their classification, correct set-up and use, and potential hazards; it should be used in conjunction with manufacturers' operator guidelines and warnings where available. This is not an exhaustive description, but the principles will be transferable to other machines of similar operation.

Set-up and use of commonly encountered automatic ventilators in UK small animal practice

The Bird Mark 7 ventilator

Classification:

- Volume controlled, pressure cycled.
- Inspiratory phase is initiated either by time (time triggered) or by the patient attempting to breathe (pressure triggered).

This ventilator (Figure 6.5) is suitable for both small and large animal use depending upon the size of bellows to which it is attached. It is driven by medical compressed gas or oxygen at approximately 4 bar and may be supplied from either the high-pressure oxygen outlet of an anaesthetic machine, or a separate cylinder with regulator. On its own, the ventilator simply produces a flow of gas and it is always used in conjunction with a separate set of bellows (e.g. as part of a Vet-Tech SAV-75). The flow of gas from the Bird pressurizes the space between the bellows and a surrounding canister or 'bottle'. The bellows, which contain the gases to be delivered to the patient, are compressed by this increase in surrounding pressure. Gas is forced from the bellows via a corrugated tube into a breathing system (circuit). Suitable breathing systems include the circle, the Bain (in both of which the attachment to the bellows simply replaces the reservoir bag), a T-piece or the Humphrey ADE in E mode. The key controls on the Bird include: inspiratory flow (up to 70 l/minute), peak (and hence cycling) pressure up to 60 cmH_2O and expiratory phase time (resulting in 4–60 breaths/minute). There is also an option to set a triggering pressure (negative 0.5–5.0 cm H_2O) at which the ventilator will cycle from expiration to inspiration in response to inspiratory effort. This overrides the setting for expiratory phase time. A pressure indicator is also provided.

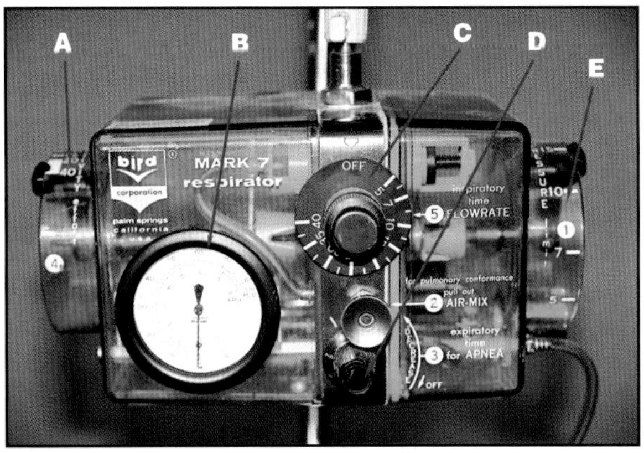

6.5 The Bird Mark 7 ventilator – a pressure cycled machine which may drive both companion and large animal ventilation systems. A = Triggering pressure control; B = Pressure indicator; C = Flow control; D = Expiratory time control; E = Inspiratory pressure control.

Set-up:

1. Attach 4 bar (400 kPa) driving gas (this does not reach the patient); oxygen or air is suitable.
2. Set the inspiratory pressure control (E) to between 15 and 20 cmH_2O. This determines when the ventilator stops inflating and is later adjusted in combination with the flow setting to optimize tidal volume.
3. Set the triggering pressure (A) to maximum to eliminate patient triggering.
4. Ensure that the expiratory valve assembly on the bellows housing is open and attached to the scavenging system – this allows escape of expired gases in the expiratory phase.
5. Connect the hose from the bellows to the reservoir bag port on the breathing system.
6. Close the adjustable pressure limiting (APL) valve ('pop off' valve) of the breathing system.
7. Increase or decrease the flow (C) from the ventilator to deliver a tidal volume in what appears to be a normal time for that animal (usually 1–2 seconds).
8. Set the expiratory phase time (D) to adjust the number of breaths per minute and hence the minute volume. Ideally adjusted to maintain normal arterial carbon dioxide based on capnography or arterial blood gases.

The Pneupac ventiPAC, paraPAC and transPAC (Smiths Medical)

The details in this section also apply to the Penlon Nuffield Series 200.

Classification:

- Volume controlled, time cycled.
- Inspiratory phase is initiated by time (time triggered).

The Pneupac ventiPAC is shown in Figure 6.6. These are simple, suitable for anaesthesia use, versatile and can be sourced cost effectively (ex-human medical use). Although some models are designed for ambulatory use and vary in terms of control over inspiratory and expiratory times, these ventilators all work on a similar principle and are considered together.

The basic unit is a control module and a patient valve that attaches directly to a suitable anaesthetic breathing attachment (see Bird ventilator) or to a bellows (bag in bottle) arrangement (Figure 6.6c). The driving gas may be air or oxygen at 4 bar (from the anaesthetic machine pressure port) and even when attached directly to the breathing attachment, this gas should not reach the patient. The control unit comprises a spool valve (Figure 6.6d) and two timers, one to control the inspiratory phase (A) and one for the expiratory phase (B). The spool valve can be in two

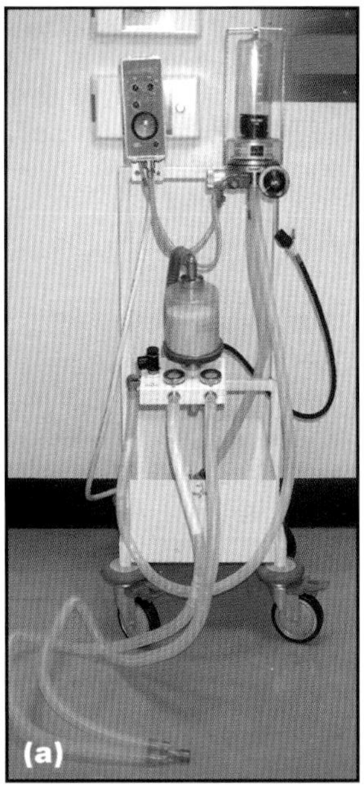

6.6 **(a)** The Pneupac ventiPAC (*in situ*). **(b)** Detail of the Pneupac ventiPAC. A = Inspiratory phase timer; B = Expiratory phase timer; C = Flow controller; D = Pressure gauge; E = On/off switch). **(c)** A typical bag in a bottle arrangement which would be attached to the Pneupac ventiPAC in volume-controlled time cycled modes. **(d)** Working principles of the Pneupac ventiPAC. A = Inspiratory phase timer; B = Expiratory phase timer; C = Flow controller; E = Gas inlet.

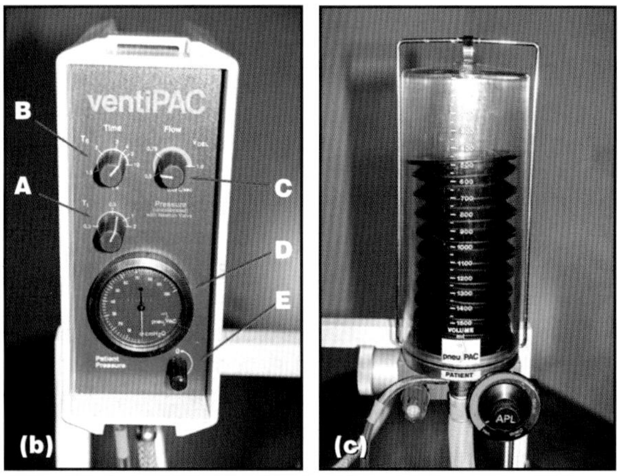

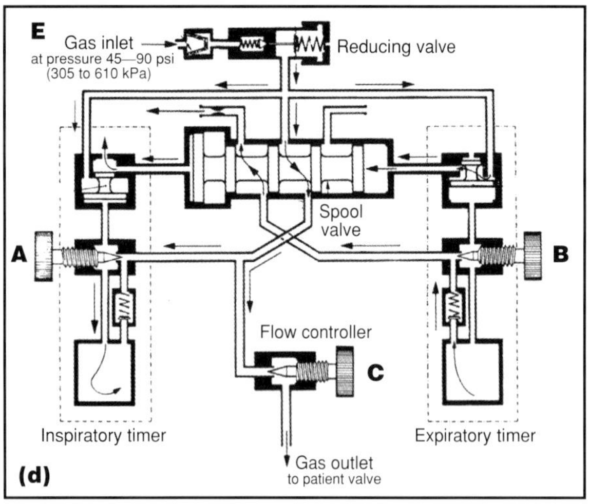

positions, one allowing driving gas to pass to the breathing attachment at a rate (C) and for a time that is set by the operator. At the end of inspiration, the valve closes and gas builds up in a capacitor until the pressure is sufficient to push the valve back into the inspiratory position. Pressure is indicated by a large gauge on the front of the control unit (D). The patient valve is a simple pneumatic valve at the base of the ventilator, through which the gases pass to the breathing attachment (this may be located on a bellows assembly where the ventiPAC is attached to a 'bag in bottle'). The valve directs all gas from the ventilator to the breathing attachment during the inspiratory phase, but allows gas returning from the patient to pass to a scavenging port during expiration.

Set-up:

1. Attach 4 bar (400 kPa) driving gas.
2. Estimate the patient's tidal volume based on 10–15 ml/kg. Set the flow and inspiratory phase time settings to achieve this volume. For example for a 30 kg dog with a tidal volume of 350 ml, a flow of 0.3–0.4 l/sec for 1 second will be suitable. Try to make this as normal for that animal as possible, judged by adequacy of chest wall movement.
3. Ensure scavenging is attached to the expiratory port of the patient valve.
4. Connect the hose from the patient valve to the breathing system.
5. Close the APL valve of the breathing system.
6. Switch on the ventilator (E).
7. Set the expiratory phase time (B) to adjust the number of breaths per minute and hence the minute volume. Ideally it should be adjusted to maintain normal arterial carbon dioxide based on capnography or arterial blood gases.

Pneupac ventiPAC used with a Newton valve

The normal patient valve can simply and quickly be replaced with an alternative (a Newton valve) (Figure 6.7) to convert the ventilator to a 'mechanical thumb' on an Ayre's T-piece or Bain. This makes it suitable for any animal down to a mass of 100 g, because the tidal volumes delivered can be very small and *any change in tidal volume of the animal will be matched by the ventilator* (similar to pressure cycling). The Newton valve connects via a corrugated tube to the bag port of a modified Ayre's T-piece (Mapleson E) or Bain (Mapleson D). The flow of gas from the ventilator, instead of going to the T-piece, acts to occlude or

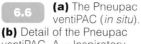

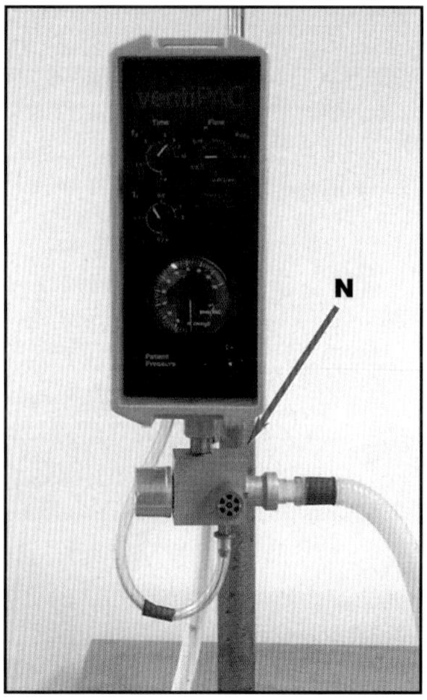

6.7 The Pneupac ventiPAC with Newton valve (N) attachment, converting this versatile ventilator into a 'mechanical thumb' or pressure generator.

partially occlude the end of the tube. This is analogous with placing a thumb over the end of the T-piece. The animal's lungs are inflated at a rate that is dependent upon the flow of fresh gas from the anaesthetic machine, and for a time dependent on how long the 'thumb' is in place. At low flows, set by the ventilator, the pressure generated is low and only partly overcomes the pressure of gas coming from the T-piece or Bain: occlusion is partial and tidal volumes are very small. As ventilator flow is increased, occlusion becomes more complete; at higher flows some driving gas is forced into the tube and the rate of lung inflation is greater than that produced just by the flow from the anaesthetic machine.

Set-up:

1. Attach 4 bar (400 kPa) driving gas.
2. Set the inspiratory phase time to be normal for that patient.
3. Ensure scavenging is attached to the expiratory port of the Newton valve.
4. Connect the hose from the patient valve to the breathing system.
5. Switch on the ventilator (E).
6. Starting with the flow on the lowest setting, increase the flow until chest wall excursion appears normal. The pressure reading (D) should peak at 15–20 cmH_2O.
7. Set the expiratory phase time (B) to adjust the number of breaths per minute (and hence minute volume). Ideally it should be adjusted to maintain normal arterial carbon dioxide based on capnography or arterial blood gases.

The Hallowell EMC Model 2000/3000 (and 2002) veterinary ventilator

Classification:

- Volume controlled, time cycled.
- Inspiratory phase is initiated by time (time triggered).

This ventilator has built-in ascending bellows and is designed for direct attachment to the reservoir bag port of a suitable breathing system (Figure 6.8). The device relies on both a driving gas supply (4 bar) and a mains power supply. The key controls include inspiratory flow (A) (up to 100 l/minute), a variable peak pressure limit (B) (up to 60 cmH_2O) and breaths per minute (C). There is also a respiratory 'hold' button (D) for maintaining inflation and overriding cycling. Low breathing-system pressure is indicated by an alarm in the event of disconnection. Bellows are interchangeable and suitable for tidal volumes from 20 ml to 3 l. The I:E ratio is fixed at 1:2. A major potential pitfall of this ventilator is that the volume control (A) regulates inspiratory flow directly and is effectively a *minute* volume setting and not a *tidal* volume setting. If the number of breaths per minute is reduced by the operator, without a concomitant decrease in the flow setting, then the tidal volume of each breath will increase: halving the breaths per minute will double the tidal volume unless the two controls are adjusted in synchrony. The pressure limiter will terminate inspiration, although if this has been set to 60 cmH_2O the potential for volutrauma exists.

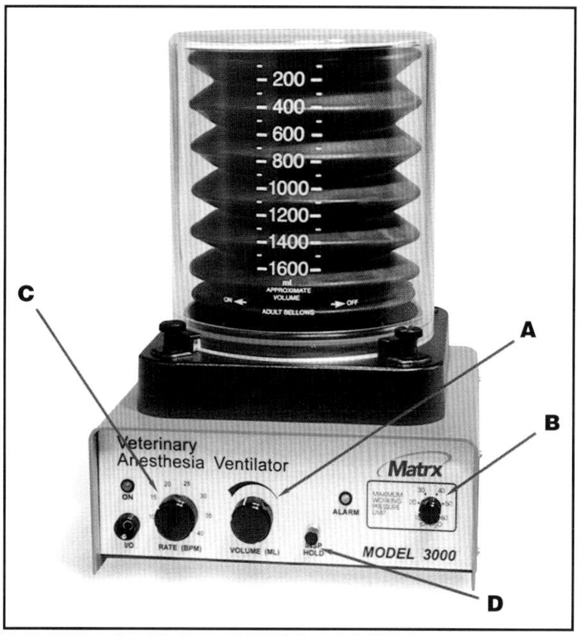

6.8 The Hallowell EMC Model 3000 veterinary ventilator. A = Inspiratory flow controller; B = Peak pressure controller; C = Breathing rate controller; D = Respiratory hold button.

The Model 2002 version is functionally equivalent to the Model 2000, with the exception that there is an additional fine needle valve that may be used to regulate flows from 0–20 l/minute. This fine control adds to the output of the coarse control and is for 'fine tuning' the tidal volume when the ventilator is active.

Set-up:

1. Attach 2–4 bar driving gas.
2. Select and attach appropriate bellows.
3. Set the maximum working pressure limit to 30 cmH_2O (or less) for normal patients.
4. Connect the corrugated tubing to breathing system.
5. Close APL valve on breathing system.
6. Switch on power and select breaths per minute.
7. Increase volume setting until each breath is of the correct tidal volume as indicated by excursion of the bellows.
8. The rate control is then used to fine tune the tidal volume of each breath.
9. The volume setting is used to control minute volume and is adjusted to maintain normal arterial carbon dioxide based on capnography or arterial blood gases.

The Manley MP2/3 and MN2

These old but still serviceable machines (Figure 6.9) are widely available and highly popular in veterinary practice. They are reliable, extremely easy to use, and require neither additional driving gas nor power supply. Second-hand, ex-human use machines can be

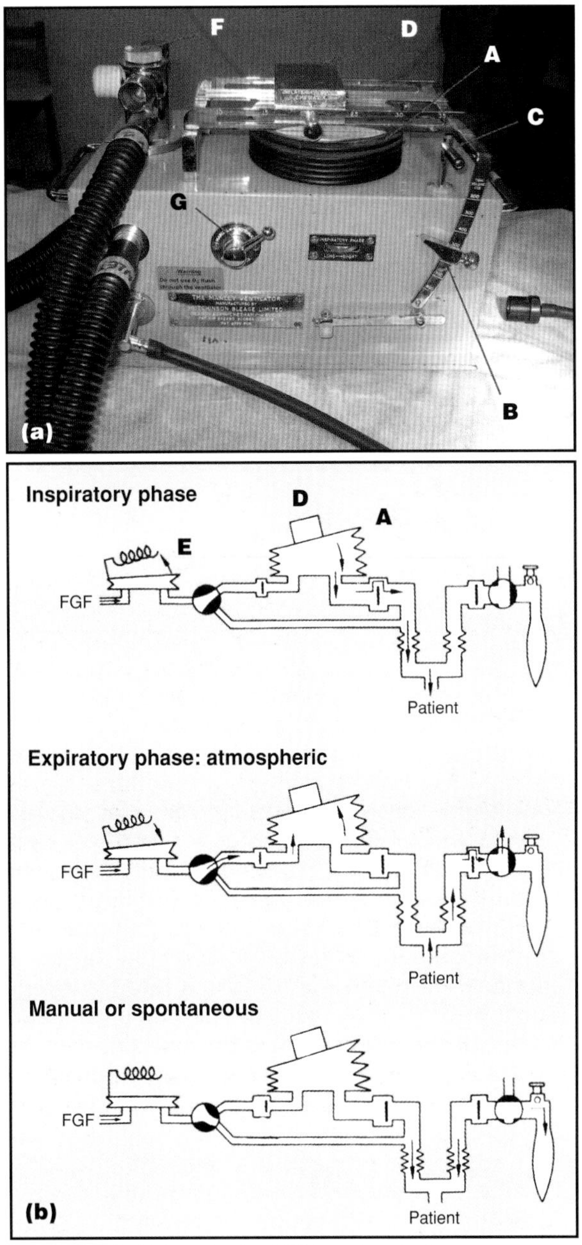

6.9 **(a)** The Manley MP2: a classic if aging machine, yet far from being a museum piece. A = Externally visible bellows; B = Volume control; C = Tidal volume catch for main bellows; D = Sliding weight; F and G = Controls to switch ventilator to automatic. **(b)** Working principles of the Manley MP2. A = Externally visible bellows; D = Sliding weight; E = Internal bellows.

sourced for little money. When purchasing a machine, the state of the bellows is critical; these devices have both external and internal black rubber bellows that may perish. If there is any sign of such deterioration, the machine should be checked and ideally serviced before first use. The description here is based on the MP2 (the MN2 has a setting for negative pressure during exhalation that has little application in veterinary use). The MP3 has an autoclavable patient connector, an airway manometer and the ability to deliver higher tidal volumes. The main limitation of these ventilators is the inability to provide lower tidal volume settings that limits their use to animals above approximately 13 kg.

Classification: These are unusual, as they do not fit into any classification explained above. They are best described as minute volume dividers in that they take the volume of gas delivered by the anaesthetic machine per minute and deliver it in breaths of a tidal volume set by the operator. All of the gas from the anaesthetic machine passes through the ventilator to the patient.

The working principle is explained in Figure 6.9b. The ventilator is attached directly to the common gas outlet from the anaesthetic machine. All gas from the machine (including nitrous oxide and other volatile agents) passes into the ventilator. During the expiratory phase, the gas accumulates in a set of bellows visible externally on the machine (A). The bellows inflate to a volume set by the operator by means of (B) at which point a mechanism is tripped (C) and the volume in A is delivered to the patient at a fixed pressure set by the operator by a sliding weight (D) – usually 20 cmH_2O. During inspiration, fresh gas from the anaesthetic machine is still flowing and accumulates in internal bellows (E). These bellows inflate to a set volume, at the end of which the expiratory phase is initiated and the gas from E is dumped into bellows A. The degree to which the internal bellows E inflate before tripping controls the inspiratory time and is determined by the setting of the inspiratory phase control. This description may make the device sound complex but in practice the operator normally simply sets the tidal volume on the ventilator and then adjusts the breaths per minute by changing the fresh gas flow on the anaesthetic machine.

Set-up:

1. Set the tidal volume to that estimated for the animal using the slider (B).
2. Check the weight (D) is at about the 20 cmH_2O mark.
3. Attach the ventilator to the fresh gas outlet of the anaesthetic machine.
4. Switch the ventilator to automatic at control knobs F and G.
5. Adjust the fresh gas flow on the anaesthetic machine until the ventilatory rate is suitable to maintain the required arterial carbon dioxide (as judged by capnography or arterial blood gases).

The Vetronic™ 'Merlin' veterinary ventilator

Classification:

- Volume controlled, time cycled, pressure cycled or volume cycled.
- Inspiratory phase is initiated either by time (time triggered) or by the patient attempting to breathe in assist mode.

This is a highly advanced ventilator specifically designed for veterinary use (Figure 6.10). It uses gases delivered from the anaesthetic machine (or room air) and can deliver tidal volumes in the range of 1–800 ml. The working principle is a precision-controlled piston that acts like a syringe to generate

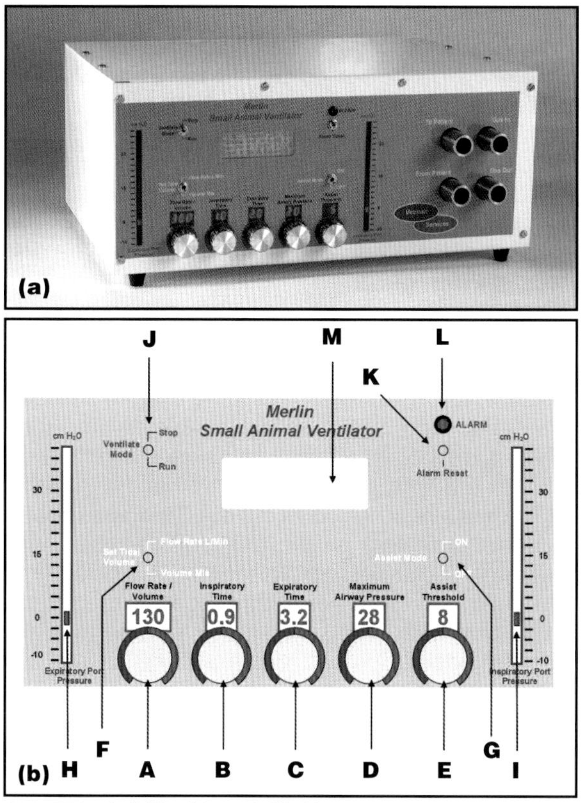

6.10 **(a)** The Vetronic™ 'Merlin' veterinary ventilator. **(b)** The Vetronic™ 'Merlin' veterinary ventilator – controls (schematic). A = Flow or volume control setting; B = Inspiratory time control setting; C = Expiratory time control setting; D = Maximum airway pressure control setting; E = Assist threshold control setting; F = Flow rate/volume selector switch; G = Assist mode on/off selector switch; H = LED indicator for expiratory port pressure; I = LED indicator for inspiratory port pressure; J = Ventilate mode stop/run selector switch; K = Alarm reset switch; L = Alarm flashing LED indicator; M = Main status LCD screen.

driving pressure. The piston can be controlled to within 0.03 ml at low volumes. It has the capacity to operate in either volume cycled (with optional time limit) or pressure cycled modes. The manufacturers claim it is suitable for animals between 50 g and 70 kg. Inspiratory and expiratory times are between 0.2 and 9 seconds. Maximum airway pressure is 57 cmH_2O and negative triggering pressures may be set from 1–10 cmH_2O. The maximum flow is relatively low at only 25 l/minute. There are audible and visual warnings for high airway pressures, blocked inlets and patient disconnection. A small display on the unit provides information on the patient's tidal volume, minute volume, respiratory rate, I:E ratio, inspiratory and expiratory times and airway pressures, triggering pressure for assist mode, cycling pressure (for pressure cycled mode) and even a calculated figure for compliance. The ventilator is normally connected to the common gas outlet of an anaesthetic machine, from which it requires a flow of above minute volume. As peak flow into the ventilator exceeds this during piston filling (in the expiratory phase), a reservoir bag must be present between anaesthetic machine and ventilator. Connections from the ventilator allow connection to either a rebreathing or non-rebreathing system.

Controls are illustrated in Figure 6.10b:

- Flow or volume control setting
- Inspiratory time control setting (seconds)
- Expiratory time control setting (seconds)
- Maximum airway pressure control setting (cmH_2O)
- Assist threshold control setting (cmH_2O)
- Flow rate/volume selector switch
- Assist mode on/off selector switch
- LED indicator for expiratory port pressure (cmH_2O)
- LED indicator for inspiratory port pressure (cmH_2O)
- Ventilate mode stop/run selector switch
- Alarm reset switch – non-latching, momentary action only
- Alarm flashing LED indicator
- Main status LCD screen.

This ventilator provides flexibility of operating modes and a wealth of settings not normally seen (or indeed necessary) on an anaesthetic ventilator. With this, however, comes a greater level of complexity and user involvement. A full description of the settings, set-up and correct use of the Merlin in all its modes of operation is therefore beyond the scope of this text and the reader is referred to the in-depth and excellent support materials provided by the manufacturer.

One mode of operation is described as an illustration. This is the volume cycled mode and is recommended by the manufacturer for less experienced users.

Set-up:

1. Set tidal volume switch to volume (F).
2. Set an inspiratory time and volume (A and B).
3. Make sure that the ventilation assist mode is set to OFF (G).
4. Set the expiratory time (C).
5. Set the maximum airway pressure to a safe level for the animal you are about to ventilate (D) and make sure there is a non-return valve somewhere in the breathing system delivering gas to the patient.
6. Ensure that the anaesthetic circuit is delivering gas and that the flow of the incoming gas at least matches the minute volume of the patient as shown on the main display or is at least half of the inspiratory phase flow.
7. Set the ventilate mode switch to run (J).
8. The Max P reading on the screen will start to increase as the pressure in the chest rises.
9. Compliance will be displayed on the screen based on the tidal volume and the pressure change.
10. The bar graph displays on either side of the unit will register the pressure measured in both limbs of the patient delivery system (H and I).
11. In normal operation, both bar graph measurements will be identical. If there is any functional blockage of the expiratory limb, this will show as a reduced pressure reading on the expiratory port pressure bar graph.

The Vetronic™ SAV03 veterinary ventilator

Classification:

- Pressure cycled ('mechanical thumb for Ayre's T-piece').
- Inspiratory phase is initiated either by time (time triggered) or by the patient attempting to breathe (pressure triggered).

  Details include:

- Trigger range: 0–40 cmH_2O
- Expiratory phase: 1–30 seconds
- Breaths per minute: 2–60.

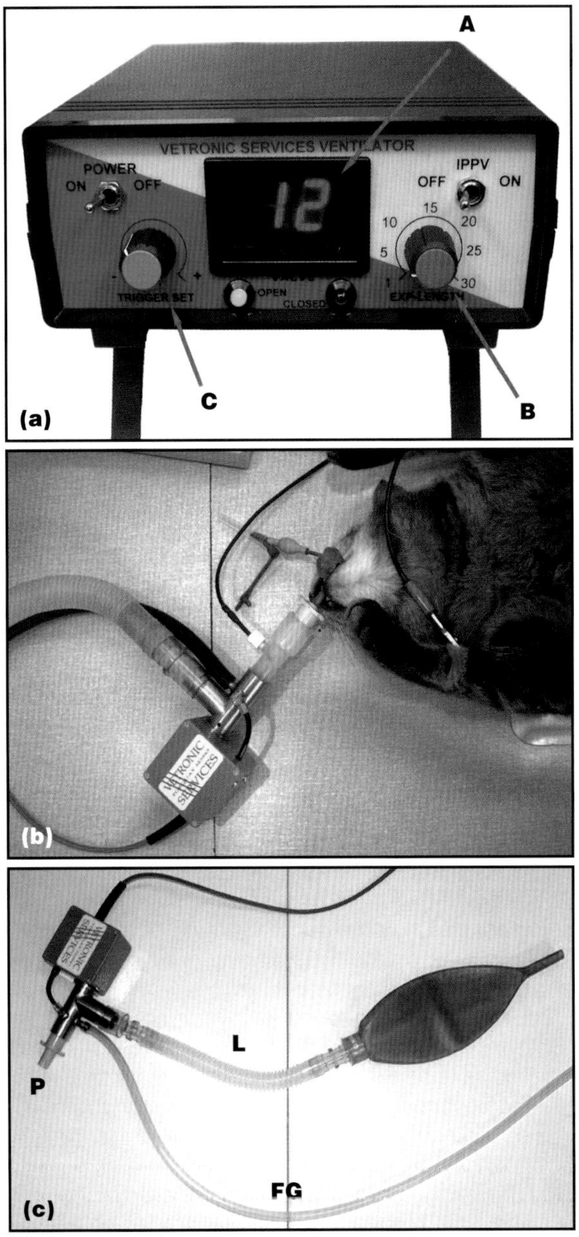

6.11 **(a)** The Vetronic™ SAV03 veterinary ventilator – a pressure cycled 'mechanical thumb' designed for patients less than 10 kg. A = Display; B = Expiratory phase time control; C = Trigger set. **(b)** The Vetronic™ SAV03 veterinary ventilator (in use). **(c)** The Vetronic™ SAV03 veterinary ventilator valve assembly. FG = Fresh gas; L = Limb; P = Patient attachment.

The SAV03 is a mains-powered, pressure cycled ventilator designed for use in animals up to 10 kg (Figure 6.11). The driving gas is taken directly from the anaesthetic machine and delivered via the valve of the ventilator to the endotracheal tube. During inspiration, gas is delivered to the patient in the inspiratory phase until a set airway pressure is reached, at which point the patient is allowed to exhale. A user-defined delay then elapses before inspiration begins again and the cycle repeats. The peak airway pressure can be adjusted to control the depth of respiration. This airway pressure is shown on a digital display, together with valve status indicators. The SAV03 is designed for use in very small animals, for which pressure cycling is more suitable.

Set-up and operation are simple. When not in ventilate mode, the valve remains open and the valve attachment acts as a T-piece; the patient, attached at P, draws gas from the limb (L). During expiration and the expiratory pause, this is replaced by fresh gas from the anaesthetic machine via FG. In 'IPPV On' mode, the valve is closed in response to attempted ventilation. The negative pressure at which the ventilator is triggered is set by the user (C). Inspiration is terminated when inspiratory pressure reaches a figure set by the operator using the same trigger set control, but before the IPPV mode is started. The display (A) will indicate the set cycle pressure at this point. The valve then opens and expired gas passes into the limb (L) and thence to scavenging. Expiratory phase time is set by the operator (B).

Preventing spontaneous ventilation during IPPV

As most anaesthetized patients hypoventilate, spontaneous ventilatory efforts during IPPV ('bucking' the ventilator) do not tend to occur. If normocapnia is maintained and spontaneous breathing attempts are made, this may cause sharp changes (negative and positive) in intrathoracic pressure. This interferes with the normal process of the thoracic venous pump and in many cases reduces ventilator effectiveness. Strategies to reduce spontaneous ventilatory attempts are listed in Figure 6.12. It is important to ensure adequate provision of analgesia and anaesthesia first.

Strategy	Comment
Increase tidal volume	The response of pulmonary stretch receptors to IPPV is to suppress spontaneous inhalation. Take care that peak airway pressure is not greater than 20 cmH_2O in healthy patients
Use of neuromuscular-blocking agents	See Chapter 15
Use of supplemental CNS depression	Low doses of an additional agent will further reduce ventilatory drive (e.g. midazolam 0.2 mg/kg i.v. dog/cat; medetomidine 1–5 µg/kg i.v. dog/cat; ketamine 1–2 mg/kg i.v. dog/cat; fentanyl 1–5 µg/kg i.v. dog/cat). NOTE: these may reduce the requirements for volatile agents

6.12 Strategies to reduce spontaneous ventilation during IPPV.

Monitoring and supporting the patient during IPPV

All the basic principles of monitoring the anaesthetized patient apply (see Chapter 7). Capnography (or arterial blood gas analysis) and, to a lesser extent, pulse oximetry are of particular value in these patients. Capnography is the simplest and most effective technique; it is a non-invasive and reliable way to show ventilatory (and hence ventilator) performance on a breath-by-breath basis. All clinics in which IPPV is more than a rarely performed novelty should consider purchasing suitable equipment. For occasional use, there are cheap, disposable, semiquantitative carbon dioxide detectors available. The other additional focus of monitoring during IPPV should be mean arterial blood pressure (MAP). This is the parameter most likely to be compromised by the effects of ventilation, especially where there is reduced cardiovascular reserve (see below).

Ventilators are known fomites in human anaesthetic practice. In-line bacterial filters (Figure 6.13) are widely available, are of low resistance and are cost effective compared to sterilization of the ventilator (where this is possible).

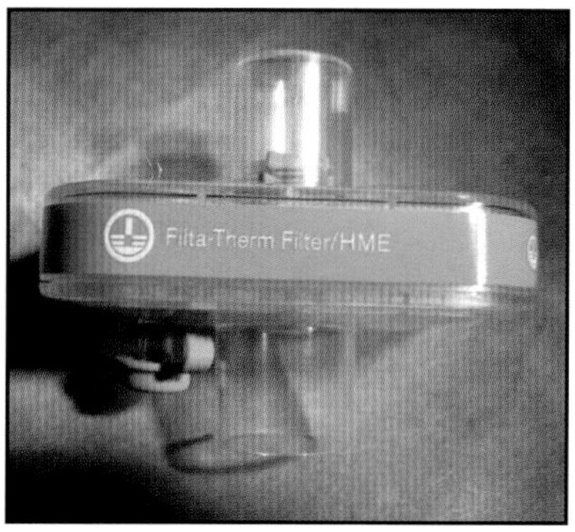

6.13 An example of an in-line bacterial filter.

Weaning from automatic ventilation

Weaning from IPPV after short periods of intraoperative use is less of a challenge than after prolonged ventilation of the ICU patient, in which ventilatory drive may be suppressed. In theory, where normocapnia is maintained, a reduction of the ventilatory rate set by the ventilator will allow a rise in arterial carbon dioxide and initiation of spontaneous ventilation. Alternatively, the patient may be removed from the ventilator and ventilated by squeezing the reservoir bag of a suitable breathing system at a reduced rate, until spontaneous ventilation returns. A very slight reduction of the tidal volume at this point may also reduce pulmonary stretch and increase respiratory drive, although care should be taken to avoid peripheral alveolar collapse. In practice, this is performed at the end of surgery where there is less surgical stimulus and often a deeper level of CNS depression. A concomitant reduction in the depth of anaesthesia may therefore be beneficial. Oxygen saturation should be monitored carefully at this time, although, with high inspired oxygen concentrations in the healthy patient undergoing some ventilation (albeit at a reduced rate), this is unlikely to fall. Hypothermia reduces ventilatory drive and attempts to correct this should be initiated at this point, if not already in progress.

The physiological effects of mechanical ventilation

Respiratory effects

The main determinants of arterial oxygen tension are inspired oxygen concentration and mean airway pressure. Mean airway pressure is altered by changes in the duration of inspiration (I:E ratio) and changes in peak airway pressure. Automatic ventilation increases mean airway pressures and, during anaesthesia, is performed with an F_iO_2 >0.21. Therefore, oxygenation is usually maintained or improved by use of an automatic ventilator. Removal of carbon dioxide is primarily determined by minute volume. Either high ventilatory rates with a concurrent low tidal volume, or low rates with a high tidal volume may therefore result in a similar minute volume and consequent arterial carbon dioxide tension. The ventilator is best set such that the ventilatory characteristics are as physiological as possible for that patient. For time or volume cycled ventilators, this is best achieved by setting the calculated tidal volume first. This is then checked by observing the animal to ensure that the excursion of the chest wall looks normal for that animal and, where available, checking that the peak airway pressure rises to between 15 and 20 cmH_20 in the healthy animal. The ventilatory rate is then set, ideally to the animal's measured arterial carbon dioxide levels, as indicated by arterial blood gas analysis or capnography. Where no measurement is available, the rate should be set to a value which is just below a normal estimated rate for that animal – IPPV is more effective than spontaneous ventilation and normal rates will result in hypocapnia, and respiratory alkalosis. Where severe hypocapnia results (P_aCO_2 <20 mmHg (2.6 kPa)), cerebral vasoconstriction and cerebral hypoxia may result. In a pressure cycled ventilator, the cycling pressure is initially set and adjusted based on observing chest wall excursion, as above. Ventilatory rate is then set as described above. Where the expiratory phase time (or I:E ratio) can be set, the expiratory phase must be long enough to allow adequate exhalation. Failure of exhalation will lead to gas trapping and potentially over-inflation. This is more likely in patients with increased small airway resistance (feline asthma) or high compliance (neonates).

During the inspiratory phase of spontaneous ventilation, gases are drawn into the lung by a drop in intrathoracic pressure. Passive expiration sees a return to baseline pressures and towards atmospheric pressure. Throughout the active phase of spontaneous ventilation, intrathoracic (intrapleural) pressures are therefore below baseline (Figure 6.14). In contrast, during IPPV inspiration occurs by an increase in intrathoracic pressure; this pressure returns to baseline but remains above atmospheric pressure throughout expiration. The distribution of ventilation (V) and

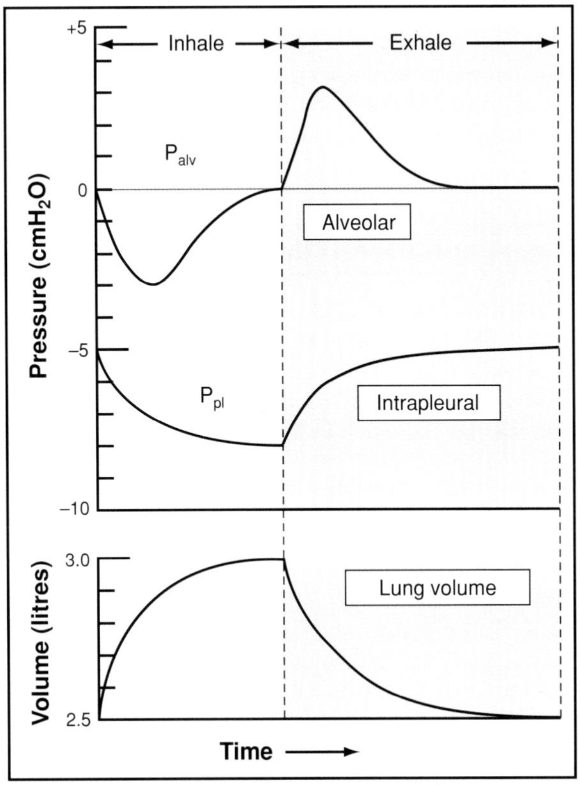

6.14 Normal respiratory pressures during spontaneous ventilation. Note that intrapleural pressure remains negative during the entire cycle – a key component of the 'thoracic pump' and the maintenance of cardiac preload.

blood perfusion (Q) in the lung depends upon the pressure and volume changes and is therefore very different for spontaneous ventilation and controlled ventilation. In a recumbent anaesthetized animal, dependent parts of the lung are less compliant due to increased tissue mass surrounding them. IPPV will therefore preferentially ventilate the more compliant non-dependent lung zones, exacerbating the V/Q mismatch already present in an anaesthetized recumbent animal. In addition, where inflation pressures achieve values greater than 30 cmH_2O, those capillaries in non-dependent lung areas (which have a relatively low capillary pressure) may be compressed. The consequent reduction in capillary blood flow further exacerbates the V/Q mismatch. IPPV is physiologically very different to spontaneous ventilation and worsens any V/Q mismatch that may be seen in an anaesthetized recumbent patient. This is usually of little clinical significance in small animal patients with no concurrent lung disease.

Cardiovascular effects

Adequate venous return relies on the maintenance of a pressure gradient between the venous reservoirs and the right atrium of the heart. During IPPV, the rise in intrathoracic pressure is transmitted through the right atrial wall, reducing this gradient and venous return. In extreme cases this mimics cardiac tamponade. The reduction in return is worsened by a long inspiratory phase time, high mean airway pressures and PEEP. The reduction in right-sided preload reduces right-sided cardiac output. This will then reduce left-sided preload, stroke volume and mean arterial pressure. This is more serious in animals with either hypovolaemia or pre-existing cardiac failure, especially diastolic failure (the cat with hypertrophic cardiomyopathy; the dog with pericardial effusion). In such cases, the use of central venous pressure (CVP) monitoring is invaluable in assessing right-sided preload, the effects of IPPV and outcomes of interventional therapy. A drop in CVP is seen in normal patients during IPPV; in animals that are hypovolaemic there is a longer time to recovery of CVP (and also MAP). This may be used as a marker of a potential problem in such cases. Increased right ventricular wall tension may also impede coronary perfusion and, when accompanied by low diastolic pressures, myocardial hypoxia may further decrease cardiac output and predispose to arrhythmias. Management strategies include optimizing ventilator set-up to provide a long expiratory phase time and pre-emptive and reactive intravenous fluid loading (titrated to CVP). Use of vasopressors is rarely indicated as they will increase afterload, which in the face of a pre-existing inadequate preload will further reduce cardiac output.

Changes in lung volume affect autonomic tone and pulmonary vascular resistance. This is seen in many species during spontaneous ventilation as a sinus arrhythmia. This pattern may be exaggerated during IPPV, especially where there is a concurrent hypovolaemia. Over-inflation leads to stimulation of pulmonary stretch receptors and a reflex increase in vagal tone (as well as inhibition of spontaneous ventilatory drive). Where over-inflation is associated with high peak airway pressures, capillary collapse also increases pulmonary vascular resistance. Heart rate in these circumstances may fall significantly, even to the point of sinus arrest with severe over-inflation.

Increased intrathoracic pressure also reduces venous drainage from the jugular veins and increases intracranial pressure. In normal patients cerebral autoregulation will prevent reduction in cerebral perfusion and oxygen delivery. In patients with CNS disease this process may be suboptimal and IPPV should be used with caution.

In summary:

- Minimize cardiovascular effects of IPPV by supporting preload and maximizing duration of the expiratory phase
- Avoid over-inflation
- Low heart rates, exaggerated sinus arrhythmia or low mean arterial blood pressures necessitate adjustment of inspiratory phase settings.

Renal and hepatic effects

A reduction in cardiac output results in a baroreceptor-mediated increase in sympathetic nervous tone and increased release of antidiuretic hormone (ADH). Reduced renal perfusion, coupled with the increased sympathetic drive, also stimulates the renin–angiotensin system, resulting in an aldosterone-mediated increase in the reabsorption of sodium and water. A reduction in atrial natriuretic peptide (ANP) release accompanies the reduction in atrial stretch due to reduced preload, again increasing the reabsorption of sodium and water. Reduced hepatic blood flow results from a reduced MAP. Reduced portal blood flow results from raised intrathoracic pressure and hepatic venous congestion. Clinically this means that patients with renal or hepatic disease may be further compromised by IPPV, although this is unlikely with the short periods of IPPV associated with routine anaesthesia.

References and further reading

Atallah MM, Demian AD, el-Diasty TA *et al.* (2000) Can we increase hepatic oxygen availability? The role of intentional hypercarbia. *Middle East Journal of Anesthesiology* **15**, 503–514

Cullen DJ and Eger EI (1974) Cardiovascular effects of carbon dioxide in man. *Anesthesiology* **41**, 345–349

Eichbaum FW and Yasaka WJ (1973) Influence of pulmonary ventilation with oxygen and carbon dioxide-oxygen mixtures upon cardiac arrhythmias. *Arquivos Brasileiros de Cardiologia* **26**, 109–123

Eisele JH, Eger EI and Muallem M (1967) Narcotic properties of carbon dioxide in the dog. *Anesthesiology* **28**, 856–865

Horwitz L, Bishop VS, Stone HL and Stegall HF (1969) Cardiovascular effects of low-oxygen atmospheres in conscious and anaesthetized dogs. *Journal of Applied Physiology* **27**, 370–373

Kil HK (2000) Hypercapnia is an important adjuvant factor of oculocardiac reflex during strabismus surgery. *Anesthesia and Analgesia* **91**, 1044

Rolf N and Cote CJ (1991) Persistent cardiac arrhythmias in pediatric patients: effects of age, expired carbon dioxide values, depth of anesthesia and airway management. *Anesthesia and Analgesia* **73**, 720–724

Useful websites

www.hallowell.com
www.pneupac.co.uk
www.surgivet.com
www.vetronic.co.uk
www.viasyshealthcare.com

7

Patient monitoring and monitoring equipment

Yves Moens and Paul Coppens

Introduction

When performing general anaesthesia, a reversible 'coma-like' state is produced. Most drugs used in anaesthesia have an inherent degree of toxicity and often produce cardiovascular and respiratory side effects. These side effects jeopardize body homeostasis and make anaesthesia a potentially dangerous procedure.

In order to limit the risks of general anaesthesia, 'controllable' problems must be prevented. Patient-related problems can be detected by the pre-anaesthetic examination (see Chapter 2). Checking equipment will help to prevent problems due to technical errors (Figure 7.1; see also Chapters 4, 5 and 6). Furthermore, basic prevention of problems involves maintaining the patient at an appropriate anaesthetic level throughout the procedure. However, even with adequate preparation, it is not possible to eliminate risk because every patient may exhibit individual and unpredictable reactions to anaesthesia. Earliest detection of any adverse reaction by the patient (by closely observing physiological functions during anaesthetic administration) is vital. Therefore, attention should be focused on the monitoring of vital systems, such as the cardiovascular and the respiratory systems, which are responsible for correct delivery of oxygen to the organs. Additionally, other parameters reflecting general homeostasis and the degree of antinociception and unconsciousness should be carefully observed. If deviations from normality outside defined limits occur, analysis of the situation is necessary and corrective measures should be taken. The results of such action must also be evaluated.

Monitoring is performed in various ways. Initially, the veterinary surgeon must always make full use of his/her own senses (vision, touch, smell, hearing) to collect clinical information, on which decisions can be made as to whether intervention is necessary. Clinical examination, although very relevant, does have limitations. The information is, in general, more qualitative than quantitative. Moreover, when staff availability is limited, or when the veterinary surgeon monitors more than one patient (or performs some adjustments to equipment), continuous collection of patient parameters will be difficult if not impossible. Therefore, monitoring can be complemented by mechanical and electronic auxiliary equipment. During the last two decades, several new devices have come on to the market and more affordable prices for these have led to their increasing popularity in veterinary anaesthesia. These devices are able to collect information on a continuous basis and can upgrade clinical observation with more sensitive information. The risk of anaesthesia in veterinary medicine remains very high compared with that of human anaesthesia. Healthy dogs and cats run a mortality risk of 0.054% and 0.112%, respectively (Brodbelt *et al.*, 2005). Actual anaesthetic mortality in humans is reported to be as low as 0.05 for every 10,000 patients (Arbous *et al.*, 2001). One should bear in mind that in human medicine (unlike veterinary medicine), anaesthesia is performed by a medical professional specially trained in anaesthesia.

Anaesthetic machine
Check **gas source**(s): • Open cylinder(s) • Check quantity • Check output pressure Check **flowmeter**(s) Check **vaporizer**(s): • Off position • Quantity Check **oxygen bypass** Choose and connect a **breathing system** Check the breathing system; carry out a **leak test**: 1. Close exhaust valve 2. Obstruct the patient extremity of the breathing system 3. Fill system with oxygen until reservoir bag is under tension (40 cmH_2O) 4. Check if pressure is kept, otherwise find and fix leak 5. Open exhaust valve If **ventilator** available: • Check function • Carry out a leak test • Preset the parameters
Monitoring equipment
• Power on • Battery state • Test • Calibration if necessary
Specific equipment
• Intravenous catheter • Intubation • Fluids • Hypothermia prevention • Ophthalmic ointment
Resuscitation equipment availability
Prepare the anaesthesia record

7.1 The preventive approach: pre-anaesthetic equipment check.

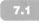

Monitoring equipment occasionally provides artefactual and wrong information. Hence, the function and limits of these devices (as well the physiological significance of the information they provide) must be very well understood if they are to be used to increase patient safety. Furthermore, this information must be used alongside clinical judgement when evaluating a situation and deciding on possible therapeutic intervention.

It is erroneous to think that monitoring may be omitted for some 'simple' or 'quick' procedures, with specific 'safe' drugs or during 'stable' episodes of anaesthesia. Unexpected events often occur during short and simple procedures on apparently healthy patients. Both clinical and technical monitoring must not be limited only to the patient but also include the anaesthetic machine.

Monitoring must not concentrate either on one clinical sign or one measured parameter. Simultaneous observation of several parameters (integrated monitoring) is necessary to build a more complete picture of vital system function in the individual animal and the function of the anaesthetic machine. In this way, monitoring is the central tool to 'pilot' anaesthesia with enhanced safety.

The main monitor: human senses

Veterinary surgeons are used to performing a clinical examination, using their senses, on a daily basis and should adapt this skill to conditions during anaesthesia (Figure 7.2). Moreover, even today, the most appropriate method for assessing the depth of anaesthesia in veterinary practice remains the assessment of clinical signs (Figures 7.3 and 7.4).

Sense	Observation	Information
Sight	**Mucous membrane colour** Pale Pink Red Brick red Blue	 Hypoperfusion, anaemia Normal Vasodilation, local congestion Haemoconcentration Cyanosis
	Surgical site Tissue colour Bleeding: colour, intensity Blood vessels: colour, turgescence	 Cardiovascular and respiratory status
	Thorax, bag of the breathing system, bellows of the ventilator Rate Amplitude Type	 Respiratory rate Tidal volume Respiratory pattern
	Eye Position Lacrimation Pupil size Degree of third eyelid protrusion	 Depth of anaesthesia
	Movement Spontaneous motor activity	 Depth of anaesthesia
Touch	**Pulse**: femoralis, sublingual, metacarpal, metatarsal arteries Tonus/amplitude Rate/rhythm Synchronicity with heart auscultation, ECG	 Cardiovascular system: heart rate/rhythm, blood pressure Autonomous response to noxious stimuli Depth of anaesthesia

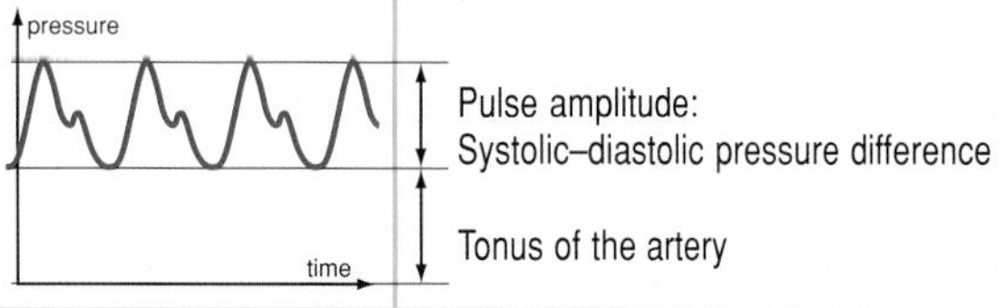

Sense	Observation	Information
Touch	**Capillary refill time**	Cardiovascular status: peripheral perfusion
	Palpebral/corneal reflex	Depth of anaesthesia
	Skin temperature	Body temperature
	Muscle relaxation Relaxation of the jaw	 Muscle tone, depth of anaesthesia
	Squeeze the bag after closing the exhaust valve Mechanical integrity of the breathing system and respiratory tract	 Leak Obstruction Pulmonary compliance Thoracic or extrathoracic resistance

7.2 Parameters that can be monitored during anaesthesia using the senses. (continues)

Sense	Observation	Information
Hearing	**Abnormal noise** Mechanical integrity of the breathing system and respiratory tract	Leak Obstruction
	Cardiac auscultation: stethoscope, oesophageal stethoscope Rate Rhythm Synchronicity with pulse, ECG Murmur	Cardiac system: heart rate, rhythm, heart integrity Autonomic responses to noxious stimuli Depth of anaesthesia
	Pulmonary auscultation: stethoscope, oesophageal stethoscope Rate Rhythm Lung sounds	Respiratory system: rate, rhythm, integrity Autonomic rsponse to noxious stimuli Depth of anaesthesia
Smell	**Presence of abnormal odour** Mechanical integrity of the breathing system and respiratory tract	Leak in the presence of halogenated anaesthetic agent

7.2 (continued) Parameters that can be monitored during anaesthesia using the senses.

Parameter	Light anaesthesia	Adequate anaesthesia	Deep anaesthesia
Eye position	Central 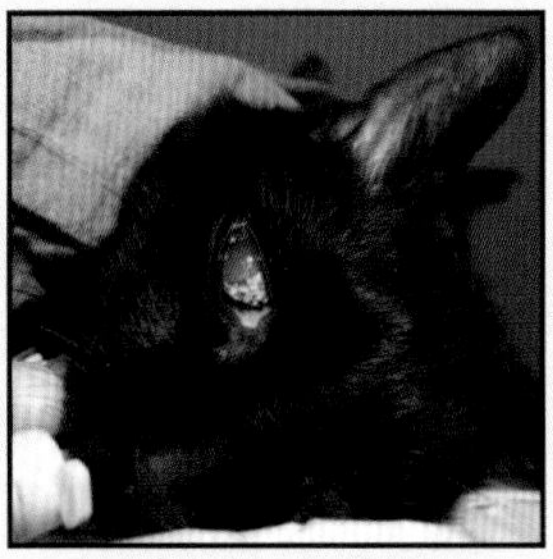	Rotated 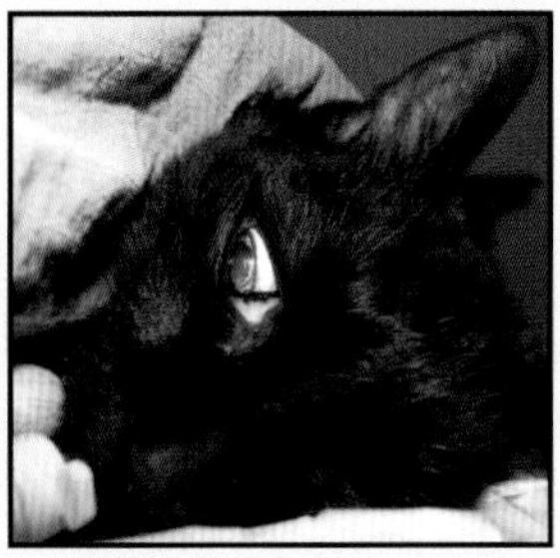	Central 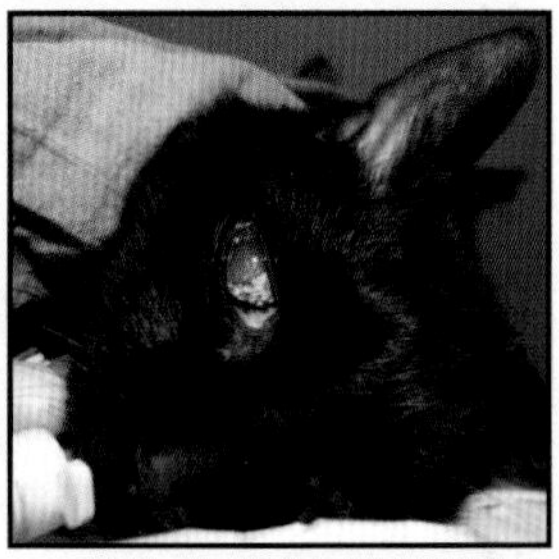
Palpebral reflex	+	–	–
Jaw tonicity	+	–	–
Movement	Possible	Absent	Absent
Cornea	Moist	Moist	Dry
Heart rate	Usually increased		Usually decreased
Respiratory rate	Usually increased		Usually decreased
Haemodynamic and/or respiratory variations following surgical stimulation	Yes	Usually no	No

7.3 Clinical signs of depth of anaesthesia. Eye position, palpebral reflex and jaw tonicity are the most accurate signs to evaluate depth of anaesthesia. Note that heart rate and respiratory rate are influenced by many other factors. These signs are not valid for anaesthesia performed with a dissociative anaesthetic agent.

Parameter	Light anaesthesia	Adequate anaesthesia	Deep anaesthesia
Eye position	Central	Central	Central
Palpebral reflex	+	+	±
Jaw tonicity	+	+	±
Movement	Possible	Possible	Possible/absent
Cornea	Moist	Moist	Moist/dry
Heart rate	Usually increased		Usually decreased
Respiratory rate	Usually increased		Usually decreased
Haemodynamic and/or respiratory variations following surgical stimulation	Yes	Usually no	No

7.4 Clinical signs of depth of anaesthesia with a dissociative anaesthetic agent. Note that heart rate and respiratory rate are influenced by many other factors.

Initially, the person in charge of anaesthesia needs to organize his/her workplace in such a way that the collection of clinical information necessary to assess depth of anaesthesia and the quality of the vital signs is easy: the concept of *ergonomics*. The aim of this concept is to be able to perform, from one location, a quick and complete assessment of all monitored parameters and machine function (Figure 7.5). The layout of the workplace will help concentration on the perception and integration of measurements from the patient, anaesthetic equipment and monitoring devices. This includes:

- Clinical parameters, such as eye position, palpebral reflex, jaw tone, mucous membrane colour, capillary refill time, sublingual pulse, chest movement, skin temperature and, during surgery, blood colour and bleeding intensity
- Indirect clinical parameters, e.g. movement of the reservoir bag
- Parameters collected from technical/electronic devices, e.g. wave forms and numeric displays on the screen
- Monitoring of the anaesthetic machine: inlet pressure (when available), flowmeters, vaporizer, breathing system and function of any other accessories like ventilators or syringe pumps.

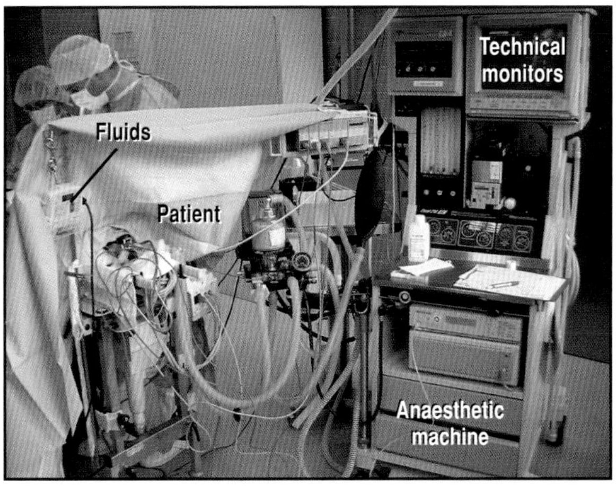

7.5 Ergonomics in the workplace.

The use of an anaesthesia 'screen' (Figure 7.6), so the patient's head can be seen, and the placement of an oesophageal stethoscope (Figure 7.7), to make cardiac and lung auscultation easier, are strongly recommended. However, the veterinary surgeon remains the main monitor; he/she is the collector of parameters, the central analyser and is responsible for all decisions (i.e. he/she is the 'pilot' on board). The limit of this 'main monitor' is that its quality (and thus safety) is dependent on qualifications, knowledge and experience.

A record of anaesthesia, even in a simple form, must be completed. This will:

- Aid appreciation of trends in observed and measured parameters
- Act as a reference for future anaesthesia in an individual animal

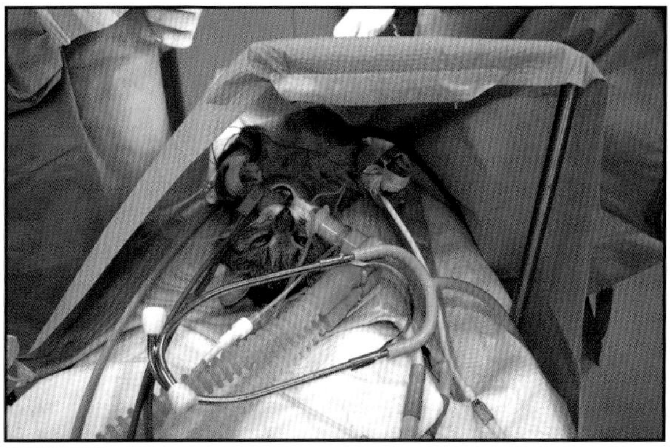

7.6 The anaesthesia 'screen'.

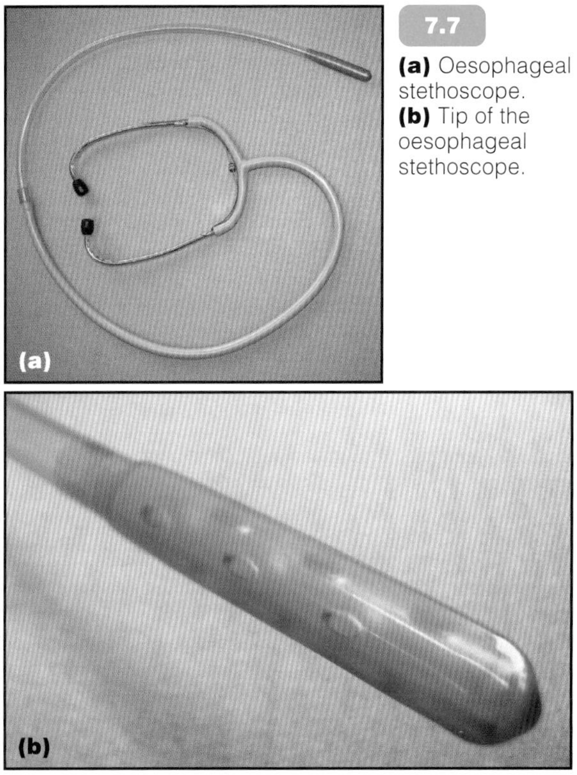

7.7 **(a)** Oesophageal stethoscope. **(b)** Tip of the oesophageal stethoscope.

- Act as a source for retrospective analysis, allowing further improvement of anaesthesia strategies
- Represent a medicolegal document, attesting the presence of an active monitoring effort of the patient during anaesthesia.

Monitoring of parameters that reflect the integration of several physiological functions

Capnometry and capnography

Capnometry is the measurement and numerical display of the carbon dioxide concentration in the respiratory gas during the whole respiratory cycle (inspiration and expiration). When a continuous graphical display (screen or paper) is available, the measurement produces typical curves (a *capnogram*) and the technique (instrument) is often referred to as *capnography* (*capnograph*).

The measuring principle relies on absorption of infrared light by carbon dioxide molecules. Capnometers are available as either *sidestream* or *mainstream* infrared analysers. Sidestream capnometers require a sampling line connected to the airway and continuously sample the respiratory gases (Figure 7.8a). Samples are then analysed in the measuring chamber of the instrument. With mainstream analysers, miniaturization allows placement of the measuring chamber directly in the airway and the measurement signal is generated here (Figure 7.8b).

The capnogram

The production of the capnogram is based on the fact that carbon dioxide is produced in cells as a result of metabolism and then carried by the circulation to the lungs, where it is removed by alveolar ventilation.

There are four distinct phases of the capnogram (Figure 7.9a):

- Phase I is the inspiratory baseline. This phase represents the analysis of the gas mixture inspired by the patient for carbon dioxide. The

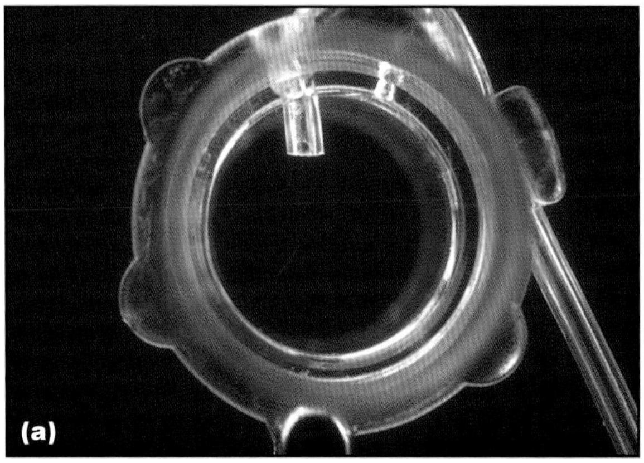

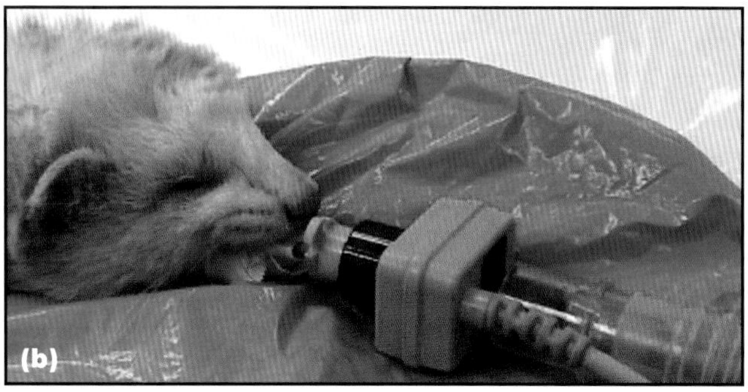

7.8 **(a)** Close-up of a connector for sampling gas (sidestream capnograph). **(b)** Adaptor and sensor of a mainstream capnograph.

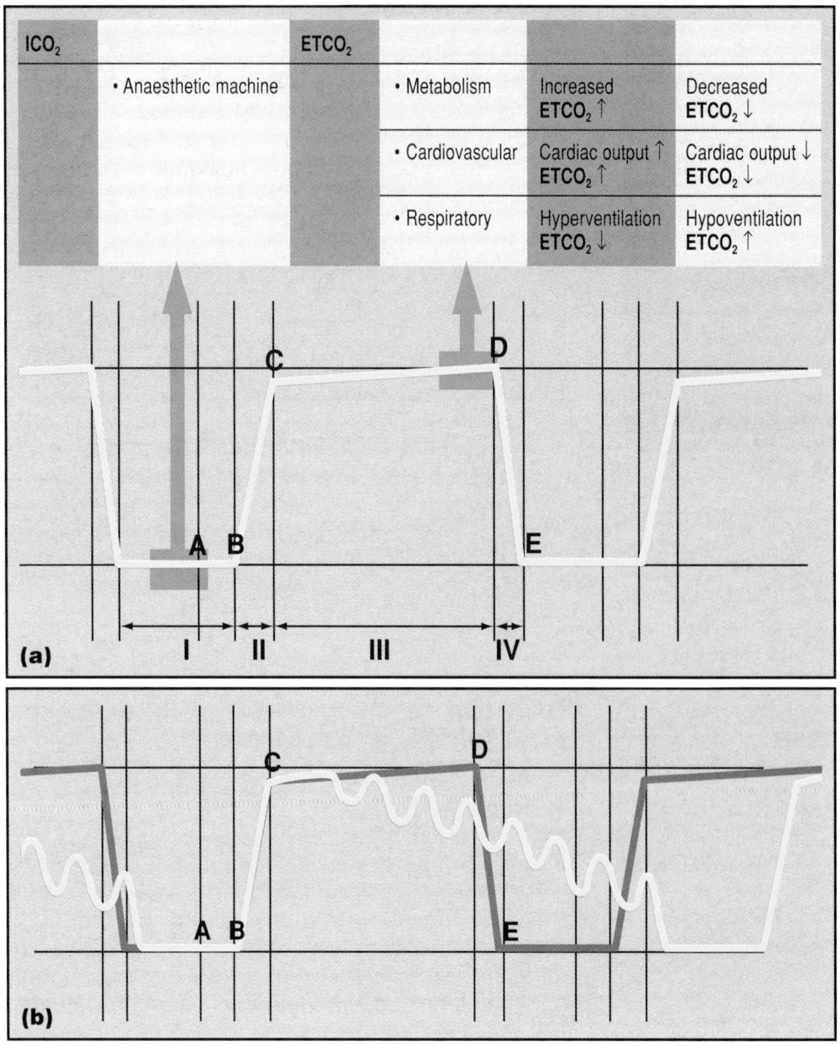

7.9 **(a)** The normal capnogram. **(b)** Cardiogenic oscillations. A–B: exhalation of carbon dioxide-free gas contained in deadspace at the beginning of expiration. B–C: respiratory upstroke, representing the emptying of connecting airways and the beginning of emptying of alveoli. C–D: expiratory (alveolar) plateau, representing emptying of alveoli. D: end-tidal carbon dioxide level – the best approximation of alveolar carbon dioxide level. D–E: inspiratory downstroke, as the patient begins to inhale fresh gas. E–A: continuing inspiration, where carbon dioxide remains at zero. $ETCO_2$ = End-tidal carbon dioxide; ICO_2 = Inspired carbon dioxide.

baseline should have a value of zero, otherwise the patient is rebreathing carbon dioxide

- Phase II is the expiratory upstroke. This represents arrival at the sampling site of carbon dioxide from the alveoli and the mixing with gas present in the conducting airways. It is usually very steep
- Phase III is the expiratory (alveolar) plateau, which represents pure alveolar gas (of emptying alveoli). Due to uneven emptying of alveoli, the slope continues to rise gradually during the expiratory pause. The peak of this exhaled carbon dioxide is called the *end-tidal* carbon dioxide
- Phase IV is the inspiratory downstroke. This is the beginning of the inhalation and the carbon dioxide curve falls steeply to zero.

During anaesthesia, with long expiratory times, phase III can show cardiogenic oscillations caused by movement of the heart and this is considered normal (Figure 7.9b).

The capnometer usually displays respiratory rate, the value of end-tidal carbon dioxide and sometimes the value for inspiratory carbon dioxide. If a capnograph is used, the presence of a normal shape of the capnographic curve indicates that the number displayed for end-tidal carbon dioxide is likely to represent a true end-expiratory sample. When grossly normal ventilation/perfusion conditions in the lungs exist, the end-tidal carbon dioxide reflects the partial pressure of carbon dioxide in arterial blood (P_aCO_2; Figure 7.10). Hence capnometry offers a continuous, non-invasive way to reflect the partial pressure of carbon dioxide in arterial blood, which is directly determined by alveolar ventilation.

End-tidal carbon dioxide is displayed as a concentration in volume percent (%) or as a partial pressure (in mmHg or kPa). Concentration can be converted into mmHg with the formula:

$$PCO_2 = (P_{bar}\text{-}47) \times \%CO_2/100$$

where P_{bar} is barometric pressure in mmHg. Capnometers can often perform the conversion because of a barometric pressure sensor in the device. End-tidal carbon dioxide concentrations between 5 and 6% (35–45 mmHg; 4.6–6 kPa) are considered normal in anaesthetized animals.

Interpreting the capnogram

The approach for proper interpretation of capnographic information is initially to check if a normal capnographic curve is present and then to note the numerical value of end-tidal carbon dioxide. One must acknowledge the possible contribution of metabolism, circulation and ventilation to the production of this number. When two functions are stable, capnometry monitors closely the third function, e.g. if metabolism and circulation are stable, the capnometer monitors ventilation. Conversely, if metabolism and ventilation are stable, the state of the circulation will be more closely reflected. Additionally, capnography will provide information about airway patency, technical faults and adequacy of gas flow in non-rebreathing systems. Capnography has become standard care for intraoperative monitoring of ventilatory efficiency and thus decreases the need for invasive arterial blood gas analysis.

Increased ETCO$_2$: Increases in end-tidal carbon dioxide concentrations (Figure 7.11a) may be due to impaired alveolar ventilation (anaesthetic-induced respiratory depression), increased metabolism (malignant hyperthermia or early sepsis), increased cardiac output or the addition of carbon dioxide to the circulatory system as a result of rebreathing carbon dioxide. In the latter case, increased inspired carbon dioxide will be associated with increased end-tidal carbon dioxide (Figure 7.11b). Increased end-tidal carbon dioxide is also observed during laparoscopy due to absorption from the peritoneum of carbon dioxide used to inflate the abdomen.

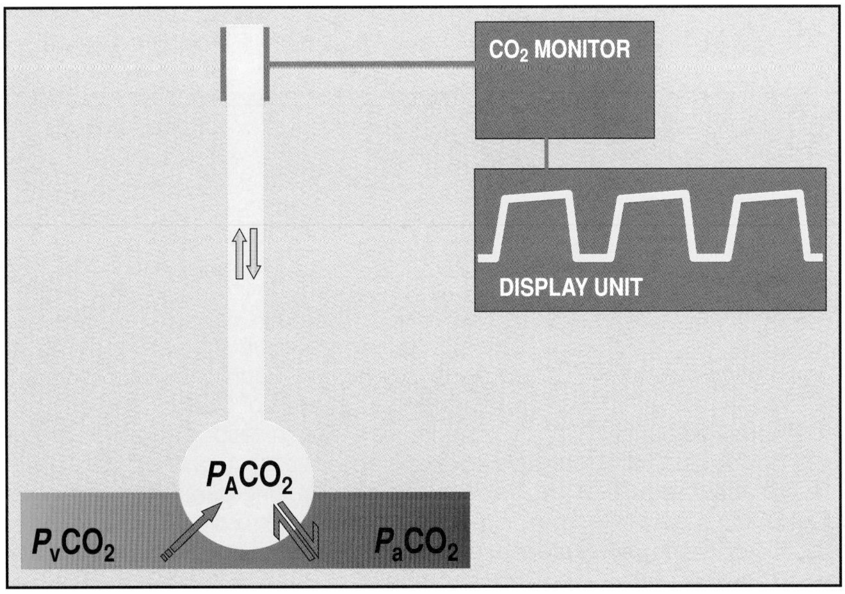

7.10 Capnography: the principle. P_ACO_2 = Alveolar carbon dioxide; P_aCO_2 = Partial pressure of carbon dioxide in arterial blood; P_vCO_2 = Partial pressure of carbon dioxide in venous blood.

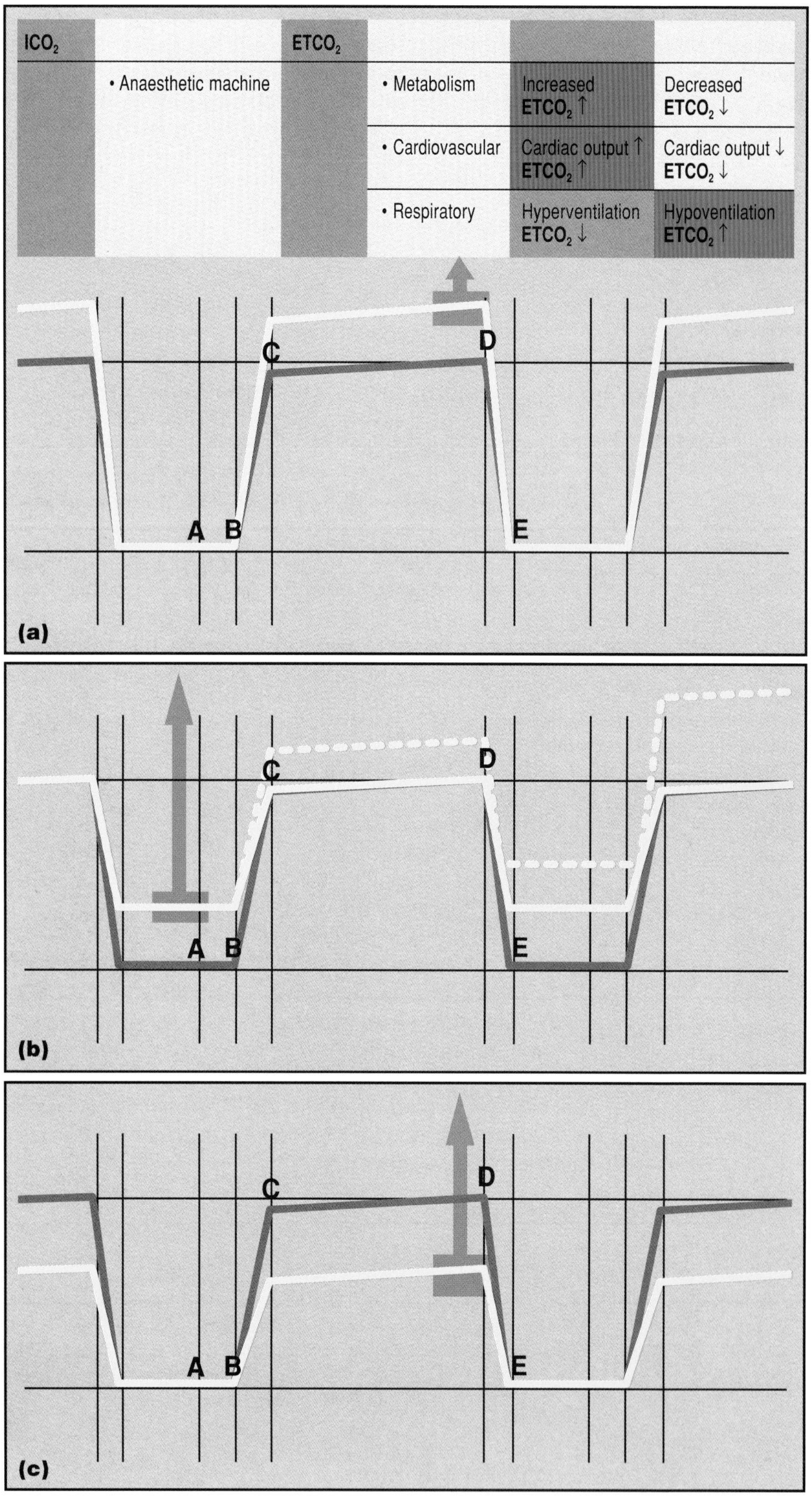

7.11 Capnographs showing **(a)** increased end-tidal carbon dioxide; **(b)** increased inspired carbon dioxide; and **(c)** decreased end-tidal carbon dioxide.

Decreased $ETCO_2$: Decreased end-tidal carbon dioxide concentrations (Figure 7.11c) may be due to hyperventilation, low cardiac output (low blood volume delivered to the lungs) or pronounced hypothermia. Rapidly falling end-tidal carbon dioxide, in the presence of respiratory movements and absence of hyperventilation, is a good indicator of failing circulation and cardiac arrest. Absent end-tidal carbon dioxide can indicate respiratory arrest (no alveolar ventilation), cardiac arrest (no circulation) or technical problems (see below). Rapid diagnosis of cardiac arrest increases the chance of a successful outcome for cardiopulmonary resuscitation. End-tidal carbon dioxide values during resuscitation and cardiac massage reflect efficiency of lung perfusion, and in human medicine have been considered to have prognostic value for successful restoration of spontaneous circulation.

Technical monitoring: Several technical aspects of breathing systems, their function and connection to the patient are also monitored by quantitative (capnometer value) and qualitative analysis (capnogram morphology). The presence of inspired carbon dioxide (rebreathing) (see Figure 7.11b) can be due to soda lime exhaustion; an incompetent expiratory valve on a circle system allowing exhaled carbon dioxide to be re-inhaled (even with normal function of soda lime); insufficient gas flow in a non-rebreathing system. An abnormal capnogram may be due to:

- A dislodged endotracheal tube
- A misplaced endotracheal tube (oesophageal intubation)
- An obstructed endotracheal tube or airway (endotracheal tube cuff hernia; Figure 7.12)
- A leak around the endotracheal tube cuff (Figure 7.13)
- Disconnection of the endotracheal tube from the breathing system.

Capnometry* versus *capnography: The drawback of a capnometer compared with a capnograph is that the former lacks the capnogram and, therefore, cannot provide a qualitative analysis and precise diagnosis from the morphological changes of exhaled carbon dioxide.

When ventilation/perfusion mismatch in the lungs becomes important, the end-tidal carbon dioxide underestimates P_aCO_2 due to an increase in alveolar deadspace (e.g. low cardiac output, pulmonary thromboembolism).

With sidestream devices, artefactually low end-tidal carbon dioxide is seen:

- When concomitant aspiration of ambient air occurs anywhere between sampling site and measuring chamber
- With rapid respiratory rates and very low tidal volumes
- When sampling at the level of fresh gas delivery in non-rebreathing systems. The sampling line can become obstructed by condensation drops or aspiration of any fluids.

With mainstream capnographs, the measuring chamber in the airway adaptor can become dirty or damaged, leading to erroneous end-tidal or inspired carbon dioxide values. Sidestream technology offers other (less important) possibilities like sampling directly from a nostril in non-intubated patients. Mainstream technology can be used only in the presence of an endotracheal tube, but copes better with rapid respiratory rates and very small tidal volumes.

Pulse oximetry

The pulse oximeter is a device that allows non-invasive measurements of the saturation of haemoglobin with oxygen (S_pO_2); in addition, it displays heart rate. The principle of measurement is as follows: a probe, which features a transmitter and receiver of red and infrared light, is positioned to transilluminate a pulsatile arteriolar bed. In small animal patients, it is usually placed on the tongue, prepuce or other unpigmented area (Figure 7.14). Computer software analyses the total absorption of the light and detects the pulsating component of the

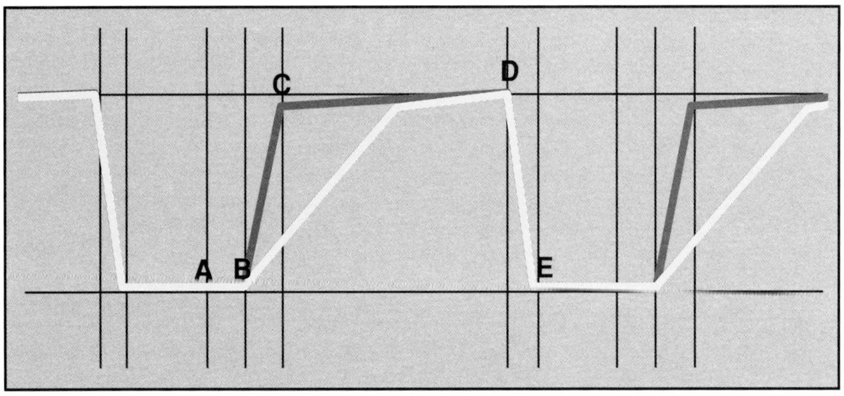

7.12 Capnograph showing increased resistance at expiration.

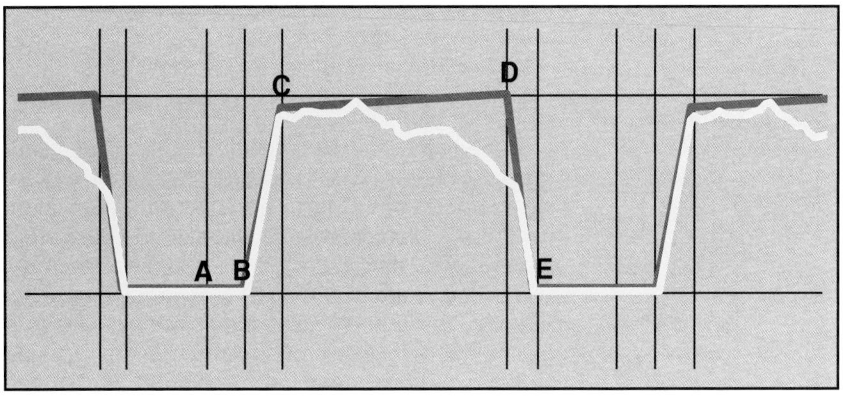

7.13 Capnograph showing leakage at the level of endotracheal tube and/or breathing system.

absorption that originates from cyclic arrival of arterial blood in the tissue. The absorption of infrared and red light by the pulsatile component is measured differentially. Because oxyhaemoglobin and reduced haemoglobin absorb more infrared and red light, respectively (Figure 7.15), a ratio is calculated that corresponds to a percentage of haemoglobin saturated with oxygen (Figure 7.16). Because maximal total light absorption corresponds to a pulse, the pulse oximeter also provides a figure for pulse rate.

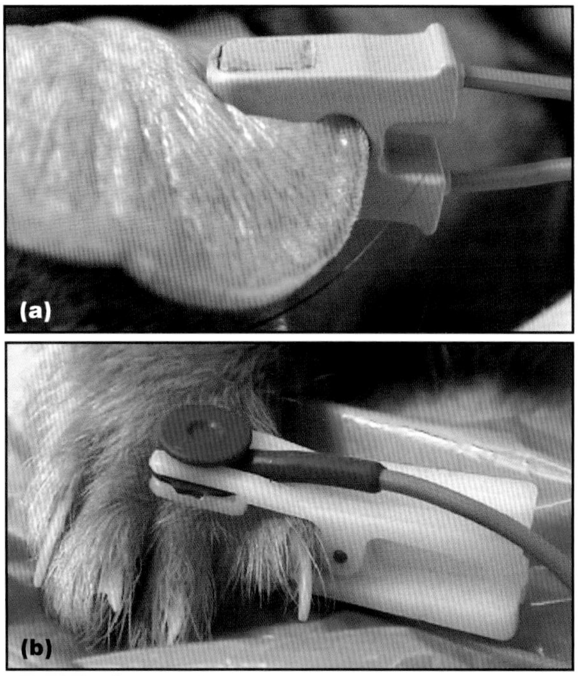

7.14 Sensor of a pulse oximeter. **(a)** On the tongue. **(b)** On a non-pigmented toe.

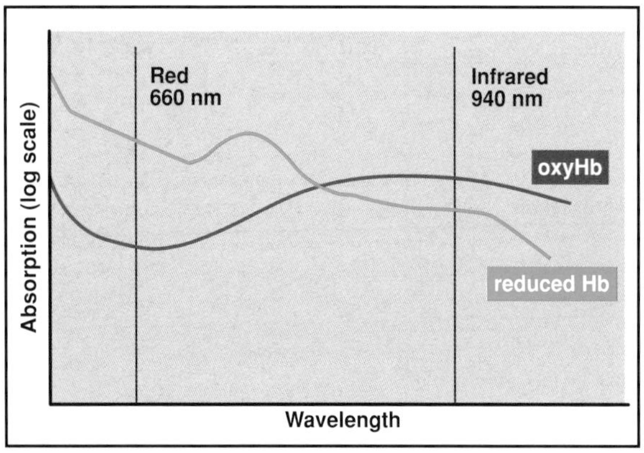

7.15 Light absorption of reduced haemoglobin and oxyhaemoglobin.

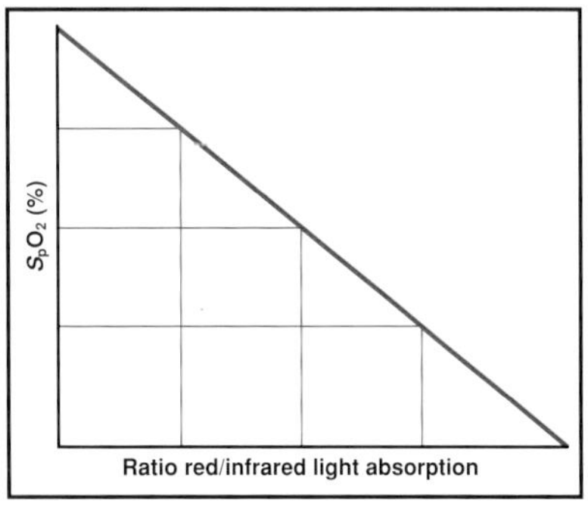

7.16 Relationship between the ratio of red to infrared light absorption and the saturation of haemoglobin with oxygen (S_pO_2).

The threshold of hypoxaemia occurs at an arterial oxygen tension of 60 mmHg (8 kPa). As shown on the dissociation curve of haemoglobin (Figure 7.17), this threshold corresponds to a saturation of 90%. During anaesthesia, therefore, oxygen saturation must be kept above 90%. When oxygen is supplied (or even in a healthy patient breathing room air), a saturation closer to 100% should be expected. The usual precision of measurement of a pulse oximeter is ± 2%. It is important to note that S_pO_2 only indicates that the patient is receiving enough oxygen; S_pO_2 can be normal in hypoventilating patients when the inspired oxygen fraction is increased (which normally should be the case during anaesthesia). In these circumstances, S_pO_2 gives no information about adequacy of ventilation. Conversely, when a patient hypoventilates whilst breathing room air, S_pO_2 will fall.

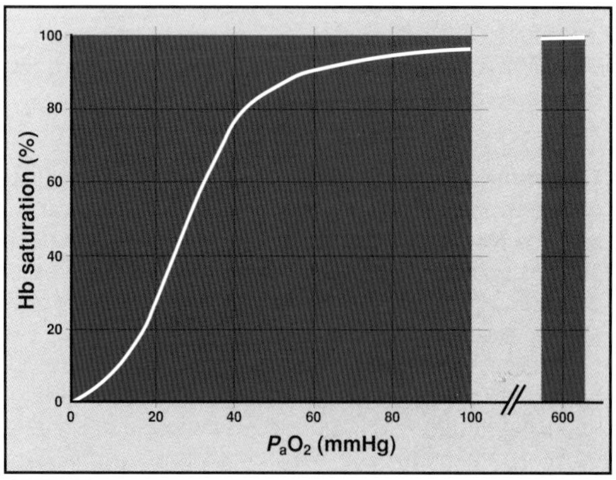

7.17 Haemoglobin–oxygen dissociation curve.

Any general cause of poor peripheral perfusion, such as vasoconstriction associated with shock, hypothermia or use of alpha-2 agonists, causes erroneously low values or failure to measure. Local hypoperfusion can also be induced by progressive pressure from the clip holding the probe; changing the position of the clip and the probe every so often temporarily solves the situation.

Other factors can also interfere with pulse oximetry readings:

- The presence of abnormal haemoglobin will affect measurement. For instance, in the presence of carboxyhaemoglobin S_pO_2 will be overestimated
- Interference from ambient light will reduce the quality of the signal received
- Motion or shivering, use of electrosurgical equipment and mucosal or skin pigmentation.

Some pulse oximeters display a photoplethysmographic waveform. The presence of a regular and distinct waveform similar to an arterial pressure waveform confirms the validity of the displayed S_pO_2 values (Figure 7.18). Moreover, this can be supported by a displayed heart rate equivalent to the true heart rate. However, the amplitude of the waveform does not necessarily reflect the quality of the signal because the gain can be automatically adapted.

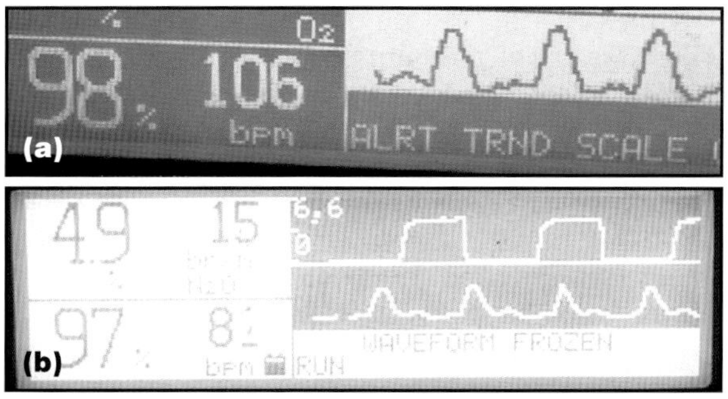

7.18 **(a)** Pulse oximeter: display of S_pO_2, heart rate and waveform. **(b)** Display of capnography and pulse oximetry.

Capnography and pulse oximetry

Capnography and pulse oximetry (see Figure 7.18b) provide complementary information. It has been shown that the proper interpretation of information received by capnography and pulse oximetry, used together, have the potential to prevent 93% of the complications during anaesthesia in human medicine (Tinker, 1989).

Blood gas analysis

Blood gas analysers measure directly the pH and the partial pressures of oxygen and carbon dioxide in a blood sample. They also calculate derived variables, such as plasma bicarbonate concentration (HCO_3^-), base excess and saturation of haemoglobin with oxygen (S_aO_2). In traditional analysers, the blood sample is aspirated into a circuit bringing the blood in contact with different electrodes to perform the measurements. These machines are expensive and require careful maintenance. Recently, portable and even handheld blood gas analysers have become available, allowing blood gas analysis to be performed in remote locations. These devices use disposable cartridges, which need only a minimal amount of blood to perform the measurement. They measure blood gas parameters but offer the option to measure additional parameters, e.g. electrolytes, glucose and lactate.

Blood gas analysis is the 'gold standard' method for evaluation of gas exchange. It provides invaluable information about the oxygenation, ventilation and acid–base status of the patient. Interpretation of the values for pH, PCO_2 and HCO_3^-, coupled to the clinical history of the patient, allows identification of respiratory and metabolic acidosis and alkalosis, as well as ongoing compensatory mechanisms. The detailed interpretation of blood gas measurements can be complex as all the results are interrelated, and interested readers are advised to consult standard textbooks on the subject. Figure 7.19 summarizes basic interpretation of blood gas analysis.

If the ability of the lungs to oxygenate blood is to be assessed, sampling of arterial blood is mandatory. The value of P_aO_2 (partial pressure of oxygen in arterial blood) on its own is not meaningful to evaluate oxygenation if the inspired oxygen fraction (F_iO_2) is not known. Classical indices of oxygenation are:

- The ratio P_aO_2/F_iO_2 (normal: >300)
- The alveolar–arterial difference for PO_2 ($(A\text{-}a)PO_2$) where $P_AO_2 = ((P_{bar} - 47) \times F_iO_2) - 1.2P_aCO_2$ (normal: 5–10 mmHg if $F_iO_2 = 0.21$, 100 mmHg if $F_iO_2 = 1.0$).

The 'gold standard' to evaluate the efficiency of ventilation is P_aCO_2. The assessment of venous blood samples does not provide straightforward information about oxygenation, but it does allow satisfactory monitoring of the ability to remove carbon dioxide by ventilation and the acid–base status.

The classic blood gas machine uses samples of heparinized blood. Failure to use the correct samples causes clotting within the circuit. To obtain accurate results, blood samples should be withdrawn anaerobically (no air bubbles) to avoid actual gas tensions being modified by gas exchange with room air. Analysis is best done promptly, but storing blood samples for less than 1 hour in iced water is acceptable. Taking an arterial blood sample is relatively easy in larger animals, but rather difficult in very small ones. Femoral and dorsal metatarsal arteries are often used. Without careful attention to technique, complications such as haematoma or bruise formation at the site of sampling can occur. In particular, pressure should be applied to the site for several minutes after sample collection to allow the vessel to seal. If it is likely that multiple samples will be required, insertion of an arterial catheter should be considered; this is often done in combination with invasive blood pressure measurement.

Blood gas analysis is useful in the management of critically ill patients and patients with ventilatory problems. Specific treatment can be planned from the results of initial blood gas analysis, and the response to this treatment can be monitored by taking further blood gas samples. The necessity of repeated blood sampling in anaesthesia is diminished when non-invasive monitors of oxygenation and ventilation are used simultaneously, e.g. pulse oximetry and capnometry.

Parameter	Normal values	Decrease	Increase
pH	7.35–7.45	Acidaemia	Alkalaemia
P_aCO_2	35–45 mmHg	Respiratory component: alkalosis	Respiratory component: acidosis
HCO_3^-	22–26 mmol/l	Metabolic component: acidosis	Metabolic component: alkalosis
P_aO_2	If oxygen level in inspired gas (F_iO_2) = 21%: 80–100 mmHg (10.7–13.3 kPa)	Hypoxaemia: <60 mmHg (8kPa)	Due to increased F_iO_2 or increased atmospheric pressure
S_aO_2	95–100%	Hypoxaemia: < 90 %	

7.19 Basic interpretation of blood gas analysis.

Cardiovascular monitoring

Heart rate indicator

Heart rate indicators exist as separate devices but more often heart rate counting is a feature of an electrocardiographic monitoring system. The heart rate is deduced using detection of the QRS complex. The number of complexes is counted over a certain time period and calculated as beats per minute. Algorithms are based on human use and in veterinary patients regularly cause the display of a double heart rate when relatively high T waves are erroneously detected as QRS complexes. The displayed heart rate must be regularly double-checked by clinical examination. There is no information about the pumping function of the heart (see Electrocardiography, below) and consequently such heart rate indicators can give a false feeling of security.

Blood pressure

Arterial blood pressure

Arterial blood pressure is one of the most useful measures of cardiovascular function available to the veterinary surgeon. Two methods of measuring blood pressure can be used: invasive (direct) and non-invasive (indirect). Invasive blood pressure measurement is less straightforward to carry out in practice conditions but, on the other hand, non-invasive blood pressure measurement might not fulfil the expectations of reliability and accuracy.

Invasive blood pressure measurement: Invasive blood pressure measurement is considered the 'gold standard' technique. A catheter must be placed in a peripheral artery. In the dog, the dorsal metatarsal artery is most commonly used, but the femoral artery or the palmar artery can also be used. In the cat, the femoral artery is the most common site. The catheter is connected to a pressure transducer via non-compliant tubing filled with heparinized saline. Pure mechanical pressure transducers have been mostly abandoned for electronic ones connected to the monitoring device. The transducer must be 'zeroed' to ambient air at the level of the right atrium. The transducer–monitor combination gives a continuous reading of blood pressure and shows the pressure waveform. Systolic and diastolic pressures are taken as the cyclic maximum and minimum pressures, respectively. Mean pressure is automatically calculated. To allow trouble-free continuous monitoring (avoiding clotting in the arterial line), the set-up is combined with a pressurized continuous flush system that does not influence the accuracy of the pressure reading (Figure 7.20). Repeated arterial blood sampling (blood gas analysis) is easy when an arterial catheter is in place.

Non-invasive blood pressure measurement: There are two methods generally used to measure blood pressure non-invasively: the oscillometric method and the Doppler method. Both methods are based on the occlusion of blood flow to an extremity by the inflation of a cuff and detection of reappearance of blood flow during deflation. Any of the limbs or the tail can be used. The ideal cuff width is usually quoted as 40% of the circumference of the limb. Wider cuffs will lead to underestimation of the true pressure, while narrow cuffs will tend to overestimate. Most cuffs have a mark that should be placed directly over the artery.

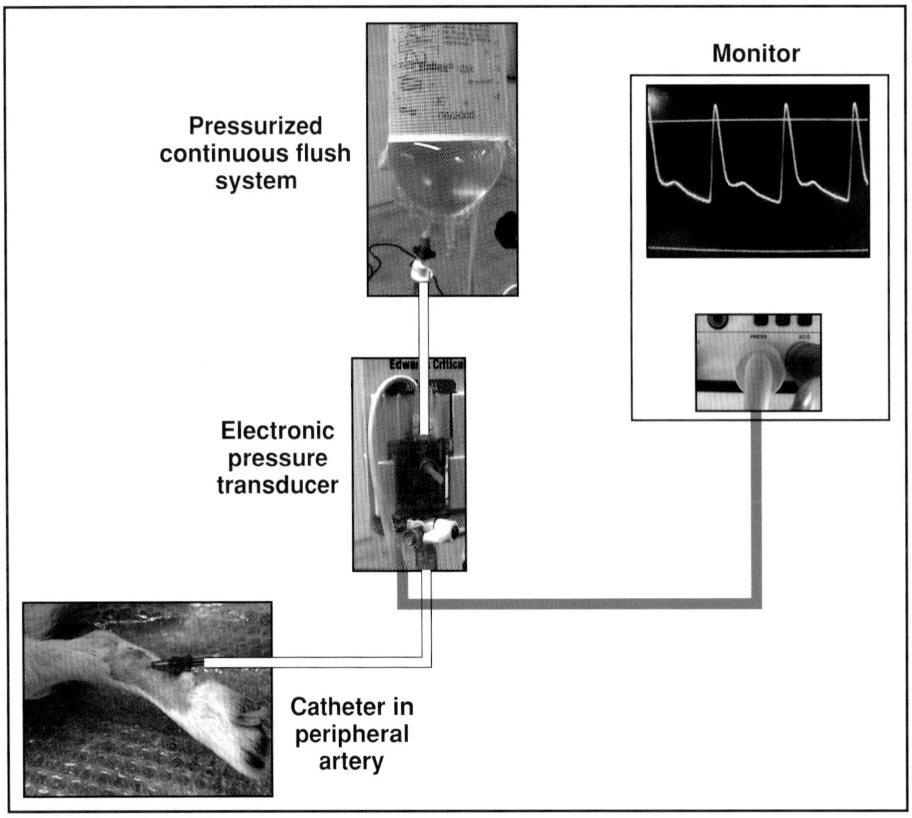

7.20 Set-up for invasive blood pressure measurement.

Using the oscillometric method, returning blood flow is detected by pulsatile pressure changes in the cuff itself. The pressure at which pulses in the cuff appear is taken as systolic blood pressure. As the cuff is further deflated, diastolic and mean blood pressure are measured. Oscillotonometric devices record mean blood pressure as the pressure at which the pulses in the cuff are maximal and diastolic pressure as the pressure below which they disappear. The option of automated function provides non-invasive blood pressure measurements at adjustable time intervals. Heart rate is also usually displayed.

Using the Doppler method, placement of an ultrasound probe over an artery distal to the cuff is necessary. The emitted ultrasound is reflected by the moving blood and a frequency shift is converted to an audible signal. The pressure at which blood flow recommences, characterized by a typical 'whoosh' sound, is taken as systolic blood pressure. Diastolic pressure is more difficult to determine. No automatic function is available but leaving the probe in place with a deflated cuff allows one to hear the blood flow continuously, hence turning it into a continuous monitor. Changes in the pitch of the tone suggest changing haemodynamics. The Doppler technique can be applied to any size of animal, including cold-blooded animals, and is relatively inexpensive. It requires more operator experience than automated oscillometric measurement and the noise it produces can be disturbing to some unless headphones are used.

Significance of information: There is a wide range in blood pressure encountered in anaesthetized dogs and cats. Ranges commonly seen are between 90 and 120 mmHg for systolic, between 55 and 90 mmHg for diastolic, and between 60 and 120 mm Hg for mean blood pressure.

Generally, arterial blood pressure gives an indication of the adequacy of cardiovascular function. The systolic blood pressure is determined by a combination of peripheral vascular resistance, stroke volume and intravascular volume, whereas diastolic blood pressure primarily arises from peripheral vascular resistance. Measurement of systolic and diastolic blood pressures allows estimation of pulse pressure, which is the difference between systolic and diastolic pressures (pulse quality). Mean blood pressure is an important factor in relation to general tissue perfusion. Blood flow to the major organs of the body is autoregulated across a range of mean blood pressures from about 60 mmHg to about 120 mmHg. When mean blood pressure falls below this range, blood flow to the major organs is jeopardized. This results in inadequate oxygen delivery and accumulation of lactic acid, leading to acidosis. On the other hand, it must be realized that a normal mean blood pressure does not necessarily equate to good overall tissue perfusion. If a normal blood pressure is generated by excessive vasoconstriction, perfusion of tissue might be insufficient. Acute hypertension can have deleterious effects on the central nervous system and the lungs.

Changes in blood pressure and heart rate can be seen with inadequate anaesthetic depth, anaesthetic agent overdose, hypovolaemia and overhydration (see also Chapters 19 and 29). Analysis of the arterial waveform with invasive blood pressure measurement allows semiqualitative estimation of ventricular contractility, hypovolaemia, cardiac output and the role of peripheral resistance, e.g. a low dichrotic notch indicates vasodilation, steepness of upstroke represents strength of contraction.

Invasive blood pressure monitoring is less practical than non-invasive techniques in the clinical setting. It requires more expensive equipment, skills in placement of a catheter (especially in smaller patients) and correct calibration. There is a risk of haematoma formation, particularly after withdrawal of the catheter, and a risk of infection.

Individual blood pressure values obtained by noninvasive methods must always be regarded cautiously. Oscillometric blood pressure measurements tend to be less accurate or the measuring devices regularly cease to function during hypotension and peripheral vasoconstriction (especially in small patients <5 kg bodyweight). The Doppler technique, in principle, only indicates systolic pressure; in cats the Doppler technique underestimates true systolic pressure and tends to be more closely related to mean blood pressure.

Central venous pressure

Central venous pressure (CVP) represents the balance between the filling of the central venous reservoir and the pumping ability of the heart. CVP is measured in the vena cava within the thoracic cavity via a long intravenous catheter. The classical approach is to position the catheter, via the jugular vein, in the thoracic portion of the cranial vena cava. Alternatively, the femoral or saphenous approach can be used to position the catheter in the thoracic portion of the caudal vena cava. CVP can be measured using the technique described for invasive arterial blood pressure. The zero reference point is the level of the right atrium. Landmarks are the manubrium (in lateral recumbency) and the scapulohumeral joint (in patients in dorsal recumbency). Instead of electronic transducers, a cheap saline manometer is often used (Figure 7.21).

A change of CVP over a short time period, in the absence of a changed fluid load suggests changes in cardiac function. A low or falling CVP suggests the presence of hypovolaemia. High or rising CVP can be due to fluid overload or to failing heart function. The administration of a fluid bolus, which is followed by a transient rise in CVP, suggests hypovolaemia but adequate cardiac function. Subsequent fluid therapy can be guided by CVP control. CVP can be a valuable aid in differentiating low arterial blood pressure due to hypovolaemia from low arterial blood pressure due to heart failure. The normal range is quite variable (3–8 cmH_2O), so single values have limited meaning. Conversely, repetitive measurements and determination of trends provide valuable information.

CVP measurement is not a routine procedure during anaesthesia. In many cases, CVP measurement may have already begun before anaesthesia. It is of particular use in critical patients who need extensive and prolonged fluid therapy and/or are being treated for haemodynamic instability. During intermittent positive pressure ventilation (IPPV), CVP is influenced by

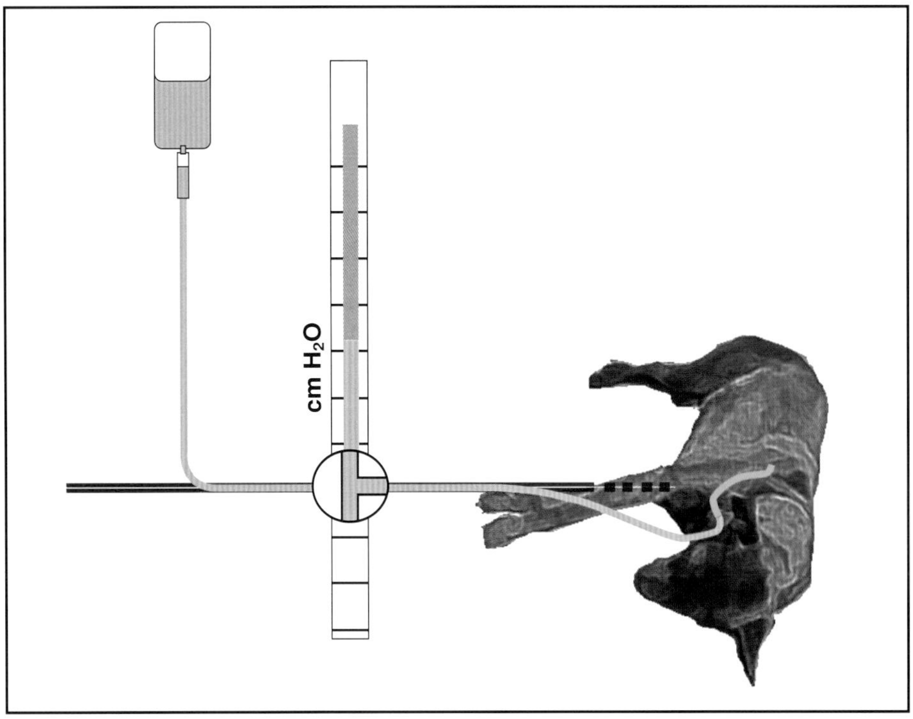

7.21 Set-up for CVP measurement. Note that the zero point on the saline manometer is set at the level of the manubrium in the laterally recumbent patient.

the elevated intrathoracic pressure, especially when positive end-expiratory pressure is used, and CVP measurements have to be corrected accordingly.

Electrocardiography

The electrocardiogram (ECG) was the first monitoring to be made compulsory in human medicine and it may be the most frequently used monitor in veterinary anaesthesia.

In veterinary practice, the three electrode system is almost exclusively used: the electrical activity of the heart is measured between two electrodes, with the third electrode acting as the ground electrode. They are normally located on left and right forelimbs and the left hindlimb. Perfect electrical contact with the skin is essential to obtain reliable and prolonged ECG tracings. This contact can be achieved with adhesive electrode patches, crocodile clips or transcutaneous needles. In general, electrode gel is recommended to improve electrical contact and is preferred to alcohol; the latter tends to evaporate and the associated loss of electrical contact can be the cause of artefacts. Placing adhesive electrode patches on the skin necessitates shaving, but this can be avoided when they are attached to the pads of the paws. Patches can be reused when fixed with self-adhesive bandage.

A normal ECG trace is shown in Figure 7.22. The three-electrode system is effective for arrhythmia analysis, but in human medicine is considered insufficient for detection of myocardial ischaemia (analysis of the ST segment). When the surgical site does not allow normal electrode placement, a base–apex derivation can be used: one electrode is placed dorsal to the base of the heart, another ventrally near the apex and the third peripherally. Transoesophageal ECG, using a special oesophageal probe or stethoscope equipped with ECG electrodes, is also a very convenient method of monitoring cardiac rhythm.

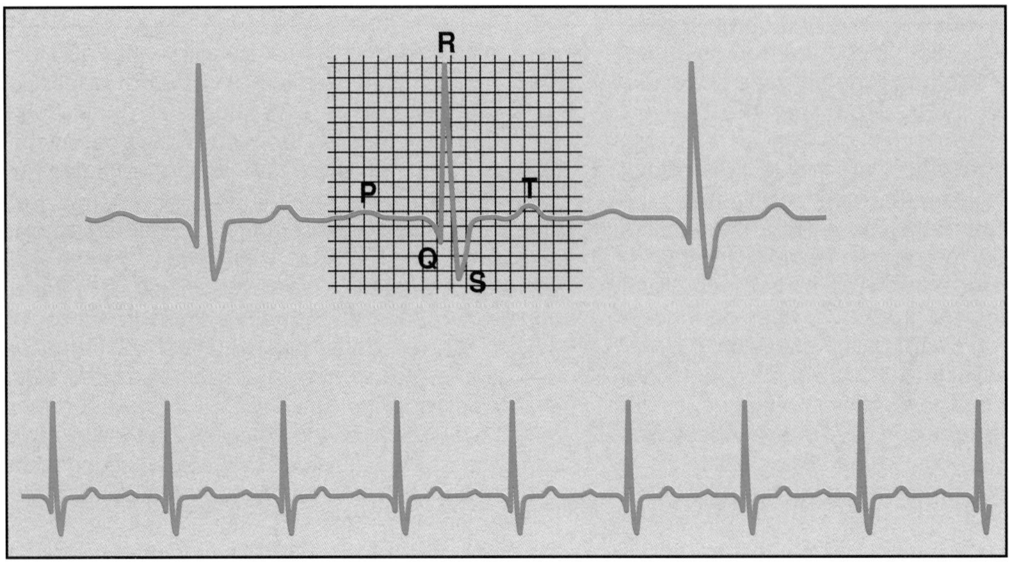

7.22 Normal ECG.

The ECG:

- Provides information limited to electrical activity of the heart. It does not provide any information about pumping function and haemodynamic consequences. An extreme example is electromechanical dissociation, where the ECG remains normal but the heart is not beating
- Allows quick diagnosis of the type of cardiac arrest (asystole, ventricular fibrillation, electromechanical dissociation) and is the only way to detect and analyse any other arrhythmias.

Examples of common ECG abnormalities during anaesthesia are shown in Figure 7.23.

Common causes of artefacts in ECG monitoring are poor electrical contact of the electrodes (insufficient gel, dirty crocodile clips), detachment of electrodes, 50/60 Hz interference, electrical interference from electrosurgical devices and movement of the patient.

Respiratory monitoring

Respiratory rate counters

One type of respiratory rate monitor uses a connector attached to the end of the endotracheal tube. This connector is equipped with a thermistor, which detects the movement of respiratory gases (expired gas is warmer than inspired gas). These monitors can emit an audible tone synchronous with the detection of movement of gas. They can also display the time in seconds since the last breath, or the respiratory frequency. They produce an alarm in case of apnoea ('apnoea detector'). However, the respiratory rate displayed should not be used as a safe indicator of the efficiency of ventilation, because no information is provided about tidal volume. A 'normal' displayed respiratory rate, and even tachypnoea, can be associated with hypoventilation. In addition, if instrument sensitivity is not properly adjusted, it is possible for these monitors to produce artefactual acoustic signals and display erroneous information.

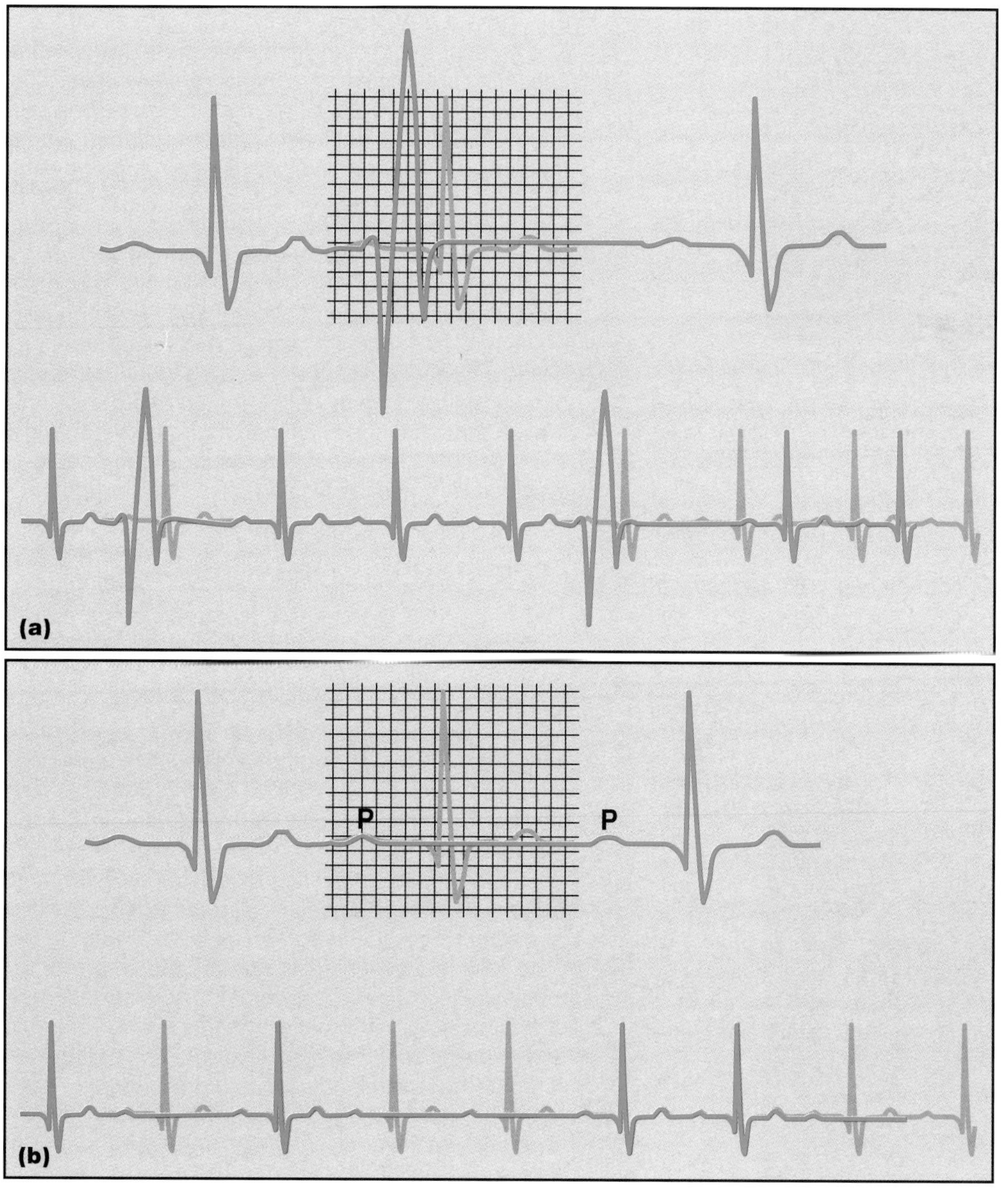

7.23 Abnormal ECGs, with normal ECG trace superimposed in grey. **(a)** Ventricular extrasystole. **(b)** Atrioventricular block, second degree.

Airway pressure gauges

It is highly desirable to have an airway pressure gauge (Figure 7.24) in an anaesthetic breathing system. This is a simple mechanical aneroid (or Bourdon-type) manometer with a scale varying from –10 to +100 cmH_2O. This instrument helps the performance of a pre-anaesthetic quantitative leak test of the anaesthetic machine and breathing system. The monitoring of the typical pressure cycles of IPPV will serve as a guide during manual ventilation and for adjustment of automatic ventilators. The absence of pressure swings indicates major leaks or disconnection of patient and anaesthetic apparatus. Airway pressure monitoring will detect dangerously high airway pressure, e.g. due to maladjustment of ventilator settings or when the exhaust valve remains inadvertently closed during spontaneous ventilation. If the delivered tidal volume is known, the ratio of tidal volume to airway pressure is an indicator of compliance of the respiratory system when IPPV is applied. Moreover, the level of positive end-expiratory pressure can be checked.

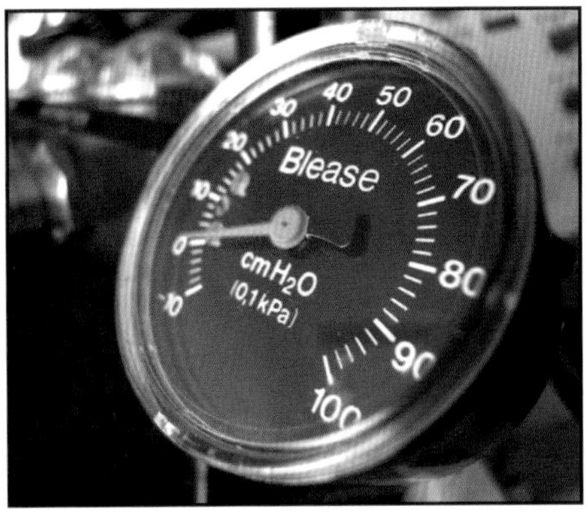

7.24 Airway pressure gauge.

Spirometers

A simple method to evaluate the efficiency of ventilation is the use of a mechanical respirometer (Figure 7.25). This instrument measures the volume of expired gases and is often fixed in the expiratory limb of a breathing system. Alternatively, it can be connected directly to an endotracheal tube or facemask. A respirometer indicates tidal volume and thus the minute volume must be calculated using a stopwatch. Some respirometers have a built-in timer and automatically display the minute volume (minute volume (MV) is the product of respiratory rate (RR) per minute and tidal volume (V_t) of the patient ($MV = V_t \times RR$/minute)).

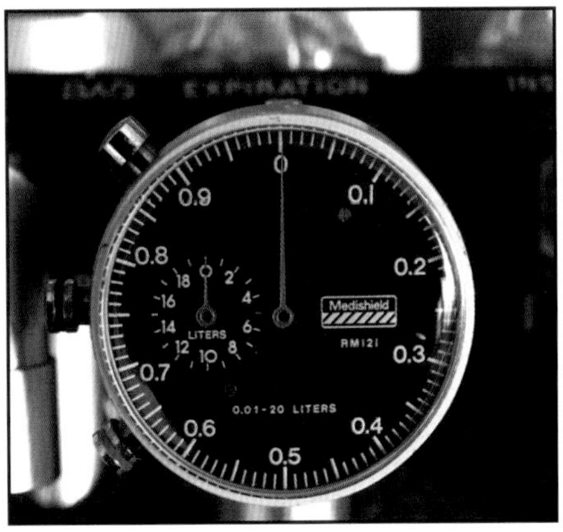

7.25 Spirometer.

Electronic spirometers exist in different forms for both research and clinical purposes and are based on different physical principles. However, they are expensive and rarely found in veterinary practice. Some devices do not provide any more information than the mechanical spirometer.

Spirometry is reliable and shows whether or not ventilation is within acceptable limits (minute volume 100–300 ml/kg/minute, tidal volume 7–15 ml/kg). However, acceptable values for ventilation are not necessarily associated with acceptable gas exchange; because the contribution of deadspace volume (about one third in normal circumstances) remains unknown, the alveolar part of the minute volume (which determines P_aCO_2) remains speculative. In this respect, capnometry and blood gas analysis are most useful.

Some spirometers allow advanced monitoring of ventilation because they use physical principles that permit measurement of respiratory flow and airway pressure, calculate compliance of the respiratory system, and provide graphic presentation of the pressure–flow and pressure–volume relationships in the form of loops.

Oxygen analyser

The measurement of oxygen concentration in inspired gas (F_iO_2) is compulsory in human anaesthesia. When several gases are used (oxygen, nitrous oxide, air), monitoring of the inspired oxygen fraction is a basic method to prevent delivery of a hypoxic gas mixture and hypoxaemia. The measurement of F_iO_2 also allows safe use of low-flow anaesthesia techniques (see Chapter 5). This measurement is often included in respiratory gas analysis performed by multiparameter anaesthetic monitors and different physical principles are used. A popular simple stand-alone device is based on a chemical reaction in a fuel cell. The lifespan of this relatively costly cell is limited and depends on the amount and time of oxygen measurement. A minimum of 30% oxygen in the inspired gas should be provided during anaesthesia of healthy patients.

Temperature monitoring

The continuous measurement of body temperature is performed by a thermistor or a thermocouple mounted on an appropriate probe. The probe can be placed in the oesophagus, nasopharynx or rectum.

Perioperative monitoring of body temperature is important to detect hypothermia, which commonly develops during anaesthesia. Among other reasons, this is due to depression of hypothalamic thermoregulation and heat loss from surgical exposure of body cavities. Hypothermia leads to reduced cellular metabolism, decreased anaesthetic requirements (danger of overdosage), delayed recovery, bradycardia and increased morbidity. It is important to take preventive measures, such as insulation of the surgical table, use of a circulating warm water mattress, warm blankets and heating pads. However, if not well controlled, there is a potential risk of inducing iatrogenic hyperthermia. Hyperthermia is also seen occasionally during low-flow anaesthesia in a warm environment, and during sepsis and malignant hyperthermia.

Inhalational anaesthetic agent monitoring

Monitors that continuously measure the concentration of inhaled anaesthetic agents in the breathing system are available. In many of these devices, infrared analysis is used, and is often combined with the measurement of oxygen and carbon dioxide.

Measurement allows control of the dosage of volatile agent administered to the patient and correlation of this with its clinical effects. The principle is that alveolar (end-tidal) concentration of an agent reflects its arterial and cerebral concentration; this value can be compared with the documented minimum alveolar concentration (MAC) value of the agent (see Chapter 14). However, a very large number of factors influence MAC value (e.g. individual variation, sedative and analgesic drugs) and measured values are indicative of the dosage of the agent but not of the depth of anaesthesia. Clinical examination remains the key factor in the assessment of anaesthetic depth.

If properly calibrated, these monitors can be used to check the accuracy of the output of vaporizers. In this case, it is imperative that sampling be done at the outlet of the vaporizer and not in the breathing system.

Monitoring depth of anaesthesia

In clinical veterinary anaesthesia, the most accurate method to assess the depth of anaesthesia is based on collection and interpretation of relevant clinical parameters (see Figure 7.3). The use of neuromuscular-blocking agents as part of a balanced anaesthesia protocol eliminates many of these important clinical parameters (see Chapter 15). In human medicine, this has occasionally led to difficulties in estimation of anaesthetic depth, resulting in awareness during anaesthesia, or undesired recall afterwards. For this reason, there is an increased use in human clinical practice of electronic devices to evaluate depth of anaesthesia. These devices are based on computerized analysis of the electroencephalogram (EEG) (bispectral analysis) or EEG reaction to auditory stimulation (middle latency auditory evoked potentials). In veterinary anaesthesia, this kind of monitoring is reserved for research purposes.

Monitoring of the neuromuscular junction

For information on monitoring of the neuromuscular junction, see Chapter 15.

Additional monitoring

When a urinary catheter is in place, the urine output can easily be measured by collecting the urine in a bag (normal 1–2 ml/kg/h). A normal urine output reflects correct cardiovascular status and normal renal perfusion. Renal perfusion can be reduced due to cardiovascular failure, hypovolaemia and shock (see Chapter 23). Urine output is part of the fluid balance evaluation comparing fluid input during anaesthesia (intravenous infusions) and fluid losses (blood, urine, transudates).

In some circumstances, the perioperative monitoring of blood glucose concentration (e.g. anaesthesia of diabetic patients and those with insulinoma) or electrolytes, haematocrit and total protein (unstable critical patients with emergency surgery) may be necessary.

Guidelines for monitoring strategy in veterinary anaesthesia

When organizing and purchasing anaesthetic monitoring equipment, there are several factors to bear in mind:

- Staff numbers and qualifications
- Costs *versus* benefits
- Case load and nature of those cases
- The anaesthetic techniques used
- The need to monitor several cases simultaneously
- The need for post-anaesthetic monitoring.

The choice of which monitoring equipment to buy depends on:

- The organization of the practice: if nobody is available to monitor anaesthesia, more equipment will be necessary to alert the surgeon, but this method has clear limits. It is far preferable to have a trained person to monitor anaesthesia, rather than rely exclusively on the use of electronic monitors. It cannot be overemphasized that the purchase and use of monitors is of no use if:
  - Clinical monitoring is not mastered
  - Artefactual information cannot be identified
  - The physiological meaning of the information provided is not understood and the right corrective steps cannot consequently be undertaken. Adequate training of staff is therefore of utmost importance, and the practice must be organized in a way that allows someone with adequate training to assess anaesthetized patients on a regular basis
- The budget: cost of the equipment is a limiting factor. Also, to invest in expensive monitoring equipment which is not properly understood (and whose information cannot be correctly interpreted) will be of no use in either improving quality of anaesthetic management or reducing the incidence of anaesthetic mishaps
- Patient condition (ASA status): patients with increased anaesthetic risk will require more complete monitoring of their vital functions so that rapid detection of abnormalities is possible and correct assessment and therapeutic decisions can be made quickly

- The chosen anaesthetic technique:
  - Capnography in non-intubated patients is difficult, whereas pulse oximetry can be used
  - High doses of alpha-2 agonists in intubated patients may increase the likelihood of unreliable pulse oximeter function, but capnography will still be reliable
  - When nitrous oxide is used, or when using low-flow techniques, there is a potential risk of administration of a hypoxic gas mixture. In this case, the use of an oxygen analyser in the breathing system and/or a pulse oximeter is recommended (S_pO_2)
- The case load and the types of surgery or diagnostic examinations: it is not obligatory to use all available monitoring equipment for very short and simple procedures on healthy patients. A pulse oximeter in non-intubated patients or a capnograph in intubated patients can suffice. Generally, the greater the disturbance in homeostasis that is anticipated, the greater the number of physiological functions that must be monitored. Invasive surgery (e.g. thoracotomy), or surgery associated with specific pathophysiology or problems (e.g. bleeding) will need appropriate monitoring.

For practices performing invasive procedures or dealing with emergency cases and postoperative care, capnography, pulse oximetry, ECG, non-invasive blood pressure measurement (with the option of invasive blood pressure measurement) and temperature monitoring are highly desirable. Nevertheless, regular clinical assessment of depth of anaesthesia remains necessary because no technical device can replace this evaluation (Figure 7.26).

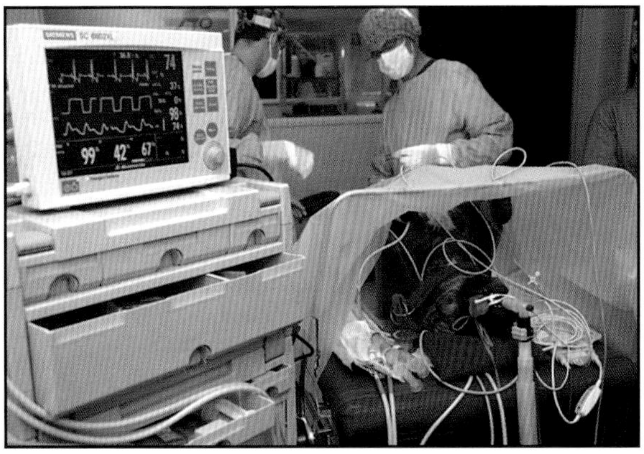

7.26 Multiparametric monitor and anaesthesia 'screen'.

The use of normal anaesthetic and monitoring equipment inside a magnetic resonance unit is not possible. The magnetic field attracts all ferrous metal and electronic functions are disturbed. Special monitoring equipment that can remain inside the room is available, but is very expensive. For respiratory gas analysis, including capnography, a simple alternative solution is to sample via a very long line while the monitor is stationed outside the room. For ECG and pulse oximetry, special sensors are necessary.

Conclusion

It is clear that monitoring equipment can never replace a suitably qualified person: it has not been proven that monitoring equipment necessarily decreases anaesthetic risk. As complexity increases, the chances for errors to occur due to artefacts and misinterpretations increase accordingly. The preparation and set-up of monitoring equipment can be time-consuming and the devices are usually expensive; such considerations could lead one to question the true benefits.

One important aspect is that the whole concept of monitoring provides continuous information about the patient, and thus becomes a kind of teacher supporting the person in charge of anaesthesia. This teacher demonstrates the physiological consequences of administered drugs and dosages, and of the complex interactions between anaesthesia, disease and surgical manipulation. In this way one can become a better veterinary surgeon, with more insight into what one is actually 'doing' to the patient.

In conclusion, 'when applied appropriately, operated properly, and interpreted correctly, however, monitors afford the patient the best possible outcome' (Lawrence, 2005).

References and further reading

Arbous MD, Grobbee DE, van Kleef JW *et al.* (2001) Mortality associated with anaesthesia: a qualitative analysis to identify risk factors. *Anaesthesia* **56**, 1141–1153

Bhavani-Shankar K http://www.capnography.com (a useful, free, website with animated capnographs)

Brodbelt D, Brearley J, Young L, Wood J and Pfeiffer D (2005) Anaesthetic-related mortality risks in small animals in the UK. *AVA Spring Meeting, Rimini, Italy 20–23 April 2005*

Lawrence JP (2005) Advances and new insights in monitoring. *Thoracic Surgery Clinics* **15**, 55–77

Tinker JH, Dull DL, Caplan RA, Ward RJ and Cheney FW (1989) Role of monitoring devices in prevention of anesthetic mishaps: a closed claims analysis. *Anesthesiology* **71**, 541–546

8

The physiology and pathophysiology of pain

Jill Price and Andrea Nolan

Introduction

Mankind has struggled to understand the nature of pain since ancient times. The conscious experience of pain defies precise anatomical, physiological and pharmacological definition; unlike any other sensory experience, pain is a subjective emotion which can be experienced even in the absence of obvious external noxious stimulation, and which can be enhanced or abolished by a wide range of behavioural experiences, including fear, memory and emotional stress. Adaptive 'physiological' pain announces the presence of a potentially harmful stimulus and thus has an essential protective function: lack of nociceptive pain sensation in humans with congenital insensitivity to pain reduces life expectancy. In contrast, maladaptive pain represents malfunction of neurological transmission and serves no physiological purpose, leading to chronic syndromes in which pain itself becomes the primary disease.

While elusive and ill defined, pain nonetheless has substance and specific characteristics. The official definition of the International Association for the Study of Pain (IASP) is *'an unpleasant sensory and emotional experience, associated with actual or potential tissue damage, or described in terms of such damage'*. Recognizing that animals (similar to nonverbal humans) are unable to verbally communicate and describe their pain experience, a widely used, more specific definition of animal pain is *'an aversive sensory and emotional experience representing awareness by the animal of damage or threat to the integrity of its tissues...producing a change in physiology and behaviour directed to reduce or avoid the damage, reduce the likelihood of recurrence and promote recovery'* (Molony and Kent, 1997).

There is no simple definition of chronic pain, but it is generally described in human medicine as pain which persists beyond the normal time of healing, or as persistent pain caused by conditions where healing has not occurred or which remit and then recur. More recently chronic pain in dogs has been described as 'pain lasting longer than one month, associated with a wide range of often subtle behavioural disturbance' (Wiseman-Orr *et al.*, 2004).

Conscious perception of pain represents the final product of a complex neurological information-processing system, resulting from the interplay of facilitatory and inhibitory pathways that communicate via an orchestra of interacting neurotransmitter systems.

Although we tend to think of pain as a single sensory entity, several distinct types exist, classified as *nociceptive, inflammatory, neuropathic* and *functional* (Woolf, 2004a). Cancer pain often displays characteristics of both inflammatory (tissue damage) and neuropathic (nerve damage) pain. As the neurobiological mechanisms responsible for these different types of pain become more clearly defined, we can better understand their distinct aetiologies, identify individuals at risk and develop analgesic strategies that target and prevent specific pain mechanisms, rather than purely treating symptoms.

Types of pain

Nociceptive pain

The conscious experience of acute pain resulting from a noxious stimulus is mediated by a high-threshold nociceptive sensory system. The basic neuroanatomy of this system is summarized in Figure 8.1 and has been recently reviewed (Usunoff *et al.*, 2006). Nociceptors are the least differentiated of the several types of sensory receptors found in body tissues. They represent the free endings of primary sensory neurons, with their cell bodies located in the dorsal root and trigeminal ganglia. The primary afferent nerve fibres, which carry information from these free nerve endings to their central location, consist of two main types: unmyelinated C fibres and myelinated Aδ fibres. Following tissue trauma, changes in the properties of nociceptors occur such that large-diameter Aβ fibres may also transmit 'pain information'.

Unmyelinated C fibres are activated by intense mechanical, chemical and thermal stimuli and conduct impulses relatively slowly at 0.5 m/s, contributing to the familiar 'slow burn' sensation of pain. Aδ fibres conduct impulses at 5–30 m/s, contributing to the rapid 'stab' of the acute pain response. There is also a population of so-called 'silent' nociceptors, which may become active during inflammation or tissue damage.

The stimulation thresholds of C fibres are substantially higher than those of other types of afferent sensory fibre, and physiologically demonstrate a direct relationship between stimulus intensity and receptor response. Under normal conditions, the greater the stimulus intensity, the more vigorous is the C fibre response. In contrast to other sensory afferent fibres, C nociceptors have no physiological background

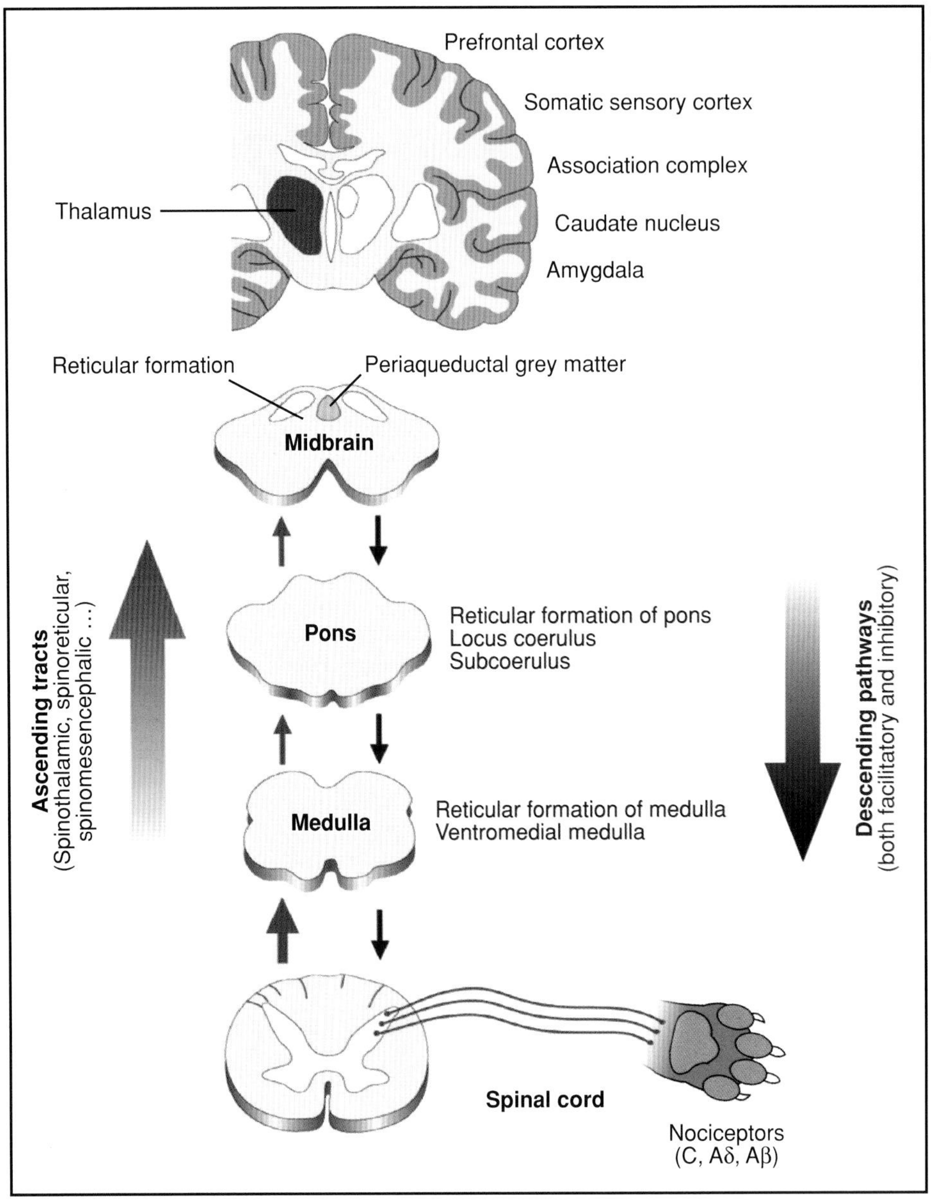

8.1 Neuroanatomical pathways involved in nociception.

pattern of discharge. Intense or repeated noxious stimulation can induce *peripheral sensitization*, in which the direct relationship between stimulus and response in peripheral nociceptors is uncoupled and tonic background activity can develop, which persists in the absence of ongoing noxious stimulation.

Primary afferent fibres carrying sensory information from nociceptors synapse in the dorsal horn of the spinal cord: Aδ fibres predominantly in laminae I and V and C fibres in superficial laminae I and II, the so-called *substantia gelatinosa*. The fibres of 'nociceptive' responsive cells of the spinal cord project to various higher centres involved in pain transmission, both ipsilaterally and contralaterally to their site of origin. Several spinal–brainstem–spinal pathways are activated simultaneously when a noxious stimulus occurs, providing widespread positive and negative feedback loops by which information relating to noxious stimulation can be amplified or diminished. Spinal tracts involved in pain transmission differ between animal species, but common pathways include the *spinomesencephalic tract* (which projects to the periaqueductal grey matter and superior colliculus), the *spinothalamic tract* (which projects to the medial and ventrobasal thalamus) and *spinoreticular fibres* (which project to the reticular formation of the midbrain). Sensory input from nociceptors located in the head travels via neuronal cell bodies located in the trigeminal ganglion and, thereafter, noxious information is conveyed to the nucleus caudalis (part of the trigeminal sensory complex). Recently, it has been recognized that there are descending spinal pathways which are facilitatory, in addition to descending inhibitory pathways.

The cerebral cortex is the seat of conscious experience of pain. A noxious stimulus activates not only several cortical areas, but also, as the intensity of the stimulus increases, an increasing number of subcortical and cortical regions. The cerebral cortex exerts powerful 'top-down' control on almost all nociceptive relays within the central nervous system (CNS), such that supraspinal cortical and subcortical mechanisms can modulate (enhancing *or* inhibiting) the sensation of pain. This 'corticofugal modulation' underlies the magnifying effects of factors, such as attention, anticipation, mood, anxiety, placebo administration and hypnosis, on pain perception. Central pain associated with a cortical or subcortical lesion can result in severe pain, which is not associated with any detectable pathology in the body.

Recognizing this complexity, the 'pain experience' is now considered to consist of three key components: a *sensory–discriminatory* component (temporal, spatial, thermal/mechanical), an *affective* component (subjective and emotional, describing associated fear, tension and autonomic responses) and an *evaluative* component, describing the magnitude of the quality (e.g. stabbing/pounding; mild/severe). Undoubtedly, an animal's pain experience is similarly composed despite the tendency to focus on pain intensity alone.

Inflammatory pain

When tissue damage occurs despite the nociceptive defence system (through trauma, surgery or inflammatory disease), the body's imperative shifts from *preventing* tissue injury to *protecting* the injured region so that it can heal. When tissue injury occurs, there is a change in the way in which the peripheral and central nervous systems process subsequent noxious (and non-noxious) stimuli.

The nociceptive sensory system is not 'hardwired', but rather is an inherently plastic system, able to change its sensitivity following intense or repeated stimulation. Following tissue damage or inflammation, the sensitivity of an injured region is enhanced so that normally innocuous stimuli are perceived as painful, thus preventing use of (or contact with) the injured tissue and promoting healing. This is inflammatory pain.

Inflammatory pain is the pain that, under normal circumstances, drives acute postoperative pain until the wound has healed and thus represents a potentially beneficial adaptive response to injury. It is evoked within minutes of tissue trauma and, in general, its extent, intensity and duration are directly related to the extent and severity of tissue damage during surgery. The changes in the nociceptive system are generally reversible and normal sensitivity of the system should be restored as tissue heals. However, if the noxious insult was severe or if a focus of ongoing inflammation persists, then the pain will persist. This is the pain experience of animals with chronic inflammatory diseases such as arthritis, otitis, gingivitis, dermatitis and back pain.

Neuropathic and functional pain

Neuropathic pain is the pain that develops following injury to peripheral or central nerves. A whole spectrum of mechanisms contribute to the neuropathic pain syndrome (Woolf, 2004b), including changes in the peripheral nervous system, spinal cord, brainstem and brain. Nerve injury can disrupt the electrical properties, neurochemistry and central conductivity of neurons so that the damaged nerves begin to generate spontaneous volleys of ectopic discharges, initiate abnormal 'crosstalk' with adjacent fibres and develop hyperresponsiveness to inflammatory and other normally innocuous stimuli.

In humans, neuropathic pain underlies post-amputation phantom limb pain, sciatica, distal limb pain associated with diabetic neuropathy and post-herpetic neuropathy, all conditions that are difficult to control using standard analgesic strategies such as non-steroidal anti-inflammatory drugs (NSAIDs) and opioids. Iatrogenic neuropathic pain is postulated to be the major cause of long-term postsurgical pain in humans (Kehlet *et al.*, 2006). It is surprising, therefore, that neuropathic pain is rarely recognized or diagnosed in animals. Many of the drugs which demonstrate efficacy against neuropathic pain act essentially as 'membrane stabilizers' able to attenuate ectopic neuronal hyperexcitability; these include anticonvulsants such as gabapentin, local anaesthetics, tricyclic antidepressants and anti-arrhythmics.

'*Functional*' or central pain is a specific type of neuropathic pain in which no peripheral injury or neurological lesion can be identified, but pain sensitivity is nonetheless amplified. Several common human conditions are believed to have a functional component, including fibromyalgia and irritable bowel syndrome, but it is rarely diagnosed in animals.

Cancer pain

Although cancer is common in domestic animals and represents a significant proportion of the veterinary surgeon's caseload, recognition of the adverse effects of neoplastic disease on pain processing and thus the key role of pain management in veterinary cancer treatment remains a neglected field. This is of real concern, since it is known that human cancer patients with unresolved or chronic pain are significantly more emotionally disturbed than those without pain, respond less well to therapy and die sooner than patients with no pain (Woodforde and Fielding, 1975; Ahles *et al.*, 1983). In human cancer patients in developed countries, several national studies have demonstrated that only slightly greater than 50% pain control is achieved; the proportion of animal cancer patients receiving adequate pain relief is unlikely to be higher. The affective component of the pain experience is often highly developed in cancer patients, and non-pharmacological strategies, such as transcutaneous nerve stimulation (TENS) and acupuncture, are often required in combination with more complicated pharmacological approaches to achieve adequate relief of cancer pain.

Postsurgical pain

In humans, despite 'routine' administration of analgesia, persistent postsurgical pain represents a major, largely unrecognized problem. Major and routine surgical procedures are often followed by significant pain, impaired organ function and prolonged hospitalization (Kehlet and Holte, 2001). Acute postoperative pain is followed by persistent pain in 10–50% of humans following common operations, with 2–10% of these patients experiencing severe chronic pain (Kehlet *et al.*, 2006). Chronic postsurgical pain in humans is believed to be primarily neuropathic in nature, associated with surgical injury to peripheral nerves, or less commonly as a result of ongoing inflammation (Kehlet *et al.*, 2006).

Although less well researched, it is likely that the risk of persistent postsurgical pain in animals undergoing surgery is similar to that reported in humans. Persistent pain and hypersensitivity cause substantial distress in human patients, and can have serious adverse effects on psychological, social and functional status and quality of life. Studies in dogs with persistent pain due to chronic inflammation have indicated that quality of life, measured by identifying patterns of altered behaviour, is adversely affected (Wiseman *et al.*, 2001; Wiseman-Orr *et al.*, 2004).

Hyperalgesia and allodynia

The clinical hallmarks of sensitization of the nociceptive system are hyperalgesia and allodynia. Hyperalgesia is an exaggerated and prolonged response to a noxious stimulus while allodynia is a pain response to a low-intensity, normally innocuous stimulus, such as light touch to the skin or gentle pressure (Figure 8.2). Hyperalgesia can develop in undamaged skin in neuropathic pain conditions, and can be a consequence of somatic referral from visceral pain and injury or pathology of internal organs (such as the heart and oesophagus) (Verne *et al.*, 2004; Chahal and Rao, 2005).

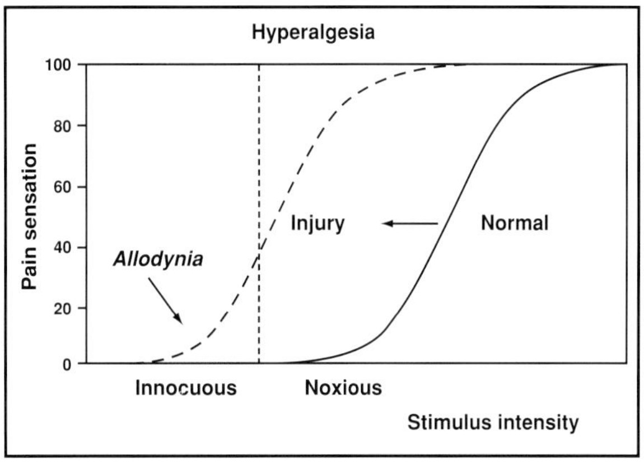

8.2 Changes in pain sensitivity associated with tissue injury.

Neuronal plasticity and pain

There is no direct relationship associated with the duration or intensity of peripheral injury that transforms acute transient pain into chronic maladaptive pain. Nociceptive plasticity is driven by two interdependent mechanisms: peripheral and central sensitization. This plasticity can be reversible, associated with changes in the 'software' of the system (e.g. neurotransmitter concentrations, receptor sensitivity), as predominates in inflammatory pain; or it can be long-lasting, associated with changes in the 'hardware' of the nociceptive system, namely the phenotype of the nociceptive cells and their expression of neurotransmitters, receptors and other proteins involved in pain processing (Woolf and Salter, 2000; Ji *et al.*, 2003; Woolf, 2004b).

Peripheral sensitization

Peripheral sensitization is the result of changes in the chemical milieu bathing nociceptor terminals as a result of tissue injury or inflammation. A barrage of chemical mediators is released by damaged cells, including hydrogen and potassium ions, histamine, purines including adenosine and adenosine triphosphate (ATP), neuropeptides including substance P and neurokinin A, bradykinin, serotonin, arachidonic acid metabolites, cytokines and growth factors (Figure 8.3). Some of these agents (such as adenosine) directly activate the nociceptor, while others (such as prostaglandins) sensitize the nerve terminal so that its response to subsequent stimuli is amplified.

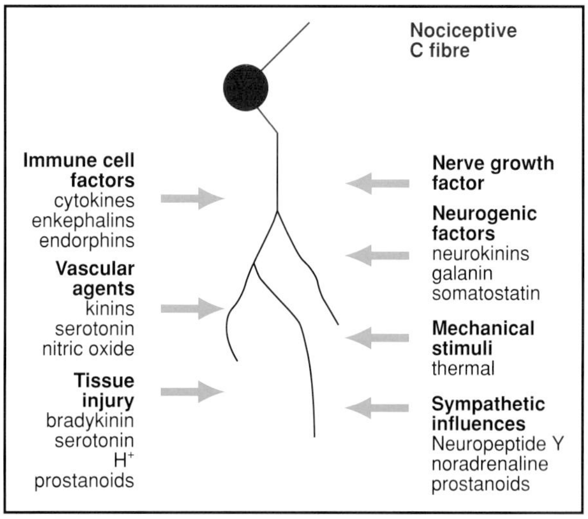

8.3 Chemical and other mediators involved in peripheral sensitization.

Inflammatory injury can also induce changes, mediated by growth factors, in intracellular signalling pathways, leading to upregulation of protein expression for synthesis of receptors, ion channels and neurotransmitters. This results in long-lasting changes in the functional properties, intrinsic excitability and analgesic sensitivity of peripheral nociceptors.

Central sensitization

Trauma and inflammation can also sensitize nociceptor transmission in the spinal cord to produce *central sensitization*. Central sensitization is a more precise description of the electrophysiological phenomenon of 'wind-up' described in the spinal cord by Mendell and Wall (1965), the first recognition of the inherent plasticity of central pain processing.

Induction of central sensitization requires a brief but intense period of nociceptor stimulation, e.g. a surgical incision, intense input from sensitized peripheral nociceptors following tissue trauma, or input from damaged sensory neurons following nerve injury. As a result of this input, the response threshold of the central neuron falls, its response to subsequent stimulation is amplified and its receptive field enlarges to recruit additional previously 'sleeping' afferent fibres into nociceptive transmission.

Key neurotransmitter pathways and neurological changes involved in central sensitization are summarized in Figure 8.4. Amino acids, nitric oxide and

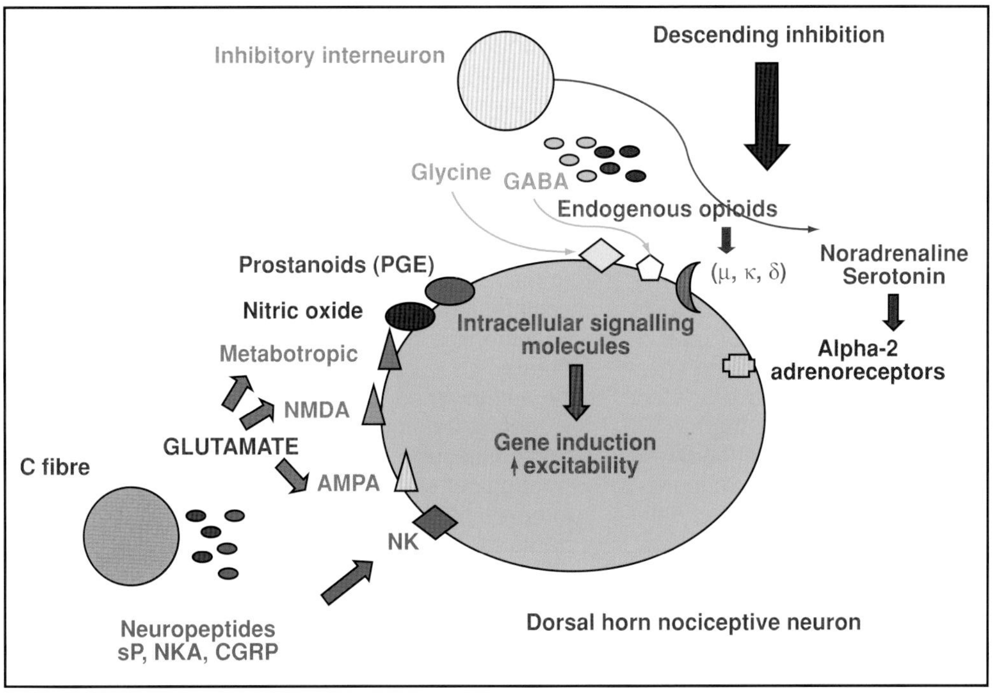

8.4

Neurotransmitters involved in modulation of central nociceptive transmission and central sensitization. AMPA = α-3-hydroxy-5-methyl-4-isoxazole propionic acid; CGRP = Calcitonin gene-related peptide; GABA = Gamma-aminobutyric acid; NK = Neurokinin; NKA = Neurokinin A; NMDA = *N*-methyl-D-aspartate; sP = Substance P.

neuropeptides, including substance P, neurokinin A and brain-derived neurotrophic factor (BDNF), released from peripheral nociceptors in the dorsal root ganglion contribute to the sensitization. Glutamate, the key excitatory neurotransmitter in the CNS, plays a key role through several receptor systems. Physiological 'nociceptive' pain is primarily mediated through glutamate acting at its AMPA (α-3-hydroxy-5-methyl-4-isoxazole propionic acid) receptor on dorsal horn neurons, instantaneously alerting the brain to noxious insult. If injury persists or if the afferent barrage is intense, then metabotropic and NMDA (*N*-methyl-D-aspartate) glutamate receptors are also activated and profoundly amplify the excitability of the central nociceptive neuron. As with peripheral sensitization, intense stimulation can alter gene expression within the neuron and thus induce the long-lasting phenotypic changes in neuronal behaviour that underlie persistent central sensitization. Some of the changes in gene expression are restricted to the region of the spinal cord that receives inputs from the injured tissue; other genes are activated more widely throughout the CNS, including those for endogenous opioids and their receptors, and cyclo-oxygenase-2 (COX-2) and its prostanoid receptors. COX-2 expression is initiated in many regions of the CNS within a few hours of a localized peripheral tissue injury, contributing to the generalized aches often associated with inflammatory disease (Samad *et al.*, 2001).

Several types of analgesic drug are able to inhibit the development of central sensitization, including NMDA receptor antagonists and nitric oxide synthase inhibitors. Central sensitization is better prevented by inhibitory or analgesic agents when they are administered before, rather than after, the initiating afferent barrage. This is the rationale used to justify pre-emptive analgesia, although the efficacy of pre-emptive analgesia has been difficult to prove in the clinical setting.

Prostanoids, cyclo-oxygenase enzyme inhibition and nociception

Prostaglandins are classic inflammatory mediators synthesized from arachidonic acid via COX enzymes. There are four subtypes of prostaglandin receptors (EP_1–EP_4) and there is evidence that all four receptors contribute to nociceptive processing, with prostaglandin E_2 (PGE_2) considered the principal sensitizing prostanoid. The principal anti-nociceptive action of NSAIDs was originally attributed to COX inhibition at the site of inflammation: prostaglandins certainly play a key role in peripheral sensitization, acting as 'sensitizing agents' that enhance the nociceptive properties of other inflammatory mediators, including bradykinin and histamine. However, prostaglandins also play a key role in central sensitization, and it has recently been proposed that prostaglandins generate hyperalgesia principally through their central, rather than their peripheral, effects (Turnbach *et al.*, 2002).

COX exists as two isoenzymes, COX-1 and COX-2. Recently, a splice variant of COX-1 (conveniently named COX-3) has also been characterized in canine and human neuronal and cerebrocortical tissues. COX-1, being found in most cells, is classically termed the constitutive 'housekeeping enzyme' responsible for production of basal physiological prostaglandins involved in gastrointestinal mucosal protection, preservation of normal renal haemodynamics and normal platelet function. The gene for COX-2 is principally a 'primary response' gene with many regulatory sites, which are induced in response to inflammatory injury. However, low levels of COX-2 are also tonically, constitutively expressed in the CNS, reproductive tissue and kidneys. COX-2 in the spinal cord plays a key role in the generation of PGE_2 levels during peripheral inflammation and is mainly responsible for central sensitization associated with inflammatory pain. However, recent findings have shown that COX-1 also plays an important role in spinal nociceptive processing and sensitization after surgery (Zhu *et al.*, 2003), suggesting that COX-1 inhibition may also be important for treatment of postoperative inflammatory and neuropathic pain.

Central inhibitory systems

Within the CNS, several endogenous receptor systems are activated by noxious stimulation or by drug administration to produce analgesia. Opioids have been used as analgesic agents for over 5000 years. Three key opioid receptor types have been characterized: delta (OR1), kappa (OR3) and mu (OR2), with a fourth opioid-like receptor, the orphan (ORL1) receptor, recently characterized. Most clinically effective opioid drugs act principally on the mu receptor (see Chapter 9). Butorphanol is primarily a kappa receptor agonist and a mu receptor antagonist. Endogenous opioid agonists, the enkephalins, act primarily on the mu and delta receptors to inhibit excitatory nociceptive transmission, while dynorphins exert complex actions on pain sensation. Opioid receptors are densely located in the dorsal horn of the spinal cord, the brainstem and midbrain. They can also be found in the forebrain and in peripheral sites, such as the synovial membrane and in the skin. In the spinal cord, opioids act both presynaptically, to inhibit excitatory neurotransmitter release from nociceptive sensory neurons, and postsynaptically, to inhibit activity of dorsal horn neurons.

Another pharmacological system that plays an important role in endogenous analgesia is the alpha-2 adrenoreceptor system. Within the CNS, alpha-2 adrenoreceptors are densely located in the dorsal horn of the spinal cord and found both pre- and post-synaptically on nociceptive (and non-nociceptive) neurons which release noradrenaline. Alpha-2 adrenoreceptors are also densely localized in the locus coeruleus of the brainstem and are also found in the periaqueductal grey matter; both are important regions involved in modulation of nociceptive neurotransmission.

Within the spinal cord, inhibition of ascending pain transmission is mediated by inhibitory neurons that act principally through releasing the neurotransmitters glycine and gamma-aminobutyric acid (GABA). In higher centres (cortex, midbrain and brainstem), monoamine systems (noradrenaline acting through alpha-2 receptors and serotonin acting through 5-hydroxytryptamine (5-HT) receptors) interact with excitatory neurotransmitters, such as glutamate, and inhibitory transmitters, such as GABA, some synergistically and some antagonistically, to produce 'top-down' modulation of pain. These pathways link pain sensation to emotional responses such as fear and anger, and also link pain to depression. Other neurotransmitter systems contributing to descending inhibition of pain transmission include adenosine (acting through the A_1 receptor) and cannabinoids.

Pain assessment

Pain assessment is the keystone of effective pain management, but the ability to measure pain in a reliable, communicable, accurate and valid fashion remains one of the most difficult challenges facing veterinary surgeons. Failure to assess animal pain competently is currently considered one of the biggest deficiencies in our understanding of animal pain.

Analysis of veterinary attitudes and working practices relating to the management of pain in dogs and cats has shown that recognition and management of pain in companion animals is suboptimal and that recognition that animals do feel pain often fails to translate into positive actions taken by veterinary surgeons to resolve that pain (Capner *et al.*, 1999). Even in articulate humans who are able to self-report, pain assessment is complicated by the multidimensional nature of the pain experience. Evaluation of pain in an animal under veterinary care is at best a 'value judgement' dominated by personal bias, perception and philosophy, where we define and evaluate pain through our subjective interpretation of those behaviours we personally consider to represent pain. In order to evaluate pain competently, we must be familiar with the full range of 'normal' behaviours displayed by the individual animal, and then be able to identify and discriminate changes from 'normal' that are attributable to pain. At present, positive response to appropriate analgesic therapy is probably the best marker for effective diagnosis of pain.

Chronic pain is even harder to define and evaluate than acute pain. Behavioural changes associated with chronic pain often develop gradually and are extremely subtle, so that they can only be detected by someone very familiar with the animal (usually the owner). It is generally recognized that chronic pain impairs 'quality of life', which in humans is represented through eight key indicators: sleep disturbance, irritability, appetite disturbance, psychomotor retardation, social withdrawal, lowered pain tolerance, constipation and abnormal illness behaviour (Sternbach, 1981; Wiseman-Orr *et al.*, 2004). Similar changes are often described by owners of dogs with chronically painful conditions such as osteoarthritis.

Assessment of acute pain

The key points in assessment of pain in companion animals are shown in Figure 8.5. Behavioural expression of pain is highly species-specific and is further influenced by age, breed, individual temperament and the presence or absence of additional stressors, such as anxiety or fear. Debilitating disease can dramatically reduce the range of behavioural indicators of pain that an animal is capable of showing. Prey animals, such as small rodents and rabbits, dramatically change their behaviour in the presence of a perceived predator, which may be another animal *or* the individual grading their pain. Many analgesic drugs, including opioids and alpha-2 agonists, have sedative properties, which make it even more difficult to distinguish sedation from adequate or inadequate analgesia.

Appreciation of the many subtle behavioural indicators of pain in any species requires familiarity with the species, breed and particular stimulus. When assessing pain in any animal, key behavioural categories which should be assessed include posture, mobility, activity, response to touch, attention to the painful area and vocalization (Holton *et al.*, 2001).

- Assume that humans and animals are closely similar in terms of pain perception and anticipation, and manage pain accordingly
- At present, response to appropriate analgesia remains the best marker for accurate diagnosis of pain
- Remember that breed, age, illness, temperament and drug administration influence behavioural responses to pain
- Since the pain experience can alter rapidly, pain assessment must be performed frequently
- Pain assessors should have experience in pain assessment and be familiar with the patient
- Compare an animal's behaviour before and after the onset of pain where this is possible (i.e. pre- and postoperatively), so that improvement or deterioration can be evaluated realistically
- Assess response to interaction with a handler in addition to simple observation in the cage
- Assess response to gentle palpation or manipulation of the affected area
- Look for subtle indicators of pain, particularly in sick patients. Remember that invasive procedures, trauma and medical illnesses cause pain, and may leave animals unable to demonstrate explicit pain behaviour. Certain animals may respond to pain through withdrawal
- Develop clinic protocols for assessment of acute and chronic pain. An ideal scoring system should be relatively easy to use by all staff, with clearly defined assessment criteria, and validated in a clinical setting
- Reassess. Re-evaluate analgesic efficacy. Re-administer analgesia appropriately as assessment requires

8.5 Key points in assessment of pain in companion animals.

Roughan and Flecknell (2001) identified some 150 specific pain-associated behavioural changes in rats associated with laparotomy.

Figure 8.6 indicates some key behaviours associated with pain in dogs and cats. While cats and dogs share many similar behavioural indicators of acute pain, cats have their own spectrum of behaviours, many responding to pain through withdrawal (Taylor and Robertson, 2004; Robertson, 2005).

Dog
Hyperalgesia or allodynia Postures: hunching, 'praying', not resting in a normal position Locomotion: stiff, no weightbearing on affected limb Vocalization: barking, growling, whining Facial expressions: ear position, eye position Attention to (or guarding of) the affected area Aggression Inappetance Weak tail wag
Cat
As for dog, with additionally: Vocalization: hissing Facial expressions: furrowed brow, ears pinned back Depression, no self-grooming Hunched immobile stance Hyperventilation Ears pulled back Sitting in back of cage or hiding under blanket Pupillary dilation Restlessness Tachypnoea or panting

8.6 Behavioural indicators of pain in companion animals. These may also indicate stress, disease or anxiety.

Physiological variables provide useful supplementary information when assessing pain but it is important to remember that they are influenced by a host of factors other than pain, including concurrent disease, drug therapy and other stressors, and thus are not consistent or reliable indicators of pain when used in isolation (Holton *et al.*, 1998). Physiological signs associated with *either* pain, anxiety or ill-health include changes in heart rate, respiratory rate, blood pressure (usually hypertension), increased body temperature and changes in serum concentrations of cortisol, adrenaline, noradrenaline and acute phase proteins.

Pain scoring systems

Until recently, the most commonly used pain scoring systems used in animals were analogous to the subjective unidimensional scoring systems used to score pain in human infants and non-verbal humans. The scales most commonly used in pain scoring are the visual analogue scale (VAS), numerical rating scale (NRS) and simple descriptive scale (SDS). All of these simple scoring systems have fundamental limitations, which are summarized in Figure 8.7.

Pain scale	Limitations
Visual analogue scale (VAS)	Significant inter-observer variability Sensitivity depends on observer training and experience Expresses summation of observer's interpretation of many different behaviours
Numerical rating scale (NRS)	Significant inter-observer variability Differences in pain severity between categories are undefined and inconsistent (uneven weighting) Expresses summation of observer's interpretation of many different behaviours
Simple descriptive scale (SDS)	Significant inter-observer variability Absence of selection criteria for behaviours assessed Low sensitivity Cannot identify small changes in the pain response In humans has been shown to artificially magnify the efficacy of analgesics
Composite scoring system	Time consuming No selection criteria for the behaviours assessed Few validated tools in small animals
Multidimensional scoring system	Time consuming No selection criteria for the behaviours assessed

8.7 Limitations of commonly used pain scoring systems.

More recently, composite and multidimensional scales have been developed for assessment of acute pain in dogs (Hellyer and Gaynor, 1998; Firth and Haldane, 1999) and also in laboratory rats (Roughan and Flecknell, 2001, 2003). These systems evaluate a collection of specific behaviours, physiological variables and contextual factors to produce a 'composite pain score'. No composite scales have yet been developed for assessment of pain in cats.

Recognizing the limitations of physiological and subjective behavioural indices, *objective* evaluation of behaviour currently provides the most sensitive means of assessing pain in animals, but is tremendously time consuming. However, as has been achieved with laboratory rats, once behavioural indices of discomfort have been identified and clearly defined it should be possible subsequently to develop, validate and optimize more rapid techniques for subjective behaviour-based clinical evaluation of animal pain.

In humans, multidimensional pain scoring systems, such as the McGill Pain Questionnaire, evaluate not only intensity but also sensory and affective qualities of pain, thus providing a more complete picture of an individual's 'pain experience'. Similar multidimensional systems have been developed for evaluation of post-operative pain in dogs undergoing surgery, including the Melbourne Pain Scale (Firth and Haldane, 1999) and the Glasgow Composite Pain scale (GCMPS) (Holton *et al.*, 2001). The GCMPS is the only scale for evaluating acute pain in dogs to have been developed and validated according to psychometric principles, and is summarized in Figure 8.8. Dogs are observed from a distance, and then their responses to interaction and wound palpation by an observer are evaluated. The GCPMS is time consuming but a shorter form (downloadable from www.gla.ac.uk/vet/research/cascience/shortform.htm) provides a practical and sensitive means of evaluating and recording patient comfort and response to analgesic therapy in a busy practice environment.

Recently, an interval level pain assessment scale has been developed from the GCMPS, in which the individual items evaluated in the composite pain scale have been weighted, providing another useful tool for evaluating and monitoring acute pain in busy clinics (Morton *et al.*, 2005).

Assessment of chronic pain

Assessment of chronic pain in companion animals is an emerging science. Presently, the best tools available to evaluate chronic pain in companion animals are structured questionnaires, similar to those used for human chronic pain patients. These aim to provide a comprehensive picture of the quality of life of animals with chronic pain. Wiseman-Orr *et al.* (2004) have identified 13 key behavioural domains, which are relevant to assessment of dogs with chronic pain, and descriptive terms used by owners to describe these domains (Figure 8.9).

Variable	Question	Descriptors
Posture	Does the dog seem...	rigid? hunched or tense? to have normal posture?
Comfort	Does the dog seem...	restless? comfortable?
Vocalization	If the dog is vocalizing, is it...	crying or whimpering? groaning? screaming? not vocalizing or none of these?
Attention to the wound area	Is the dog...	chewing the wound? licking, looking at or rubbing the wound? ignoring the wound?
Demeanour	Having interacted with the dog, does the dog seem to be...	aggressive? depressed? uninterested? nervous, anxious or fearful? quiet or indifferent? happy and content? happy and bouncy?
Mobility (in some instances, this assessment is not possible because of the type of surgery)	After walking the dog for a short distance (if possible), did the dog seem to be...	stiff? slow or reluctant to rise or sit? lame? able to move with normal gait? assessment not carried out?
Response to touch	When gentle, even pressure was applied to the area approximately 5 cm around the surgical wound (or near the area of the wound if it was inaccessible) did the dog...	cry? flinch? snap? growl or guard wound? have no adverse response to touch?

8.8 Prototype composite pain assessment system. (Adapted from Holton *et al.*, 2001).

Domain	Negative descriptors	Positive descriptors
Activity	Apathetic, apprehensive, lacklustre, lethargic, listless, reluctant, sleepy, slowed, sluggish, tired, weary	Active, boisterous, bouncy, energetic, lively, playful, tireless
Comfort	Complaining, groaning, moaning, pained, sore, stoic, uncomfortable	Comfortable, stretching
Appetite	Off food, picky (with regard to food)	Enthusiastic about food, greedy, interested in food, thirsty
Extroversion/introversion	Detached, quiet, subdued, unresponsive, unsociable, withdrawn	Affectionate, bold, curious, eager, excitable, friendly, fun loving, nosy, outgoing, sociable
Aggression	Aggressive, grumpy, irritable, territorial or protective	Good natured, even tempered, placid
Anxiety	Anxious, cautious, distressed, frightened, nervous, panicky, strained, uneasy, upset	Accepting, easygoing, laid back
Alertness	Depressed, dull, confused, uninterested	Alert, bright, inquisitive, interested, keen, obedient
Dependence	Attention seeking, clingy, comfort seeking, pathetic or pitiful	Confident, independent
Contentment	Miserable, sad, sorrowful, resigned, unhappy	Contented, happy
Consistency	Inconsistent	Consistent
Agitation	Agitated, crying, disturbed, panting, restless, unsettled, whining	Calm, at ease
Posture–mobility	Awkward, limping, stiff	Athletic, fit, relaxed
Compulsion	Compulsive	No terms

8.9 Behavioural domains relevant to the assessment of dogs with chronic pain and descriptive terms used by owners to describe those domains. (Adapted from Wiseman-Orr *et al.*, 2004).

Summary

Although great progress has been made in the ability to assess pain in companion animals over recent years, many challenges remain. Current assessment tools provide a framework from which, with time, veterinary surgeons and nurses/technicians should be able to improve their ability to identify different types of pain in all of the companion animal species under their care.

References and further reading

Ahles T, Blanchard EB and Ruckdeschel JC (1983) The multidimensional nature of cancer-related pain. *Pain* **17**, 277–288

Capner CA, Lascelles BDX and Waterman-Pearson AE (1999) Current British veterinary attitudes to peri-operative analgesia for dogs. *Veterinary Record* **145**, 95–99

Chahal R and Rao S (2005) Functional chest pain: nociception and visceral hyperalgesia. *Journal of Clinical Gastroenterology* **39**, S204–210

Firth AM and Haldane SL (1999) Development of a scale to evaluate postoperative pain in dogs. *Journal of the American Veterinary Medical Association* **214**, 651–659

Hellyer P and Gaynor J (1998) Acute post-surgical pain in dogs and cats. *Compendium on Continuing Education for the Practicing Veterinarian (Small Animals)* **20**, 140–153

Holton LL, Reid J, Scott EM, Pawson P and Nolan AM (2001) Development of a behaviour-based scale to measure acute pain in dogs. *Veterinary Record* **148**, 523–531

Holton LL, Scott EM, Nolan AM, Reid J and Welsh E (1998) Relationship between physiological factors and clinical pain in dogs scored using a numerical rating scale. *Journal of Small Animal Practice* **39**, 469–474

Ji R-R, Kohno T, Moore KA and Woolf CJ (2003) Central sensitisation and LTP: do pain and memory share similar mechanisms? *Trends in Neuroscience* **26**, 696–705

Kehlet H and Holte K (2001) Effect of postoperative analgesia on surgical outcome. *British Journal of Anaesthesia* **87(1)**, 62–72

Kehlet H, Jensen TS and Woolf CJ (2006) Persistent post-surgical pain: risk factors and prevention. *Lancet* **367**, 1618–1625

Mendell LM and Wall PD (1965) Response of single dorsal cord cells to peripheral cutaneous unmyelinated fibres. *Nature* **206**, 97–99

Miranda C, Di Virgilio M, Selleri S *et al.* (2002) Novel pathogenic mechanisms of congenital insensitivity to pain with anhidrosis genetic disorder unveiled by functional analysis of neurotrophic tyrosine receptor kinase type 1/nerve growth factor receptor mutations. *Journal of Biological Chemistry* **277**, 6455–6462

Molony V and Kent JE (1997) Assessment of acute pain in farm animals using behavioural and physiological measurements. *Journal of Animal Science* **75,** 266–272

Morton CM, Reid J, Scott EM, Holton LL and Nolan AM (2005) Application of a scaling model to establish and validate an interval level pain scale for assessment of acute pain in dogs. *American Journal of Veterinary Research* **66**, 2154–2166

Robertson SA (2005) Managing pain in feline patients. *Veterinary Clinics of North America: Small Animal Practice* **35**, 129–146

Roughan J and Flecknell P (2001) Behavioural effects of laparotomy and analgesic effects of ketoprofen and carprofen in rats. *Pain* **90**, 65–74

Roughan J and Flecknell P (2003) Evaluation of a short duration behaviour-based post-operative pain scoring system for rats. *European Journal of Pain* **7**, 397–405

Samad TA, Moore KA, Sapirstein A *et al.* (2001) Interleukin-1beta-mediated induction of COX-2 in the CNS contributes to inflammatory pain hypersensitivity. *Nature* **410**, 425–427

Sternbach R (1981) Chronic pain as a disease entity. *Triangle* **20**, 20–37

Taylor PM and Robertson SA (2004) Pain management in cats – past, present and future. Part 1. The cat is unique. *Journal of Feline Medicine and Surgery* **6**, 313–320

Turnbach ME, Spraggins DS and Randich A (2002) Spinal administration of prostaglandin E2 or prostaglandin F2-alpha primarily produces mechanical hyperalgesia that is mediated by nociceptive specific spinal dorsal horn neurons. *Pain* **97**, 33–45

Usunoff KG, Popratiloff A, Schmitt O and Wree A (2006) Functional neuroanatomy of pain. *Advances in Anatomy, Embryology, and Cell Biology (Berlin)* **184**, 1–115

Verne GN, Robinson ME and Price DD (2004) Representations of pain in the brain. *Current Rheumatology Reports* **6**, 261–265

Wiseman ML, Nolan AM, Reid, J and Scott EM (2001) Preliminary study on owner-reported behaviour changes associated with chronic pain in dogs. *Veterinary Record* **149(14)**, 423–424

Wiseman-Orr M, Nolan AM, Reid J and Scott EM (2004) Development of a questionnaire to measure the effects of chronic pain on health-related quality of life in dogs. *American Journal of Veterinary Research* **65**, 1077–1084

Woodforde J and Fielding J (1975) Pain and cancer. In: *Pain, Clinical and Experimental Perspectives*, ed. M Weisenberg, pp. 326–335. Mosby, St Louis

Woolf CJ (2004a) Pain: moving from symptom control toward mechanism-specific pharmacologic management. *Annals of Internal Medicine* **140**, 441–451

Woolf CJ (2004b) Dissecting out mechanisms responsible for peripheral neuropathic pain: Implications for diagnosis and therapy. *Life Sciences* **74**, 2605–2610

Woolf CJ and Salter MW (2000) Neuronal plasticity: increasing the gain in pain. *Science* **288**, 1765–1768

Zhu X, Conklin D and Eisenach JC (2003) Cyclo-oxygenase-1 in the spinal cord plays an important role in post-operative pain. *Pain* **104**, 15–23

9

Pain management I: systemic analgesics

Carolyn Kerr

Introduction

Most agents used for analgesia in small animal patients fall into the opioid or non-steroidal anti-inflammatory (NSAID) groups. Recently, however, *N*-methyl-D-aspartate (NMDA) antagonists, local anaesthetics and alpha-2 adrenergic agonists have also been used for analgesia. Traditionally, opioid analgesics have been used to treat acute pain while NSAIDs have been reserved for chronic pain management. Fortunately, newer drugs and new formulations of older drugs have expanded the potential of these drug groups.

The different categories of drugs influence pain processing through different mechanisms, and can therefore be used in combination to maximize analgesia (multimodal analgesia). In addition to the selection of appropriate analgesics, the timing of drug administration is important as it influences the efficacy of analgesic drugs. Administration of analgesics prior to the initial painful stimulus (e.g. elective neutering) optimizes pain control during surgery, and less analgesic drug is required postoperatively (pre-emptive analgesia). In the sections below, the general properties of analgesic drugs are reviewed and followed by descriptions of individual drugs within each category.

Opioid analgesics

Opioids are generally considered the most efficacious drugs for acute pain. The term 'opiate' refers to drugs derived from either opium or thebaine (a derivative of opium) and includes morphine, codeine and derived semi-synthetic congeners. Opioid analgesic (or 'opioid') is a more general term and refers to any naturally occurring, semi-synthetic or synthetic substance with morphine-like activity. Because opioids can be abused, all countries legally regulate the purchase, storage and use of opioids. The severity of regulation is dependent on opioid class scheduling (see Chapter 1). Opioids available to veterinary surgeons with the greatest potential for abuse are Schedule 2 drugs, while opioid drugs with less abuse risk are Schedule 3 drugs. In Canada, all opioids fall under Narcotic Control Regulations and scheduling does not apply.

Pharmacology

Morphine is an alkaloid derived from opium. Due to its complex synthesis, morphine is still derived from opium obtained from poppy seeds. Several newer opioids are synthesized from morphine and are called semi-synthetic. Considerable variability in lipophilicity exists between different opioids. In general, more lipophilic agents, such as fentanyl, have a shorter duration of action compared with more hydrophilic opioids, such as morphine. All opioid analgesics are metabolized in the liver prior to excretion; the metabolites of some drugs may possess analgesic properties.

Most opioids are well absorbed following intramuscular or subcutaneous administration. The intravenous route is also suitable for the majority of opioids, except for morphine and pethidine (meperidine). These two drugs produce mast cell degranulation, histamine release and a significant decrease in systemic arterial blood pressure. Morphine can be administered slowly intravenously with few clinically significant effects on haemodynamics, although the intravenous route is not recommended in patients with mast cell neoplasia. The preservatives found in most opioid formulations have not been reported to cause any adverse consequences when they are administered parenterally.

Although most opioids are well absorbed from the gastrointestinal tract, only a few can be administered enterally due to limited bioavailability. After absorption, most opioids are extensively metabolized during their first pass through the liver. With some agents, the mucous membrane route (oral, nasal and buccal) can bypass hepatic metabolism and produce effective plasma concentrations. Transcutaneous delivery is a novel approach suitable for long-term administration of some opioids.

The goal of opioid administration is to achieve plasma concentrations associated with analgesia. The plasma half-life of the drug is used to determine the duration of action and dosing intervals. With some opioid analgesics, such as morphine, there is often a discrepancy between plasma concentrations and duration of clinical or experimental analgesia; this discrepancy probably occurs because plasma concentrations do not always reflect drug concentrations at the site of action within the central nervous system (CNS). It is also possible that an active metabolite exists and contributes to analgesia. Recommended dosing intervals are also based on analgesia trials or, in some cases, clinical experience.

Mechanism of action

The desirable and undesirable effects of opioid analgesics are derived from activity at opioid receptors within the CNS. Currently there are three major classes of opioid receptors recognized, designated *mu*, *delta* and *kappa*. These receptors differ in their binding properties, functional activity and distribution. For example, mu and delta receptors are located supraspinally and spinally, while kappa receptors are primarily located in the spinal cord. Within each class, several subtypes may exist. Despite these differences, all opioid receptors are couple to G-proteins and subsequently inhibit adenylate cyclase, decreasing the conductance of voltage-gated calcium channels, and/or open inwardly rectifying potassium channels. As a result, neuronal activity is decreased, neurotransmitter release is reduced and postsynaptic membranes are hyperpolarized, thereby decreasing the propagation of action potentials.

Drugs acting on opioid receptors are classified as agonists, partial agonists, mixed agonist/antagonists and antagonists:

- Agonist drugs have high affinity and intrinsic activity for mu receptors and include morphine, pethidine (meperidine), hydromorphone, methadone, fentanyl, sufentanil, alfentanil, remifentanil and codeine
- Partial agonists, which by definition are only partly as effective as agonists, include buprenorphine
- Mixed agonist/antagonists, such as butorphanol, are agonists at some receptors and antagonists at others depending on their affinity and intrinsic activity at the receptor site. Mixed agonist/antagonists can reverse the effects of pure mu agonists, so they should not be administered with mu agonists unless the goal is to reverse the mu receptor effects
- Antagonists, e.g. naloxone and nalmefene, can reverse the effects of mu and kappa agonists because of their high affinity and low intrinsic activity.

Analgesic effects

In general, opioids are considered more effective for continuous dull pain rather than sharp intermittent pain. However, effects of mu agonist opioids are dose dependent and it is possible to reduce the intensity of most types of pain with their use. The analgesic effect is produced rapidly, but is of relatively short duration (<12 hours). Opioids specifically act on nociception; touch, pressure and proprioception are mostly unaffected. In humans, there is considerable inter-individual variation in opioid requirements for postoperative analgesia. The same is probably true for cats and dogs. Therefore, to optimize the effect, patient response to opioid treatment should be continuously assessed and treatment adjusted accordingly. Fortunately, opioids can be titrated to effect and have a wide therapeutic index, so that doses can be safely adjusted over a wide range.

All three classes of opioid receptor mediate analgesia. The different opioid drugs produce characteristic patterns of analgesia, due partly to differences in receptor affinity and location. For example, systemically administered mu agonists produce analgesia through receptors located in the brain (centrally mediated or supraspinal analgesia). Analgesia produced by kappa agonists is mediated through activity at receptors located in the spinal cord (spinally mediated analgesia).

In general, mu agonists produce the most profound analgesia and are recommended for moderate to severe pain and anaesthetic-sparing effects. Mixed agonist/antagonists are generally recommended for mild to moderate pain and are suitable for minor surgical procedures. A 'ceiling effect' on the quality of analgesia produced by mixed agonist/antagonists has been described and refers to a plateau effect in the level of analgesia despite increased doses. The relative potency of different agents is generally compared with the potency of morphine and this is shown in Figure 9.1. Potency, however, refers to the dose required to produce similar effects and is not necessarily indicative of overall efficacy in relieving pain.

Drug	Classification (potency relative to morphine)	Dosage forms	Dose	Duration of effect of one bolus
Morphine	Mu agonist (1)	Injectable: 0.5–50 mg/ml	0.1–1.0 mg/kg i.m. or s.c. CRI: 0.1–0.2 mg/kg/h Epidural: 0.1–0.2 mg/kg	4–6 hours
Pethidine (meperidine)	Mu agonist (0.2–0.3)	Injectable: 10–100 mg/ml	3–5 mg/kg i.m. or s.c.	1–1.5 hours
Methadone	Mu agonist (1)	Injectable: 10 mg/ml	0.1–0.5 mg/kg i.v., i.m. or s.c.	4 hours
Hydromorphone	Mu agonist (5)	Injectable: 2–100 mg/ml	0.05–0.1 mg/kg i.v., i.m. or s.c.	4 hours
Fentanyl	Mu agonist (100)	Injectable: 50 and 78.5 µg/ml Transdermal: 25, 50, 75 and 100 µg/h	5–20 µg/kg CRI: 3–5 µg/kg bolus followed by 3–6 µg/kg/h i.v. 4 µg/kg	20–30 minutes
Sufentanil	Mu agonist (500)	Injectable: 50 µg/ml	3–5 µg/kg (bolus) followed by CRI: 2.6–3.4 µg/kg/h	10–20 minutes
Alfentanil	Mu agonist (25)	Injectable: 500 µg/ml	CRI: 0.5–1 µg/kg/minute	10–20 minutes

9.1 Opioid analgesics used in dogs. (continues) ▶

Drug	Classification (potency relative to morphine)	Dosage forms	Dose	Duration of effect of one bolus
Remifentanil (not available in Canada)	Mu agonist (50)	Injectable: 1 mg/ml	CRI: 0.1 µg/kg/minute	
Tramadol (not available in Canada)	Mu agonist (0.1)	Injectable: 50 mg/ml Tablet: 50mg	1–4 mg/kg orally	6–12 hours
Butorphanol	Mu antagonist–kappa agonist	Injectable: 10 mg/ml	0.2–0.4 mg/kg i.v., i.m. or s.c.	1.5–2 hours
Buprenorphine	Partial mu agonist	Injectable: 0.3 mg/ml	0.01–0.02 mg/kg i.v., i.m. or s.c.	4–12 hours
Naloxone	Antagonist	Injectable: 0.4 and 1 mg/ml	0.002–0.04 mg/kg i.v., i.m. or s.c.	30 minutes–1 hour

9.1 (continued) Opioid analgesics used in dogs.

CNS effects

Classically, mu opioid agonists produce euphoria and kappa agonists produce dysphoria, although some authors use these behavioural descriptions interchangeably. Euphoria in dogs is described as excessive wakefulness and vocalization. In cats, euphoria produces rolling, grooming, 'kneading' and extreme friendliness. Dysphoria in dogs is typified by agitation, excitement, restlessness, excessive vocalization and disorientation. In cats, fearful behaviour, open-mouth breathing, agitation, vocalization, pacing and apparent hallucinations are described. Both behaviours are typically observed with high doses of mu agonists or mixed agonist/antagonists. Fortunately, these behaviours can be managed by administering sedatives/tranquillizers and/or opioid antagonists.

In healthy, dogs without pain, most mu agonists produce mild to moderate sedation while the kappa agonists result in little change or mild sedation. In healthy, cats without pain, mu agonists produce mild euphoric behaviour. In cats or dogs in pain it is rare for euphoric or dysphoric behaviours to occur with either mu or kappa agonists.

Mu and kappa agonists potentiate sedation produced by sedatives or tranquillizer drugs when given in combination. High doses of mu agonists, such as hydromorphone or fentanyl, in combination with a benzodiazepine can produce a light plane of anaesthesia in dogs.

Respiratory effects

Depression of the respiratory centre response to hypercapnia and hypoxaemia are well recognized side effects of opioids. At equi-analgesic doses, the different mu agonists exhibit a similar degree of respiratory depression. Respiratory depression should be expected when administering opioids in combination with other CNS depressants, such as volatile anaesthetics, or with respiratory disease, especially when there is increased work of breathing. The veterinary surgeon should therefore be watchful for apnoea or severe hypoventilation. In cats or dogs without respiratory disease, respiratory depression is not clinically significant at recommended doses. Some opioids also depress the cough reflex, independent of their respiratory depressant effect. Cough suppression is dependent on the individual opioid rather than receptor affinity. For example, both butorphanol and fentanyl are considered potent cough suppressants.

A change in respiratory pattern can be observed following opioid administration. In healthy, pain-free dogs, panting is a frequent observation with pure mu agonists. This occurs secondary to a change in the central thermoregulation set-point. In cats, open-mouth breathing may be observed and is probably due to dysphoria.

Cardiovascular effects

At analgesic doses, especially with pure mu agonists, decreased heart rate secondary to increased vagal tone is common. However, the resulting bradycardia is responsive to anticholinergics. When mu agonists are used alone for analgesia, the decreased heart rate rarely requires treatment. When administered with other cardiodepressant drugs, such as volatile anaesthetics, administration of an anticholinergic may significantly improve haemodynamic status. In general, the effect of the opioids on systemic blood pressure is minimal.

Gastrointestinal effects

Vomiting and defecation in dogs without pain are common following administration of some mu agonists. However, when administered to patients in pain, or postoperatively, these side effects are uncommon. The incidence of vomiting is lower in cats and dogs after intravenous injection compared with the intramuscular route. Vomiting can be reduced if acepromazine is administered 15 minutes prior to intramuscular morphine or hydromorphone. In cats, excessive salivation and vomition are frequently observed following mu agonists, although defecation is rarely observed.

Decreased gastric emptying time and intestinal propulsive motility have been demonstrated in dogs, and therefore increased gastrointestinal transit time should be anticipated following opioid administration. An increase in pyloric sphincter tone has been reported following mu agonists; they are not, therefore, recommended prior to duodenal endoscopy. Similarly, mu agonists increase the tone of the biliary sphincter of Oddi, resulting in a decrease in biliary secretions. Mu agonists are therefore not recommended in cats or dogs with biliary obstruction.

Ocular effects

The mu agonists produce miosis in dogs, while mydriasis is observed in cats. The miotic effect is a consideration for intraocular surgery, otherwise it has little clinical significance. Miosis is produced through opioid-mediated stimulation of cell bodies in the oculomotor nuclear complex. In cats, mydriasis occurs secondary to an opioid-induced increase in circulating catecholamines. Mydriasis impairs normal vision and increases sensitivity to light; these alterations should be considered when handling and exposing the cat to light.

Urinary effects

Mu agonists increase urethral sphincter tone and inhibit the voiding reflex. This may be manifested as a short-term decrease in urination, although urine production is otherwise not decreased significantly by opioid analgesics.

Thermoregulation

In dogs, opioids decrease the thermoregulatory set point in the CNS and cause panting, When opioids have been used perioperatively in dogs, it is common to observe decreased body temperature. In cats, however, postoperative hyperthermia is a relatively common adverse side effect of mu agonists. Hyperthermia appears to be dose related, with higher doses associated with greater probability of hyperthermia. The mechanism for this observation is currently unknown, but body temperature should be closely monitored in cats given mu agonists.

Auditory sensitivity

Certain opioids, such as fentanyl, increase noise sensitivity in cats and dogs and the environment should be as quiet as possible.

Opioid mu agonists

Morphine

Morphine has been used in Western medicine since the mid 19th century and remains the 'gold standard'. It has high affinity for mu receptors, but also has mild affinity for kappa and delta receptors. It is relatively hydrophilic compared to more potent mu agonists. It is generally administered intramuscularly or subcutaneously; rapid intravenous administration is associated with histamine release, causing vasodilation, decreased blood pressure and urticaria. The final effect is dependent on the dose and rate of administration; a slow intravenous infusion can be administered either alone, or combined with other analgesics, to produce continuous analgesia. Morphine may also be given via the epidural route (see Chapter 10).

The reported half-life of intravenous morphine is approximately 60 minutes in dogs and 75 minutes in cats. Bioavailability is 100% following intramuscular injection. Orally administered sustained or extended release formulations have 5–20% bioavailability with considerable individual variability. Reduced bioavailability is attributed to first-pass metabolism by the liver and intestinal mucosa following absorption from the gastrointestinal tract. Based on the individual variability and low bioavailability, oral formulations are currently not recommended.

Using a thermal device to determine pain threshold, onset of analgesia following 0.2 mg/kg morphine i.m. in cats was reported to be 4 hours with duration of effect lasting 2 hours. Using this particular model, morphine was found to have lower efficacy relative to hydromorphone or buprenorphine. To achieve target serum concentrations for analgesia in dogs, 0.5 mg/kg i.v. every 2 hours has been recommended, although this dosing regime has not been validated in clinical settings. Clinical trials using doses ranging from 0.3–0.8 mg/kg i.m. resulted in good postoperative analgesia following orthopaedic surgery in over 70% of dogs for 4 hours after termination of anaesthesia. A single dose of morphine (0.3 mg/kg i.m.) or buprenorphine (0.01 mg/kg i.m.) for premedication prior to arthrotomy in dogs resulted in similar postoperative analgesia for 7 hours. Following thoracotomy in dogs, doses of 1.0 mg/kg i.m. or intrapleurally provided similar postoperative pain control to intercostal nerve blocks with bupivacaine. Morphine and nerve blocks can be used together to facilitate pain management following thoracotomy. In summary, duration of effective analgesia is approximately 2–6 hours in cats and dogs at the doses shown in Figures 9.1 and 9.2, and this interval is used for repeat dosing. As previously mentioned, in the healthy dog or cat without pain, high doses of morphine, or any other opioid, should be combined with a sedative/tranquillizer to prevent dysphoria or euphoria.

Drug	Classification	Dosage forms	Dose	Duration of effect of one bolus
Morphine	Mu agonist	Injectable: 0.5–50 mg/ml	0.1–1.0 mg/kg i.m. or s.c. Epidural: 0.1–0.2 mg/kg	4–6 hours
Pethidine (meperidine)	Mu agonist	Injectable: 10–100 mg/ml	3–5 mg/kg i.m. or s.c.	1–1.5 hours
Methadone	Mu agonist	Injectable: 10 mg/ml	0.1–0.3 mg/kg i.v., i.m. or s.c.	4 hours
Hydromorphone	Mu agonist	Injectable: 2–100 mg/ml	0.05–0.1 mg/kg i.v., i.m. or s.c.	4 hours
Fentanyl	Mu agonist	Injectable: 50 and 78.5 µg/ml Transdermal: 25 µg/h	5–10 µg /kg i.v. CRI: 2–3 µg/kg bolus followed by 2–3 µg/kg/h i.v. 4 µg/kg	20–30 minutes

9.2 Opioid analgesics routinely used in cats. (continues) ▶

Drug	Classification	Dosage forms	Dose	Duration of effect of one bolus
Butorphanol	Mu antagonist–kappa agonist	Injectable: 10 mg/ml	0.2–0.4 mg/kg i.v., i.m. or s.c.	1.5–2 hours
Buprenorphine	Partial mu agonist	Injectable: 0.3 mg/ml	0.01–0.02 mg/kg i.v., i.m. or s.c.	4–12 hours
Naloxone	Antagonist	Injectable: 0.4 and 1 mg/ml	0.002–0.04 mg/kg i.v.	30 minutes–1 hour

9.2 (continued) Opioid analgesics routinely used in cats.

Morphine can be administered to dogs as a constant rate infusion (CRI) for prolonged analgesia. This technique provides consistent levels of analgesia and minimizes adverse side effects following intermittent boluses, and less morphine is administered overall. For example, following laparotomy, dogs were reported to have similar levels of analgesia when receiving morphine either at 0.12 mg/kg/h i.v. or at 1.0 mg/kg i.m. every 4 hours. In general, both groups exhibited good postoperative analgesia with minimal adverse side effects. Despite the CRI group receiving half the amount of morphine used in the intermittent bolus group, it appeared that the dosing techniques provided equipotent analgesia. The target plasma concentrations achieved using the CRI technique were lower than previously reported plasma concentrations in other species. However, it is feasible that following more invasive surgery, such as thoracotomy or major orthopaedic intervention, higher infusion rates would be necessary in dogs. Currently recommended rates of infusion are shown in Figure 9.1. Recommended infusion rates for cats have not been published at this time.

Morphine at recommended doses also produces mild sedation; administration with acepromazine or medetomidine improves the quality of sedation and analgesia. When administered at recommended doses during inhalational anaesthesia, morphine has an anaesthetic-sparing effect. The minimum alveolar concentration (MAC) of isoflurane is decreased by 50% using morphine at 2 mg/kg i.v. in dogs, and by 25% using 1 mg/kg i.v. in cats.

Using morphine and atropine for premedication in dogs can make duodenal endoscopy more difficult to perform compared with premedication with pethidine (meperidine) (with or without an anticholinergic). Morphine is also reported to increase biliary sphincter tone more than fentanyl, pethidine or butorphanol in humans. Morphine administered prior to anaesthesia in dogs without pain can increase the incidence of gastro-oesophageal reflux, but the clinical significance remains to be determined. Administration (intramuscular or subcutaneous) typically induces emesis in most healthy cats and dogs without pain. The rate of emesis is lower with the intravenous route. It is rare for emesis to occur when intravenous or intramuscular morphine is administered postoperatively at analgesic doses. If necessary, the pharmacological effects can be reversed with naloxone or butorphanol.

Pethidine (meperidine)

Pethidine is a semi-synthetic mu agonist with one third to one fifth of the potency of morphine. It should only be administered intramuscularly or subcutaneously because intravenous administration results in profound hypotension secondary to histamine release. It has a short half-life following intramuscular administration and the duration of action is approximately 1–2 hours in cats and dogs.

It is not as efficacious as morphine or hydromorphone for treating severe pain. Due to its short duration of action, it is only recommended for procedures associated with mild discomfort. At analgesic doses (3–5 mg/kg), pethidine is associated with mild sedation and a low incidence of vomiting. It can therefore be used as a premedicant in those patients requiring light sedation, or where emesis is undesirable, and other pure mu agonists can be given to 'top-up' analgesia during anaesthesia if necessary.

Methadone

Methadone is a synthetic pure mu agonist with similar analgesic properties to morphine, but with less sedation. It rarely induces emesis, unlike morphine, and is therefore useful in those cases where vomiting is undesirable (e.g. those cases with increased intraocular or intracranial pressure). However, it is more likely to cause dysphoria than morphine, and clinical experience suggests that cats and dogs are less 'happy' after receiving methadone than they are after morphine. Doses of 0.1–0.5 mg/kg i.m. or i.v. in dogs, and 0.1–0.3 mg/kg i.m. in cats have been recommended.

Hydromorphone

Hydromorphone is also a semi-synthetic opioid derived from morphine. It is a pure mu agonist and its physiochemical properties, such as hydrophilicity, are similar to morphine. It has five to ten times the potency of morphine and can be administered intramuscularly, subcutaneously or intravenously. The characteristics and efficacy of hydromorphone and oxymorphone are similar, but hydromorphone is less expensive. Since oxymorphone is now unavailable in North America, hydromorphone has gained popularity in veterinary medicine.

Similar to other pure mu agonists, it produces dose-dependent analgesia. When administered intravenously, onset of analgesia and sedation is more rapid than with morphine. At doses of 0.05–0.1 mg/kg i.m., the duration of analgesic effects is 3–7 hours in cats and dogs. In cats, 0.1 mg/kg i.m. or i.v. has been reported to result in an increase in pain threshold, using a thermal testing device within 15 minutes of administration, which lasted 5–7 hours. Hyperthermia following hydromorphone administration in cats has been reported, although this has also been reported following high doses of morphine or fentanyl.

The incidence of vomiting following intramuscular administration in dogs ranges from 0% to 10%. If acepromazine is administered prior to intramuscular hydromorphone, or if hydromorphone is administered intravenously, the incidence of vomiting is reduced.

Mydriasis is observed in cats, but miosis is common in dogs. When administered in combination with acepromazine, intraocular pressure does not increase in normal dogs, although the effect of hydromorphone alone on intraocular pressure in the dog or cat has not been reported.

Fentanyl

Fentanyl is a synthetic pure mu agonist, but with 100 times the potency of morphine. Fentanyl can be administered intramuscularly, subcutaneously, intravenously or via the transdermal route. When administered intravenously, the elimination half-life is reported to be 3–6 hours in dogs and 2 hours in cats. Clinically, intravenous administration results in rapid onset (1–2 minutes) and a short duration of action (20–30 minutes in dogs). Fentanyl may be administered using a bolus technique to control acute, severe pain (10–20 μg/kg i.v.), but can also be given by intravenous CRI or a transdermal delivery system. Other routes of administration, such as topical and intranasal, have recently been evaluated, but further development is required prior to their clinical use.

In the healthy dog without pain, bolus doses in the range used to control pain will generally result in recumbency and sedation. Healthy, cats without pain receiving a bolus (10 μg/kg i.v.) are reported to be easy to handle and quiet with mild signs of euphoria. Fentanyl infusion rates in dogs and cats are presented in Figures 9.1 and 9.2. Trials evaluating the analgesic effects in cats and dogs found plasma concentrations in the order of 1–3 ng/ml to be associated with analgesia. Specifically, in cats, the thermal threshold was increased by 2–12°C for 110 minutes following a 10 μg/kg i.v. bolus of fentanyl. Fentanyl administered as an intravenous bolus produces bradycardia, but has minimal direct depressant effects on the myocardium or vasculature. Bradycardia is due to increased vagal tone and is responsive to anticholinergics. Anticholinergics can be used to increase heart rate and improve cardiac output, although this is rarely necessary but might be considered when fentanyl is used in combination with anaesthetic drugs.

Transdermal administration of fentanyl has become popular as a method of providing prolonged analgesia for patients. Transdermal fentanyl patches are available in four different sizes based on the delivery rate to the systemic circulation across human skin. The patch itself is composed of a drug reservoir, a rate-limiting membrane and an adhesive perimeter for attaching the patch to skin. The rate of absorption of fentanyl is dependent on the surface area of the patch exposed to skin. Therefore, only partially removing the protective cover will reduce the exposed surface area, lower the rate of fentanyl absorption and reduce plasma concentration. The transdermal bioavailability of fentanyl is approximately 64% in dogs and 36% in cats and the dose required for analgesia is approximately 4 μg/kg/h. The size of patch recommended for cats and dogs is given in Figure 9.3. In cats weighing between 1.6 and 4.3 kg, it has been shown that exposure of 50% of the patch to skin results in decreased plasma concentrations compared with full exposure. However, although plasma fentanyl concentrations were below theoretical therapeutic concentrations in the 'partial exposure' group, analgesia following ovariohysterectomy was comparable to analgesia in the 'full exposure' group. Some authors recommend using partial patch exposure in cats weighing <4 kg, but the invasiveness of the procedure and the degree of analgesia required should be considered when selecting amount of patch exposure.

Patient size	Recommended fentanyl patch size
Cats and dogs <10 kg	25 μg/h
Dogs 10–20 kg	50 μg/h
Dogs 20–30 kg	75 μg/h
Dogs >30 kg	100 μg/h

9.3 Recommended fentanyl patch size for cats and dogs.

The recommended location for patch placement includes the dorsal or lateral thorax. The tarsal area or dorsum (possibly using the area clipped for a previous epidural injection) has also been used. An *in vitro* study using canine cadaver skin revealed faster absorption rates from the groin region compared with the thoracic and neck regions, although this has not been tested *in vivo*.

The area selected should be clipped of hair and the skin cleaned with mild soap (not alcohol), and allowed to dry prior to patch placement. The protective cover is removed, and the patch applied to the skin and held in place for 60 seconds. If necessary, a light bandage can be placed over the patch to prevent its removal. Therapeutic plasma concentrations of fentanyl are reached in approximately 24 hours in dogs, and within 12 hours in cats. Plasma fentanyl concentrations are generally maintained within the analgesic range for up to 72 hours following patch application in cats and dogs. Removal or replacement of the patch at 72 hours is recommended because plasma concentrations begin to fall at this time. Once the patch is removed, plasma concentrations decrease to below the analgesic range within 4–6 hours in dogs and 6–20 hours in cats. In cats and dogs, studies have revealed relatively large individual variations in plasma fentanyl concentrations, although the concentrations were still in the desired therapeutic range in dogs. Therefore, the veterinary surgeon should attempt to assess degree of analgesia in each patient following patch application to verify that adequate analgesia is provided.

Studies evaluating the analgesic efficacy of transdermal fentanyl in dogs undergoing orthopaedic surgery have shown that early postoperative analgesia (0–6 hours) from patches was not as profound as the analgesia from epidurally or systemically administered pure mu agonists. However, overall analgesia over a 48-hour assessment period was better with transdermal fentanyl. For 24 hours following ovariohysterectomy in dogs transdermal fentanyl was reported to result in similar behavioural and analgesic effects to oxymorphone. In cats undergoing onychectomy (not permitted in the UK), transdermal fentanyl has compared favourably with butorphanol.

Few adverse effects have been reported with use of transdermal fentanyl alone. Cutaneous irritation at the site of patch placement can be common. Mild sedation, bradycardia and anorexia have been reported in dogs, and hyperthermia, euphoria and dysphoria have been reported in cats. Respiratory depression during patch application has not been shown to be clinically significant in the awake dog. However, if plasma fentanyl concentrations have reached analgesic levels in the preoperative period, further respiratory depression is possible during general anaesthesia. Skin temperature can influence rate of absorption of fentanyl from the patch: external warming devices such as heating pads and water blankets may dramatically increase plasma concentrations and lead to severe respiratory depression. Halothane anaesthesia and surgery have not been shown to influence plasma fentanyl concentrations in cats. Hypothermia in isoflurane-anaesthetized cats, and halothane- and isoflurane-anaesthetized dogs, however, significantly reduced plasma fentanyl concentrations.

Sufentanil/alfentanil/remifentanil

Sufentanil, alfentanil and remifentanil are all short-acting, potent derivatives of fentanyl. In humans, they have fewer side effects with less variability in cardiovascular responses than are observed with fentanyl. Due to their short duration of action, these mu agonists are primarily administered as an infusion to provide analgesia during general anaesthesia. Unfortunately, they are more expensive than fentanyl and there are few studies evaluating their relative efficacy compared with fentanyl in cats and dogs. A long-acting form of sufentanil has recently been reported to provide sedation and analgesia for approximately 24 hours in dogs although this formulation is not yet commercially available.

Codeine

Codeine is a synthetic opioid agonist that exerts its analgesic effects through its metabolism to morphine. In humans, codeine has an oral bioavailability of approximately 60% and it is most commonly administered in an oral formulation. In cats and dogs, it has been shown to have poor oral bioavailability and a lower conversion rate to morphine. Codeine at 4 mg/kg s.c. was shown to be equivalent to 0.2 mg/kg s.c. of morphine in dogs during an analgesia study. To date, there are no studies evaluating the analgesic efficacy of orally administered codeine in cats or dogs and its poor bioavailability may limit its use.

Partial agonists

Buprenorphine

Pharmacologically, buprenorphine is classified as a partial mu agonist with little or no effect at kappa receptors. Because of this, it needs to occupy a greater fraction of the available pool of functional mu receptors (compared with a full mu agonist) in order to induce a response of similar magnitude. However, buprenorphine has high receptor affinity and can displace morphine from the mu receptor and its reversal using naloxone is difficult. Buprenorphine can be administered intravenously, intramuscularly and subcutaneously and has excellent bioavailability following oral/transmucosal administration in cats.

One of the major benefits of its use is the long duration of action, which has made it a popular analgesic for laboratory animals, cats and dogs. The reported duration of analgesia varies from 4–12 hours. However, the onset time of analgesia is longer compared with that for hydromorphone, ranging from 30 minutes to 2 hours. If given for postoperative analgesia, it must be administered pre- or intraoperatively to provide immediate postoperative analgesia.

In the past, doses of buprenorphine were often restricted because early studies showed a 'bell shaped' dose-response curve, where administration of higher doses led to a reduced analgesic effect. However, the doses that result in a reduction in efficacy are much higher than the doses used clinically. In dogs, several studies have found that doses of buprenorphine (0.007–0.02 mg/kg i.m.) have similar analgesic efficacy to morphine (0.3–0.8 mg/kg i.m.) following orthopaedic surgery. Interestingly, in cats, buprenorphine (0.01 mg/kg i.m.) produces increased analgesia from 4–12 hours (using a thermal testing device) compared with a duration of only 4–6 hours in cats receiving morphine (0.2 mg/kg i.m.).

Mixed opioid agonist/antagonists

Butorphanol

Butorphanol has agonist activity at the kappa receptor and antagonist activity at the mu receptor, for which it has high affinity. It is considered effective for mild to moderate visceral pain and is a popular pre-anaesthetic and postoperative analgesic for minor elective surgical procedures. For analgesia, the intravenous, intramuscular or subcutaneous routes of administration are used. In some countries, an oral formulation is available as an anti-tussive, but this has low oral bioavailability and high doses are required for analgesia. The duration of analgesia in cats and dogs ranges from 30–120 minutes with intravenous administration.

Although butorphanol is a commonly used analgesic in dogs, the literature suggests that, alone, it is not an effective analgesic compared with pure mu agonists or newer non-steroidal analgesic drugs. In dogs following laparotomy, 0.4 mg/kg i.m. provided inadequate postoperative analgesia to half the dogs in the study. Meloxicam has been demonstrated to provide superior analgesia for 12 hours compared with butorphanol following ovariohysterectomy in bitches. When used as an analgesic for pain resulting from orthopaedic procedures, butorphanol has consistently been demonstrated to result in inadequate analgesia.

Butorphanol is considered a good visceral but a poor somatic analgesic in cats. Using doses ranging from 0.1–0.4 mg/kg i.v. or 0.2–0.8 mg/kg s.c., somatic analgesia was only reported at the dose of 0.8 mg/kg s.c. Visceral analgesia was reported with 0.1 mg/kg i.v. and 0.4 mg/kg s.c. and duration of visceral analgesia was longer using the higher dose. Minimal analgesic effects were produced using a thermal stimulus with 0.2 mg/kg i.m., and were limited to the 5-minute period following administration. Another study demonstrated analgesic effects for 15–165 minutes following 0.4 mg/kg i.m. These results would suggest that somatic analgesia requires a dose of at least 0.4 mg/kg i.m. This has been confirmed in cats undergoing onychectomy and/or ovariohysterectomy, demonstrating that a dose of 0.4 mg/kg i.v. or s.c. is required to improve analgesia, although the non-steroidal analgesic meloxicam was better for cats undergoing onychectomy.

Butorphanol administered alone results in mild sedation and is an effective anti-tussive. Therefore, it is a useful addition to the pre-anaesthetic medication of animals undergoing airway examination and bronchoscopy. As part of pre-anaesthetic medication butorphanol does not impair passing of an endoscope through the pyloric sphincter, unlike pure mu agonists. It is therefore a suitable premedication agent for duodenal endoscopy.

Although butorphanol is associated with some respiratory depression, it is less profound than depression obtained with pure mu agonists. The degree of respiratory depression is characterized by a 'ceiling effect' as with its analgesic effects. With increasing doses respiratory depression and analgesia do not become more profound.

Butorphanol can be used to reverse the effects of a pure mu agonist. This technique is often used to reverse a relative overdose of a pure mu agonist in a patient exhibiting dysphoric behaviour or profound respiratory depression. In these situations, the goal is to reverse the undesirable effects of the pure mu agonist without reversing kappa receptor-mediated analgesia. It is recommended that 0.1–0.4 mg/kg of butorphanol is diluted in a large volume (10 ml) of saline and administered in small intravenous increments every 2–5 minutes until adequate reversal has occurred.

Miscellaneous opioid drugs

Tramadol

Tramadol is classified as an atypical, centrally acting opioid analgesic. Tramadol has one tenth the potency of morphine. It is now considered a controlled drug in many countries and is under regulatory control as with other opioids. Central analgesic effects are produced through activity of both the parent drug and its metabolites at the mu receptor. Tramadol also inhibits serotonin and noradrenaline uptake, which may contribute to a reduction in nociceptive transmission within the spinal cord. Tramadol is available in oral and parenteral formulations.

It is metabolized in the liver via demethylation and glucuronidation prior to excretion through the kidney. Pharmacokinetic data on orally administered tramadol is not yet available for cats and dogs, so bioavailability is unknown. To date, few clinical trials are available to evaluate its analgesic efficacy in cats or dogs. A dose of 2.0 mg/kg i.v. resulted in similar postoperative analgesia over a 6-hour period to morphine (0.2 mg/kg i.v.). The dose recommended for dogs is 1–4 mg/kg i.v., or orally every 6 hours for acute severe pain, or 1–4 mg/kg orally every 12 hours for treatment of osteoarthritis.

Opioid antagonists

Naloxone

Naloxone is considered an opioid antagonist with least agonist effects (pure antagonist). It can be used to reverse the effects of mu agonists or mixed agonist/antagonists, since it has higher affinity for the mu and kappa receptors, but no intrinsic activity. Naloxone does not effectively reverse buprenorphine because this partial mu agonist has greater affinity for the mu receptor than pure antagonists. If using naloxone to reverse excessive opioid-induced respiratory depression in an animal in pain, administer naloxone slowly in small intravenous increments to achieve the desired effect. Ideally, the goal is to reverse undesirable side effects while maintaining analgesia. Fortunately, naloxone has a rapid onset of action (1–2 minutes) facilitating this titration technique. Naloxone can also be administered intramuscularly. Duration of action is reported to be 30–60 minutes, therefore when used to reverse long-acting opioid mu agonists, close monitoring for return of undesirable mu agonist side effects is necessary. For example, when naloxone was used to reverse oxymorphone sedation, dogs showed clinical signs of renarcotization, such as sedation, 2 hours after naloxone administration. The dose range for naloxone is shown in Figures 9.1 and 9.2.

Nalmefene

Like naloxone, nalmefene is a rapid-onset opioid antagonist. It is, however, approximately four times more potent than naloxone with a duration of effect approximately twice that of naloxone. A dose of 0.03 mg/kg i.v. was shown effectively to reverse oxymorphone-induced sedation in dogs.

Nalorphine and diprenorphine

Nalorphine and diprenorphine are mu antagonists but partial kappa agonists. They have mild sedative effects when administered alone. They are primarily used to antagonize the effects of mu agonists used in wildlife immobilization, where prolonged duration of action is required.

Naltrexone

Naltrexone is a synthetic opioid antagonist that is available in oral formulation. It is primarily used for the treatment of behavioural disorders in cats and dogs.

Non-steroidal anti-inflammatory drugs

Use of NSAIDs for acute and chronic pain management has dramatically increased over the past 10 years with the introduction of newer, less toxic agents. Although not reversible and with a much lower therapeutic index than opioids, they have some advantages:

- Long duration of effect
- Anti-inflammatory properties
- No behaviour modifying effects
- Lack of respiratory and cardiovascular side effects
- Availability in oral formulation
- No regulatory control due to the lack of abuse potential.

NSAIDs are indicated for postoperative pain, inflammatory conditions, osteoarthritis, panosteitis, hypertrophic osteodystrophy, pain from cancer and dental pain. Marked species differences exist in the efficacy and toxicity of NSAIDs, and therefore considerable care must be exercised to ensure appropriate drug and dose selection in cats or dogs. Some NSAIDs are available without prescription and owners should be questioned whether they have given an NSAID to their pet. Without this information, inadvertent overdose of NSAIDs may occur.

Pharmacology

Chemically, the NSAIDs are a heterogenous group of compounds, although they do share considerable similarities in their pharmacokinetic and pharmacodynamic properties. The majority of older NSAIDs are weak acids, while the newer agents may be neutral, but they are all highly protein bound with a small volume of distribution. NSAIDs have different half-lives between species, so dosing should be based on individual drug data for the species. Duration of anti-inflammatory effects is considerably longer than the measured plasma half-life. This is partly because the plasma concentrations do not reflect tissue concentrations. In particular, inflamed tissue has a pH that tends to result in NSAID accumulation at the site of action.

Most NSAIDs primarily undergo hepatic metabolism with the metabolites excreted through the kidney. Enterohepatic recycling may occur with some NSAIDs and conjugated metabolites excreted in bile are reabsorbed from the gastrointestinal tract. This recycling results in a prolonged half-life. Cats have a limited ability to metabolize drugs through glucuronidation, and the half-life of some NSAIDs may be prolonged. Increased half-lives contribute to the risk of toxicity when NSAIDs are used in cats. If the appropriate dose and dosing interval are selected, however, NSAIDs can be useful for pain management in cats.

Patients with hepatic or renal disease may have greater and more prolonged peak plasma concentrations of the NSAID (and metabolites) due to reduced metabolism and/or elimination of both parent drug and metabolites. Therefore, NSAIDs are not recommended in patients with underlying hepatic or renal disease.

Mechanism of action

The majority of desirable and undesirable effects from NSAIDs stem from their inhibitory action on the COX enzyme. COX is responsible for conversion of arachidonic acid (a byproduct of membrane phospholipids) into prostaglandins (PGE_2, PGF_2, PGD_2), prostacyclin (PGI_2) and thromboxanes. Figure 9.4 illustrates the synthesis of mediators from membrane phospholipids. These compounds are synthesized from arachidonic acid throughout the body and have many diverse functions. For example, many prostaglandins regulate blood flow in peripheral tissues such as the gastric mucosa, kidney and intestinal tract. Thromboxanes play a key role in platelet aggregation. Byproducts of arachidonic acid are also involved in the initiation and propagation of inflammation, hyperalgesia and allodynia. Prostaglandins are released from peripheral nerves at sites of injury causing vasodilation and neutrophil chemotaxis, leading to increased vascular permeability and cellular influx.

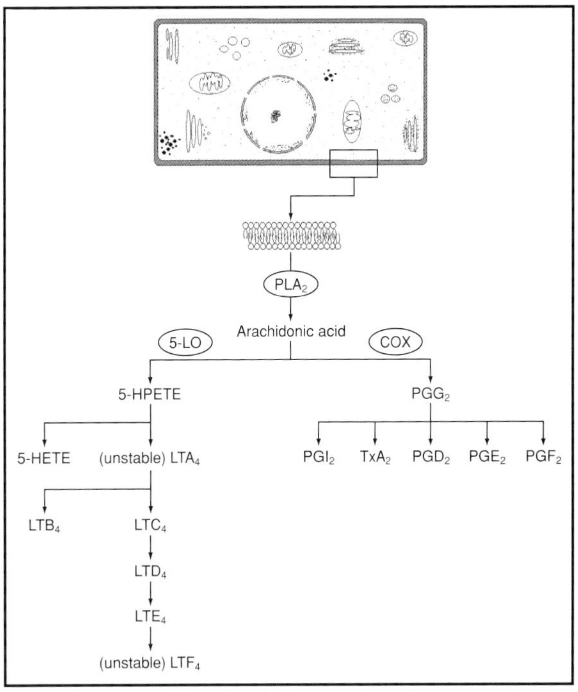

9.4 Formation of inflammatory mediators from membrane phospholipids. COX = Cyclo-oxygenase; 5-HETE = 5-hydroxyeicosatetraenoic acid; 5-HPETE = 5-hydroperoxyeicosatetraenoic acid; 5-LO = 5-lipoxygenase; LT = Leukotriene; PG = Prostaglandin; PGG_2 = Hydroperoxide; PGI_2 = Prostacyclin; PLA_2 = Phospholipase A_2; TxA_2 = Thromboxane A_2.

The COX enzyme is not identical throughout the body. It has isoforms, which have been numbered COX-1 and COX-2. Conventional NSAIDs, such as aspirin, are non-specific inhibitors of the COX enzyme, inhibiting both COX-1 and COX-2 isoforms. The COX-1 isoform was initially thought to be the sole constitutive enzyme, produced in consistent quantities throughout the body and responsible for producing byproducts important for normal homeostasis, such as regional tissue and organ blood flow, and platelet function. Conversely, the COX-2 isoform was thought to be an inducible enzyme, produced in response to stimuli such as cytokines and other inflammatory mediators released following tissue injury. Therefore, it was hypothesized that drugs that inhibited only the COX-2 enzyme would be effective inhibitors of inflammation, but free of side effects. Although COX-2 is the sole isoform involved in producing prostaglandins associated with inflammation, it is also produced constitutively in some tissues such as the kidney to maintain renal blood flow. It may also play a role in the repair of gastrointestinal erosions. The newer COX-2-specific drugs are as effective as general COX-1 and

COX-2 inhibitors at limiting inflammation, yet are associated with fewer gastrointestinal and bleeding dysfunctions. However, they are still not completely free of adverse effects.

Different NSAIDs vary in the way they block the COX enzyme. Most agents produce either competitive, reversible inhibition, or a time-dependent inhibition of the active site on the enzyme. Aspirin is an exception, as it forms a covalent bond with the active site of the enzyme, resulting in irreversible inhibition. In addition, some NSAIDs have been shown to inhibit the enzyme lipoxygenase, thereby decreasing formation of leukotrienes in addition to prostaglandins.

Analgesic effects

Prostaglandins increase the sensitivity of nociceptors and nociceptive neurons to stimuli capable of producing pain. High concentrations of prostaglandins in peripheral tissues also result in changes to pathways involved in transmitting nociceptive stimuli within the CNS. NSAIDs block the COX-2 enzyme, reduce prostaglandins and/or leukotrienes in peripheral tissues, and minimize subsequent alteration of pain processing pathways. NSAIDs may also inhibit prostaglandin synthesis within the CNS. Both non-specific COX and COX-2-specific inhibitors block the COX-2 enzyme, and all are effective analgesic/anti-inflammatory agents.

Gastrointestinal effects

The COX-1 isoform is mainly responsible for the production of prostaglandins that influence mucosal blood flow, epithelial cell turnover and mucus and bicarbonate secretion in the gastrointestinal tract. Conventional, general COX inhibitors have a low gastrointestinal margin of safety, with side effects of vomiting, diarrhoea, anorexia, abdominal pain and gastrointestinal ulceration. In severe cases, gastrointestinal perforation may occur. The risk of adverse gastrointestinal events is increased with high doses of NSAIDs, prolonged use, multiple NSAID use, underlying gastrointestinal disease and concurrent glucocorticoid administration. The COX-2-selective drugs are clearly associated with fewer gastrointestinal side effects, although inappropriate dosing or patient selection can still result in similar adverse events.

Gastric ulcer prophylaxis may be recommended in some high-risk patients. Misoprostol (synthetic prostaglandin E_1) has been shown to reduce the incidence of gastrointestinal ulcers in dogs. A dose of 2–5 μg/kg orally is recommended at 12-hour intervals. Sucralfate may also play a role in the prevention of gastrointestinal ulcers in dogs and can be administered concurrently with misoprostol. Sucralfate must be administered either 1 hour after or 2 hours before misoprostol. The recommended dose of sucralfate for prevention of ulcers is 0.5–1.0 g orally every 8 hours in dogs, and 0.25 g orally every 8–12 hours in cats. Anti-ulcer therapy may be necessary in patients that have developed clinical signs associated with gastrointestinal ulcers during NSAID treatment. NSAID administration should be stopped and current treatment options for gastric or duodenal ulceration include:

- Sucralfate at double the listed doses above
- Famotidine at 0.5 mg/kg i.v. every 12 hours in cats or dogs
- Omeprazole at 0.7 mg/kg i.v. every 24 hours in cats or dogs (<20 kg), or 20 mg orally every 24 hours in dogs (>20 kg).

Renal effects

When renal blood flow is reduced, locally produced prostaglandins in the kidney produce afferent arteriolar vasodilation to restore renal blood flow. Prostaglandins are also involved in the control of renin release and tubular function. By blocking prostaglandin formation, NSAIDs adversely affect renal perfusion when blood flow to the kidney is reduced. The COX-2 as well as the COX-1 isoform is expressed constitutively in the kidney, so even COX-2-selective agents may have adverse renal effects. In the well hydrated patient with normal renal function, the probability of NSAID-related renal dysfunction is low. In patients with renal disease or with cardiovascular dysfunction leading to reduced renal blood flow (including anaesthetic-induced hypotension), there is increased risk of NSAID-induced acute ischaemic renal failure and/or renal papillary necrosis. When administering NSAIDs that are licensed for perioperative use, intravenous fluid therapy and haemodynamic monitoring are recommended intraoperatively to prevent periods of low renal blood flow. Some NSAIDs have also been reported to impair prostaglandin inhibition of antidiuretic hormone (ADH), leading to decreased urine output and dilutional hyponatraemia. In this case, renal injury is not present.

Effects on coagulation

Inhibition of COX-1, which is responsible for the formation of thromboxane, leads to platelet dysfunction and prolonged bleeding. The non-selective COX inhibitors are therefore not recommended for use preoperatively because of increased risks of intraoperative haemorrhage. Patients receiving conventional NSAIDs should have treatment withdrawn for a period (10–14 days) before elective surgery to allow NSAID elimination and restoration of platelet function. The COX-2-specific inhibitors are associated with a significantly reduced bleeding risk in humans. In healthy dogs, COX-2 inhibitors have been shown to have minimal effect on platelet function, although they have not been assessed in animals with pre-existing platelet disorders.

Hepatic effects

NSAIDs are metabolized in the liver and hepatotoxicity is a risk following overdose with any of these agents. Idiosyncratic hepatotoxicity has been reported with numerous different NSAIDs in humans and in small animal patients. Idiosyncratic hepatotoxicity is not dose dependent and frequently occurs within a few weeks after starting NSAID therapy. Clinical signs of vomiting and inappetance are observed with a marked increase in hepatic enzymes.

Reproductive effects

Prostaglandins are involved in normal labour, closure of the ductus arteriosus in the neonate, ovulation and embryo implantation. The safety of the currently available NSAIDs has not been assessed in pregnant animals; they are, therefore, not recommended for pregnant, lactating or breeding animals, until there is evidence of their safety.

Effects on cartilage

The effects of NSAIDs on cartilage are controversial and appear to be dependent on the specific NSAID and the method used to evaluate cartilage status. Some NSAIDs decrease proteoglycan synthesis and possibly contribute to chondrocyte death, while others may have chrondroprotective effects. Of the NSAIDs currently licensed for use in dogs for treatment of osteoarthritis, there is no evidence to support clinically significant deleterious effects on cartilage, hyalurate or proteoglycan homeostasis and some literature suggests they may offer a chondroprotective effect.

Contraindications for non-steroidal anti-inflammatory drugs

Based on known side effects of NSAIDs, these drugs should not be used in patients with the following conditions:

- Impaired renal or hepatic function
- Dehydration or hypovolaemia
- Coagulopathies
- Animals receiving other NSAIDs or corticosteroids
- Gastrointestinal ulcers or erosions
- Conditions associated with low circulating blood volume, such as congestive heart failure
- Pregnant, lactating or breeding animals.

When switching from one NSAID to another, it is recommended that a 5–7-day washout interval is allowed to prevent adverse drug interactions. If NSAID withdrawal is due to adverse side effects, the patient should be fully recovered prior to starting treatment with an alternative NSAID.

Veterinary approved non-steroidal anti-inflammatory drugs

Several different NSAIDs are currently authorized for use in cats and dogs, while others, although not approved, have been used in veterinary patients off-label for many years. Due to the physiological roles of the different COX isoforms, interest has primarily been given to developing COX-2-specific inhibitors. Unfortunately, *in vitro* studies have produced highly variable results with respect to relative COX-1 and COX-2 inhibitory actions of various NSAIDs. Furthermore, although COX-2 agents are relatively less likely to induce gastrointestinal and haemostatic abnormalities, they are not completely without side effects *in vivo*. The selection of a specific NSAID should take into consideration:

- The reported COX-2 selectivity
- Reported efficacy and safety in clinical trials
- Suitable dosing format
- The individual's response to the drug.

Suitable doses for use in dogs and cats are shown in Figures 9.5 and 9.6.

Drug	Dosage forms	Dose
Carprofen	Injectable: 50 mg/ml	4 mg/kg s.c.
	Capsules (not available in UK): 25, 75 and 100 mg Chewable tablets: 20, 50, 100 mg in UK (25, 75, 100 mg in USA and Canada)	UK: 2–4 mg/kg/day orally in 2 equally divided doses Dose may be reduced to 2 mg/kg/day orally as a single dose after 7 days, subject to clinical response USA and Canada: 4.4 mg/kg orally q24h or 2.2 mg/kg orally q12h
Meloxicam	Injectable: 5 mg/ml	0.2 mg/kg i.v. or s.c. on day 1, 0.1 mg/kg i.v. or s.c. on subsequent days
	Oral Suspension: 1.5 mg/ml	0.2 mg/kg orally on day 1, 0.1 mg/kg orally q24h on subsequent days
Ketoprofen	Injectable: 100 mg/ml Tablets: 5 and 20 mg	2 mg/kg i.v., i.m., s.c. or orally on day 1, followed by 1 mg/kg i.v., i.m., s.c. or orally q24h
Tolfenamic acid	Injectable: 40 mg/ml Tablets: 6, 20 and 60 mg	4 mg/kg orally or s.c. q24h for 3 days, followed by a minimum of 4 days with no administration, then repeat
Deracoxib (USA and Canada)	Chewable tablets: 25 and 100 mg	Postoperative: 3–4 mg/kg orally q24h for maximum of 7 days Chronic treatment: 1–2 mg/kg orally q24h
Etodolac (USA)	Tablets: 150, 300 and 500 mg	10–15 mg/kg orally q24h
Firocoxib	Tablets: 57 and 227 mg	5 mg/kg orally q24h
Tepoxalin	Tablets: 30, 50, 100 and 200 mg	10–20 mg/kg orally on day 1 followed by 10 mg/kg orally q24h

9.5 Non-steroidal anti-inflammatory drugs licensed for use in dogs.

Drug	Dosage forms	Dose
Carprofen	Injectable: 50 mg/ml	4 mg/kg s.c.(licensed for single dose only)
Meloxicam	Injectable: 5 mg/ml	0.1–0.2 mg/kg i.v. or s.c.(licensed for single dose only) 0.1 mg/kg orally can be administered once a day for 3–4 days, followed by 0.025 mg/kg (or total 0.1 mg per cat) orally 2–3 times a week (unlicensed use)
Ketoprofen	Injectable: 100 mg/ml	2 mg/kg s.c. single dose followed by oral administration or 2 mg/kg s.c. q12h for a maximum of 3 days
	Tablets: 5 and 20 mg	1 mg/kg orally q24h for a maximum of 5 days
Tolfenamic acid	Injectable: 40 mg/ml Tablets: 6, 20 and 60 mg	4 mg/kg orally or s.c. q24h for maximum of 3 days, followed by a minimum of 4 days with no administration, then repeat

9.6 Non-steroidal anti-inflammatory drugs licensed for use in cats.

Carprofen

Carprofen is considered to be a relatively COX-2-specific NSAID. It is licensed for use in cats and dogs in Europe, Canada and the USA. It is available as injectable and oral formulations. The injectable formulation is licensed for cats and dogs. It can be administered intravenously or subcutaneously preoperatively or postoperatively. The oral formulation is only licensed for dogs, although there are reports of use in cats. In cats and dogs the oral bioavailability of carprofen is over 90%, and peak plasma concentrations are achieved between 1 and 3 hours after administration. The plasma half-life of injectable carprofen is reported to be 10 hours in dogs. In cats, the half-life is reported to be approximately 20 hours, although considerable variability exists with a reported range of 9–49 hours. Time to onset of action following administration of injectable carprofen (intravenously) is <1 hour and its duration of action in dogs is reported to be 12–18 hours (considerably longer than most opioid analgesics).

A dose of 4.0 mg/kg i.v. has been shown to be a very effective postoperative analgesic in dogs undergoing orthopaedic and soft tissue surgery. One study evaluated its use preoperatively and postoperatively in dogs with favourable results, and preoperative administration resulted in superior postoperative analgesia compared with postoperative administration. Its efficacy in the immediate postoperative period is unlikely to be as profound as that of potent mu opioid agonists. However, carprofen (4.0 mg/kg orally) was shown to be superior to butorphanol (0.2 mg/kg i.v.) in an acute synovitis laboratory model.

Carprofen has been shown to be an effective analgesic for osteoarthritis in numerous studies and has relatively good gastrointestinal tolerance when administered to dogs for long periods of time. Although carprofen can be given orally twice a day in dogs, administration once daily may still provide adequate analgesia because of its long half-life. Hepatotoxicity has been reported in dogs following carprofen administration and a large proportion of the dogs in the study were Labrador Retrievers. However, the study did not evaluate the relative breed prevalence of dogs with adverse effects, and it is not possible to determine if true breed sensitivity exists. Data from the US Food and Drugs Administration suggest the incidence of hepatotoxicity (<0.05%) associated with carprofen is similar to that of other NSAIDs.

Clinically important alterations in renal function have not been demonstrated in dogs given carprofen prior to anaesthesia and surgery. However, maintenance of renal blood flow by optimizing fluid status, as well as ensuring adequate systemic arterial blood pressure is recommended with preoperative administration of any NSAID. Carprofen (4 mg/kg i.v. or s.c.) does not inhibit formation of thromboxane and has not been shown to have any significant effect on mucosal bleeding time in healthy dogs or in dogs requiring fracture repair.

Carprofen injectable is licensed at 4 mg/kg s.c. in cats, although it has also been shown to be effective at 2 mg/kg s.c. It is an effective postoperative analgesic, comparable to pethidine (meperidine) but with a duration of analgesia lasting approximately 20 hours. Due to its variable half-life in cats, close monitoring for toxicity should accompany long-term use (it is not licensed for chronic use in cats).

Meloxicam

Meloxicam is a COX-2-specific inhibitor available in injectable and oral liquid formulations. The parenteral formulation is licensed for use in cats and dogs in Europe, Canada and the USA. It can be administered intravenously and subcutaneously, and is used both preoperatively and postoperatively. The oral formulation is only licensed for use in dogs, although it is widely used off-label in cats because it is easy to dispense and cats find it palatable. It has a long elimination half-life in dogs (20–30 hours), and therefore is administered once a day. The reported half-life in cats is 11–21 hours following parenteral and oral administration.

Preoperative or postoperative administration at a dose of 0.2 mg/kg i.v. or s.c. has repeatedly been shown to produce effective postoperative analgesia for soft tissue and orthopaedic surgery. Similar to carprofen, the degree of analgesia in the immediate postoperative period is not as profound as that provided by pure mu opioid agonists. Analgesia from meloxicam, however, is superior to that obtained from partial agonists or mixed agonist/antagonists and meloxicam has a prolonged duration of effect. Fortunately, opioids and NSAIDs can be combined to improve overall analgesia. Studies in dogs comparing different NSAIDs have found comparable analgesia with the perioperative administration of carprofen (4.0 mg/kg s.c.) and meloxicam (0.2 mg/kg s.c.) following ovariohysterectomy. Meloxicam also performed similarly to ketoprofen in dogs following orthopaedic surgery.

No adverse effects on renal function have been demonstrated in dogs when meloxicam has been administered preoperatively, even when periods of mild hypotension were created. Also, it has not been shown to impair platelet function or lead to any haemostatic alterations when administered preoperatively.

Meloxicam is also an effective analgesic for chronic osteoarthritis. The recommended dose is 0.2 mg/kg on day 1, followed by 0.1 mg/kg once daily thereafter. It has been shown to be effective and well tolerated by dogs with osteoarthritis receiving recommended doses chronically. In one large study, the most common adverse clinical signs reported in dogs on chronic therapy included vomiting, diarrhoea and inappetance.

A dose of 0.1–0.3 mg/kg has been shown to be an effective postoperative analgesic in cats. In one study evaluating several NSAIDs, it was shown to provide good analgesia for 24 hours postoperatively, although all cats still had some incisional tenderness. A dose of 0.2–0.3 mg/kg has compared favourably to buprenorphine in cats undergoing ovariohysterectomy, or to butorphanol in cats undergoing onychectomy with or without neutering.

Most studies report a 24-hour duration of analgesia from meloxicam in dogs and cats. Although repeated administration is not licensed in cats, its continuous use has been reported. Following an initial dose of 0.1–0.2 mg/kg, 0.1 mg/kg orally can be administered once a day for 3–4 days, followed by 0.025 mg/kg (or total 0.1 mg per cat) orally 2–3 times a week. Cats should be closely monitored for adverse effects during treatment.

Ketoprofen

Ketoprofen is a non-specific COX inhibitor available in injectable and oral formulations. The injectable formulation can be administered intravenously, intramuscularly or subcutaneously. It is approved for chronic administration and for immediate postoperative use in dogs in Europe and Canada. It has a long duration of effect despite a relatively short half-life (0.5–1.5 hours) and is therefore administered once every 24 hours. It has been shown to have high oral bioavailability, with rapid absorption from the gastrointestinal tract.

A dose of 2.0 mg/kg i.v. has been shown to be an effective postoperative analgesic for dogs undergoing soft tissue and orthopaedic procedures. The quality of analgesia provided with ketoprofen is similar to that with carprofen and meloxicam in dogs. Due to its lack of COX selectivity, ketoprofen inhibits platelet aggregation and increases the incidence of gastrointestinal ulceration compared with placebo. Ketoprofen should only be administered postoperatively in patients with normal haemostatic profiles.

The dose of ketoprofen for chronic pain management should be reduced to 1.0 mg/kg once a day for dogs. These animals should be closely monitored for signs of gastrointestinal dysfunction as a relatively high rate of gastrointestinal erosions has been reported with prolonged use of this agent.

A dose of 2.0 mg/kg s.c. or i.m. has been shown in several studies to be an effective postoperative analgesic in cats. It has compared favourably to the opioids buprenorphine and oxymorphone following onychectomy, or onychectomy and neutering. As with dogs, the dose should be reduced to 1.0 mg/kg once a day for repeated treatment. Treatment should, however, be limited to a total of 5 days.

Tolfenamic acid

Tolfenamic acid is considered a specific COX-2 NSAID, although it also has anti-thromboxane activity. It is available in injectable and oral formulations and is licensed for use in cats and dogs in Europe and Canada for the treatment of postoperative and chronic pain. It is reported to have excellent antipyretic and anti-inflammatory properties, and has a long half-life in cats and dogs. Due to its antithromboxane activity, it is not recommended preoperatively or in patients with haemostatic disorders. Unfortunately, there are few clinical studies comparing its analgesic efficacy to other currently available NSAIDs. Tolfenamic acid has been shown to provide similar postoperative analgesia to carprofen, ketoprofen or meloxicam following ovariohysterectomy in cats.

Deracoxib

Deracoxib is a specific COX-2 inhibitor licensed in Canada and the USA for treatment of postoperative pain and inflammation associated with orthopaedic surgery, and for control of pain and inflammation associated with osteoarthritis in dogs. It is reported to inhibit the COX-2 enzyme irreversibly, a unique feature for this class of drug. It is currently only available in an oral formulation. It has high oral bioavailability and an elimination half-life of approximately 6 hours. Similar to other NSAIDs, because of its long duration of action, deracoxib is administered every 24 hours.

It has been shown to be an effective analgesic in an acute synovitis model in dogs. In this model, it was superior to carprofen in alleviating lameness and pain associated with synovitis. In a study evaluating pain and lameness following stifle surgery, deracoxib was also shown to reduce pain and improve range of motion. The efficacy of deracoxib compared with other NSAIDs administered postoperatively remains to be determined.

When prescribing deracoxib for chronic pain management, the recommended dose is 1–2 mg/kg orally once daily. At this dose, in dogs suffering from osteoarthritis, it has been shown to reduce lameness and improve quality of life when assessed by the owner. The most commonly reported side effects associated with chronic deracoxib administration are vomiting and diarrhoea. The recommended dose for acute postoperative pain is shown in Figure 9.5.

Etodolac
Etodolac is a selective COX-2 inhibitor available in an oral formulation. It is approved for use in dogs in the USA for treatment of inflammation and pain associated with osteoarthritis. It has an elimination half-life of approximately 14 hours and is administered once daily at a dose of 10–15 mg/kg orally. As with other NSAIDs, gastrointestinal erosions and bleeding dysfunction have been reported when doses exceed those recommended.

Firocoxib
Firocoxib is available in an oral formulation in Europe and the USA for treatment of osteoarthritis in dogs. It is one of the newly released selective COX-2 NSAIDs. The recommended dose is shown in Figure 9.5.

Tepoxalin
Tepoxalin is reported to be a COX-1, COX-2 and lipoxygenase inhibitor. It is licensed for treatment of osteoarthritis in dogs in Europe and the USA, and is available as a dissolvable tablet. As with firocoxib, this drug has only relatively recently received approval and clinical studies comparing its efficacy with other currently available NSAIDs are not yet available. The dose is shown in Figure 9.5.

Non-conventional or adjunctive analgesics

Recommended doses are shown in Figure 9.7.

Drug	Dosage forms	Dose
Gabapentin	Capsules: 100, 300 and 400 mg Tablets: 600 and 800 mg	Dog: 5–25 mg/kg orally 8qh Cat: 5–25 mg/kg orally 8qh
Ketamine	Injectable: 100 mg/ml	Dog: 0.2–4.0 mg/kg i.v. bolus followed by CRI of 2–60 µg/kg/minute Cat: 0.2–4.0 mg/kg i.v. bolus followed by CRI of 2–60 µg/kg/minute
Lidocaine	Injectable: 20 mg/ml	Dog: 1–4 mg/kg i.v. bolus followed by 1–3 mg/kg/h
Medetomidine	Injectable: 1 mg/ml	Dog: 1–5 µg/kg i.v. or i.m. or 1–5 µg/kg/h i.v. as a CRI Cat: 1–5 µg/kg i.v. or i.m. or 1–5 µg/kg/h i.v. as a CRI

9.7 Adjunctive analgesics.

Gabapentin
Gabapentin is primarily used as an anticonvulsant in humans, although it has also been shown to have analgesic properties in humans with neuropathic pain, and postoperatively following abdominal surgery. The exact mechanism of action is unclear, although it is thought to produce its clinical effects secondary to an increase in synthesis of the inhibitory neurotransmitter, gamma-aminobutyric acid (GABA). Analgesia may also be mediated through blockage of membrane calcium channels. Although no controlled clinical trials evaluating the analgesic efficacy of gabapentin exist, it is currently recommended for control of neuropathic pain in cats and dogs. In an acute pain phase or for postoperative use, it should be used in combination with other traditional analgesics such as opioids or NSAIDs. The major side effect is sedation. It does not undergo significant hepatic metabolism, but is excreted through the kidney, and therefore patients should have normal renal function. It is only available in an oral formulation and the recommended dose range is wide. Currently recommended doses range from 5–25 mg/kg orally every 8 hours. A dose of 10 mg/kg is given initially, with subsequent dose adjustments made according to the response.

Ketamine
Ketamine is a non-competitive NMDA receptor antagonist routinely used as an anaesthetic in veterinary medicine. Its analgesic properties, however, have more recently been recognized and understood. By inhibiting NMDA receptors, ketamine has been shown to reduce the activity of neurons in the spinal cord in response to nociceptive stimuli and reduce sensitization of these neurons. Other proposed mechanisms for analgesic effects include interaction at opioid receptors and/or activation of noradrenergic and serotonergic neurons.

When administered as a CRI at 10 µg/kg/minute to dogs, ketamine has been has been shown to reduce isoflurane anaesthetic requirements. In dogs presented for forelimb amputation, ketamine has been administered first as an intravenous bolus (0.5 mg/kg) followed by an intravenous infusion intraoperatively (10 µg/kg/minute), continued into the postoperative period (2 µg/kg/minute) for 18 hours. Adequate analgesia was demonstrated with no adverse side effects. These dogs also received morphine preoperatively and fentanyl postoperatively (CRI). To date, no controlled clinical studies evaluating ketamine as a postoperative analgesic have been reported. Recommended doses for conscious cats and dogs as an adjunct to traditional analgesia are a 0.2–4.0 mg/kg i.v. bolus, followed by an infusion of 2–60 µg/kg/minute based on patient response. Side effects may include dysphoria, increased blood pressure and ventricular arrhythmias.

Local anaesthetics
Local anaesthetics are routinely administered locally to block nerve conduction. When administered as an intravenous infusion, they are thought to inhibit modulatory nociceptive processing. In experimental studies, lidocaine has been shown to provide analgesia for neuropathic pain and to possess MAC reducing properties. A pilot study in dogs reported that lidocaine administered intraoperatively as an infusion provided some postoperative analgesia. Several authors also report the use of lidocaine as a CRI to control pain in dogs and cats refractory to other traditionally used analgesics. In dogs, a 1–4 mg/kg i.v. bolus followed by 1–3 mg/kg/h is suggested, while in cats recommended doses are not currently available. Nausea and vomiting are observed in awake dogs when infusion rates >4.5 mg/kg/h are given, which may limit its use. In the dog, these infusion rates have been shown to induce minimal cardiopulmonary alterations.

Alpha-2 adrenergic agonists

The alpha-2 adrenergic agonist medetomidine is licensed in the dog and cat as a sedative. However, it has potent analgesic properties that are primarily mediated via alpha-2 adrenergic receptors located in the dorsal horn of the spinal cord. These receptors modulate the release of neurotransmitters responsible for transmission of nociceptive signals to higher centres. Alpha-2 receptors located in the periphery may also play a role in the mediation of nociception. Alpha-2 adrenergic agonists also have effects on the cardiovascular system such as increased systemic vascular resistance and, therefore, increased systemic arterial blood pressure. Decreased heart rate occurs from increased vagal tone (triggered by increased blood pressure). Cardiac output is decreased as a result of reduced myocardial contractility, reduced heart rate and increased systemic vascular resistance. In patients where sedative and cardiopulmonary effects are not clinically significant, low doses of medetomidine can be administered either as a bolus (1–5 μg/kg i.v. or i.m.) or as an intravenous infusion (1–5 μg/kg/h) for pain refractory to other analgesics.

References and further reading

Bergmann HM, Nolte IJ and Kramer S (2005) Effects of preoperative administration of carprofen on renal function and hemostasis in dogs undergoing surgery for fracture repair. *American Journal of Veterinary Research* **66**, 1356–1363

Booth DA (2001) Control of pain in small animals: opioid agonists and antagonists and other locally and centrally acting analgesics. In: *Small Animal Clinical Pharmacology and Therapeutics*, ed. DA Booth, pp. 405–424. WB Saunders Company, Philadelphia

Borer LR, Peel JE, Seewald W, Schawalder P and Spreng DE (2003) Effect of carprofen, etodolac, meloxicam, or butorphanol in dogs with induced acute synovitis. *American Journal of Veterinary Research* **64**, 1429–1437

Brodbelt DC, Taylor PM and Stanway GW (1997) A comparison of preoperative morphine and buprenorphine for postoperative analgesia for arthrotomy in dogs. *Journal of Veterinary Pharmacology and Therapeutics* **20**, 284–289

Carroll GL, Howe LB and Peterson KD (2005) Analgesic efficacy of preoperative administration of meloxicam or butorphanol in onychectomized cats. *Journal of the American Veterinary Medical Association* **226**, 913–919

Caulkett N, Read M, Fowler D and Waldner C (2003) A comparison of the analgesic effects of butorphanol with those of meloxicam after elective ovariohysterectomy in dogs. *The Canadian Veterinary Journal* **44**, 565–570

Davidson CD, Pettifer GR and Henry JD (2004) Plasma fentanyl concentrations and analgesic effects during full or partial exposure to transdermal fentanyl patches in cats. *Journal of the American Veterinary Medical Association* **224**, 700–705

Dobbins S, Brown NO and Shoefer FS (2002) Comparison of the effects of buprenorphine, oxymorphone hydrochloride, and ketoprofen for postoperative analgesia after onychectomy or onychectomy and sterilization in cats. *Journal of the American Animal Hospital Association* **38**, 507–514

Dyson DH, Doherty T, Anderson GI and McDonell WN (1990) Reversal of oxymorphone sedation by naloxone, nalmefene, and butorphanol. *Veterinary Surgery* **19**, 398–403

Gassel AD, Tobias KM, Egger CM and Rohrback BM (2005) Comparison of oral and subcutaneous administration of buprenorphine and meloxicam for pre-emptive analgesia in cats undergoing ovariohysterectomy. *Journal of the American Veterinary Medical Association* **227**, 1937–1944

Karnik PS, Johnston S, Ward D, Broadstone R and Inzana K (2006) The effects of epidural deracoxib on the ground reaction forces in an acute stifle synovitis model. *Veterinary Surgery* **35**, 34–42

Kukanich B, Lascelles BDX and Papich MG (2005) Pharmacokinetics of morphine and plasma concentrations of morphine-6-glucuronide following morphine administration to dogs. *Journal of Veterinary Pharmacology and Therapeutics* **28**, 371–376

Kyles AE, Hardie EM and Hansen BD (1998) Comparison of transdermal fentanyl and intramuscular oxymorphone on post-operative behaviour after ovariohysterectomy in dogs. *Research in Veterinary Science* **65**, 245–251

Lascelles BD, Cripps PJ, Jones A and Waterman-Pearson AE (1998) Efficacy and kinetics of carprofen, administered preoperatively or postoperatively, for the prevention of pain in dogs undergoing ovariohysterectomy. *Veterinary Surgery* **27**, 568–582

Lascelles BD and Roberston SA (2004) Antinociceptive effects of hydromorphone, butorphanol, or the combination in cats. *Journal of Veterinary Internal Medicine* **18**, 190–195

Lucas AN, Firth AM, Anderson GA, Vine JH and Edwards GA (2001) Comparison of the effects of morphine administered by constant rate intravenous infusion or intermittent intramuscular injection in dogs. *Journal of the American Veterinary Medical Association* **218**, 884–891

MacPhail CM, Lappin MR, Meyer DJ *et al.* (1998) Hepatocellular toxicosis associated with administration of carprofen in 21 dogs. *Journal of the American Veterinary Medical Association* **212**, 1895–1901

Mastrocinque S and Fantoni DT (2003) A comparison of preoperative tramadol and morphine for the control of early postoperative pain in canine ovariohysterectomy. *Veterinary Anaesthesia and Analgesia* **30**, 220–228

Mathews KA (2000) *The Veterinary Clinics of North America Small Animal Practice: Management of Pain.* WB Saunders Company, Philadelphia

Mathews KA, Paley DM, Foster RA, Valliant AE and Young SS (1996) A comparison of ketorolac with flunixin, butorphanol, and oxymorphone in controlling postoperative pain in dogs. *The Canadian Veterinary Journal* **37(9)**, 557–567

McCann ME, Andersen DR, Zhang D *et al.* (2004) In vitro effects and in vitro efficacy of a novel cyclooxygenase-2 inhibitor in dogs with experimentally induced synovitis. *American Journal of Veterinary Research* **65(4)**, 503–512

Millis DL, Weigel JP, Moyers T and Buonomo FC (2002) Effect of deracoxib, a new COX-2 inhibitor, on the prevention of lameness induced by chemical synovitis in dogs. *Veterinary Therapeutics* **3(4)**, 453–464

Polis I, Moens Y, Gauthuys F, Hoenben D and Tshamala M (2004) Antinociceptive and sedative effects of sufentanil long-acting during and after sevoflurane anaesthesia in dogs. *Journal of Veterinary Medicine* **51**, 242–248

Robertson SA (2005) Assessment and management of acute pain in cats. *Journal of Veterinary Emergency and Critical Care* **15(4)**, 261–272

Robertson SA, Lascelles BDX, Taylor PM and Sear JW (2005) PK-PD modeling of buprenorphine in cats: intravenous and oral transmucosal administration. *Journal of Veterinary Pharmacology and Therapeutics* **28**, 453–460

Robertson SA, Taylor PM and Sear JW (2003) Systemic uptake of buprenorphine by cats after oral mucosal administration. *Veterinary Record* **152**, 675–678

Robinson TM, Kruse-Elliot KT, Markel MD *et al.* (1999) A comparison of transdermal fentanyl versus epidural morphine for analgesia in dogs undergoing major orthopedic surgery. *Journal of the American Animal Hospital Association* **35**, 95–100

Sawyer DC and Rech RH (1987) Analgesia and behavioral effects of butorphanol, nalbuphine and pentazocine in the cat. *Journal of the American Animal Hospital Association* **23**, 438–446

Skingle M and Tyers MB (1980) Further studies on opiate receptors that mediate antinociception: tooth pulp stimulation in the dog. *British Journal of Pharmacology* **70**, 323–327

Slingsby LS and Waterman-Pearson AE (2000) Postoperative analgesia in the cat after ovariohysterectomy by use of carprofen, ketoprofen, meloxicam or tolfenamic acid. *Journal of Small Animal Practice* **41**, 447–450

Slingsby LS and Waterman-Pearson AE (2002) Comparison between meloxicam and carprofen for postoperative analgesia after feline ovariohysterectomy. *Journal of Small Animal Practice* **43**, 286–289

Smith LJ, Bentley E, Shih A and Miller PE (2004) Systemic lidocaine infusion as an analgesic for intraocular surgery in dogs: a pilot study. *Veterinary Anaesthesia and Analgesia* **31**, 53–63

Stanway GW, Taylor PM and Brodbelt DC (2002) A preliminary investigation comparing preoperative morphine and buprenorphine for post-operative analgesia. *Veterinary Anaesthesia and Analgesia* **29**, 29–35

Stobie D, Caywood DD, Rozanski EA *et al.* (1995) Evaluation of pulmonary function and analgesia in dogs after intercostal thoracotomy and use of morphine administered intramuscularly or intrapleurally and bupivacaine administered intrapleurally. *American Journal of Veterinary Research* **56**, 1098–1109

Trepanier LA (2005) Potential interactions between non-steroidal anti-inflammatory drugs and other drugs. *Journal of Veterinary Emergency and Critical Care* **15(4)**, 248–253

Wagner AE, Walton JA, Hellyer PW, Gaynor JS and Mama KR (2002) Use of low doses of ketamine administered by constant rate infusion as an adjunct for postoperative analgesia in dogs. *Journal of the American Veterinary Medical Association* **221**, 72–75

10

Pain management II: local and regional anaesthetic techniques

Kip A. Lemke

Introduction

Local and regional anaesthetic techniques are gaining widespread acceptance in the management of perioperative pain in both cats and dogs. In recent years, a clearer understanding of the pathophysiology of perioperative pain has provided the conceptual framework for a more rational use of these techniques. Surgical trauma and inflammation produce sensitization of the peripheral nervous system, and the subsequent barrage of nociceptive input produces sensitization of neurons in the dorsal horn of the spinal cord. Because local and regional anaesthetic techniques are the only analgesic techniques that produce complete blockade of peripheral nociceptive input, they are the most effective way to prevent sensitization of the central nervous system (CNS) and the development of pathological pain.

The neuroendocrine or stress response to surgical trauma compromises haemostatic, metabolic and immunological function, which increases perioperative morbidity and mortality. Preoperative use of local and regional anaesthetic techniques, in particular epidural techniques, attenuates the neuroendocrine response and dramatically reduces the incidence of major complications in human patients. Preoperative use of these techniques also reduces inhalant anaesthetic requirements and autonomic responses to noxious surgical stimuli. These reductions improve cardiopulmonary function intraoperatively, and facilitate a rapid smooth recovery from anaesthesia postoperatively.

Local and regional anaesthetic techniques are often used perioperatively in combination with opioids, alpha-2 adrenergic agonists, dissociative anaesthetics and anti-inflammatory drugs as part of a multimodal strategy to manage pain. They can be easily incorporated into anaesthetic and pain management plans for dogs and cats undergoing most types of surgical procedure. Branches of the maxillary and inferior alveolar nerves can be blocked in patients undergoing dental procedures. The brachial plexus and more distal nerves of the thoracic limb can be blocked in patients undergoing forelimb procedures. Intercostal nerves can be blocked in patients undergoing thoracic procedures, and lumbar nerves can be blocked by epidural administration of local anaesthetics in patients undergoing abdominal and hindlimb procedures. A clear understanding of the clinical pharmacology of local anaesthetics, as well as relevant canine and feline anatomy, is required to use these techniques safely and effectively.

Clinical pharmacology

Chemistry

Local anaesthetics are weak bases that are classified as aminoesters (procaine) or aminoamides (lidocaine, bupivacaine). All local anaesthetics have an aromatic group that is connected to a tertiary amine group by either an ester or an amide linkage. As a general rule, the structure of the aromatic group determines the lipid solubility of the drug, while the structure of the tertiary amine group determines the water solubility of the drug. At physiological pH (7.4), the tertiary amine group readily accepts protons, and local anaesthetic molecules exist in equilibrium as a neutral, lipid-soluble base, and a positively charged, water-soluble acid. The dissociation constant, or pKa, is the pH at which concentrations of neutral base and positively charged acid are equal. Most local anaesthetics have pKa values in the 7.5–8.5 range. As the pKa value decreases, a greater fraction of the drug exists as neutral base, more molecules penetrate lipid membranes and the onset of action tends to be more rapid. Conversely, as the pKa value increases, a greater fraction of the drug exists as positively charged acid, fewer molecules penetrate lipid membranes and the onset of action tends to be slower.

Mechanism of action

Peripheral nerves are composed of different types of myelinated (Aα, Aβ, Aγ, Aδ) and unmyelinated (C) nerve fibres that are surrounded by connective tissue sheaths. Local anaesthetics are injected near peripheral nerves and the drug must penetrate these connective tissue sheaths before reaching the neuronal membranes. Diffusion of local anaesthetics away from the injection site is a function of tissue binding and uptake into the systemic circulation. Local anaesthetics block the generation and conduction of nerve impulses by inhibiting voltage-gated sodium channels in neuronal membranes. The binding site for local anaesthetics is located on the cytoplasmic or intracellular surface of the sodium channel. The neutral base must diffuse across the lipid membrane and dissociate from the membrane to gain access to this site. Once inside the cell, the tertiary amine group is protonated and the charged acid binds to the sodium channel. Local anaesthetics stabilize inactive conformational states of the sodium channel and delay reactivation of the channel rather than physically blocking the pore. Only moderately lipid-soluble local anaesthetics with pKa values close to the physiological pH can penetrate connective tissue sheaths and neuronal membranes, gain access to the cytoplasmic binding site and inactivate sodium channels.

The onset and duration of local anaesthetic blockade differs by anatomical location, fibre type and frequency of stimulation. As a general rule, fibres innervating more proximal regions are located more superficially in peripheral nerve bundles than those innervating more distal regions. Consequently, local anaesthetics penetrate superficial nerve fibres first and proximal areas are blocked sooner than more distal areas. Fibre type also influences the onset and duration of local anaesthetic blockade. The conventional understanding has been that small sensory fibres, specifically myelinated (Aδ) and unmyelinated (C) nociceptive fibres, are blocked before larger sensory (Aβ) and motor (Aα) fibres. However, recent experimental evidence shows that small unmyelinated (C) fibres are more resistant to local anaesthetic blockade than previously thought, and are blocked after larger sensory and motor fibres. Based on these findings, it appears that nociceptive transmission mediated by unmyelinated C fibres can persist even after motor blockade has been established. Frequency of stimulation also influences the onset of local anaesthetic blockade. Nociceptive fibres from areas of tissue trauma discharge at higher rates than those in normal tissue, and are more susceptible to local anaesthetic blockade than other types of fibres. This increase in susceptibility at high discharge rates is called use-dependent or frequency-dependent blockade.

Absorption and metabolism

Systemic absorption of local anaesthetics is determined by dose, volume and route of administration. Absorption from mucosal, pleural and peritoneal surfaces is rapid and complete, and peak plasma concentrations are reached within 10 minutes. Plasma concentrations achieved after interpleural or intercostal administration are comparable to those achieved after intravenous administration. Local anaesthetics are also absorbed quickly from epidural injection sites and peak plasma concentrations are reached in approximately 30 minutes. Absorption from subcutaneous sites is slower and peak plasma concentrations are approximately half those achieved after interpleural or intercostal administration.

Binding to tissue proteins and vascularity of the injection site also influences systemic absorption of local anaesthetic drugs. Moderately lipid-soluble drugs (e.g. lidocaine) do not bind extensively to tissue proteins and are rapidly absorbed, while highly lipid-soluble drugs (e.g. bupivacaine) bind extensively to tissue proteins and are more slowly absorbed. All commonly used local anaesthetics cause vasodilation, which accelerates systemic absorption of the drug. Vasoconstrictors (adrenaline) can be added to local anaesthetic solutions to delay absorption and reduce systemic toxicity, but they can also cause localized ischaemia. Vasoconstrictors are added to prolong the duration of action of short-acting drugs (e.g. lidocaine), but they have little effect on the duration of action of long-acting drugs (e.g. bupivacaine). Given the potential for localized ischaemia as well as the availability of long-acting local anaesthetics with inherently slow systemic absorption, the addition of vasoconstrictors to local anaesthetic solutions has limited clinical utility.

Once absorbed into the systemic circulation, local anaesthetics bind reversibly to plasma proteins (α-1 acid glycoprotein, albumin) and red blood cells. The degree of tissue and protein binding influences the onset and duration of action, as well as the toxicity of local anaesthetic drugs. Aminoesters tend to be less lipid-soluble and protein-bound, and tend to have a faster onset and shorter duration of action. Conversely, aminoamides tend to be more lipid-soluble and protein-bound, and tend to have a slower onset and longer duration of action. Consequently, doses of local anaesthetics, especially aminoamides, should be calculated carefully for patients with significant anaemia or hypoproteinaemia.

Aminoesters and aminoamides are metabolized by distinctly different pathways and at very different rates. Aminoesters are rapidly hydrolysed by tissue and plasma esterases, and metabolites are excreted by the kidneys. Aminoamides are metabolized primarily in the liver by cytochrome P450 enzymes at a relatively slow rate. The major routes of hepatic metabolism are hydroxylation, *N*-dealkylation and hydrolysis, with subsequent elimination of metabolites by the kidneys. Some metabolism of the aminoamides also occurs extrahepatically in the lungs and kidneys. Consequently, doses of aminoamides should be calculated carefully for patients with advanced liver disease to avoid toxic plasma concentrations associated with hypoproteinaemia and delayed metabolism.

Local and systemic toxicity

Local anaesthetics are relatively safe drugs if they are used with reasonable care. Dosage calculations should be based on lean bodyweight, and total doses should be calculated carefully to avoid systemic toxicity – especially in small patients (<5 kg). Administration of an incorrect dose and inadvertent intravascular administration are probably the most common causes of systemic toxicity in dogs and cats. Interpleural or intercostal administration of large doses is also a potential cause of systemic toxicity. Recently, mixtures of lidocaine and bupivacaine have become popular for some local anaesthetic techniques. Unfortunately, toxicity of local anaesthetics is additive, and administration of lidocaine–bupivacaine mixtures produces little change in onset time and a significant decrease in duration of action when compared with administration of bupivacaine alone. Most commonly used local anaesthetic solutions also cause some degree of local tissue irritation, and inappropriate administration of concentrated solutions consistently causes local tissue toxicity and nerve damage. Aminoesters have the potential to cause allergic reactions but they are used infrequently in veterinary medicine. Conversely, allergic reactions to aminoamide local anaesthetics are extremely rare, although some preservatives (methylparaben) can cause allergic reactions.

Concentrated local anaesthetic solutions produce local tissue irritation and are directly neurotoxic. Application of 5% lidocaine to peripheral nerves causes irreversible conduction block within minutes. Even standard concentrations of commonly used local anaesthetics (2% lidocaine) produce localized tissue irritation and significant histological changes. Because of the tissue damage associated with administration of standard concentrations of most local anaesthetic solutions, regional blockade of nerves proximal to the surgical field is preferred to local infiltration of tissues within the field. Dilution of local anaesthetics at the site of injection also plays an important role in reducing local tissue toxicity, and some preservatives (sodium bisulphite) used in local anaesthetic solutions are potentially neurotoxic. Consequently, only low concentrations (2% lidocaine, 0.5% bupivacaine) of preservative-free local anaesthetic solutions should be administered by the intrathecal or epidural route.

In cats and dogs, the relative potency and systemic toxicity of bupivacaine are approximately four times those of lidocaine. As a result, a 0.5% solution of bupivacaine is equivalent to a 2% solution of lidocaine in terms of both potency and toxicity. Systemic reactions to local anaesthetics involve primarily the CNS, but the cardiovascular system can be affected if very large doses are given (Figure 10.1). Initial signs of CNS toxicity include sedation, disorientation and ataxia. Muscle tremors, convulsions and respiratory depression can occur after administration of large doses. The intravenous dose of lidocaine that produces convulsions in cats (12 mg/kg) is approximately 40% lower than that in dogs (20.8–22.0 mg/kg), while the intravenous dose of bupivacaine that produces convulsions in cats (3.8 mg/kg) is only 20% lower than that in dogs (4.3–5.0 mg/kg). Initial signs of CNS toxicity (sedation, ataxia) become apparent after administration of approximately half of the convulsive dose. Furthermore, moderate respiratory acidosis (P_aCO_2 = 60–80 mmHg (8–10.7 kPa)) increases cerebral blood flow and the proportion of free drug available for diffusion across neuronal membranes, and decreases the convulsive dose of lidocaine and bupivacaine by approximately 50%. As a result, adequate ventilatory support, in addition to anticonvulsant therapy, is critically important in the management of systemic toxicity.

Clinical signs of cardiovascular toxicity occur at doses that are approximately four times higher than those required to produce CNS toxicity (see Figure 10.1). Local anaesthetics produce direct effects on the heart and blood vessels, and indirect effects mediated by blockade of the autonomic nervous system. Toxic doses of local anaesthetics depress myocardial contractility, and cause peripheral vasodilation and profound hypotension. Conduction abnormalities and arrhythmias are rarely observed after administration of large doses of short-acting local anaesthetics (e.g. lidocaine, mepivacaine). However, administration of large doses of long-acting local anaesthetics (e.g. bupivacaine) can produce ventricular arrhythmias and cardiovascular collapse in cats and dogs. New long-acting local anaesthetics (e.g. ropivacaine, levobupivacaine) have recently been developed, and these drugs appear to be slightly less cardiotoxic than bupivacaine at equipotent doses.

A summary of the clinical pharmacology of selected aminoamide local anaesthetic drugs is given in Figure 10.2.

Drug	CNS toxic dose (convulsions)	CV toxic dose (ventricular tachycardia and fibrillation)	CV/CNS toxicity ratio	Comments
Lidocaine Cat (Chadwick, 1985) Dog (Liu *et al.*, 1982, 1983; Feldman *et al.*, 1989)	 11.7 mg/kg i.v. 22.0 mg/kg i.v. 20.8 mg/kg i.v.	 47.3 mg/kg i.v. 76.2 mg/kg i.v.	 4.0 3.5	The total dose of lidocaine should not exceed 6–8 mg/kg in healthy cats and dogs. For example, a healthy 3 kg cat should not be given more than 1 ml of the 2% (20 mg/ml) solution or 0.2 ml of the 10% (100 mg/ml) spray Ventricular tachycardia and fibrillation occur at doses that are approximately ten times those used clinically and four times those that produce convulsions
Mepivacaine Dog (Liu *et al.*, 1982)		 80.4 mg/kg i.v.		CNS and CV toxicity are comparable to lidocaine
Bupivacaine Cat (Chadwick, 1985) Dog (Liu *et al.*, 1982, 1983; Feldman *et al.*, 1989)	 3.8 mg/kg i.v. 5.0 mg/kg i.v. 4.3 mg/kg i.v.	 18.4 mg/kg i.v. 20.4 mg/kg i.v.	 4.8 4.1	The total dose of bupivacaine should not exceed 1.5–2.0 mg/kg in healthy cats and dogs. For example, a healthy 3 kg cat should not be given more than 1 ml of the 0.5% (5 mg/ml) solution Ventricular tachycardia and fibrillation occur at doses that are approximately ten times those used clinically and four times those that produce convulsions
Ropivacaine Dog (Feldman *et al.*, 1989)	 4.9 mg/kg i.v.			CNS and CV toxicity are comparable to bupivacaine at equipotent doses

10.1 Central nervous system (CNS) and cardiovascular (CV) toxicity of aminoamide local anaesthetic drugs.

Drug	pKa	Protein binding (%)	Onset time (minute)	Duration of action (hours)	Relative potency (lidocaine = 1)	Indications	Formulations	Comments
Lidocaine	7.7	55–65	5–15	1–2	1	Topical Local infiltration Peripheral and central (epidural) neural blockade	2% (20 mg/ml) solution 10% (100 mg/ml) topical spray	Used in cats and dogs for a wide variety of minor surgical and diagnostic procedures The 2% solution is approved for use in cats and dogs in Canada, the UK and the USA
Mepivacaine	7.6	75–80	5–15	1.5–2.5	1	Local infiltration Peripheral and central (epidural) neural blockade	2% (20 mg/ml) solution	Used in cats and dogs for a wide variety of minor surgical and diagnostic procedures Approved for use in dogs in Canada
Bupivacaine	8.1	85–95	10–20	4–6	4	Local infiltration Peripheral and central (epidural) neural blockade	0.5% (5 mg/ml) solutions with and without preservative	Used perioperatively in cats and dogs for a variety of major surgical procedures Not approved for use in animals
Levobupivacaine	8.1	97	10–20	4–6	4	Local infiltration Peripheral and central (epidural) neural blockade	0.5% (5 mg/ml) solution without preservative	Not approved for use in animals
Ropivacaine	8.1	94	10–20	3–5	3	Local infiltration Peripheral and central (epidural) neural blockade	0.75% (7.5 mg/ml) solution without preservative	Not approved for use in animals

10.2 Pharmacology of aminoamide local anaesthetic drugs.

General techniques

Local and regional anaesthetic techniques are usually safer and easier to perform in cats and dogs that have been sedated or anaesthetized. Patients are easier to position, anatomical landmarks are easier to identify, specific nerves and blood vessels are easier to isolate and needle placement is more precise and less traumatic. Healthy cats and dogs can be sedated with acepromazine–opioid or medetomidine–opioid combinations, and fractious cats can be immobilized with low doses of ketamine. In anaesthetized patients, local and regional anaesthetic techniques are usually performed shortly after induction of anaesthesia and at least 10–20 minutes before the start of surgical, dental or diagnostic procedures.

A clear three-dimensional understanding of relevant anatomical landmarks and the location of nerves, vessels and anatomical spaces is required to perform local and regional anaesthetic techniques in a safe and effective manner. Many superficial nerves can be easily palpated, and others can be located by identifying specific anatomical landmarks. Often, traditional anatomy texts provide the best descriptions and illustrations to review anatomical landmarks and the location of specific nerves and blood vessels.

Topical anaesthesia

Topical application of local anaesthetics is used primarily for minor surgical procedures, and to facilitate placement of endotracheal tubes, nasal oxygen lines and urinary catheters. Most local anaesthetic solutions will not penetrate intact skin, and high concentrations are required to penetrate and desensitize mucous membranes. Lidocaine spray (5–10%, 50–100 mg/ml; 2% in the UK) can be used to desensitize oral, nasal and urogenital mucous membranes in most patients. However, systemic toxicity can be a problem in small patients (<5 kg) if the spray is not applied carefully. Topical application (splash blocks) of standard concentrations of lidocaine (2%) or bupivacaine (0.5%) to abraded or cut skin is ineffective. Splash blocks before incision closure are essentially subcutaneous injections with significant drug loss and may not be effective. In human paediatric patients, mucous membranes and abraded or cut skin are desensitized with a mixture of lidocaine (4%, 40 mg/ml), adrenaline (0.0005%, 5 μg/ml) and tetracaine (0.5%, 5 mg/ml), but this mixture has not been used widely in veterinary medicine. A eutectic mixture of lidocaine (2.5%, 25 mg/ml) and prilocaine (2.5%, 25 mg/ml) can be used to desensitize intact skin, but the mixture must be applied under an occlusive dressing for 60 minutes.

Infiltration anaesthesia

Infiltration of local anaesthetics can be used to desensitize dermal and subcutaneous tissues for minor diagnostic and surgical procedures. After aseptic preparation of the skin, local anaesthetic solution is injected as a subcutaneous bleb to desensitize small areas, or in a linear, triangular or rectangular pattern to desensitize larger areas. The needle should always be withdrawn to a point just below the dermis before it is redirected. Attempting to redirect without first withdrawing the needle simply bends the needle and causes unnecessary tissue trauma. When large areas need to be desensitized, the potential for systemic toxicity should be considered, and local anaesthetic solutions diluted if necessary.

Interpleural anaesthesia

Local anaesthetics can be administered interpleurally through chest tubes or specialized catheters. The interpleural technique has been very popular in veterinary and human medicine in recent years, and is easy to perform in conscious patients once a chest tube or catheter has been placed. However, the quality of analgesia is variable and the efficacy of the technique for post-thoracotomy pain has been questioned in human medicine. Further, uptake of local anaesthetics from the pleural space into the systemic circulation is rapid, plasma concentrations are extremely high, and the risk of systemic toxicity (convulsions) is considerable. Given these findings, the clinical efficacy and toxicity of interpleural administration of local anaesthetics needs to be more critically evaluated in veterinary patients. Local anaesthetic solution is administered through a chest tube or interpleural catheter using aseptic technique with the patient positioned 'incision side down' for 10 minutes. The block can be performed with either 2% lidocaine or 0.5% bupivacaine, and the total dose of local anaesthetic should be calculated carefully to avoid systemic toxicity.

Intra-articular anaesthesia

Intra-articular anaesthesia is used infrequently in cats and dogs. The technique has been used for stifle surgery (cruciate repair) in recent years and is relatively easy to perform. Local anaesthetic solution is administered intra-articularly after closure of the stifle joint and before closure of the skin. Intra-articular administration of bupivacaine appears to improve analgesia for several hours postoperatively. The stifle joint can be blocked in most patients by placing a 22 gauge (0.7 mm) needle aseptically into the joint on either side of the patellar tendon and administering a total dose of 1–2 ml of 2% lidocaine or 0.5% bupivacaine. The potential for local tissue toxicity should be considered before using this technique, and the total dose of local anaesthetic should be calculated carefully to avoid systemic toxicity.

Intravenous regional anaesthesia

Intravenous regional anaesthesia is rarely used in cats and dogs. Although the technique is relatively easy to perform, a large amount of local anaesthetic is required and the risk of systemic toxicity is high. For this reason, the use of intravenous regional anaesthesia should be avoided in small patients (<5 kg). Techniques that selectively block specific nerves are usually safer and more effective for most patients than intravenous regional techniques.

Peripheral neural blockade

Guidelines for peripheral neural blockade are as follows:

- Identify key anatomical landmarks
- Note the location of blood vessels that lie in close proximity to target nerves
- Use aseptic and atraumatic technique
- Aspirate syringes before injections are made to avoid inadvertent intravascular administration
- Calculate the total dose of local anaesthetic carefully for each patient to avoid systemic toxicity
- Base total dose calculations on lean bodyweight, not on actual bodyweight
- Dilution of standard solutions to 1% lidocaine or 0.25% bupivacaine may be required for cats and small dogs.

Techniques in the dog

Cranial nerves: Selective blockade of the *maxillary and mandibular branches of the trigeminal nerve* can be used for a variety of surgical and dental procedures (Figure 10.3). Most nerves can be blocked by injecting 0.5–1 ml of 2% lidocaine or 0.5% bupivacaine using a 22 gauge (0.7 mm), 1 inch (2.5 cm) needle.

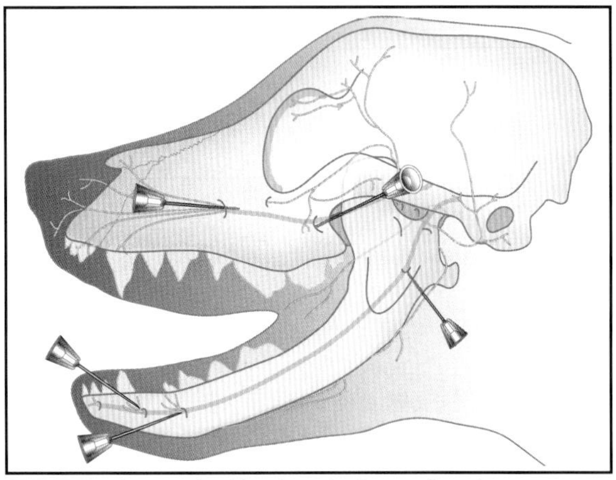

10.3 Anatomical landmarks for performing maxillary, infraorbital, inferior alveolar and mental nerve blocks in dogs.

The *maxillary nerve* and its branches provide sensory innervation to the upper dental arcade, soft and hard palates and muzzle. The maxillary nerve is blocked proximally before it enters the infraorbital canal by inserting a needle under the rostral portion of the zygomatic arch, and directing it towards the maxillary foramen. The infraorbital nerve provides sensory innervation to the rostral portion of the maxilla. The nerve is blocked by palpating the infraorbital foramen, inserting a needle transorally or transcutaneously above the third premolar, and directing it towards the infraobital foramen.

The *mandibular nerve* and its branches provide sensory innervation to the lower dental arcade, tongue and chin. The inferior alveolar nerve can be blocked proximally before it enters the mandibular foramen on the medial surface of the mandible just rostral to the angular process. The foramen and nerve are easily palpated from inside the mouth on the medial surface of the mandible. The nerve is blocked by inserting a needle transcutaneously below the rostral portion of the angular process and directing it towards the foramen along the medial surface of the mandible. The nerve can also be blocked distally as it exits the mental foramina.

Chronic otitis externa is an extremely painful condition that often requires aggressive medical and surgical intervention. Blockade of the *auriculotemporal (mandibular) nerve* and *great auricular nerve (cervical nerve II)* can be used to facilitate medical and surgical procedures involving the inner surface of the auricular cartilage and the external ear canal (Figure 10.4). The *auriculotemporal nerve* is blocked by inserting a needle rostral to the vertical ear canal, and directing it towards the base of the 'V' formed by the caudal aspect of the zygomatic arch and the vertical canal. The *great auricular nerve* is blocked by inserting a needle ventral to the wing of the atlas and caudal to the vertical ear canal, and directing it parallel to the vertical canal.

Cervical and thoracic nerves: Selective blockade of cervical and thoracic nerves can be used for surgical procedures involving the forelimb and thorax. Most nerves can be blocked by injecting 1–3 ml of 2% lidocaine or 0.5% bupivacaine using a 22 gauge (0.7 mm), 1 inch (2.5 cm) needle. Particular attention should be paid to the location of major blood vessels that lie in close proximity to the brachial plexus as well as the intercostal nerves.

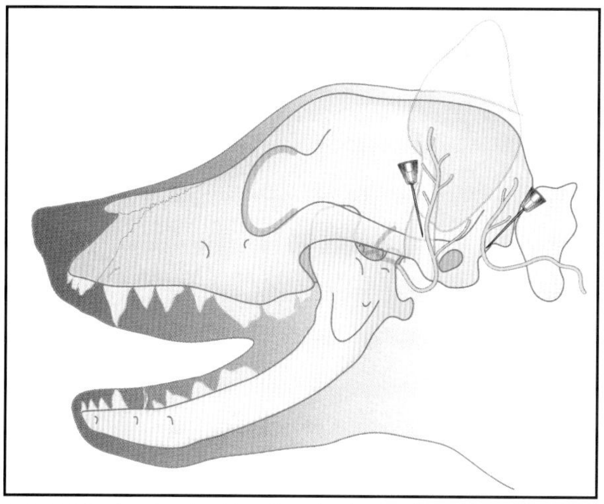

10.4 Anatomical landmarks for performing auriculotemporal and great auricular nerve blocks in dogs.

Blockade of the nerves of the brachial plexus can be used to manage perioperative pain associated with forelimb injuries and fractures (Figure 10.5). The block has traditionally been performed by injecting local anaesthetic into the axillary space at the level of the shoulder (similar to the technique for the cat shown in Figure 10.10). Although this technique is relatively easy to perform, large amounts of local anaesthetic solution are required, the shoulder and proximal humerus are not anaesthetized, and incomplete blockade is relatively common. An alternative technique, the *paravertebral brachial plexus* block, has been used at the Atlantic Veterinary College for several years. The nerves of the brachial plexus (C6, C7, C8, T1) are blocked as close as possible to their respective intervertebral foramina rather than in the axillary space. To perform the paravertebral block, the scapula is shifted caudally to expose the large transverse process of the sixth cervical vertebra and the first rib. Ventral branches of C6 and C7 are blocked as they cross the dorsal surface of the transverse process of the sixth cervical vertebra by inserting a needle dorsal to the process, and directing it towards the cranial and caudal margins, respectively. Ventral branches of C8 and T1 are blocked at their juncture on the lateral surface of the first rib by directing the needle to the cranial and also ventral border of the dorsal part of the first rib, close to the articulation with the vertebra. When blocking the ventral branches of C6 and C7, the needle should be directed caudally to avoid epidural or intrathecal administration. The vertebral artery and branches of the costocervical artery run in close proximity to the nerves as they exit intervertebral foramina and care should be taken to avoid intravascular injection. Unilateral blockade of the phrenic nerve and hemiparalysis of the diaphragm can occur with either the axillary or paravertebral technique, and these blocks should not be performed bilaterally. Pneumothorax is also a potential complication with both techniques.

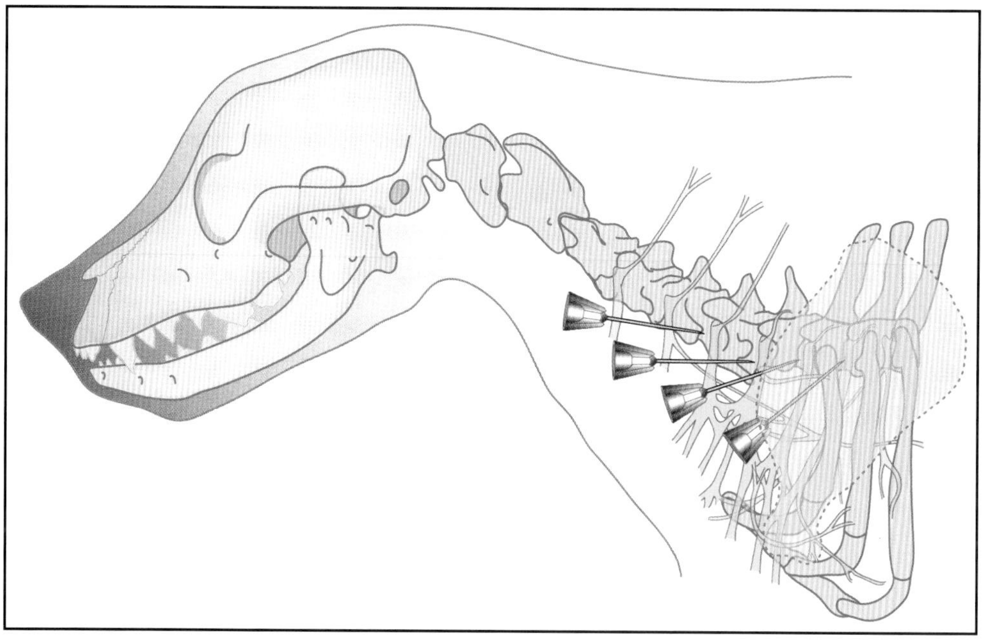

10.5 Anatomical landmarks for performing paravertebral blockade of the brachial plexus in dogs (dotted line shows normal anatomical position).

Perioperative pain associated with injuries or fractures distal to the elbow can be managed by selectively blocking the *radial*, *ulnar*, *median* and *musculocutaneous nerves* (RUMM block) (Figure 10.6). The *radial nerve* is blocked by inserting a needle proximal to the lateral epicondyle of the humerus and directing it between the brachialis and the lateral head of the triceps. The radial nerve can be palpated between these muscles over the distal third of the humeral shaft. The *ulnar*, *median* and *musculocutaneous nerves* are blocked by inserting a needle proximal to the medial epicondyle of the humerus and directing it between the biceps brachii and the medial head of the triceps. Pulsation of the brachial artery can be used to locate these nerves, and they can be palpated between these muscles over the distal third of the humerus. Because of the proximity of the brachial artery and vein, care should be taken to avoid intravascular injection.

Intercostal nerve blocks can be used to manage pain in animals with fractured ribs, or to manage perioperative pain in patients undergoing lateral thoracotomy (Figure 10.7). Intercostal nerves and vessels lie adjacent to the caudal border of each rib, and two or three nerves on either side of the fracture or incision site must be blocked. Needles are inserted distal to the angle of the rib near the insertions of the epaxial (longissimus, iliocostalis) muscles, and are directed dorsally along the caudal border of each rib. Pneumothorax can occur if the needle enters the interpleural space, and patients should be watched closely for 20–30 minutes after performing the block.

Lumbar and sacral nerves: Selective blockade of lumbar and sacral nerves can be used for surgical procedures involving the hindlimb. Most nerves can be blocked by injecting 1–2 ml of 2% lidocaine or 0.5% bupivacaine using a 22 gauge (0.7 mm), 1 inch (2.5 cm) needle.

Perioperative pain associated with injuries and fractures distal to the stifle can be managed by selectively blocking the *saphenous*, *common peroneal* and *tibial nerves* (Figure 10.8). The *saphenous nerve* is a branch of the femoral nerve, and runs through the femoral triangle on the medial surface of the thigh. The nerve lies cranial to the femoral artery and vein, and pulsation of the artery can be used to facilitate correct placement of the needle. The saphenous nerve is blocked by placing a needle cranial to the femoral artery within the femoral triangle. Because of the proximity of the femoral artery and vein, care should be

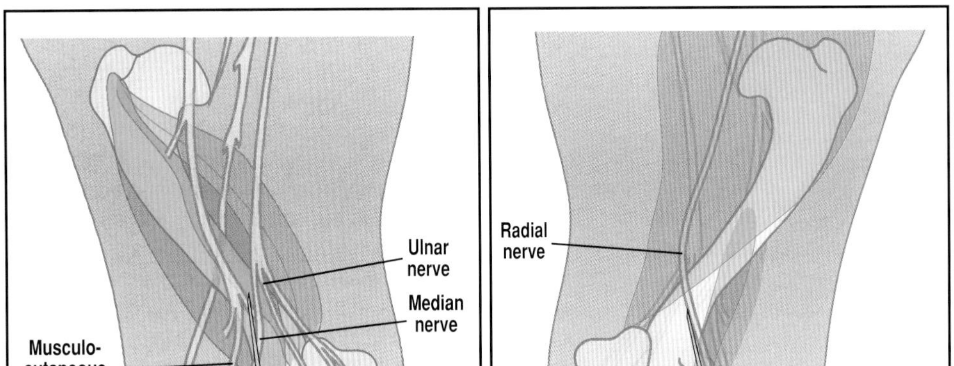

10.6 Anatomical landmarks for performing radial, ulnar, median and musculocutaneous nerve blocks in dogs. **(a)** Medial view. **(b)** Lateral view.

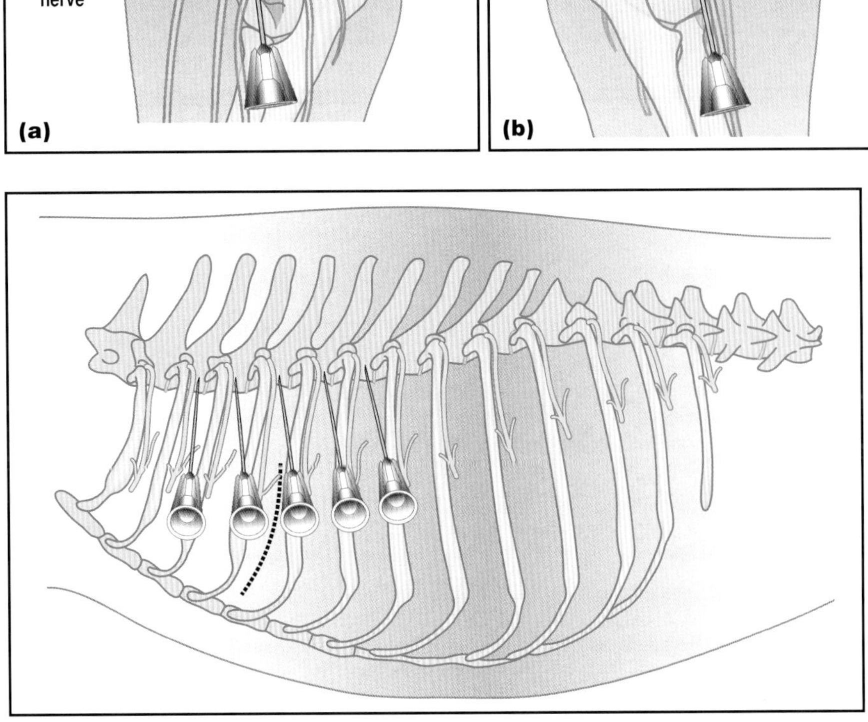

10.7 Anatomical landmarks for performing intercostal nerve blocks in dogs (dotted line shows position of surgical incision).

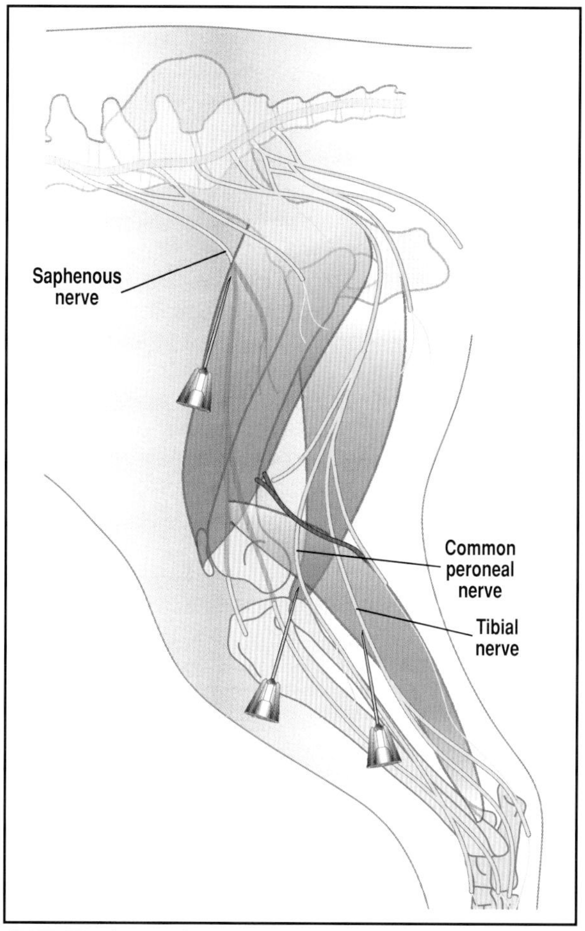

10.8 Anatomical landmarks for performing saphenous, common peroneal and tibial nerve blocks in dogs (medial view).

taken to avoid intravascular injection. The *common peroneal nerve* is a branch of the sciatic nerve, and runs laterally over the gastrocnemius and across the lateral surface of the fibular head. The nerve is easily palpated and blocked by inserting a needle distal to the fibular head and directing it towards the nerve. The *tibial nerve* is also a branch of the sciatic nerve, and runs deep to the medial and lateral heads of the gastrocnemius and then between the superficial digital flexor tendons and the long digital extensor tendon. The nerve is blocked by placing a needle deep to the medial and lateral heads of the gastrocnemius, or by placing a needle between the superficial digital flexor tendons and the long digital extensor tendon distal to the lateral saphenous vein.

Techniques in the cat

Cranial nerves: Selective blockade of the *maxillary and mandibular branches of the trigeminal nerve* can be used for a variety of surgical and dental procedures (Figure 10.9). Most nerves can be blocked by injecting 0.1–0.3 ml of 2% lidocaine or 0.5% bupivacaine using a 25 gauge (0.5 mm), 0.6 inch (1.6 cm) needle.

The *infraorbital nerve* and its branches provide sensory innervation to the rostral upper dental arcade, hard palate and muzzle. The nerve is blocked as it exits the infraorbital foramen, which is located ventral to the eye at the junction of the zygomatic arch and the maxilla.

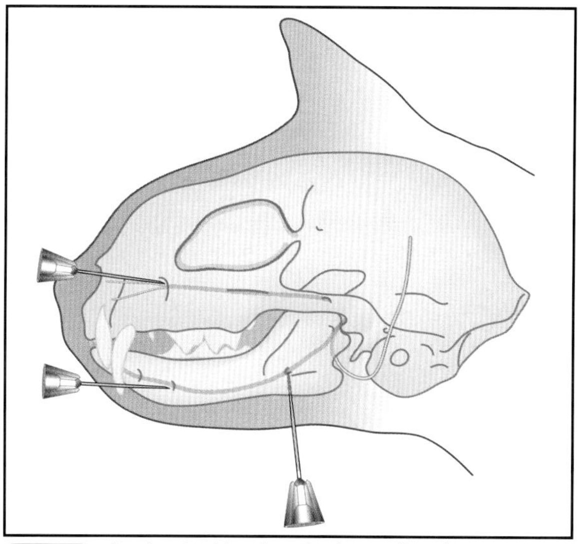

10.9 Anatomical landmarks for performing infraorbital, inferior alveolar and mental nerve blocks in cats.

Unlike the dog, the cat's infraorbital foramen is recessed and cannot be palpated, although the ridge is obvious. The nerve is blocked by inserting a needle transorally or transcutaneously above the premolars and directing it towards the infraorbital foramen.

The *inferior alveolar nerve* and its branches provide sensory innervation to the lower dental arcade, tongue and chin. The nerve can be blocked proximally before it enters the mandibular foramen. The nerve is blocked by inserting a needle transcutaneously below the rostral portion of the angular process and directing it towards the foramen along the medial surface of the mandible. The nerve can also be blocked distally as it exits the mental foramina.

Cervical and thoracic nerves: Selective blockade of cervical and thoracic nerves can be used to manage perioperative pain associated with surgical procedures of the forelimb and thorax. The *brachial plexus* is blocked by injecting approximately 1 ml of 2% lidocaine or 0.5% bupivacaine using a 22 gauge (0.7 mm), 1 inch (2.5 cm) needle. Most other nerves can be blocked by injecting 0.1–0.3 ml of 2% lidocaine or 0.5% bupivacaine using a 25 gauge (0.5 mm), 0.6 inch (1.6 cm) needle.

Blockade of the nerves of the brachial plexus can be used to manage perioperative pain associated with forelimb injuries and fractures below the elbow (Figure 10.10). Nerves of the brachial plexus (C6, C7, C8, T1) are blocked as they enter the axillary space. The block is performed by inserting a needle into the axillary space at the level of the shoulder, and directing it towards the first rib. The brachial plexus is located just cranial to the first rib within the axillary space. The axillary artery and vein run in close proximity to the brachial plexus and syringes should be aspirated before injection. Unilateral blockade of the phrenic nerve and hemiparalysis of the diaphragm can also occur, and this block should not be performed bilaterally. Although the technique is easy to perform, large amounts of local anaesthetic solution are required, and the shoulder and proximal humerus are not anaesthetized.

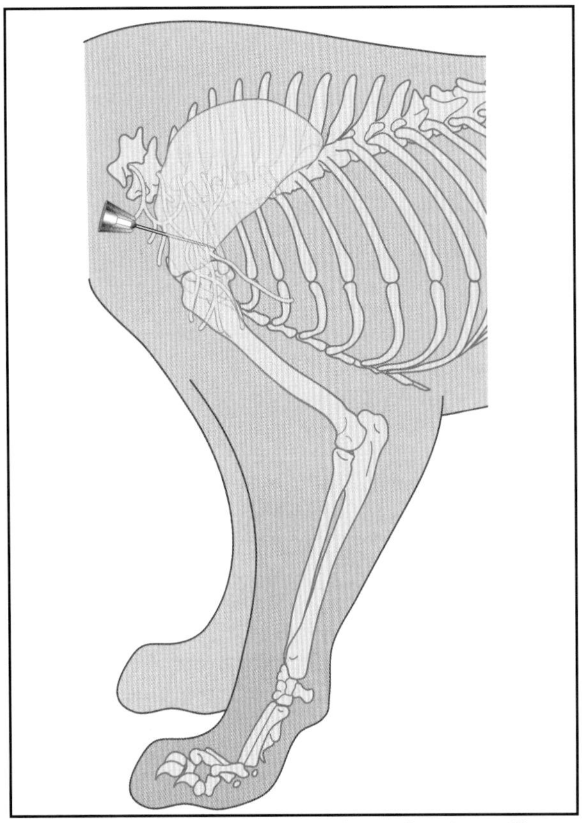

10.10 Anatomical landmarks for performing axillary blockade of the brachial plexus in cats.

Selective blockade of the distal branches of the *radial*, *ulnar* and *median nerves* can be used to manage perioperative pain associated with surgical procedures of the front paw (Figure 10.11). The *radial nerve* is blocked by placing a needle subcutaneously dorsomedial to the carpus just proximal to the joint. The *median* and *ulnar nerves* are blocked by placing needles subcutaneously medial and lateral to the accessory carpal pad on the ventral surface of the paw. Care should be taken to avoid entering the joint spaces when making these injections.

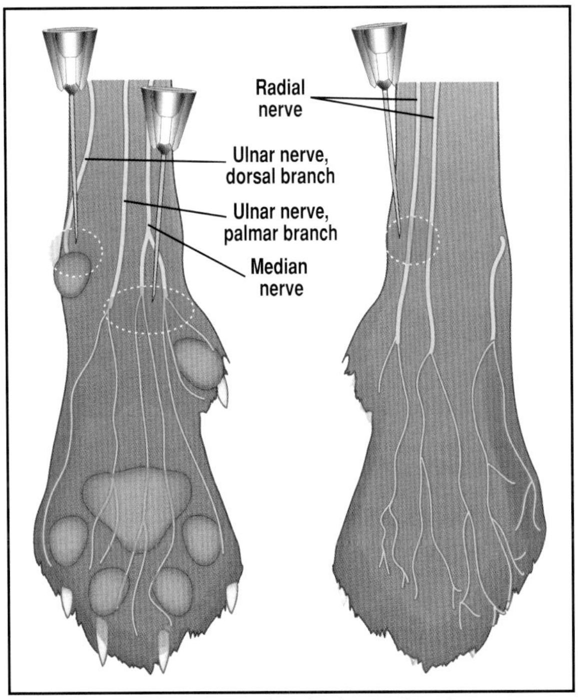

10.11 Anatomical landmarks for performing nerve blocks of the distal branches of the radial, ulnar and median nerves in cats. Shaded areas within dotted lines show areas to be blocked.

Intercostal nerve blocks can be used to manage pain in animals with fractured ribs, or to manage pain in patients undergoing lateral thoracotomy. As in dogs, intercostal nerves and vessels lie adjacent to the caudal border of each rib, and two or three intercostal nerves on either side of the fracture or incision site must be blocked. Needles are inserted distal to the angle of the rib near the insertions of the epaxial (longissimus, iliocostalis) muscles, and are directed dorsally along the caudal border of each rib. Pneumothorax is a potential complication and patients should be watched closely for 20–30 minutes after the block is performed.

Lumbar and sacral nerves: Selective blockade of lumbar and sacral nerves can be used to manage perioperative pain associated with surgical procedures of the hindlimb. Most nerves can be blocked by injecting 0.1–0.3 ml of 2% lidocaine or 0.5% bupivacaine using a 25 gauge (0.5 mm), 0.6 inch (1.6 cm) needle.

Perioperative pain associated with injuries and fractures distal to the stifle can be managed by selectively blocking the *saphenous*, *common peroneal* and *tibial nerves*. The *saphenous nerve* is a branch of the femoral nerve, and runs through the femoral triangle on the medial surface of the thigh. As in dogs, the nerve lies cranial to the femoral artery and vein, and pulsation of the artery can be used to facilitate correct placement of the needle. The saphenous nerve is blocked by placing a needle cranial to the femoral artery within the femoral triangle. Because of the proximity of the femoral artery and vein, care should be taken to avoid intravascular injection. The *common peroneal nerve* is a branch of the sciatic nerve, and runs laterally over the gastrocnemius and across the lateral surface of the fibular head. The nerve is easily palpated and blocked by inserting a needle distal to the fibular head and directing it towards the nerve. The *tibial nerve* is also a branch of the sciatic nerve, and runs deep to the gastrocnemius and then between the superficial digital flexor tendons and the long digital extensor tendon. The nerve is blocked by placing a needle between the superficial digital flexor tendons and the long digital extensor tendon.

Central neural blockade

Epidural anaesthesia and analgesia in dogs

Epidural administration of local anaesthetics or opioids can be used to manage perioperative pain associated with injuries and fractures of the hindlimb (Figure 10.12). The term 'epidural anaesthesia' refers to the complete sensory, motor and autonomic blockade produced by epidural administration of local anaesthetics. Lumbosacral epidural administration of local anaesthetics produces segmental blockade of lumbar and sacral nerve roots. Cranial spread of the blockade is dependent on the volume of local anaesthetic

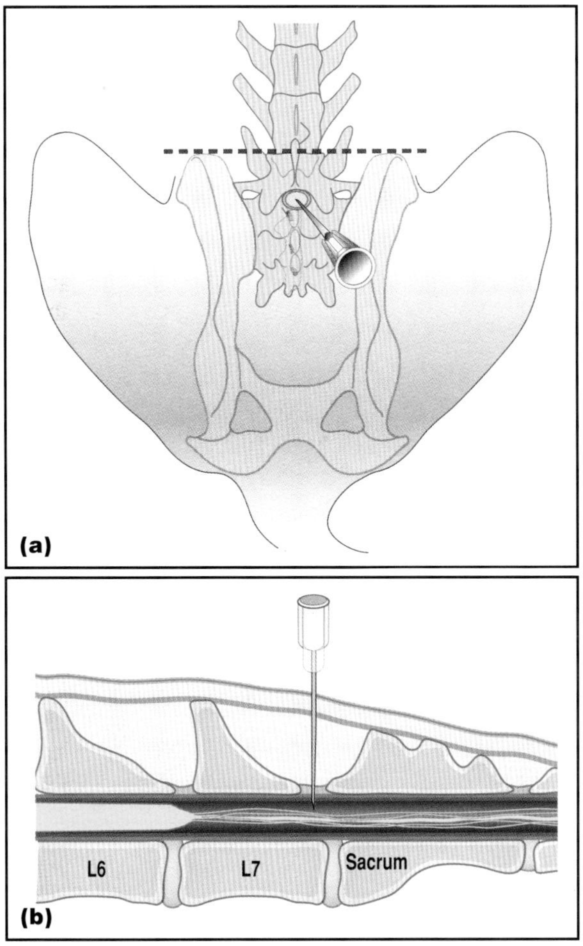

10.12 Anatomical landmarks for performing lumbosacral epidural anaesthesia and analgesia in dogs. **(a)** Dorsal view. **(b)** Lateral view. The lumbosacral space can be found caudal to a line drawn between the cranial borders of the ilia (marked with a dotted line).

administered. Small volumes (1 ml/10 kg) produce blockade of the immediate lumbosacral area while larger volumes (1 ml/5 kg) produce blockade up to the level of the umbilicus. Epidural anaesthesia is frequently used in combination with general anaesthesia as part of a balanced technique designed to reduce anaesthetic requirements, improve analgesia and muscle relaxation and reduce the incidence of major complications. Epidural administration of 2% lidocaine typically provides 1–2 hours of 'anaesthesia' while epidural administration of 0.5% bupivacaine provides 4–6 hours of regional 'anaesthesia'.

The term 'epidural analgesia' refers to the analgesia produced by epidural administration of opioids. Epidural administration of morphine (preservative-free preparation; 0.1–0.3 mg/kg) produces longer lasting analgesia with fewer side effects than administration of more lipid-soluble opioids, such as fentanyl or hydromorphone. Epidural administration of morphine produces analgesia for hindlimb as well as abdominal, thoracic and forelimb procedures. Unlike epidural administration of local anaesthetics, cranial spread is not dependent on volume but on diffusion of morphine from the epidural space into the cerebrospinal fluid and the dorsal horn of the spinal cord. Morphine is often given in combination with local anaesthetics. Preoperative epidural administration of 0.5% bupivacaine with morphine provides 4–6 hours of intraoperative and postoperative 'anaesthesia', and 12–24 hours of postoperative 'analgesia' with a single injection.

Unlike other domestic species, the spinal cord in dogs ends at the level of the sixth lumbar vertebra, and the meninges end at the level of the seventh lumbar vertebra. The epidural space surrounds the spinal cord and meninges, and is limited dorsally by the vertebral laminae and the ligamentum flavum. The epidural space communicates with the paravertebral space and spinal nerve roots via intervertebral foramina. Epidural injections are usually made at the lumbosacral junction or space. Patients are placed in sternal or lateral recumbency and the cranial edges of the wings of the ilia are palpated. The lumbosacral space is caudal to a line connecting these two points. The indentation over the lumbosacral space is bordered cranially by the dorsal spinous process of the seventh lumbar vertebra and caudally by the sacral ridge. After aseptic preparation of the site, a 20 gauge (0.9 mm), 1.5 inch (3.8 cm) spinal needle is placed in the centre of the indentation perpendicular to the plane of the pelvis, and advanced slowly towards the lumbosacral space. Longer needles may be required in large dogs, but these needles are more difficult to stabilize once the epidural space has been entered.

An increase in resistance followed by an abrupt loss of resistance, commonly referred to as a 'pop', is encountered as the needle passes through the ligamentum flavum and enters the epidural space. The needle is stabilized with one hand and the stylet is removed with the other, and a test injection of 1–3 ml of air is made to verify correct placement of the needle. Absence of resistance to injection of air indicates correct placement of the needle. The 'hanging drop' technique can also be used to identify correct placement, but the technique is not as reliable in dogs as it is in larger domestic animals and patients must be placed in sternal recumbency. Preservative-free 2% lidocaine or 0.5% bupivacaine is administered slowly over 10–20 seconds at a dose of 1 ml/5 kg (lean bodyweight). Addition of 1–2 ml of air to the syringe helps to confirm correct placement of the spinal needle during injection. Collapse of the air space within the syringe indicates an increase in resistance and movement of the needle. After injection, the patient can be rotated to facilitate migration of the local anaesthetic solution towards the nerve roots supplying the surgical site. Alternatively, preservative-free morphine (0.2 mg/kg) can be given alone in an equivalent volume of saline, or in combination with lidocaine or bupivacaine. At the Atlantic Veterinary College, a concentrated (25 mg/ml) morphine solution is preferred to avoid dilution of local anaesthetic solutions when the drugs are mixed together. As always, dosage calculations should be based on lean bodyweight, and total doses should be calculated carefully to avoid systemic toxicity. Syringes should also be labelled clearly and strict aseptic technique should be followed when administering drugs epidurally.

Complications are infrequent if epidural techniques are performed carefully. Identification of landmarks can be difficult in obese patients or in those with pelvic injuries. Epidural techniques should not be used if a localized skin infection is present at the injection site. Coagulopathy and septicaemia are potential contraindications and epidural injections are usually avoided in these patients. Sympathetic blockade produced by epidural administration of local anaesthetics can cause significant peripheral vasodilation and hypotension. Consequently, local anaesthetics should not be given epidurally to patients that are volume depleted or haemodynamically unstable. Even in healthy anaesthetized patients, vaporizer settings should be reduced, blood pressure should be monitored closely, and intravenous fluids should be given to maintain adequate perfusion pressures. Postoperatively, urine retention can be a problem, so all patients should be checked periodically for bladder distension.

Epidural anaesthesia and analgesia in cats

Epidural administration of local anaesthetics and opioids can be used to manage perioperative pain associated with injuries and fractures of the hindlimb. Unlike in the dog, the spinal cord ends at the level of the seventh lumbar vertebra and the meninges extend into the sacral region. Patients are placed in sternal or lateral recumbency and the cranial edges of the wings of the ilia are palpated. Anatomical landmarks for lumbosacral injection are more distinct in cats than in dogs, but the epidural space is much smaller. Because the spinal cord and meninges extend into the lumbosacral region the potential for intrathecal injection or direct injury to the spinal cord is higher than in dogs.

After aseptic preparation of the site, a 22 gauge (0.7 mm), 1.5 inch (3.8 cm) spinal needle is placed in the centre of the indentation between the sacral ridge and the dorsal spinous process of the seventh lumbar vertebra, and advanced slowly towards the epidural space. Techniques for needle placement are similar to those for dogs, but a smaller volume of air (0.5 ml) is used to verify correct placement. If cerebrospinal fluid is observed when the stylet is removed, the needle should be withdrawn slightly so the distal end is within the epidural space, before making the injection. Preservative-free 2% lidocaine or 0.5% bupivacaine is administered slowly over 10–20 seconds at a dose of 1 ml/5 kg. As always, dosage calculations should be based on lean bodyweight, and total doses should be calculated carefully to avoid systemic toxicity. After injection, the patient can be rotated to facilitate migration of the local anaesthetic solution towards the nerve roots supplying the surgical site. Alternatively, preservative-free morphine (0.2 mg/kg) can be given alone in an equivalent volume of saline, or in combination with lidocaine or bupivacaine. Contraindications and complications are similar to those for dogs.

Summary

Local and regional anaesthetic techniques are usually the safest and most effective way to improve the quality of anaesthesia and analgesia for patients undergoing surgical, dental and diagnostic procedures. Currently, lidocaine and bupivacaine are the local anaesthetics used most commonly in dogs and cats. Bupivacaine has a slightly slower onset of action but lasts 3–4 hours longer than lidocaine. Consequently, bupivacaine is usually a better choice than lidocaine for the management of perioperative pain. Local and regional anaesthetic techniques are relatively safe if they are performed with reasonable care. Relevant anatomy should be reviewed, and doses of local anaesthetics, especially those for cats and small dogs, should be calculated carefully to avoid systemic toxicity. Preoperative use of local and regional anaesthetic techniques reduces anaesthetic requirements, improves analgesia, attenuates the stress response to surgical trauma and reduces the incidence of major complications. In short, these techniques can dramatically improve the quality of care provided to most patients undergoing a wide variety of surgical, dental and diagnostic procedures.

References and further reading

Chadwick HS (1985) Toxicity and resuscitation in lidocaine- or bupivacaine-infused cats. *Anesthesiology* **63**, 385–390

Feldman HS, Arthur GR and Covino BG (1989) Comparative systemic toxicity of convulsant and supraconvulsant doses of intravenous ropivacaine, bupivacaine, and lidocaine in the conscious dog. *Anesthesia and Analgesia* **69(6)**, 794–801

Foster RH and Markham A (2000) Levobupivacaine: a review of its pharmacology and use as a local anesthetic. *Drugs* **59**, 551–579

Gokin AP, Philip B and Strichartz GR (2001) Preferential block of small myelinated sensory and motor fibers by lidocaine: in vivo electrophysiology in the rat sciatic nerve. *Anesthesiology* **95**, 1441–1454

Kehlet H and Dahl JB (1993) The value of multimodal or balanced analgesia in postoperative pain treatment. *Anesthesia and Analgesia* **77**,1049–1056

Kehlet H and Wilmore DW (2002) Multimodal strategies to improve surgical outcome. *American Journal of Surgery* **183**, 630–641

Lamont LA (2002) Feline perioperative pain management. *Veterinary Clinics of North America: Small Animal Practice* **32**,747–763

Lemke KA (2000) Local and regional anesthesia. *Veterinary Clinics of North America: Small Animal Practice* **30**, 839–857

Lemke KA (2004) Understanding the pathophysiology of perioperative pain. *Canadian Veterinary Journal* **45**, 405–413

Liu PL, Feldman HS, Covino BM *et al.* (1982) Acute cardiovascular toxicity of intravenous amide local anesthetics in anesthetized ventilated dogs. *Anesthesia and Analgesia* **61**, 317–322

Liu PL, Feldman HS, Giasi R *et al.* (1983) Comparative CNS toxicity of lidocaine, etidocaine, bupivacaine, and tetracaine in awake dogs following rapid intravenous administration. *Anesthesia and Analgesia* **62**, 375–379

McClure JH (1996) Ropivacaine. *British Journal of Anaesthesia* **76**, 300–307

Muir WW and Woolf CJ (2001) Mechanisms of pain and their therapeutic implications. *Journal of the American Veterinary Medical Association* **219**, 1346–1356

Reiestad F and Stromskag KE (1986) Interpleural catheter in management of postoperative pain: a preliminary report. *Regional Anesthesia* **11**, 89–91

Rodgers A, Walker N, Schug S *et al.* (2000) Reduction of post-operative mortality and morbidity with epidural or spinal anesthesia: Results from an overview of randomized trials. *British Medical Journal* **321**, 1493–1504

Rosenburg PH, Scheinin BM, Lepantalo MJ *et al.* (1987) Continuous intrapleural infusion of bupivacaine for analgesia after thoracotomy. *Anesthesiology* **67**, 811–813

11

Pain management III: ancillary therapies

Shauna Cantwell

Introduction

This chapter provides an introduction to non-pharmacological means of providing analgesia or preventing pain. More common modalities such as acupuncture and transcutaneous electrical nerve stimulation (TENS) therapy are discussed. Some less common or scientifically unvalidated therapies are also introduced, but it should be remembered that evidence-based medicine is the standard to which medical practice should aspire. Ancillary methods of pain management are many and varied, but besides those of physical therapy in humans, most are not yet well documented and poor methodology limits the usefulness of many studies. Much of the therapy available to veterinary surgeons is a compilation of clinically used techniques from veterinary medicine, and those extrapolated from human medicine. This chapter is an introduction to many forms of therapy that are available. Most require further training and it is beyond the scope of this text to teach the application. Further information on alternative therapies can be obtained from the reference list.

Nursing care

In addition to pharmacological and invasive or manipulative techniques for pain management, basic nursing care must first be considered. Good surgical technique, infection control and wound management are paramount. Bandaging, joint immobilization or mobilization (as needed) and general comfort must be addressed. Muscle spasms secondary to pain can be controlled not only through muscle relaxants such as diazepam, but also with thick bedding, hot or cold applications and manipulative therapy.

Appropriate knowledge of patient behaviour is necessary to understand the effects of therapy, and to know when to intervene. Controlling anxiety is important to decrease fear and its potentiation of pain. This can be done with quiet handling, interaction with socialized animals and minimal handling of non-socialized animals. Provision of basic needs will reduce anxiety and allow rest. These needs include nutritional support, facilitation of timely urination and defecation, and provision of seclusion for reclusive animals such as cats. Distraction of attention has been shown to reduce pain awareness in human cancer pain studies and can be an effective, although time-consuming, therapy. If nursing care does not manage to reduce anxiety, acupuncture and herbal treatment can also be useful.

Alternative and complementary therapy

In humans, the factors leading to the desire for non-pharmacological treatment are high-intensity pain, aching pain and cutting/stabbing pain. In a study of patients with spinal cord injury, acupuncture, massage and TENS were the treatments most often sought by patients. Massage and heat have also been reported to result in appreciable alleviation of chronic pain. Ice massage over an acupuncture point has also been shown to reduce pain. Neuropathic pain responds poorly to traditional analgesics and so requires a long-term commitment to complex management strategies, which can include non-traditional approaches. For cancer pain in humans, a combination of pharmacological and non-pharmacological treatment modalities is the standard of care recommended by the World Health Organization. Complementary and alternative therapies are also becoming recognized by major research agencies, and are now acknowledged as useful tools in veterinary medicine.

Manipulative therapies

Physical modalities can be used to augment pain treatment plans. Veterinary physical therapy entails the use of non-invasive means for the rehabilitation of injuries. Optimizing range of motion, strength and neuromuscular control can reduce instability and pain associated with disuse.

Temperature

Application of heat or cold is helpful. Cold is often applied to acute postoperative sites to decrease inflammation; ice packs can be covered with a towel and applied to an inflamed area for no more than 20 minutes at a time. Heat can improve circulation, aid removal of tissue waste products and promote healing, especially of chronic lesions. Caution must be used when applying heat to patients with lack of sensation, poor perfusion, or open ulcers and wounds. Local heat may also promote growth of neoplasms so should not be applied over such areas.

Massage

Massage is a very broad term which includes many types of muscle manipulation. It can be used to improve range of motion, reduce muscle tension and improve circulation. Massage can function in a similar way to muscle relaxants, such as benzodiazepines, through interruption of positive feedback loops that create further pain and sympathetic stimulation. Muscle spindle cells and Golgi tendon organs are the effective receptors in this cycle. Massage also functions to inhibit nociceptive transmission by stimulation of Aβ fibres. These fibres are low-threshold sensory fibres and can modulate and inhibit nociceptive pathways via the gate control theory.

Animals with chronic painful disorders also have muscle spasms, tender points and trigger points. A trigger point is a localized tense area of muscle which when palpated causes radiating pain. Many types of physical therapy and even acupuncture are often directed to trigger point therapy. Veterinary surgeons or nurses/technicians can gently assess muscle zones for tenderness or rigidity. Manipulating accessible muscle origins and insertions can provide significant relief and owners can be taught to provide treatment of trouble spots at home. Common zones to be examined in dogs include the triceps, gluteals, semimembranosus/semitendinosus and longissimus dorsi over the lumbar region. Dogs with weak or painful backs and hindquarters will routinely have muscle spasm in both brachiocephalicus muscles as well as the caudal scapular muscles. They are usually very amenable to massage as well as heat therapy. Internal disorders must be ruled out as a source of referred pain to muscle regions, such as back pain with cystitis.

Alternative techniques: Techniques such as orthobionomy and Bowen therapy are muscle manipulations that are considered 'alternative'. The Bowen technique uses light pressure applied to specific and prescribed locations to stimulate the body's return to normal function. It can be helpful in alleviating pain unresponsive to standard treatment. Historically, physical therapy has been developed to rehabilitate and return people and animals to structural function. Of course function and pain can be closely linked, but perhaps physical manipulation can be used to stimulate and drive the nervous system to cause anti-nociception directly. Stimulation of the motor cortex for refractory neuropathic pain is used in humans, though the mechanism of action is not yet known. Sensitized patients (with allodynia) seem to be more responsive to this form of treatment. The use of muscle stimulation (or stimulation in specific ways of somatic sensory afferent neurons proximally along the nerve pathways) may become a method of anti-nociception.

Chiropractic

Chiropractic therapy (also known as veterinary spinal manipulative therapy) is another physical manipulative therapy that is becoming increasingly popular, especially for working dogs such as police, hunting and agility show dogs. For those unfamiliar with chiropractic therapy, the most important thing to realize is that the term 'subluxation' has a different meaning compared with the term used in traditional veterinary medicine. The lesions are called subluxations, which in chiropractic terms are areas of hypomobility in joints, usually of the spine. The hypomobility causes a segmental dysfunction, which can place undue strain on the intervertebral foramina, ligaments, muscles and other components surrounding the joints. 'Subluxations' can cause kinesiopathological changes (biomechanical problems) and neuropathology due to direct or indirect pressure on the dorsal and ventral nerve roots as well as the spinal nerves exiting the intervertebral foramen. Subsequent myopathological changes occur, manifested as muscle weakness, myofasciitis and pain. Inflammatory changes can also occur, and somatic–visceral or somatic–autonomic neural relationships can be affected. Rapid thrusts to the spinal articular joints will produce a relative separation of the joint, break down adhesions and reset the muscle spindle cells and Golgi tendon organs of the paraspinal musculature. The resulting sensory afferent stimulation can interfere with nociceptive pathways, and may alter nervous system plasticity. Stimulation of joint *versus* cutaneous sensory afferent nerves will decrease hyperalgesia, and this may be one neural mechanism of action of analgesia through chiropractic adjustments. Many prospective double-blind studies have been performed to demonstrate clinical effectiveness of chiropractic therapy, especially with lower back pain in humans.

Osteopathy

Osteopathy is a form of manipulative therapy similar to chiropractic therapy. Osteopathy may produce cannabimimetic effects rather than effects relating to endogenous opioid release. Endorphins cannot be consistently shown to increase with either chiropractic or osteopathic treatment. The 'cannabimimetic tetrad' includes changes in locomotor activity, hypothermia, catalepsy and anti-nociception. One study compared osteopathy with sham (no treatment), and found most of the above descriptors in the osteopathy group. Endogenous cannabinoids were measured, and were suggestive of an increase in the osteopathy-treated group. Osteopathy is also considered an alternative therapy.

Electrical and vibrational

Scientific data on analgesic electrical and vibrational therapy is beginning to accumulate, but conclusive information is still scant. Transcutaneous electrical nerve stimulation, pulsed electromagnetic fields, ultrasound, cold laser therapy, shock wave, iontophoresis, short-wave, microwave and infrasound vibrations represent other therapeutic options. However, most are chosen based on personal experience of the therapist. Indications for use of one *versus* the other are not yet well documented.

Acupuncture

Acupuncture is a form of traditional Chinese medicine, which aids in 'rebalancing' the body through the movement of 'chi'. The premise is that a 'rebalanced' body is pain-free. The basis of Chinese medicine is the meridian system named after internal organs. Connecting pathways throughout the body, as yet undefined as neural, humoral, fascial or otherwise, allow the chi to flow in a healthy body. Small gauge needles (28–35 gauge) can be inserted into points along the meridian system to create local, distant and systemic effects. Electrical stimulus is often applied to paired needles for more intense and longer duration of effect. Depending on the patient history, pulse quality and meridian palpation, prescribed points can suppress nausea, stop seizures, reverse bronchoconstriction, raise or lower blood pressure and alleviate pain, but there are many other actions. The metaphors of Chinese medicine are not easily adapted to Western paradigms. Western trained practitioners may be more apt to use acupuncture to stimulate trigger points, tender areas or segmental areas in order to augment musculoskeletal physical therapy (Figure 11.1).

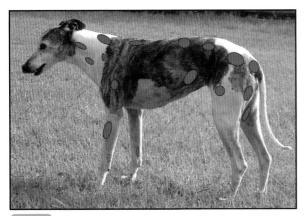

11.1 Acupuncture trigger points in the dog.

Studies have shown that some of the effects are mediated by central endorphin release, but this is not the sole mechanism of action. Electroacupuncture reduces halothane requirements in dogs, and this effect cannot be reversed with the opioid antagonist naltrexone. Electroacupuncture can also decrease the inflammation of colitis through beta adrenoreceptor activity. Acupuncture may contribute to inhibitory pain pathways by stimulating Aβ fibres. In most cases the needles do not hurt as they are inserted and the Aβ (sensory fibre) stimulation may reduce nociception via the gate control theory of pain. Many different mechanisms of action are possible, but the exact way acupuncture works is unlikely to be known for some time. The basis is most likely to be neurophysiological, but the subsequent cascade of effects is currently difficult to define. The complex physiological interactions that promote homeostasis are difficult to categorize for each treatment, but research is growing exponentially in this field.

A trained veterinary acupuncturist can be extremely effective in providing analgesia. Postoperative analgesia can be augmented in the recovery phase (Figure 11.2), but as with conventional analgesic therapy, one must remember to protect the surgical sites of animals who can suddenly feel better. While there are points that alone may contribute to pain management, use with other points in a traditional Chinese medical approach may be very beneficial in alleviating pain and discomfort, and in promoting patient well-being.

The meridian system and application of acupuncture can be studied through various teaching organizations. Skill and caution must both be used in the application of acupuncture: it is contraindicated in animals with severe clotting disorders and severe immunodeficiency, and needle placement is avoided in areas of infection. Electroacupuncture should not be used

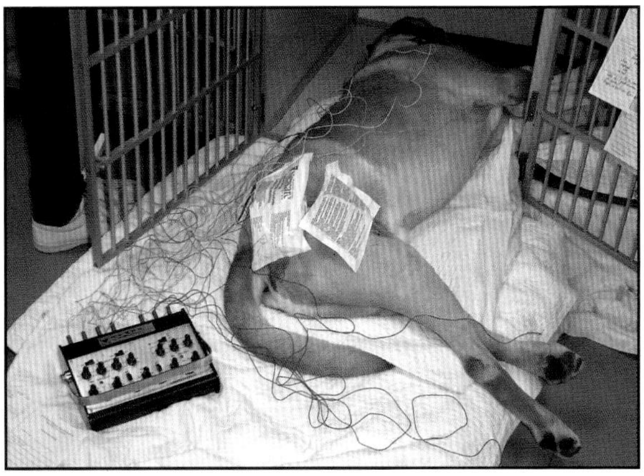

11.2 Electroacupuncture and cold therapy applied during the recovery phase of orthopaedic surgery.

around the abdomen of pregnant animals because abortion can be precipitated, nor across tumours because tumour growth may be augmented. It should also not be used near the heart in dogs with pacemakers. With repeated sessions using similar points, tolerance can develop to acupuncture. With these caveats, however, an experienced acupuncturist can be a tremendous provider of analgesia and well-being to veterinary patients.

Transcutaneous electrical nerve stimulation (TENS)

TENS is the application of electricity through superficial electrodes to promote analgesia. The electrodes can be positioned across painful joints, over large muscle masses or in the general area of discomfort. TENS is easy to use and devoid of major side effects. Clinically, TENS can be used at either low frequency (<10 Hz) or high frequency (>50 Hz), as with electroacupuncture. The intensity of the stimulus (amplitude) is set to just at or below that which will create a motor response. At higher amplitudes, it can actually cause pain. When applied under general anaesthesia, TENS can still be effective. TENS can also be useful in the postoperative period. Use in human medicine is very common, but the analgesic mechanism of action is not fully understood. The gate control theory is thought to be the mechanism of action for many of the therapies using electricity, although other studies indicate that release of neurotransmitters is also important. Opiate, serotonergic and muscarinic receptors are activated through the use of TENS and it may also be indirectly acting at the level of the spinal cord.

Electrical fields

Electrical fields, magnetic fields and electromagnetic fields are thought to have healing or curative effects. Electric fields have been shown to alleviate several types of pain (headaches, stomach aches) in numerous human patients. In one study, an electrical field of 50 Hz with intensity of 17.5 kV/m was applied to dogs with brain tumours and with spinal cord injuries, as well as to healthy dogs. The comparison yielded significant results. The degree of pain was not measured, but beta endorphin concentrations in the non-healthy dogs almost doubled with multiple treatments.

The intriguing aspect of this study is that the concentrations in normal dogs did not change with application of the electrical field. This concurs with the often noted premise that many alternative therapies cause the individual to return towards a normal or physiologically optimal state, and in that regard may not cause changes in normal animals. Electric and electromagnetic fields may be applied through use of skin patches, or magnets which can be placed in collars or on bandages or wraps. The use of electric fields may play a further role in provision of analgesia in veterinary patients in the future.

Laser

Laser light is a source of light of a single wavelength. Therapeutic lasers are usually sold with wavelengths ranging between 630 and 904 nm and the effective power range starts at 1–3 mW. Battery-operated units will provide an inconsistent source of power, but newer units have computer processing which maintains a more consistent and useful output. The effect is not thermal, but related to photochemical reactions within cells. The effect for chronic pain appears to be significant but short lasting. Low-intensity laser light has been shown to promote healing in chronic wounds and very low intensity laser light (<3 mW) over acupuncture points has been shown to decrease oedema, pain and hyperalgesia in acute inflammatory, chronic inflammatory and neuropathic pain conditions in rats. Laser light can be applied over wounds, joints, trigger points and muscle adjacent to nerve roots for pain relief.

Herbal therapy

Botanical medicine (also called phytotherapy) is routinely practised in some areas of the world. Antimicrobial and anti-inflammatory effects have been described and used to treat allergies and infections, as well as to promote wound healing and provide pain relief. Phytotherapy may be considered a form of pharmacological medicine, although most of these agents are considered to be supplements and nutraceuticals rather than traditional medicines. Because these treatments are administered for effect over a period of time, they tend to be used for chronic pain syndromes rather than acute pain.

More interest is being directed toward validation of this type of therapy through scientific studies. For instance, green tea has been administered to mice with chronic pain caused by osteoarthritis, and diminished the incidence and severity of the arthritis and subsequent pain. Antipeptide enzymes and the inflammatory mediators COX-2, interferon-γ and TNF-α were decreased significantly in the group given green tea. A comprehensive discussion of this type of therapy cannot be presented here, but some reviews of veterinary herbal therapy have been made and a review of the efficacy of analgesic herbs in human medicine has also been written. Caution must be exercised when using herbs perioperatively; for example, garlic, ginkgo and ginseng may increase surgical bleeding. Care must be taken when considering herbal therapy for species in which the use and side effects have not been documented.

Homoeopathy

Homoeopathy is a form of therapy not routinely utilized alone in Western medicine, but is often a component of integrative medicine utilizing both Western and holistic approaches. The principle of homoeopathy is that disease and symptoms are cured by using diluted and potentized forms of substances that produce symptoms similar to the illness in healthy individuals. Numerous laboratory studies, clinical trials and observational studies have been performed, but no single model has been widely validated. The most convincing model is one of a change in solvent after many dilutions of the parent compound, as the dilutions may have almost no original compound, but are still active. A positive outcome of pain management has been shown using *Arnica montana* in trauma and postoperative situations. *Ruta graveolens* has been used for pain associated with extended immobility or structural injury (ligamentous or skeletal), although no studies validate its use. Homoeopathy might be an alternative for pain management with minimal intervention, as there are no known or documented side effects, and it is thought to potentiate the individual's capacity to self-heal.

Interventional techniques

Pain management is difficult in chronic pain situations, such as metastatic neoplasia. When conventional and pharmacological therapies provide inadequate relief, alternative surgical or other interventional techniques can be considered. Radiotherapy is thought to decrease cancer pain by not only decreasing the activity of the neoplasm but by diminishing the activity of the local nociceptive neurons; radio-ablation is similar. Rhizotomies cut the nerves returning to the spinal cord, and hence diminish nociception. Vertebral stabilization diminishes nerve root pain.

Summary

Analgesia can be provided in many ways beyond pharmacological means. Some, such as acupuncture and physical therapy, are becoming better described and starting to be introduced into regular veterinary undergraduate curricula. As well as being providers of traditional Western medicine, veterinary surgeons should be trained to evaluate critically and apply novel ways to improve their medical approach; for example, surgeons are now electrically stimulating the spinal cord to relieve pain unresponsive to pharmacological analgesia. The recently discovered fact that oral sugar solutions provide analgesia in neonates, possibly by causing release of endogenous opioids, could be used clinically. One must grasp the subtle relationships between previously reported and apparently unrelated information. One must also assess this information and examine ways that it could be applied in practice; only by using this critical approach can advances be made.

Resources

McTimoney Chiropractic Association
Wallingford
Oxfordshire
OX10 8DJ
Phone: +44 (0)1491 829211
Fax: +44 (0)1491 829492
Email: admin@mctimoney-chiropractic.org

Association of British Veterinary Acupuncturists (ABVA)
ABVA Hon. Secretary
66A Easthorpe
Southwell
Notts
NG25 OHZ
Email: johnnyboyvet@hotmail.com

Association of Chartered Physiotherapists specializing in Animal Therapy
52 Littleham Road
Exmouth
Devon
EX8 2QJ
Email: bexsharples@hotmail.com

American Veterinary Chiropractic Association
442154 E 140 Road
Bluejacket, OK 74333
USA
Phone: (918)-784-2231

References and further reading

Ang-Lee MK, Moss J and Yuan CS (2001) Herbal medicines and perioperative care. *Journal of the American Medical Association* **286(2)**, 208–216

Bliddal H, Rosetzsky A, Schlichting P *et al.* (2000) A randomized, placebo-controlled, cross-over study of ginger extracts and ibuprofen in osteoarthritis. *Osteoarthritis and Cartilage* **8(1)**, 9–12

Borchers AT, Keen CL, Stern JS *et al.* (2000) Inflammation and native American medicine: the role of botanicals. *American Journal of Clinical Nutrition* **72**, 339–347

Brosseau L, Robinson V, Wells G *et al.* (2005) Low level laser therapy (Classes I, II, III) for treating rheumatoid arthritis. *The Cochrane Database of Systematic Reviews* 4: Art.No.: CD002049.DOI: 10.1002/14651858.CD002049.pub2.

Carter B (2002) Clients' experiences of frozen shoulder and its treatment with Bowen technique. *Complement Therapies in Nursing and Midwifery* **8(4)**, 204–210

Chaitow L (1988) *Soft-Tissue Manipulation: A Practitioners Guide to the Diagnosis and Treatment of Soft Tissue Dysfunction and Reflex Activity, 3rd edn.* Healing Arts Press, Rochester, Vermont

Ernst E and Chrubasik S (2000) Phyto-anti-inflammatories: a systematic review of randomized placebo controlled double-blind trials. *Rheumatic Diseases Clinics of North America* **26(1)**, 13–27

Giuliani A, Fernandez M, Farinelli M *et al.* (2004) Very low level laser therapy attenuates edema and pain in experimental models. *International Journal of Tissue Reactions* **26(1-2)**, 29–37

Haqqi TM, Anthony DD, Gupta S *et al.* (1999) Prevention of collagen-induced arthritis in mice by a polyphenolic fraction from green tea. *Proceedings of the National Academy of Science USA* **96**, 4524–4529

Harakawa S, Doge F and Saito A (2002) Exposure to electric field: its palliative effect on some clinical symptoms in human patients. *Research Bulletin Obihiro University* **22**, 193–199

Harakawa S, Takagi K, Inoue N *et al.* (2005) Effects of an electric field on plasma levels of ACTH and beta-endorphin in dogs with tumors or spinal cord injuries. *Journal of Alternative and Complementary Medicine* **11(5)**, 788–791

Haussler K (1999) Chiropractic evaluation and management. *Veterinary Clinics of North America: Equine Practice* **15(1),** 195–209

Huang KC (2000) *The Pharmacology of Chinese Herbs.* CRC Press, Boca Raton

Kastler B, Boulahdour H, Barral FG *et al.* (2005) Pain management in bone metastasis of pulmonary origin: new interventional and metabolic techniques. *Revue des Maladies Respiratoires* **22(6-2)**, 94–100

Keoung-Woo K, Tae-Wan K, Jun-Ho L *et al.* (2004) Electroacupuncture ameliorates experimental colitis induced by acetic acid in the rat. *Journal of Veterinary Science* **5(3)**, 189–195

Kracke GR, Tthoff KA and Tobias JD (2005) Sugar solution analgesia: the effects of glucose on expressed mu opioid receptors. *Anesthesia and Analgesia* **101(1)**, 64–68

Linderof B and Foreman RD (2006) Mechanisms of spinal cord stimulation in painful syndromes: role of animal models. *Pain Medicine* May-Jun (Suppl 1), S14–26

Lucroy MD, Edwards BF and Madewell BR (1999) Low-intensity laser light-induced closure of a chronic wound in a dog. *Veterinary Surgery* **28(4)**, 292–295

McPartland JM, Giuffrida A, King J *et al.* (2005) Cannabimimetic effects of osteopathic manipulative treatment. *Journal of American Osteopathy* **105(6)**, 283–291

Melzack R and Wall PD (1982) *The Challenge of Pain.* Penguin Books, London

Menefee LA and Monti DA (2005) Nonpharmacologic and complementary approaches to cancer pain management. *Journal of the American Osteopathy Association* **105(11)**, 15–20

Millis DL, Levine D and Taylor RA (2004). *Canine Rehabilitation and Physical Therapy, 1st edn.* WB Saunders, St. Louis

Norrbrink C and Lundeberg T (2004) Non-pharmacological pain-relieving therapies in individuals with spinal cord injury: a patient perspective. *Complementary Therapies in Medicine* **12(4)**, 189–197

Nuti C, Peyron R, Garcia-Larrea L *et al.* (2005) Motor cortex stimulation for refractory neuropathic pain: Four year outcome and predictors of efficacy. *Pain* **118**, 43–52

Pauls AL (2002) *The Philosophy and History of Ortho-Bionomy.* ALP Publishing, Rossland, BC, Canada

Radhakrishnan R and Sluka K (2003) Spinal muscarinic receptors are activated during low or high frequency TENS-induced antihyperalgesia in rats. *Neuropharmacology* **45**, 1111–1119

Radhakrishnan R and Sluka KA (2005) Deep tissue afferents, but not cutaneous afferents, mediate transcutaneous electrical nerve stimulation-induced antihyperalgesia. *Journal of Pain* **6(10)**, 673–680

Schoen AM (2001) *Veterinary Acupuncture: Ancient Art to Modern Medicine, 2nd edn.* Mosby, London

Smith PB, Compton DR, Welch SP *et al.* (1994) The pharmacological activity of anandamide, a putative endogenous cannabinoid, in mice. *Journal of Pharmacological Experimental Therapeutics* **270**, 219–227

Skarda RT, Tejwani GA and Muir WW (2002) Cutaneous analgesia, hemodynamic and respiratory effects, and beta-endorphin concentration in spinal fluid and plasma of horses after acupuncture and electroacupuncture. *American Journal of Veterinary Research* **63(10)**, 1435–1442

Tay AA, Tseng CK, Pace NL *et al.* (1982) Failure of narcotic antagonist to alter electroacupuncture modification of halothane anesthesia in the dog. *Canadian Anaesthesia Society Journal* **29(3)**, 231–235

Thomson M, Al-Quattan KK, Al-Sawan SM *et al.* (2002) The use of ginger (Zingiber officinale Rosc.) as a potential anti-inflammatory and antithrombotic agent. *Prostaglandins, Leukotrienes, and Essential Fatty Acids* **67**, 475–478

Walach H, Jonas W, Ives J *et al.* (2005) Research on homeopathy: state of the art. *Journal of Alternative and Complementary Medicine* **11(5)**, 813–829

Waters B and Raisler J (2003) Ice massage for the reduction of labor pain. *Journal of Midwifery and Women's Health* **48(5)**, 317–321

Wirth JH, Hudgins JC and Paice JA (2005) Use of herbal therapies to relieve pain: a review of efficacy and adverse effects. *Pain Management Nursing* **6(4)**, 145–167

Wynn SG and Marsden S (2003) *Manual of Natural Veterinary Medicine: Science and Tradition, 1st edn.* Mosby, London

12

Premedication and sedation

Joanna C. Murrell

Introduction

Premedication and sedation are common procedures carried out on a daily basis in small animal practice. The majority of animals are premedicated before induction of anaesthesia, yet the important role of premedication in the anaesthetic regimen as a whole is often forgotten: the choice of premedicants will have a major impact on the characteristics of the ensuing general anaesthetic. The appropriate selection of premedication drugs can significantly improve intraoperative cardiovascular stability, perioperative analgesia and quality of recovery. In order to optimize the advantages of premedication it is important to select drugs based upon the needs of the individual patient, rather than using a single regimen for all animals.

Sedation is often used as an alternative to general anaesthesia for minor procedures. There is a general perception, particularly amongst pet owners, that sedation is safer and therefore preferable to general anaesthesia. However, drugs used for sedation and premedication also have cardiovascular and respiratory side effects, while options for the monitoring and support of sedated patients are limited compared with those for animals under general anaesthesia. In this context general anaesthesia may be safer than heavy sedation for some high-risk patients.

The drugs used for premedication and sedation are identical and are discussed interchangeably in this chapter. Dosage schedules are discussed later in the chapter.

Aims of premedication and sedation

- Sedation and anxiolysis: quieten or immobilize an animal sufficiently to allow a procedure, such as intravenous catheterization, to be carried out. Reduce stress before and during induction of anaesthesia.
- Facilitate animal handling: this increases safety for animal and personnel during restraint.
- Contribute to a balanced anaesthetic technique: reduce the dose of other anaesthetic agents required for induction and maintenance of anaesthesia.
- Provision of analgesia.
- Counter the effects of other anaesthetic drugs, e.g. co-administration of atropine with opioids to prevent bradycardia.
- Contribute to a smooth and quiet recovery.

Pharmacology

The drugs used should ideally have the following properties:

- Produce reliable sedation and anxiolysis
- Have minimal effects on the cardiovascular system
- Cause minimal respiratory depression
- Produce analgesia
- Reversibility: the ability to reverse the effects of sedation may be desirable in some circumstances.

No individual drug used for premedication and sedation possesses all of these characteristics, and therefore combinations of drugs with different properties are employed. Provision of 'balanced' premedication and sedation using combinations of drugs with different specific effects allows the dosages of individual drugs to be reduced, minimizing side effects while maximizing the reliability of the sedation achieved. These combinations commonly utilize the synergism that occurs between different groups of sedative drugs, such as between alpha-2 adrenoreceptor agonists and opioids, or phenothiazines and opioids (neuroleptanalgesia).

Route of administration

Drugs may be given by the intravenous, intramuscular, subcutaneous and oral routes. The advantages and disadvantages of each route are shown in Figure 12.1. The route of administration will also influence the time to peak effect: this is shown in Figure 12.2 (along with duration of effect).

Drugs commonly used for sedation and premedication

See Figure 12.2. The classes of drug used are as follows:

- Phenothiazines, e.g. acepromazine, propionylpromazine
- Alpha-2 adrenoreceptor agonists, e.g. xylazine, medetomidine, dexmedetomidine

Route of administration	Advantages	Disadvantages
Intravenous	Reliable drug absorption Immediate onset of action	Animal is not sedated before handling and drug administration – stressful for the animal and animal handlers Some drugs should not be given intravenously
Intramuscular	Minimal handling required for administration Drug absorption is more reliable than by subcutaneous route Route of choice for most premedicants	May be painful when drug volume is large Administration may be difficult in very aggressive animals Delay before onset of peak sedation
Subcutaneous	Easy to administer drugs single handedly Administration of a large volume of drug is not painful	Delay before onset of peak effect is greater than for intramuscular route and more variable
Oral	Owners are able to administer sedative drugs orally Only oral preparations of acepromazine and diazepam are readily available	Variable onset and duration of action Sedation achieved following oral administration of diazepam or acepromazine is unpredictable Dose range is unpredictable and dependent on the individual patient

12.1 Advantages and disadvantages of different routes of administration of premedicant and sedative drugs.

Drug	Time to peak sedation or effect	Duration of action	Reversible?	Analgesia?
Acepromazine	35–40 minutes i.m. 15–20 minutes i.v.	4–6 hours	No	No
Medetomidine	15–20 minutes i.m. 2–3 minutes i.v.	Sedation: 2–3 hours Analgesia: 1 hour	Yes – with atipamezole	Yes
Midazolam	10–15 minutes i.m. 5 minutes i.v.	1–1.5 hours	Yes – with flumazenil	No
Diazepam	10–15 minutes i.m. 5 minutes i.v.	2 hours	Yes – with flumazenil	No
Atropine	20–30 minutes i.m. 1–2 minutes i.v.	Vagal inhibition: 2–3 hours	No	No
Glycopyrronium	20–30 minutes i.m. 2–3 minutes i.v.	Vagal inhibition: 2–3 hours	No	No
Methadone, hydromorphone	20–30 minutes i.m. 2–5 minutes i.v.	2–4 hours	Yes – with naloxone	Yes
Morphine	20–30 minutes i.m. Not recommended i.v.	2–4 hours	Yes – with naloxone	Yes
Pethidine (meperidine)	20–30 minutes i.m. Contraindicated i.v.	1–1.5 hours	Yes – with naloxone	Yes
Buprenorphine	30–45 minutes i.m. 12–15 minutes i.v.	6 hours	Yes – with naloxone	Yes
Butorphanol	20–30 minutes i.m. 2–5 minutes i.v.	1–1.5 hours	Yes – with naloxone	Yes

12.2 Characteristics of drugs used for sedation and premedication. Note that the duration of action of many of these drugs will vary between species and will depend on the dose administered. The times given are approximate guidelines only.

- Benzodiazepines, e.g. diazepam, midazolam
- Opioids, e.g. morphine, methadone, pethidine (meperidine), hydromorphone, butorphanol, buprenorphine
- Anticholinergics, e.g. atropine, glycopyrronium.

Phenothiazines

Phenothiazines are dopamine (D1 and D2) receptor antagonists, having calming, anti-psychotic, mood-altering effects. Acepromazine is the phenothiazine most commonly used for premedication in small animal practice.

Sedation

Acepromazine causes sedation and anxiolysis that is initially dose-dependent. Increasing the dose from 0.01 mg/kg to 0.05 mg/kg will usually improve sedation. With larger doses the degree of sedation is unchanged, whereas side effects are increased and duration of action prolonged. In comparison with the sedation produced by alpha-2 adrenergic agonists, sedation from acepromazine alone is generally less reliable. However, the quality and reliability of sedation can be improved by combination with an opioid (neuroleptanalgesia). Addition of an opioid also provides analgesia, which is advantageous since acepromazine itself is not an analgesic. In order to maximize sedation, the animal should be left undisturbed for 30–40 minutes after administration. In common with most sedative drugs, animals that appear sedated after acepromazine will often wake up if roused or excited and therefore quiet handling during induction of anaesthesia is necessary.

Other pharmacological effects

Cardiovascular system

Acepromazine is an antagonist at alpha-1 adrenoreceptors. Administration can therefore cause peripheral vasodilation and potentially a fall in arterial blood pressure. This is usually well tolerated in healthy animals, and changes in heart rate after acepromazine administration to normal animals are minimal, reflecting a limited effect on blood pressure. However, in animals with shock or cardiovascular disease this vasodilation can be disastrous, leading to cardiovascular collapse. Aggressive fluid therapy with a balanced electrolyte solution is the primary treatment of phenothiazine-induced hypotension. Acepromazine is long lasting and non-reversible: it is therefore advisable to avoid administration to animals where hypotension or cardiovascular compromise is anticipated as a potential complication of anaesthesia and surgery.

Heart rhythm: Acepromazine is considered to have anti-arrhythmic properties caused primarily by acting as an antagonist at alpha-1 adrenoreceptors in the heart. The clinical relevance of this anti-arrhythmic effect in small animals is unknown.

Respiratory system

Clinical doses have little effect on respiratory function, although higher doses can cause respiratory depression, particularly when given in combination with opioids.

Body temperature

Acepromazine is associated with a fall in body temperature due to a resetting of thermoregulatory mechanisms, combined with increased heat loss from the periphery due to peripheral vasodilation. Measures to support body temperature should be initiated immediately after administration of acepromazine in order to minimize changes in body temperature.

Seizure threshold

The effect of acepromazine on seizure threshold is contentious. Some people recommend that acepromazine be avoided in animals with epilepsy, or in those at an increased risk of convulsions, such as patients undergoing myelography. There are limited data in animals to support these recommendations.

Other

Giant breeds of dog are considered to be 'more sensitive' to the effects of acepromazine. This is probably a reflection of relative overdosing of large dogs when dose is calculated according to bodyweight rather than to allometric scaling.

Some Boxers are uniquely sensitive to even small doses of acepromazine, which has been attributed to orthostatic hypotension or vasovagal syncope in this breed. Although acepromazine is not contraindicated in Boxers, it is not the premedicant of choice in this breed. A very low dose (≤0.01 mg/kg) is recommended and animals should be monitored carefully after administration.

Acepromazine has an anti-emetic action and a recent study in dogs demonstrated that acepromazine given prior to opioid administration decreased the incidence of vomiting. This is attributed to a central depressant effect on the chemoreceptor trigger zone and vomiting centre. Acepromazine has weak anti-histamine effects, so its use for premedication prior to intradermal skin testing is not recommended.

Alpha-2 adrenoreceptor agonists

Alpha-2 adrenoreceptor agonists are potent sedative and analgesic drugs. Xylazine was the first to be used in veterinary practice but it has now been largely superseded by medetomidine, the most selective alpha-2 adrenoreceptor agonist currently available. Compared with medetomidine, xylazine is relatively unselective for the alpha-2 receptor (alpha-2:alpha-1 receptor selectivity binding ratios of medetomidine and xylazine are 1620:1 and 160:1 respectively); the agonist effect of xylazine at alpha-1 receptors in the heart is suggested to account for the reduced cardiovascular safety of xylazine compared with medetomidine. The superior selectivity of medetomidine makes it the alpha-2 agonist of choice for use in small animals.

Medetomidine is an equal mixture of two optical enantiomers, dexmedetomidine and levomedetomidine. The dextrorotatory isomer is the active ingredient and has gained more interest in human anaesthesiology over medetomidine. Dexmedetomidine is likely to become available on the veterinary market in the near future. Proposed advantages of dexmedetomidine over medetomidine include improved analgesia and a reduced requirement for drug metabolism because only active enantiomer is presented to the liver for metabolism. It is currently uncertain if it is clinically advantageous to use dexmedetomidine instead of medetomidine in small animals.

Sedation

Medetomidine sedation is profound and dose-related. However, similar to acepromazine, a plateau effect is reached and beyond this point further increases in dose prolong the duration of effect rather than increase the intensity of sedation. Synergism between alpha-2 agonists and opioids or benzodiazepines means that combining medetomidine with either of these agents will lead to more profound sedation, allowing the dose of medetomidine to be reduced.

Characteristics of general anaesthesia following premedication with alpha-2 agonists

Premedication with alpha-2 agonists has a significant influence on the characteristics of the ensuing anaesthesia. This must be remembered in order to use these drugs safely and the following points should be recognized:

- Significant drug-sparing effect: the dose of induction agent required after premedication with medetomidine is dramatically reduced. Failure to recognize this can easily lead to anaesthetic overdose. The concentration of inhalant agent required for maintenance of anaesthesia is similarly reduced (by up to 70% for halothane and isoflurane)
- Intravenous induction agents must be given slowly and to effect: medetomidine slows the injection site to brain blood circulation time such that it takes longer to see the peak central nervous system (CNS) depressant effect of the intravenous agent. This can inadvertently lead to anaesthetic overdose if the intravenous agent is given too quickly
- Alpha-2 agonists have potent analgesic properties: premedication with medetomidine can contribute significantly to intraoperative analgesia. This can result in a very stable plane of anaesthesia during the maintenance phase, reducing swings in depth of anaesthesia associated with changes in the level of intraoperative surgical stimulation.

Other pharmacological effects

Cardiovascular system

Medetomidine produces a biphasic effect on blood pressure (initial increase followed by a return to normal or slightly below normal values). Heart rate is decreased throughout the period of alpha-2 agonist administration, and normal expected heart rates are 45–60 and 100–115 beats per minute for dogs and cats, respectively.

Heart rate: The characteristic changes in heart rate result from the stimulation of alpha-2 adrenoreceptors located around peripheral blood vessels and in the CNS and can be divided temporally into two phases. It is important to understand the origin of these changes in order to use alpha-2 agonists safely and effectively for sedation and pre-anaesthetic medication.

Phase 1: The immediate response of the cardiovascular system to medetomidine is an increase in blood pressure, caused by peripheral vasoconstriction via activation of alpha-2 receptors located in the peripheral vasculature. The mechanism of vasoconstriction is similar to that caused by activation of the sympathetic nervous system during the 'fight or flight' (stress) response. The increase in blood pressure, however, causes a reflex reduction in heart rate, mediated by the baroreceptor reflex.

Phase 2: The peripheral vasoconstriction induced by medetomidine lasts for approximately 20 minutes and in phase 2 blood pressure returns to normal or slightly below normal. Despite the reduction in blood pressure back to approximately normal values, heart rate remains low throughout the period of medetomidine administration. Phase 2 bradycardia is mediated centrally as a result of the reduction in sympathetic nervous system tone. Medetomidine causes a fall in sympathetic tone via an effect at presynaptic alpha-2 adrenoreceptors located in the CNS and this causes a prolonged reduction in heart rate.

Cardiac output: Alpha-2 agonists cause a reduction in cardiac output. The precise aetiology of this reduction is unknown and is considered to be multifactorial. The increase in afterload resulting from peripheral vasoconstriction is thought to be a contributing factor. In animals with a healthy, normally functioning cardiovascular system, the reduction in cardiac output is not associated with reduced oxygen delivery to central organs, namely the CNS, heart, kidney and liver. However, in animals with limited cardiovascular reserve, the reduction in cardiac output following medetomidine may have detrimental consequences for organ function due to reduced oxygen delivery. Alpha-2 agonists have a very limited margin of cardiovascular safety and therefore are only suitable for use for sedation or premedication in animals with a normally functioning cardiovascular system.

Respiratory system

Minimal effects on the respiratory system are seen in healthy animals and arterial oxygen and carbon dioxide tensions (concentrations) remain within normal limits. Profound sedation after medetomidine can lead to upper airway obstruction in brachycephalic dogs.

Renal system

Urine production is increased due to a reduction in vasopressin and renin secretion. This is not of clinical significance in healthy animals.

Pancreas

Endogenous insulin secretion is reduced, leading to a transient hyperglycaemia. This is not of sufficient magnitude to result in an osmotic diuresis in dogs and cats.

Liver

Both hepatic blood flow and the rate of metabolism of other drugs by the liver are reduced. This is not of clinical significance in healthy animals, but medetomidine should be avoided in animals with liver disease.

Body temperature

Although medetomidine has a direct depressant effect on the thermoregulatory centre, peripheral vasoconstriction tends to reduce peripheral heat loss. As a consequence it can be easier to maintain normothermia during the perioperative period than in animals given acepromazine. In the author's experience, animals tend to stay warmer during medetomidine/isoflurane anaesthesia.

Emesis

Vomiting is frequently seen in cats and dogs after intramuscular or subcutaneous administration due to activation of central alpha-2 receptors. Alpha-2 agonists are contraindicated in animals with a suspected oesophageal foreign body where emesis may result in further tissue damage.

Reversal of alpha-2 agonists with atipamezole

Alpha-2 agonist sedation and analgesia are rapidly reversed by the administration of a specific alpha-2 adrenoreceptor antagonist such as atipamezole. Recoveries following intramuscular administration of atipamezole are generally smooth and of good quality. Intravenous administration of atipamezole usually produces a very rapid, excitable recovery from anaesthesia or sedation and this route is not recommended. It is important to ensure that analgesia is supplemented, if necessary, with different classes of drugs (such as opioids and non-steroidal anti-inflammatory drugs) before reversal by atipamezole. Preliminary findings from a recent study into anaesthetic-related mortality and morbidity in small animal practice (Confidential Enquiry into Perioperative Small Animal Fatalities – CEPSAF) have identified the recovery period to be of relatively high risk because animals are often poorly monitored and observed, despite still being under the influence of the cardiovascular and respiratory depressant effects of anaesthetic agents. Shortening the length of the recovery period using atipamezole can contribute to improved patient safety during the perioperative period. Yohimbine and tolazoline are commercially available (in some countries) alpha-2 antagonists that may also be used as reversal agents after medetomidine or other alpha-2 agonist sedation. Compared with atipamezole, these antagonists have a lower alpha-2:alpha-1 receptor selectivity.

Patient selection

Medetomidine affords many advantages for premedication and sedation, but in order to use the drug safely and effectively in small animals, it should only be administered to healthy animals. It should *not* be used in the following patient groups:

- Cardiovascular disease (e.g. mitral regurgitation)
- Systemic disease causing deterioration in cardiovascular function (e.g. toxaemia)
- Liver disease
- Geriatric animals: these patients do not have the normal functional organ reserve of healthy adult animals
- Very young animals: the physiological effects of medetomidine in puppies and kittens are unknown. Medetomidine is not the premedicant or sedative agent of choice in animals less than 12 weeks of age
- Diabetes mellitus: such patients often have multiple organ disease, which, in combination with the effect of medetomidine on blood glucose concentration, means that medetomidine is not the ideal premedicant or sedative drug for animals with diabetes mellitus.

Routine co-administration of atropine and medetomidine

When alpha-2 agonists were first introduced into small animal practice, there was a trend for the routine co-administration of atropine to offset the bradycardia. It is now recognized that the routine co-administration of atropine and medetomidine is detrimental. The initial reduction in heart rate is physiological and a response to an increase in blood pressure. Obtunding this normal physiological response results in tachycardia and greater hypertension. The heart is required to beat faster against a vasoconstricted peripheral vascular bed, increasing myocardial oxygen consumption. There is also less diastolic time for adequate myocardial perfusion. This can lead to ventricular arrhythmias and potential cardiovascular collapse.

Management of extremely 'low' heart rates during anaesthesia following medetomidine

Atropine

Heart rates during anaesthesia after premedication with medetomidine are lower than after premedication with other sedatives such as acepromazine. However, should the heart rate fall below the 'expected' range following medetomidine (45–60 and 100–115 beats/minute for dogs and cats, respectively) and clinical monitoring suggests that the bradycardia is having a negative impact on blood pressure, action should be taken to increase the heart rate back to within the expected range. Many factors can contribute to a low heart rate during anaesthesia and therefore other causative factors, such as 'too-deep' anaesthesia due to overdose of a volatile agent, should first be addressed. However, in cases where the excessive bradycardia appears to be primarily medetomidine mediated, a low dose of atropine (2.5–5 μg/kg, slowly i.v.) can be used to shift the heart rate back into the expected normal range for medetomidine patients.

Ketamine

Administration of a low dose of ketamine is an alternative strategy to manage extremely low heart rates during anaesthesia following medetomidine: ketamine has sympathomimetic properties. Therefore, in phase 2 of the cardiovascular response to medetomidine, when the bradycardia is primarily due to a central reduction in sympathetic tone, a low dose of ketamine (0.1–0.2 mg/kg, slowly i.v.) can also be effective to increase heart rate. It is important first to exclude other causative factors of a low heart rate. Ketamine may also be used as a second-line approach in patients where atropine has been ineffective. It is important to allow sufficient time for a response to atropine (3–4 minutes) before ketamine is given.

Partial reversal of medetomidine during anaesthesia by the administration of a low dose of atipamezole

Administration of a low dose of atipamezole (5–20 μg/kg to effect, i.v.) is an alternative technique to reduce any adverse effects of medetomidine during anaesthesia, such as an excessive reduction in heart rate.

Atipamezole will concurrently antagonize medetomidine sedation and analgesia, and therefore administration may be associated with a reduction in depth of anaesthesia. Intraoperatively, this must be managed promptly by co-administration of an intravenous anaesthetic agent such as propofol. There are no clinical studies to support the use of atipamezole intraoperatively and this technique should be used with caution.

Benzodiazepines

Diazepam and midazolam are the benzodiazepines used most commonly in small animal practice. A comparison of the physical properties and pharmacological effects of these two drugs is shown in Figure 12.3. They exert their main sedative effects through depression of the limbic system. Their action is thought to be through activation of a specific benzodiazepine receptor, part of the gamma-aminobutyric acid (GABA) receptor complex. GABA is a major inhibitory neurotransmitter in the CNS. These drugs do not have analgesic properties, except to reduce skeletal muscle spasm. Zolazepam is a benzodiazepine derivative that is only available in combination with tiletamine. This preparation (Telazol® or Zoletil®) is a short-acting anaesthetic agent in cats and dogs. The pharmacological effects of zolazepam and tiletamine are similar to ketamine combined with diazepam (see Chapter 13).

Property	Midazolam	Diazepam
Preparation	Water-soluble, can be injected intramuscularly and intravenously without causing pain or irritation	Insoluble in water, usually solubilized in propylene glycol, although an emulsion formulation is available Propylene glycol preparation causes pain on injection and thrombophlebitis when given intravenously. Unpredictable absorption after intramuscular administration
Length of action and metabolism	Metabolized in liver; metabolites are inactive, so midazolam is shorter acting than diazepam with less risk of accumulation	Metabolized in liver; metabolites are active, so risk of accumulation and prolonged action when given repeatedly
Clinical use	Benzodiazepine of choice for use in small animals	Give propylene glycol preparation slowly intravenously, preferably with free-running fluids

12.3 Comparison of midazolam and diazepam.

Sedation

Benzodiazepines administered alone produce minimal or no sedation in healthy cats and dogs, and may even cause excitation due to loss of learned inhibitory behaviour. Benzodiazepines are therefore given in combination with other sedatives. Many of these protocols combine a benzodiazepine with an opioid because both classes of drugs have few negative effects on haemodynamics.

Other pharmacological effects

Cardiovascular and respiratory systems

Benzodiazepines have minor effects on both of these systems. This is one of their major advantages and these drugs tend to be used as premedicants in animals with cardiovascular compromise. Synergism between benzodiazepines and other sedative drugs may enhance respiratory depression from other drugs when used in combination.

Anticonvulsant effects

Benzodiazepines are commonly used to manage convulsions, particularly as a first-line intervention for animals presenting in status epilepticus.

Reversal of benzodiazepines with flumazenil

The CNS effects of benzodiazepines can be effectively antagonized by the administration of the benzodiazepine receptor antagonist flumazenil. When given intravenously it will rapidly reverse all agonist effects of benzodiazepines. This drug is expensive, but low doses (0.01–0.03 mg/kg) are often adequate to reverse sedation in animals that are slow to recover after receiving high doses of benzodiazepines for sedation.

Opioids

Opioids are commonly incorporated into premedication regimens to provide analgesia and to improve the reliability and intensity of the sedation achieved following combination with the primary sedative drug. The choice of opioid will depend on the degree of analgesia needed, the speed of onset of the drug's action and the length of action required. Generally, longer-acting opioid agents, such as morphine, methadone, hydromorphone and buprenorphine, are used as premedicants. Butorphanol provides poor analgesia compared with that provided by these other opioids, but is useful to enhance sedation provided by either acepromazine or medetomidine (e.g. for diagnostic imaging).

Pharmacological effects

A more detailed description of opioid pharmacology can be found in Chapter 9.

Analgesia

Depending on the opioid chosen, different intensities of analgesia can be obtained. Opioids are a key element of perioperative pain control.

Sedation

The sedative effect of opioids is usually dose- and drug-dependent. Sedation from phenothiazines and alpha-2 agonists is enhanced when they are combined with opioids.

Other pharmacological effects

Cardiovascular system

Opioids have few negative effects on haemodynamics. They can cause a reduction in heart rate through stimulation of the vagal nerve, which can be managed by co-administration of an anticholinergic.

Respiratory system

Opioids such as methadone, morphine, hydromorphone and buprenorphine do not cause clinically significant respiratory depression in animals at the dose rates normally used.

Gastrointestinal system

Morphine and hydromorphone directly stimulate the vomiting centre and animals sedated or premedicated with morphine and hydromorphone often vomit shortly after their administration. This effect is less apparent (or not evident at all) when morphine or hydromorphone is used postoperatively for management of perioperative pain.

Opioids stimulate the sphincters of the gastrointestinal tract causing an overall action that is constipating; increased intestinal peristalsis tends to combat this effect. When animals are anaesthetized for gastrointestinal endoscopy, pyloric constriction after opioid premedication may make passage of an endoscope through the pylorus from the stomach to the duodenum more challenging.

Anticholinergic agents

Anticholinergic agents antagonize the muscarinic effects of acetylcholine and historically have been used in premedication regimens to prevent the unwanted effects of stimulation of the parasympathetic nervous system by anaesthetic agents or surgery. The two agents commonly used in small animal practice are atropine and glycopyrronium, and a comparison of their properties is shown in Figure 12.4.

Aims of premedication with an anticholinergic are as follows:

- Reduction of salivary and bronchial secretions
- Blockage of the effects of vagal stimulation
- Blockage of the effects of drugs that stimulate the parasympathetic nervous system, such as opioids.

Routine premedication with an anticholinergic is unnecessary in current anaesthetic practice. Modern volatile agents are not irritant to the airway and do not cause excessive salivary and bronchial secretions. Pre-emptive administration of an anticholinergic before stimulation of the vagal nerve may cause tachycardia. Although high doses of opioids may cause bradycardia, it is not always necessary to manage this by administration of an anticholinergic. Therefore, anticholinergics are normally given if required rather than routinely as a part of the premedication protocol.

Drug combinations

Acepromazine + opioid

- Commonly used for premedication of both cats and dogs.
- Degree of sedation is dose-dependent, but usually only light sedation is achieved.
- Sedation is usually inadequate for complex radiography or minimally invasive procedures.
- Consider cardiovascular effects of acepromazine: unsuitable for animals that are in shock or have severe cardiovascular compromise.

Medetomidine + opioid

- Potent, reliable sedation in both cats and dogs.
- Premedication prior to general anaesthesia.
- Suitable for sedation for invasive procedures (such as ear examination) and radiography where the animal needs to be immobile.
- Consider cardiovascular effects of medetomidine – any evidence of cardiovascular or systemic disease is a contraindication for use.

Property	Atropine	Glycopyrronium
CNS action	Able to cross the blood–brain barrier and placenta	A quaternary ammonium compound and highly polar, therefore limited diffusion across the blood–brain barrier and placenta
Routes of administration	Intravenous, intramuscular, subcutaneous Following intravenous administration atropine may cause an initial increase in vagal tone associated with a reduction in heart rate. The classic parasympatholytic action occurs secondarily	Intravenous, intramuscular, subcutaneous Initial increase in vagal tone following intravenous injection is less likely to occur compared with atropine
Action on the pupil	Pupil dilation – may impair vision which can contribute to poor recoveries in cats	No effect on the pupil
Duration of action	Varies between species and dose-dependent. Vagal inhibition will last for approximately 1–2 hours	Longer duration of action than atropine. Vagal inhibition lasts 2–3 hours. Antisialogogue effect may persist for up to 7 hours

12.4 Comparison of atropine and glycopyrronium.

Medetomidine + benzodiazepine

- More potent sedation than when medetomidine is given alone.
- Useful combination for sedation for procedures such as hip radiography.

Medetomidine + ketamine

- Medetomidine prevents CNS excitation from ketamine.
- Depending on the dose of ketamine administered, this combination will provide heavy sedation/general anaesthesia for invasive short procedures.
- Addition of an opioid, such as buprenorphine, to this combination will allow doses of the other drugs to be reduced.
- Recoveries from anaesthesia following this combination can be very excitable in dogs.
- The effects of ketamine during recovery are present in the cat but usually acceptable.
- Following short procedures it is important to wait at least 45 minutes before reversing the effects of medetomidine, otherwise the excitation effects of ketamine are unmasked.
- See also Chapter 13 (intravenous anaesthetics).

Opioid + benzodiazepine

- Minimal negative effects on the cardiovascular system, useful for premedicating or sedating dogs with cardiovascular compromise.
- Degree of sedation is dependent on the dose and individual patient – animals with severe systemic disease usually become more sedated than healthier patients.
- Very young animals tend to become more sedated than adults.
- Combination is not optimal for use in cats. Sedation is unreliable and excitation may occur.

Benzodiazepine + ketamine

- Benzodiazepine prevents CNS excitation from ketamine.
- Useful for sedating cats when heavy sedation is required.
- With higher doses of ketamine, general anaesthesia can be induced (see Chapter 13).
- Combination is cardiovascularly stable and is useful for cats in which the administration of acepromazine or medetomidine is undesirable. Caution should be exercised in cats with hypertrophic cardiomyopathy. The positive chronotropic effects of ketamine may result in inadequate myocardial perfusion in the presence of a hypertrophic myocardium.
- Difficult to avoid ketamine-induced behavioural changes in recovery. Animals are often disorientated for the first few hours of the recovery period.

Tiletamine + zolazepam (Telazol® or Zoletil®)

- Preparation is an equal mixture (weight to weight) of tiletamine and zolazepam.
- Similar to a diazepam or midazolam and ketamine combination.
- See above and Chapter 13 for guidelines on clinical use.

Propofol

- Low doses of propofol intravenously can be used to provide 'sedation' in cats and dogs for short procedures.
- Sedation produced by propofol, although dose-dependent, is significant and the distinction between propofol sedation and propofol anaesthesia is minimal.

Maximizing the sedation achieved by a particular drug combination

- Ensure that the animal is left in a quiet environment following drug administration.
- Ideally place cats and dogs in separate rooms.
- Do not disturb the animal until sufficient time has elapsed for drugs to have reached their peak effect.
- Darkening the environment can lead to improved sedation.
- When the animal is sedated, ensure that it is handled gently and quietly during the procedure or induction of anaesthesia. This helps to prevent sudden arousal from sedation.

Choosing the right premedicant combination for the patient

Factors that influence the choice of premedicants include:

- American Society of Anesthesiologists (ASA) classification of the patient (see Chapter 2)
- Species and breed of the patient
- Temperament of the patient
- Age of the patient
- Reason for anaesthesia and procedure to be carried out
- Degree of pain expected from the procedure.

The ASA status of the patient can be used as a basis to build protocols for premedication and sedation of animals in clinical practice. It can be a practical way to introduce some standardization into premedication and sedation regimens in a busy practice setting while still taking the needs of individual patients into consideration. The following section describes premedication or sedation protocols that are suitable for dogs or cats of different ASA classification status. Dosage schedules are shown in Figures 12.5 and 12.6.

Drug combination		Route of administration	Species	Patient selection
Drug 1	*Drug 2*			
Acepromazine (0.03–0.05 mg/kg)	/ Methadone (0.2–0.5 mg/kg) / Morphine (0.2–0.5 mg/kg) / Hydromorphone (0.05–0.15 mg/kg) / Pethidine (meperidine) (4–5 mg/kg) / Buprenorphine (20 μg/kg) / Butorphanol (0.2–0.4 mg/kg)	i.m. or i.v. i.m. i.m. or i.v. i.m. i.v., i.m., s.c. i.v., i.m., s.c.	Cat and dog Cat and dog Cat and dog Cat and dog Cat and dog Cat and dog	ASA 1–3 patients depending on assessment of cardiovascular function. Use lower dose of acepromazine in ASA 2–3 patients. Use lower dose range of drugs when given intravenously
Medetomidine (10–20 μg/kg)	/ Buprenorphine (20 μg/kg) / Butorphanol (0.2–0.4 mg/kg) / Hydromorphone (0.1 mg/kg) / Morphine (0.1– 0.2 mg/kg) / Methadone (0.1–0.2 mg/kg)	i.m. or i.v. i.m. or i.v. i.m. or i.v. i.m. i.m. or i.v. Use lower doses i.v.	Cat and dog Cat and dog Cat and dog Cat and dog Cat and dog	ASA 1–2 patients. Cardiovascular function must be normal
Medetomidine (10–20 μg/kg)	/ Midazolam (0.2–0.3 mg/kg) / Diazepam (0.2–0.3 mg/kg)	i.m. or i.v. – use lower dose i.v.	Dog Dog	ASA 1–2 patients. Cardiovascular function must be normal. Useful for non-painful procedures such as diagnostic imaging
Midazolam (0.3–0.4 mg/kg)	/ Methadone (0.2–0.5 mg/kg) / Morphine (0.2–0.5 mg/kg) / Hydromorphone (0.05–0.15 mg/kg)	i.m. or i.v. i.m. i.v. or i.m.	Dog Dog Dog, rarely cat	ASA 3–5 Good cardiovascular stability
Midazolam (0.2–0.3 mg/kg)	/ Ketamine (5–10 mg/kg)	i.m. or i.v. – use lower dose i.v.	Cat	ASA 2–4. Avoid in patients with hypertrophic cardiomyopathy. Higher dose of ketamine will induce anaesthesia
Zolazepam + tiletamine	Available as a proprietary mixture (Telazol® or Zoletil®) Dose range for premedication 3–6 mg/kg	i.m. or i.v. – use lower dose i.v.	Cat and dog	As above for midazolam/ ketamine mixture. Recovery can be stormy in dogs
Morphine (0.2–0.5 mg/kg) Methadone (0.2–0.5 mg/kg) Hydromorphone (0.05–0.1 mg/kg)		i.m. i.m. or i.v. i.m. or i.v.	Cat and dog Use lower end of dose range and intramuscular route in cats	ASA 4–5 Young animals

12.5 Drug combinations used for premedication in cats and dogs.

Drug combination		Route of administration	Species notes	Sedation notes
Drug 1	*Drug 2*			
Acepromazine (0.03–0.05 mg/kg)	/ Methadone (0.2–0.5 mg/kg) / Morphine (0.2–0.5 mg/kg) / Pethidine (4–5 mg/kg) as above / Buprenorphine (20 μg/kg) / Butorphanol (0.2–0.4 mg/kg) / Hydromorphone (0.1–0.2 mg/kg)	i.v. or i.m. i.m. i.m. i.m. or i.v. i.m. or i.v. i.m. or i.v. Use lower doses i.v.	Dogs: higher doses of opioids will provide greater sedation Cats: use low to mid dose range of opioids	Will provide light sedation in cats and dogs. Do not expect animals to become recumbent
Medetomidine (20–40 μg/kg)	/ Buprenorphine (20 μg/kg) / Butorphanol (0.2–0.4 mg/kg) / Hydromorphone (0.1 mg/kg)	i.m. or i.v. Use lower doses i.v.	Dogs and cats	Higher doses of medetomidine will provide more reliable and profound sedation. Expect animals to become recumbent. Useful for invasive painful procedures such as removal of grass seeds from the ear canal

12.6 Drug combinations used for sedation in dogs and cats (see Figure 12.5 for information regarding route of administration and patient selection). (continues) ▶

Drug combination		Route of administration	Species notes	Sedation notes
Drug 1	*Drug 2*			
Medetomidine (20–40 µg/kg)	/ Midazolam (0.3 mg/kg) / Diazepam (0.3 mg/kg)	i.m. or i.v. Use lower doses i.v.	Dogs	Higher doses of medetomidine will provide more reliable and profound sedation. Expect animals to become recumbent. Degree of analgesia is less than when medetomidine is combined with an opioid
Midazolam (0.4–0.5 mg/kg)	/ Methadone (0.2–0.5 mg/kg) / Morphine (0.2–0.5 mg/kg) / Hydromorphone (0.1–0.15 mg/kg)	i.m. or i.v. i.m. i.m. or i.v.	Dogs	Degree of sedation will depend on the health and temperament of the patient. May be able to carry out some invasive procedures if the animal is handled patiently and quietly
Midazolam (0.2–0.3 mg/kg)	/ Ketamine (5–10 mg/kg)	i.m. or i.v. – use lower doses i.v.	Cats	Expect profound sedation/light general anaesthesia
Zolazepam + tiletamine	Available as a proprietary mixture (Telazol® or Zoletil®) Dose range for sedation/short duration general anaesthesia 9–13 mg/kg	i.m. or i.v. – use lower doses i.v.	Dogs and cats	As above for midazolam/ ketamine mixture. Recovery can be stormy in dogs
Morphine (0.2–0.5 mg/kg) Methadone (0.2–0.5 mg/kg) Hydromorphone (0.1–0.2 mg/kg)		i.m. i.m. or i.v. i.m. or i.v.	Dogs and cats Use lower end of dose range and intramuscular route in cats	Mild sedation only. Do not expect animal to become recumbent

12.6 (continued) Drug combinations used for sedation in dogs and cats (see Figure 12.5 for information regarding route of administration and patient selection).

Dogs

ASA 1

- Combination of either acepromazine or medetomidine with an opioid: the choice of opioid is determined by the requirement for intraoperative analgesia. Medetomidine is a potent analgesic, so combination with buprenorphine, a partial agonist, usually provides adequate supplementary intraoperative analgesia. Medetomidine and hydromorphone is also a good choice. Full agonists, such as morphine and methadone, should be combined with acepromazine for procedures that are expected to be painful. The comparative properties of acepromazine and medetomidine are shown in Figure 12.7.

Property	Acepromazine	Medetomidine
Sedation	Less reliable than medetomidine, improved by addition of an opioid	Reliable sedation, improved by combination with an opioid
Analgesia	No analgesia	Potent analgesia
Cardiovascular system	Vasodilation and possible hypotension, minimal significance in healthy animals	Decrease in cardiac output that is of minimal significance in healthy animals. Significantly reduced margin of safety for the cardiovascular system compared with acepromazine
Respiratory system	Minimal effect	Minimal effect
Drug-sparing effect	Limited (approx. 25%)	Potent drug-sparing effect: improved balance of anaesthesia
Background 'anaesthesia/analgesia'	Limited	Tends to prevent big swings in depth of anaesthesia in response to changing surgical stimulation
Body temperature	Rapid drop in body temperature due to peripheral vasodilation	Fall in body temperature is less rapid due to peripheral vasoconstriction
Reversibility	Not reversible. Length of action approx .6 hours	Reversible (atipamezole)

12.7 Comparison of acepromazine and medetomidine.

ASA 2

- Combination of acepromazine and an opioid.
- Medetomidine combined with an opioid is appropriate for some ASA 2 animals, depending on the underlying reason for this ASA classification (see under 'Patient selection' in medetomidine section).

ASA 3

- Acepromazine (low dose) and opioid combination may be appropriate as long as there is no underlying cardiovascular disease.
- Benzodiazepine and opioid combination: useful for premedication and sedation of dogs with either cardiovascular disease or systemic abnormalities that affect cardiovascular function. Better sedation can be expected in animals showing greater clinical signs of disease.

ASA 4

- Benzodiazepine and opioid combination.

ASA 5

It is unlikely that sedation will be needed. Low doses of opioids or benzodiazepines prior to anaesthesia are desirable to reduce the concentration of anaesthetic agents needed for induction and maintenance of anaesthesia, but a distinct premedication phase is not usually necessary in very sick patients.

Cats

ASA 1

Recommendations are as for dogs. The profound sedation caused by medetomidine can be advantageous in aggressive cats where intravenous access can be challenging unless good sedation is achieved. In feral or extremely aggressive cats the addition of ketamine to this combination will ensure heavy sedation/short-term general anaesthesia. High-dose morphine (0.6 mg/kg) with acepromazine (0.1 mg/kg) also works well in aggressive ASA 1 cats.

ASA 2

Recommendations are as for dogs.

ASA 3

- Acepromazine and opioid combination (low dose): as with dogs, will depend on evaluation of the cardiovascular system. The addition of a benzodiazepine to this combination can be helpful.
- Benzodiazepine and opioid combination: unlike in dogs, this combination does not produce reliable sedation in adult cats. However, although some cats do not appear to be very sedated they can be remarkably tolerant of intravenous catheter placement.
- Benzodiazepine and ketamine combination: this is an alternative to the benzodiazepine/opioid protocol used in dogs. Low doses of ketamine (5 mg/kg i.m. with midazolam 0.3 mg/kg) will usually provide profound sedation allowing easy intravenous access for induction of anaesthesia. Higher doses of ketamine (10 mg/kg i.m.) will result in anaesthesia, allowing intubation and a direct progression to inhalant maintenance of anaesthesia. Ketamine should be avoided in cats with hypertrophic cardiomyopathy because of its positive chronotropic effects (see Chapter 13). Premedication with ketamine will usually cause behavioural changes during recovery.

ASA 4

- Benzodiazepine and ketamine combination.
- Benzodiazepine and opioid combination.
- Opioid alone: in cats that have a quiet temperament, sedation with an opioid alone (e.g. buprenorphine or morphine) may be adequate to provide mild sedation. This can be useful in cats with hypertrophic cardiomyopathy where ketamine is contraindicated.

ASA 5

Recommendations are as for dogs. Administration of a low dose of a benzodiazepine and opioid close to the time of induction of anaesthesia will contribute to a balanced anaesthetic technique.

Other specific patient groups

Geriatric animals

Geriatric animals tend to have a higher incidence of concurrent disease than younger animals, which may increase their risk for anaesthesia and affect ASA classification status (see Chapter 28). It is also likely that the normal organ reserve of geriatric animals is decreased compared with that of younger animals. This is particularly relevant for the cardiovascular system: although no abnormalities may be found on pre-anaesthetic examination, cardiovascular function may be decreased under stress, such as during anaesthesia. It is advisable to avoid medetomidine in geriatric patients because of the reduced reserve functionality in the cardiovascular system.

Young animals

Cats and dogs older than 12 weeks have normal liver function and can therefore be considered as adults in terms of anaesthetic drug metabolism. In younger patients with immature liver function, the effects of anaesthetic drugs may be prolonged and, therefore, it is advisable to avoid long-acting agents such as acepromazine. There are limited data regarding use of medetomidine in very young cats and dogs. Medetomidine combined with ketamine has been used successfully for early neutering in cats, although haemodynamic monitoring in those cases was limited. An opioid and benzodiazepine combination can be used very effectively in both puppies and kittens, which seem to be more susceptible to the sedative effects of these drugs than adults. An opioid (low dose) administered alone is also suitable, especially in sick animals where sedation will be more profound.

Animals at risk of respiratory obstruction and brachycephalic breeds

Sedation caused by premedicants can exacerbate respiratory obstruction caused by anatomical conformation or by laryngeal paralysis, although sometimes this can be offset by the calming effect of sedatives leading to a more normal breathing pattern. These animals must be carefully observed and monitored for respiratory distress after premedication or sedation, and provision of supplemental oxygen is advisable. Acute and complete respiratory obstruction is an indication to proceed directly to general anaesthesia. In this situation, opioids and benzodiazepines can be given intravenously after induction to provide a balanced anaesthetic technique.

Monitoring and support of the sedated and premedicated patient

Most of the drugs used for sedation and premedication of cats and dogs are associated with varying degrees of cardiovascular and respiratory depression. As well as the direct effects of some drugs on the respiratory system, brachycephalic dogs are predisposed to a degree of respiratory tract obstruction after sedation. The effects of sedation prevent the animal from effectively maintaining a clear airway. Sedated animals can also easily become hypothermic due to decreased muscle activity and impairment of the thermoregulatory system. Although it is clear that adequate monitoring and 'support' must be provided for sedated and premedicated patients, the logistics of this can be difficult. Animals are usually placed in a kennel following administration of sedative drugs, so that supplemental oxygen may be difficult to administer. Animals that are being moved between a kennel and diagnostic areas can be difficult to keep warm unless intensive efforts are made. Unless portable monitoring equipment is available, 'kennel side' monitoring can be difficult. Monitoring and support of sedated and premedicated patients should begin as early as possible and this support continued until the patient is fully awake. The level of support and monitoring provided should be determined by the ASA status of the patient and the reason for sedation/premedication.

Monitoring

Depth of sedation/CNS depression

This is useful to assess if the level of sedation is adequate for the procedure and should be monitored intermittently throughout the period of sedation. The following can be assessed:

- Heart and respiratory rate
- Presence of an eyelid/blink reflex
- Response to toe pinch
- Response of the animal to arousal with voice or touch.

Cardiovascular system

The level of cardiovascular system monitoring will be determined by the cardiovascular status of the animal. Monitoring the pulse rate and pulse quality is mandatory in all animals. Use of pulse oximetry is useful to monitor oxygen saturation and a probe can easily be placed on the tongue of most lightly sedated and premedicated animals. Other sites of placement include the non-pigmented and hairless vulva or prepuce, the ear pinna or interdigital skin. Pulse oximetry is often unreliable following premedication with medetomidine due to the peripheral vasoconstriction induced by this agent. This should not be of concern since oxygen concentrations are usually well maintained in healthy animals following medetomidine administration. Supplementation of oxygen is still advisable in these patients. Electrocardiographic monitoring is beneficial in higher-risk patients and patients with cardiovascular disease, particularly heart rhythm abnormalities.

Respiratory system

Observation of the respiratory rate and depth of respiration is mandatory in all sedated animals. In brachycephalic breeds it is important that the head and neck are kept extended to prevent upper respiratory obstruction from the soft tissues. Placing animals in sternal recumbency also assists maintenance of a clear airway and maximizes lung function. Monitoring airway gases (inspired and expired carbon dioxide and oxygen concentrations) is possible in animals that are not intubated, depending on the type of capnography and oxygen monitoring equipment available. With side-stream capnography the gas sampling tube can be placed in the nasal cavity of the animal, allowing reasonably accurate measurement of expired carbon dioxide concentration. Although severe respiratory depression is unusual after administration of clinically used sedation and premedication protocols, always be ready to induce anaesthesia and intubate a sedated patient to allow support of ventilation if necessary.

Body temperature

Monitoring body temperature is vital in order to support body temperature adequately in sedated patients. Practically this can be achieved using a rectal thermometer.

Blood glucose

It may be appropriate to monitor blood glucose in some patients in order to prevent hypoglycaemia. This is particularly the case in young puppies and kittens that have limited glucose reserves and are therefore at risk of hypoglycaemia during sedation and anaesthesia.

Supportive measures

Oxygen

Oxygen can be easily supplemented via an anaesthesia breathing system and facemask placed on or near the nose of the animal. Pre-oxygenation prior to induction of anaesthesia will help prevent hypoxaemia should a period of apnoea occur immediately after induction of anaesthesia. Increasing the concentration of oxygen in the inspired gas mixture to >30% in sedated animals breathing room air will prevent hypoxaemia as a result of respiratory depression, and should be implemented during sedation of all animals. Alternative techniques to increase the inspired oxygen concentration are placing sedated animals in an oxygen cage or administration of oxygen through a nasal catheter. The oxygen cage can be useful for dyspnoeic cats after premedication and before induction of anaesthesia, or while an animal is recovering from the effects of sedation. Use of nasal catheters is appropriate for animals that require longer-term sedation and oxygen supplementation.

Support of body temperature

Sedated animals quickly become hypothermic and preventing a fall in body temperature is important. The following measures can be implemented to help maintain body temperature:

- Ensure adequate ambient temperature
- Provide warm bedding in the kennel/cage of the animal
- Ensure that the animal is not lying directly on a cold surface
- Wrap the animal in reflective foil or bubble wrap as insulation
- Place 'hot packs' or latex gloves filled with warm water ('hot hands') around the animal. Be aware that a sedated animal is unable to move away from a heat source that is too hot and capable of causing skin damage.

Fluid therapy

Indications for fluid therapy during sedation will depend on the reason for sedation and the health status of the animal. One should remember that sedated animals are not capable of regulating their own fluid balance and therefore some animals will benefit from supportive fluid therapy. Examples include patients with chronic renal failure and very young puppies and kittens who may require support to maintain a normal blood glucose concentration. Higher risk (ASA 3, 4 and 5) patients for anaesthesia will probably benefit from administration of fluids intraoperatively, therefore it can be advantageous to place an intravenous catheter and begin the fluid support early, at around the time of premedication. This contributes to optimal stabilization of the patient before induction of anaesthesia.

Summary

Sedation and premedication are part of the daily routine in small animal practice. It is important to understand the pharmacology of the different drugs used so that the most appropriate combination for each individual can be chosen. Implementation of practice protocols based on ASA classification can be helpful to improve uniformity in a busy clinic, while ensuring that the requirements of individual patients are met. Monitoring and support of premedicated patients should be initiated early; the intensity of this 'peri-premedicant' support should be adjusted to the ASA status of the patient and the procedure to be carried out.

References and further reading

Alibhai HI, Clarke KW, Lee YH and Thompson J (1996) Cardiopulmonary effects of combinations of medetomidine hydrochloride and atropine sulphate in dogs. *Veterinary Record* **138**, 11–12

Brodbelt DC, Young LE, Pfeiffer DU and Wood JLN (2006) Update Results from the Confidential Enquiry into Perioperative Small Animal Fatalities (CEPSAF). *Proceedings of the Association of Veterinary Anaesthetists, Liverpool, April 2006*, 119–122

Hall LW, Clarke KW and Trim CM (2001) *Veterinary Anaesthesia, 10th edn.* WB Saunders, London

Hall TL, Duke T, Townsend HG, Caulkett NA and Cantwell SL (1999) The effect of opioid and acepromazine premedication on the anesthetic induction dose of propofol in cats. *Canadian Veterinary Journal* **40**, 867–870

Ilkiw JE, Suter CM, Farver TB, McNeal D and Steffey EP (1996) The behaviour of healthy awake cats following intravenous and intramuscular administration of midazolam. *Journal of Veterinary Pharmacology and Therapeutics* **19**, 205–216

Kuusela E, Raekallio M, Anttila M *et al.* (2000) Clinical effects and pharmacokinetics of medetomidine and its enantiomers in dogs. *Journal of Veterinary Pharmacology and Therapeutics* **23**, 15–20

Murrell JC and Hellebrekers LJ (2005) Medetomidine and dexmedetomidine: a review of cardiovascular and antinociceptive effects in the dog. *Veterinary Anaesthesia and Analgesia* **32**, 117–127

Mutoh T, Nishimura R and Sasaki N (2002) Effects of medetomidine-midazolam, midazolam-butorphanol, or acepromazine-butorphanol as premedicants for mask induction of anesthesia with sevoflurane in dogs. *American Journal of Veterinary Research* **63**, 1022–1028

Pypendop B and Verstegen J (1999) Cardiorespiratory effects of a combination of medetomidine, midazolam, and butorphanol in dogs. *American Journal of Veterinary Research* **60**, 1148–1154

Pypendop BH and Verstegen JP (1998) Hemodynamic effects of medetomidine in the dog: a dose titration study. *Veterinary Surgery* **27**, 612–622

Rishniw M, Tobias AH and Slinker BK (1996) Characterization of chronotropic and dysrhythmogenic effects of atropine in dogs with bradycardia. *American Journal of Veterinary Research* **57**, 337–341

Robinson KJ, Jones RS and Cripps PJ (2001) Effects of medetomidine and buprenorphine administered for sedation in dogs. *Journal of Small Animal Practice* **42**, 444–447

Thurmon JC, Tranquilli WJ and Benson GJ (1996) *Lumb & Jones Veterinary Anaesthesia, 3rd edn.* Williams and Wilkins, Baltimore

13

Intravenous anaesthetics

Sabine B.R. Kästner

Introduction

Injectable anaesthetics are used for induction of anaesthesia followed by maintenance with a volatile agent, or as the sole anaesthetic agents to maintain general anaesthesia. For minor procedures of short duration, a single injection will suffice. Repeated boluses or infusion of an anaesthetic in conjunction with analgesics defines total intravenous anaesthesia (TIVA). Infusion of certain anaesthetics can be used for seizure control (tetanus, status epilepticus) or to provide long-term sedation in intensive care units. For some injectable anaesthetics, there is a dose-dependent transition from sedation to general anaesthesia. Dose rates required for induction and maintenance of anaesthesia depend on the premedication given and individual sensitivity. Therefore, fragmented dosing of the calculated amount of anaesthetic is recommended to prevent overdosing. For proper administration of potent anaesthetics, it is crucial to choose an appropriately sized syringe. Placing small volumes in a large syringe inevitably leads to overdose. In cats, syringe size rarely needs to exceed 1–2 ml. In the case of very potent, highly concentrated drugs such as medetomidine or acepromazine, prior dilution with saline (e.g. 1:10) will improve accuracy of dosing.

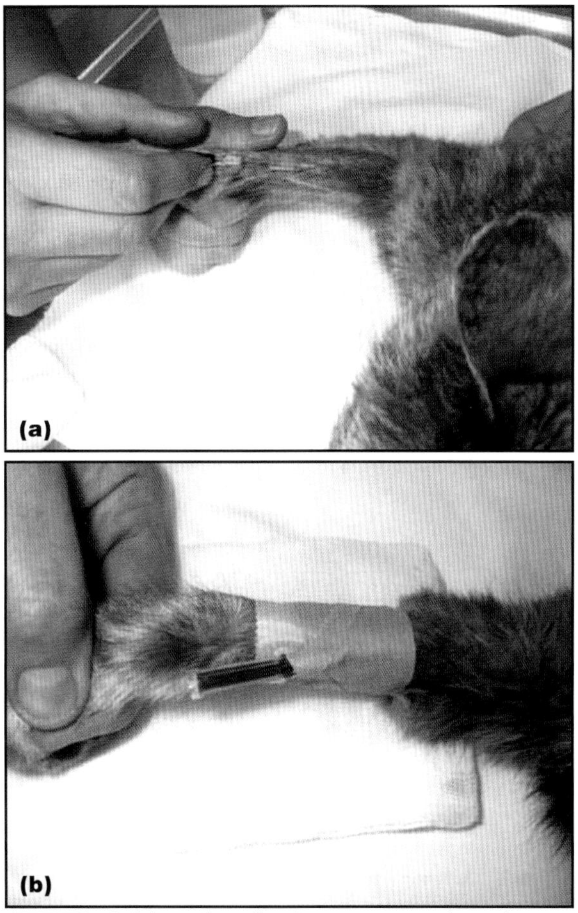

13.1 **(a)** Insertion of an intravenous catheter into the cephalic vein in a cat. **(b)** Fixation of the catheter to the limb with tape.

Venous access

Safe venous access is necessary for careful and effective administration of anaesthetics.

Proper premedication and handling usually allows placement of an intravenous catheter without forceful restraint in the majority of dogs and cats.

Catheter site

Accessible veins in the dog and the cat are the *cephalic vein* on the dorsomedial aspect of the foreleg (Figure 13.1) and the *recurrent tarsal vein* running across the lateral aspect of the hindleg above the hock. Restraint and catheter fixation are more difficult on the hindlegs. In cats, the *(medial) saphenous vein* on the medial aspect of the hindleg is easily localized if intravenous access to both cephalic veins is impossible. In large-eared dogs, external ear veins might be accessible for catheterization. For prolonged placement of venous catheters (central venous catheters) or in very small animals, the *external jugular vein* can be used.

Catheter types

Various indwelling catheters using an 'over-the-needle' technique are suitable for the peripheral veins and choice depends on animal size and personal preference (Figure 13.2). Because of the flexibility of the neck, short catheters will easily dislodge from the jugular vein and a length of at least 6 cm is required to avoid this. Conventional 'over-the-needle' catheters of this length can be difficult to introduce in the neck area and a 'through-the-needle' technique might be necessary for insertion of a jugular catheter after induction of anaesthesia. Commercial human catheter kits are suitable for placement of a central venous catheter intended for long-term use.

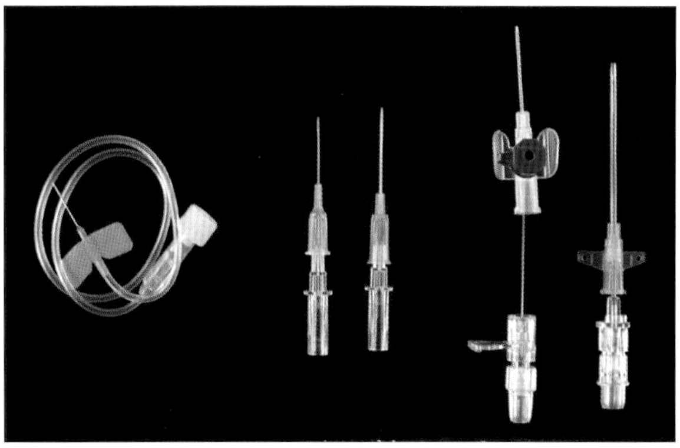

13.2 Different types of intravenous catheters.

In the well hydrated animal, percutaneous placement of peripheral catheters is possible. In older uncastrated male cats and dog breeds with very thick skin, initial perforation of the skin with a hypodermic needle is advisable to avoid damage to the catheter tip. In very small animals or in dehydrated, hypovolaemic animals, a cut-down to the vein with prior subcutaneous local anaesthesia might be necessary.

Preparation

Preparation of the catheter area depends on the type of catheter used and intended duration of catheter placement. The hair should be clipped over a wide area around the vessel to be catheterized to avoid inadvertent contamination of the catheter during insertion. The clipped area is prepared with an antiseptic solution (1–2% iodine tincture, iodophors, chlorhexidine or 70% alcohol). When using a cut-down technique or inserting long catheters using guide wires (Seldinger technique), surgical draping of the area and sterile gloves should be used to avoid contamination. After placement, the catheter is fixed by tape (limb, see Figure 13.1b) or sutured to the skin (neck). The catheter is flushed with heparinized saline (2 units heparin/ml) and capped, or an intravenous fluid infusion instituted immediately to avoid plugging of the catheter. To prevent accidental dislodgement of the catheter, the infusion line should also be fixed to the animal's body. For provision of unrestricted access to the vein with concurrent fluid administration, different catheter types and connecting pieces are available (Figure 13.3).

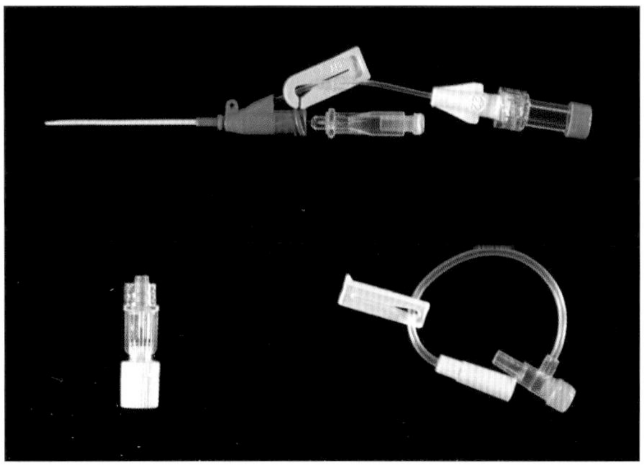

13.3 Catheter with side port, a connecting Y-piece and check valve for intravenous infusions.

Accidental perivascular injection

Accidental perivascular injection of highly irritant drugs such as thiopental leads to cellulitis, phlebitis or tissue sloughing (Figure 13.4). Immediate infiltration of the affected area with normal saline dilutes the drug and prevents tissue necrosis. Using 2% lidocaine instead of normal saline helps to neutralize the pH (especially after thiopental), prevent vasospasm, and reduce inflammation and pain reactions. Topical treatment with an ointment dressing containing heparin or an anti-inflammatory drug, in conjunction with systemic therapy using a non-steroidal anti-inflammatory drug, further reduces tissue inflammation.

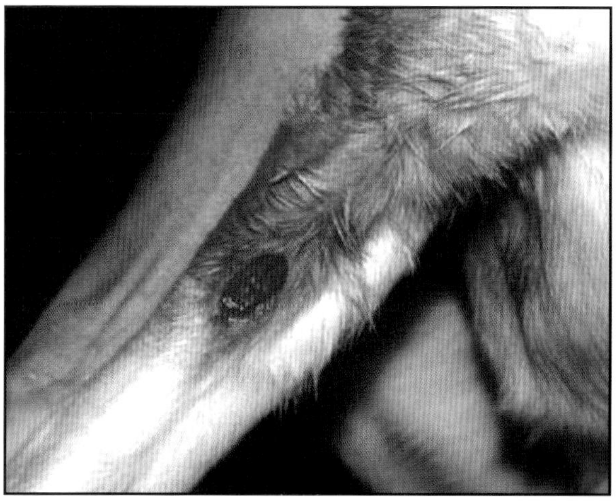

13.4 A skin slough caused by perivascular injection of thiopental.

Anaesthetics

A comparison of physicochemical and clinical properties of commonly used intravenous anaesthetics is given in Figures 13.5 and 13.6.

Barbiturates

Short-acting barbiturates have been the classical injectable anaesthetics in veterinary medicine for several decades. Barbiturates produce hypnosis with minimal analgesia and high doses are required to produce surgical anaesthesia when used as the sole anaesthetic agent. Barbiturates are also used for their anticonvulsant and sedative properties. The principal effect of barbiturates is depression of the central nervous system (CNS) by enhanced inhibition and inhibited excitation at the level of synaptic neurotransmission, mainly by interaction with the gamma aminobutyric acid A ($GABA_A$) receptor.

Rapidity of action and dose requirements depend on the amount of the unbound and unionized form of the drug in the bloodstream, because only this form can penetrate cell membranes and enter the CNS. A decrease in blood pH and hypoproteinaemia caused by disease can increase the percentage of free and unionized (active) drug and thereby dose requirements can be dramatically decreased in severely debilitated patients.

Drug concentration	Physicochemical properties	Induction/recovery	Haemodynamic effects	Respiratory effects	CNS effects	Other
Thiopental 1% (w/v) 2.5% (w/v)	Yellow crystalline powder Solution pH 11–14 Irritating, precipitates with many acidic drugs	Rapid (30 seconds), smooth induction; not suitable for repeated dosing	HR ↑↑, tachyarrhythmia MAP ↓ CO ↓↔ SVR ↔	RR ↓ VT ↓ Apnoea after rapid injection	Anticonvulsant Cerebral metabolism ↓ ICP ↓ CBF ↓	IOP ↓ Poor analgesia
Propofol 1% (w/v)	White emulsion pH ~7 Promotes bacterial growth	Smooth induction and recovery, excitatory signs can occur during induction and recovery	HR ↔↑ MAP ↓↓ CO ↓ SVR ↓↓	RR ↓ VT ↓ Apnoea after rapid injection	Anticonvulsant Cerebral metabolism ↓ ICP ↓ CBF ↓	IOP ↓ Poor analgesia
Ketamine 1% (w/v) 5% (w/v) 10% (w/v)	Clear, stable solution pH 3.5–5.5	Increased muscle tone, spasms, seizures, excitatory recovery without premedication	HR ↑↑ MAP ↑↑ CO ↑ SVR ↔	Apneustic, irregular breathing Apnoea with high doses	Stimulation Cerebral metabolism ↑↑ ICP ↑↑ CBF ↑↑	IOP ↑ Somatic analgesia NMDA receptor antagonist
Ketamine 1–10% (w/v)/ diazepam 0.5% (w/v)	Mixed immediately before use, clear solution with yellow tinge	Smooth induction Excitatory recovery	HR ↑ MAP ↑ CO ↑↔ SVR ↔	Apneustic, irregular breathing More depression than with ketamine alone Apnoea with high doses	Stimulation Cerebral metabolism ↑ ICP ↑ CBF ↑	Somatic analgesia NMDA receptor antagonist
Tiletamine/ zolazepam 250 mg/250 mg	Lyophilized powder Solution pH 2–3.5 1:1 mixture	Smooth induction, Excitatory recovery mainly in dogs	HR ↑↔ MAP ↑↓ CO ↑↔↓ SVR ↑↔	RR ↓ VT ↓ Depression with high doses	Stimulation Cerebral metabolism ↑ ICP ↑ CBF ↑	IOP ↑ Somatic analgesia
Etomidate 0.2% (w/v)	Propylene glycol preparation hyperosmolar (4640 mOsm/l) Emulsion promotes bacterial growth	Myoclonus without premedication	HR ↔ MAP ↔↓ CO ↔↓ SVR ↔	RR ↑ VT ↓ Depression with high doses	Anticonvulsant ICP ↓ CBF ↓ CPP ↔	IOP ↓ Adrenal suppression Poor analgesia
Alfaxalone (Alfaxan®)	Alfaxalone is solubilized in 2-hydroxypropyl-beta-cyclodextrin to make a clear 10 mg/ml solution at pH ~7	Smooth induction and recovery Excitatory signs can occur upon recovery although these can be decreased with proper premedication	HR (dog) ↑ HR (cat) ↓ MAP (dog) ↔ MAP (cat) ↓ CO (dog/cat) ↔/↓ SVR ↔ (dog and cat)	RR (dog) ↓ RR (cat) ↓ VT (dog) ↔ VT (cat) ↔ The risk of apnoea increases if Alfaxan® is injected rapidly	Anticonvulsant ICP ↓ CBF ↓ CPP ↔ Cerebral metabolism ↓ (these central effects are reported for alfaxalone/ alfadolone/ Cremophor EL combination (Saffan®))	Rapid clearance and does not accumulate No stinging upon injection

13.5 Comparison of some properties of commonly used intravenous anaesthetics. ↑ = Mild increase; ↑↑ = Moderate increase; ↓ = Mild decrease; ↓↓ = Moderate decrease; ↔ = No change; CBF = Cerebral blood flow; CO = Cardiac output; CPP = Cerebral perfusion pressure; HR = Heart rate; ICP = Intracranial pressure; IOP = Intraocular pressure; MAP = Mean arterial blood pressure; NMDA = *N*-methyl-D-aspartate; SVR = Systemic vascular resistance; RR = Respiratory rate; VT = Tidal volume.

Drug	Species	Elimination half-life (minutes)	Total body clearance (Cl_B) (ml/kg/minute)	Volume of distribution (Vd_{ss}) (l/kg)	Reference
Thiopental	Dog Cat	182.4	3.4	0.81(Vc 0.038)	Ilkiw *et al.*, 1991
Propofol	Dog Cat	90 322 55	58.6 50.1	4.9 6.5 1.3	Nolan *et al.*, 1993 Nolan and Reid, 1993 Adam *et al.*, 1980
Ketamine	Dog Cat	61 78.66	39.5 21.33	1.95 2.12	Kaka and Hayton, 1980 Hanna *et al.*, 1988
Etomidate	Dog Cat	86.4 59.66 173.4	 40.1 41.2	 Vc 0.108 4.88 (Vc 1.17)	Zhang *et al.*, 1998 McIntosh *et al.*, 2004 Wertz *et al.*, 1990
Alfaxalone (Alfaxan®)	Dog (2 mg/kg) Cat (5 mg/kg)	24 (harmonic) 45 (harmonic)	59 25	2.4 1.8	Ferré *et al.*, 2006 Heit *et al.*, 2004

13.6 Pharmacokinetic variables of commonly used intravenous anaesthetics. Vc = Volume of the central compartment.

Thiopental

Physicochemical properties: Thiopental is a thiobarbiturate. It is a weak organic acid provided as a sodium salt (yellow, crystalline powder) in sealed vials. Anhydrous sodium bicarbonate is added to prevent precipitation of the free acid with atmospheric carbon dioxide. After reconstitution with sterile water the solution is very alkaline (pH in the range of 11–14), which makes it extremely irritant at concentrations greater than 2.5%. Reduction of alkalinity of the solution results in precipitation of the free acid. Therefore, thiopental will not dissolve in lactated Ringer's (Hartmann's) solution and it precipitates with many other acidic drugs; care must therefore be taken to avoid occlusion of the intravenous line. The prepared solution should be tightly capped and refrigerated at 5–6°C to prolong shelf-life (approximately 1 week). When the solution becomes turbid, it loses activity and must be discarded.

Clinical properties: Thiopental causes rapid loss of consciousness (approximately 30 seconds). The time to onset of action is influenced by the circulation time to the brain, which might be prolonged by prior preanaesthetic sedation (especially alpha-2 agonists).

Thiopental is classified as an ultra short-acting barbiturate and recovery is fast (10–15 minutes) after a single injection. Recovery after a single injection is mainly governed by redistribution of the drug from the bloodstream to other tissues. Initially, well perfused tissues (brain, heart, kidney) will take up the drug, resulting in a rapid decline in plasma concentrations after a single thiopental bolus. A further decrease in plasma thiopental concentrations occurs when moderately perfused tissues, such as muscle, take up the drug. At that time, brain concentrations begin to fall and recovery occurs. Poorly perfused tissue, such as body fat, will take up thiopental slowly; however, adipose tissue has a high 'storage' capacity for lipid-soluble drugs such as thiopental. Repeated doses of thiopental will lead to an accumulation of the drug, because tissue sites become saturated and liver metabolism is slow. Successive doses lead to an exponential increase in anaesthesia time. Therefore, thiopental is unsuitable for maintenance of anaesthesia as accumulation can lead to serious cardiorespiratory depression and delayed recovery.

Thiopental induces respiratory depression and initial apnoea commonly occurs after rapid intravenous injection. Thiopental causes dose- and rate-dependent cardiovascular depression (high plasma concentrations after rapid injection). Hypotension caused by peripheral vasodilation and reduction in cardiac output from direct myocardial depression and tachyarrhythmias (e.g. ventricular extrasystole, bigeminy, ventricular tachycardia) are the main effects. In response to hypotension, persistent tachycardia can occur after thiopental injection. Drugs used concurrently (sedatives, opioids) and the animal's body condition will influence the overall effects. Cardiac arrhythmias can be accentuated by xylazine, halothane and adrenaline, whereas lidocaine and acepromazine attenuate arrhythmic effects.

In Greyhounds and other sighthounds, thiopental must be used with care. Because of their body disposition (low body fat) and decreased liver metabolism, very high plasma concentrations can occur. This can cause severe cardiovascular depression and prolonged recovery in these dog breeds. With the availability of alternative induction agents (e.g. propofol, ketamine–diazepam) it might be safer to avoid the use of thiopental in sighthounds.

Thiopental reduces the metabolic rate and oxygen requirements of the brain by depressing cellular activity. With the reduction in metabolic demands, a parallel reduction in cerebral blood flow and intracranial pressure (ICP) occurs. A reduction in ICP is desirable in head trauma or intracranial tumour patients. However, thiopental-induced hypoventilation has to be avoided because hypercapnia will increase ICP. Thiopental is an effective anticonvulsant, for example in benzodiazepine-resistant seizures, but its cardiorespiratory effects have to be closely monitored.

Practical use:

- Use as induction agent or as the sole anaesthetic for very short procedures only.
- Prepare 1–2.5% solution for small animals (as dilute as possible; consider reasonable injection volume).
- Discard turbid solution.
- Best used with intravenous catheter (perivascular injection leads to tissue necrosis).
- Give to effect (Figures 13.7 and 13.8):
  - Consider premedication
  - Consider physical status of the animal
  - Slow injection (30–60 seconds)
  - Give half of calculated dose and await maximum effect, proceed further with increments until desired effect (endotracheal intubation)
  - Decreased blood pH (e.g. uraemia) reduces required dose.
- Flush catheter before and after thiopental use.
- Avoid in hypovolaemic patients.
- Avoid in cardiac arrhythmia.
- Poor analgesia (use with analgesic).

Methohexital

Before the advent of propofol, the oxybarbiturate methohexital was used as an alternative to thiopental in Greyhounds and other sighthounds. In many countries it is no longer available, and propofol or ketamine–diazepam are considered to be better alternatives for thiopental in sighthounds.

Pentobarbital

Physicochemical properties: Pentobarbital is an oxybarbiturate. Its sodium salt occurs as white crystalline powder or granules. As an anaesthetic it is provided as an aqueous, alkaline (approximate pH 9–10.5), 5% or 10% solution, which is stable at room temperature. Preparations with higher concentrations (30–40%) are available as euthanasia solutions. In some countries (including the UK) the low-concentration pentobarbital for anaesthetic purposes is no longer available.

Drug	Premedication	Dose	Comment
Thiopental	– +	20–25 mg/kg i.v. 8–12.5 mg/kg i.v.	Give to effect
Methohexital	– +	6–10 mg/kg i.v. 5 mg/kg i.v.	Give to effect
Propofol	– +	6–8 mg/kg i.v. 2–4 mg/kg i.v.	Give to effect
Ketamine	+ +	2–5 mg/kg i.v. 5–10 mg/kg i.m.	Intramuscularly only in very uncooperative dogs
Ketamine and diazepam Ketamine and diazepam Ketamine and midazolam	± ± ± ±	5 mg/kg i.v. 0.25 mg/kg i.v. 10 mg/kg i.v. 0.5 mg/kg i.v. 5 mg/kg i.v. 0.25 mg/kg i.v.	Mix ketamine (10%) and diazepam (0.5%) at 1:1 (v:v); give 0.05–0.1 ml/kg of this mixture in increments to effect. Lower dose suitable for dogs with gastric dilatation–volvulus Mixed in one syringe given to effect
Tiletamine/zolazepam	– +	5 mg/kg i.v. 1–2 mg/kg i.v. 4–8 mg/kg i.m.	
Etomidate	– +	1–3 mg/kg i.v. 0.5–2 mg/kg i.v.	
Alfaxalone (Alfaxan®-CD RTU)	– +	3 mg/kg i.v. 2 mg/kg i.v.	

13.7 Anaesthesia induction doses in the dog. Note that induction doses can vary with type and dose of premedication; xylazine and medetomidine premedication reduces induction doses significantly (50–80%). – = Without premedication; + = With premedication.

Drug	Premedication	Dose	Comment
Thiopental	– +	10–(20) mg/kg i.v. 2–10 mg/kg i.v.	Give to effect
Propofol	– +	4–8 mg/kg i.v. 4–6 mg/kg i.v.	Give to effect
Ketamine	+ +	2–10 mg/kg i.v. 10–20 mg/kg i.m.	
Ketamine and diazepam Ketamine and diazepam Ketamine and midazolam	± ± ± ±	5 mg/kg i.v. 0.25 mg/kg i.v. 10 mg/kg i.v. 0.5 mg/kg i.v. 5 mg/kg i.v. 0.25 mg/kg i.v.	Mix ketamine (10%) and diazepam (0.5%) at 1:1 (v:v); give 0.05–0.1 ml/kg of this mixture in increments to effect Mixed in one syringe given to effect
Tiletamine/zolazepam	– +	4–5 mg/kg i.v. 1–2 mg/kg i.v. 4–8 mg/kg i.m.	
Etomidate	– +	1–3 mg/kg i.v. 0.5–2 mg/kg i.v.	
Saffan®	– +	6–9 mg /kg i.v. 3–6 mg/kg i.v.	
Alfaxalone (Alfaxan®-CD RTU)	– +	5 mg/kg i.v. 2–3 mg/kg i.v.	

13.8 Anaesthesia induction doses in the cat. Note that induction doses can vary with type and dose of premedication; xylazine and medetomidine premedication reduces induction doses significantly (50–80%). – = Without premedication; + = With premedication.

Clinical properties: Pentobarbital causes fairly rapid loss of consciousness (approximately 40–120 seconds). Pentobarbital is classified as a short-acting barbiturate and duration of action is 1–2 hours after a single injection (10–20 mg/kg).

Recovery depends on liver metabolism. In the past it was the principal agent for general anaesthesia, although it provides minimal analgesia and muscle relaxation and has a very narrow safety margin. Therefore, pentobarbital as an anaesthetic agent in small animals has been superseded by other anaesthetics.

Nowadays, the main indications for pentobarbital are the treatment of intractable seizures caused by convulsants or CNS toxins (it is an effective anticonvulsant), long-term sedation in an intensive care unit (ICU) setting to allow mechanical ventilation, and euthanasia (Figure 13.9).

Drug	Dose	Indication
Diazepam	Repeated boluses (0.2–0.5 mg/kg i.v.) to effect In case of repeated seizures 0.2–0.5 mg/kg/h constant rate infusion (CRI) to effect Diazepam CRI can induce phlebitis (use long catheter)	Seizure control
Midazolam	Repeated boluses (0.2–0.5 mg/kg i.v.) to effect In case of repeated seizures 0.3–0.9 mg/kg/h CRI to effect	Seizure control
Pentobarbital	2–15 mg/kg slowly i.v. to effect, then 0.2–1.0 mg/kg/h to effect 2–4 mg/kg i.v. initial bolus, followed by 0.5–2 mg/kg/h CRI to effect	Uncontrollable seizures Long-term sedation for ventilatory support
Propofol	4–6 mg/kg slowly i.v. to effect, then 0.1–0.4 mg/kg/minute to effect Requires intubation (risk of aspiration) and monitoring of ventilation	Uncontrollable seizures
Fentanyl Diazepam	0.5–4 µg/kg/minute and 0.2–0.5 mg/kg/h given to effect, alone or in combination with pentobarbital 0.5–2 mg/kg/h Fentanyl and diazepam are not mixed in one infusion; they must be given separately	Long-term sedation for ventilatory support

13.9 Long-term sedation and seizure control.

Recovery after pentobarbital infusions is prolonged and associated with hyperexcitability after short-term use (<2 days). After medium-term use (3–7 days) withdrawal dysphoria can occur and after long-term use (>1 week) recovery is associated with seizures, which require anticonvulsant treatment with phenobarbital before the pentobarbital is withdrawn. Switching to a propofol infusion (see later) before planned recovery may help to reduce recovery dysphoria and seizures.

Pentobarbital produces very rapid unconsciousness and cardiovascular depression, which qualifies it as an agent suitable for euthanasia. For this purpose, it is used at a high concentration (30–40%) at a dose of 80–100 mg/kg i.v. (in dogs) and 100–200 mg/kg i.v. (in cats). It is advisable to colour the solution (e.g. methylene blue) to avoid confusion with other anaesthetics.

Non-barbiturate anaesthetics

Propofol

Physicochemical properties: Propofol is a hypnotic alkyl phenol (2,6 diisopropylphenol) occurring as an oil at room temperature. It is insoluble in aqueous solutions but highly lipid soluble. To allow intravenous injection, propofol is currently formulated as a white oil-in-water emulsion containing Intralipid (1% w/v soya bean oil, 1.2% w/v purified egg phosphatide, 2.25% w/v glycerol). This formulation has a pH of 7 and appears as a slightly viscous, milky white liquid. The veterinary product usually comes at a concentration of 1% (w/v). A 2% (w/v) formulation is available as a human product. The emulsion is an ideal culture medium for bacteria; open vials should be used within 24 hours. Intramuscular injection does not induce anaesthesia at reasonable dose rates, but inadvertent perivascular injection is non-irritating. Propofol is compatible with 5% dextrose in water if a dilute solution is required.

Clinical properties: Propofol is primarily a hypnotic agent with a rapid onset (60–90 seconds) and short duration of action after a single dose (approximately 10 minutes). The hypnotic action is mainly mediated by interaction with the $GABA_A$ receptor subunit, potentiating the GABA-induced chloride current.

The half-life of equilibration between CNS effects and plasma concentrations is about 2 minutes. Therefore, an injection time of 2 minutes is recommended for induction doses to enable titration to effect and to avoid overdose and apnoea. In contrast to dogs, in cats the induction dose of propofol seems unaffected to a significant extent by acepromazine premedication. However, opioids and alpha-2 agonists reduce propofol requirements significantly and induction doses need to be adapted.

The pharmacokinetic properties of propofol (see Figure 13.6) contribute to its clinical advantages. After a single bolus injection, propofol blood levels decrease rapidly due to redistribution of the drug to highly perfused tissues. After the initial rapid distribution phase, propofol is metabolized rapidly and further slow distribution to fat occurs. This is followed by prolonged terminal elimination, which reflects slow release from fat tissue, although this has little effect on clinical recovery from anaesthesia. Clearance rates exceed hepatic blood flow and extrahepatic metabolism has been demonstrated. A high first-pass extraction of propofol in the lung has been demonstrated. Propofol is metabolized to sulphate and glucuronide conjugates, which are inactive. Propofol conjugates are mainly excreted via the urine. Hepatic and renal disease does not appear to influence propofol pharmacokinetics. In dogs, premedication with medetomidine or maintenance of anaesthesia with halothane and nitrous oxide do not alter propofol kinetics to a significant extent. In dogs, propofol doses required to induce anaesthesia seem to decrease with age.

Rapid metabolism of propofol results in minimal accumulation after repeated doses and this makes propofol suitable for administration by infusion for maintenance of anaesthesia (TIVA) with excellent results in dogs. However, in Greyhounds recovery is prolonged after propofol infusions because of their higher proportion of lean body mass to fat and lower microsomal activity. Cats have a reduced capacity for glucuronide conjugation, which is required for metabolism of phenolic compounds. This leads to prolonged recoveries in cats after propofol infusions that last longer than 30 minutes. In addition, propofol infusion of more than 30 minutes in cats leads to clinically significant reductions in packed cell volume (PCV). Therefore, propofol TIVA in cats should be kept at a low dose rate and be as short as possible. In addition, feline haemoglobin is prone to oxidative injury by phenolic compounds. Repeated propofol anaesthesia (more than 3 consecutive days) results in significant Heinz body formation, anorexia, diarrhoea, facial oedema, depression and delayed recovery from anaesthesia.

The most prominent haemodynamic effect is moderate hypotension due to reductions in cardiac output and systemic vascular resistance, which can become severe in hypovolaemic patients or patients with a low cardiac reserve. Hypotension is most severe 2 minutes after an induction dose of propofol and after rapid injection. In patients with pre-existing bradycardia (e.g. sick sinus syndrome), refractory bradycardia or asystole can occur. Bradycardia can be severe if high doses of opioids are combined with propofol, although this can be prevented by prior administration of a parasympatholytic drug. Rapid injection of propofol can result in apnoea. Respiratory depression with hypercapnia and a drop in arterial oxygen saturation occurs after repeated or continuous propofol dosing; oxygen supplementation is therefore advisable during prolonged propofol administration.

Propofol has both proconvulsant and anticonvulsant properties, by different mechanisms. Propofol has been used successfully as an anti-epileptic drug for seizure control (see Figure 13.9). On the other hand, excitatory signs, such as myoclonus, paddling, opisthotonus and nystagmus can occur during the induction period and to a lower extent during recovery. Premedication reduces the incidence of excitatory signs but cannot completely prevent their occurrence. In most cases excitatory signs cease when inhalation anaesthetics are commenced. Refractory excitations have been treated successfully with ketamine (1 mg/kg i.v.), diazepam (0.2 mg/kg i.v.) or pentobarbital (2 mg/kg i.v.).

Propofol decreases cerebral metabolic requirements for oxygen, cerebral perfusion pressure and causes a corresponding decrease in ICP (in both normal animals and those with intracranial pathology) and intraocular pressure. The reactivity of cerebral vessels to changes in P_aCO_2 seems to be maintained during propofol anaesthesia. The rapid recovery characteristics and lack of cerebrovascular dilation (in contrast to volatiles) make propofol TIVA an alternative to volatile anaesthetics in neurosurgery in dogs (see Chapter 26).

Propofol has poor analgesic properties and the doses required for induction and maintenance of anaesthesia are significantly reduced by analgesic premedications (alpha-2 agonists, opioids).

Propofol readily crosses the placenta and may affect neurological and cardiorespiratory variables in puppies and kittens. Therefore, propofol should not be used for maintenance of anaesthesia in bitches and queens undergoing Caesarean section. Clinical experience has shown that propofol is suitable for induction of anaesthesia in the mother prior to an inhalant, as long as she is haemodynamically stable. An interval of approximately 20 minutes between induction of anaesthesia and delivery of the puppies or kittens minimizes respiratory depression by residual propofol effects (see Chapter 24).

Disorders of lipid metabolism could potentially be aggravated by the lipid emulsion formulation of propofol, in particular after long-term infusion. Therefore, propofol should be used with caution in patients with diabetic hyperlipidaemia or pancreatitis.

Propofol for induction and maintenance should be titrated to effect, similar to a volatile agent, because of the variable influence of premedicants, concurrent analgesics and surgical stimulation.

Practical use:

- Induction and maintenance agent (see Figures 13.7 and 13.8).
- Keep TIVA in cats as short as possible (<30 minutes).
- Discard open vials after 24 hours (refer to manufacturer's data sheets).
- Supplement oxygen when using repeated doses or infusion.
- Give to effect:
  - Consider premedication (20–80% reduction depending on premedication)
  - Consider physical status of the animal
  - Slow injection (60–120 seconds)
  - Give half of calculated dose and await maximum effect, proceed further with increments until desired effect (e.g. deep sedation, endotracheal intubation).
- Poor analgesia (use with analgesic).
- Avoid in hypovolaemic patients.
- Avoid in heart failure.
- Avoid in hyperlipidaemia and pancreatitis.
- Avoid repeated (more than 3 consecutive days) propofol anaesthesia in cats.

Etomidate

Physicochemical properties: Etomidate is an imidazole derivative. It exists as a racemate, but only the S(+) isomer has hypnotic activity. Etomidate is water soluble at an acidic pH and becomes lipid soluble at physiological pH. Therefore, several formulations exist. The 'classic' etomidate 0.2% (v/v) preparation, which appears as clear solution, contains propylene glycol (35% v/v), has a pH of 6.9 and a high osmolarity (4640 mOsm/l). Perivascular injection causes tissue necrosis and phlebitis. A newer preparation is formulated as a lipid emulsion (Etomidate-Lipuro®, Braun Melsungen, Germany). This formulation contains Intralipid, has a pH of approximately 7 and appears as a slightly viscous, milky white liquid like propofol. The emulsion promotes bacterial growth and open ampoules should be refrigerated and be discarded within 24 hours.

Clinical properties: Etomidate is a hypnotic agent with fast penetration of the blood–brain barrier and peak brain concentrations are reached within 1 minute. Its hypnotic activity is partly related to interaction with the GABA system, by increasing the availability of GABA receptors. Recovery after a single bolus injection is rapid (10–20 minutes).

After a single bolus injection in cats, etomidate blood levels initially decrease rapidly followed by a slower distribution phase and an elimination half-life of approximately 3 hours. Total body clearance rates are high. Etomidate is rapidly hydrolysed to inactive metabolites by hepatic and plasma esterases. Drugs reducing hepatic blood flow (e.g. alpha-2 agonists) will reduce etomidate elimination. The pharmacokinetic profile (see Figure 13.6) makes etomidate suitable for repeated dosing or continuous infusion.

Etomidate alone produces minimal cardiovascular changes in healthy and hypovolaemic dogs, making it an ideal induction agent in patients with a low cardiac reserve and hypovolaemia. However, etomidate should not be used without premedication because of a high incidence of myoclonus and pain on injection (propylene glycol preparation). Therefore, the choice of premedication rather than the etomidate itself will influence the cardiovascular status. Combinations of etomidate either with diazepam or midazolam, or with fentanyl or morphine (and other opioids) have been used successfully in high-risk patients.

Etomidate induces dose-dependent respiratory depression. A slower injection rate results in less depression or apnoea, similar to thiopental and propofol.

Etomidate reduces cerebral metabolic oxygen requirements and cerebral blood flow and decreases elevated ICP. Because of the minimal influence on systemic blood pressure, cerebral perfusion pressure is well maintained. Etomidate decreases intraocular pressure. Etomidate has no analgesic properties.

The major drawback or concern with the use of etomidate is its inhibition of adrenal steroid synthesis. The production of cortisol, aldosterone and corticosterone is decreased by inhibition of 11-α and 11-β hydroxylases, and the cholesterol side-chain cleavage enzyme. A major problem (Addisonian crisis) can occur after infusion of etomidate over prolonged periods of time (constant sedation in ICU). After a single induction bolus, adrenocortical responses and cortisol are suppressed for 2–6 hours in cats and dogs. The lack of stress response to anaesthesia and surgery seems to have no detrimental effects after a single intravenous bolus, but care has to be taken in animals with pre-existing adrenal insufficiency.

The propylene glycol preparation induces acute haemolysis after rapid injection or prolonged continuous infusion, mediated by a massive increase in plasma osmolarity.

Overall, etomidate is a suitable agent for high-risk patients. The high cost and packaging in glass ampoules, which restricts repeated use after opening, are reasons for its limited use in veterinary practice.

Practical use:

- Induction agent, short infusion.
- Pain on injection and phlebitis (propylene glycol preparation).
- Refrigerate open ampoules (lipid emulsion).
- Discard open ampoules after 24 hours (lipid emulsion).
- High incidence of myoclonus when used as sole agent.
- Best used with premedication.
- Give to effect (see Figures 13.7 and 13.8):
  - Consider premedication
  - Consider physical status of the animal
  - Slow injection (60 seconds).
- Poor analgesia (use with analgesic).
- Good cardiovascular stability (high-risk patients).
- Avoid in animals with known adrenal insufficiency (supplement).

Dissociative agents

Ketamine

Physicochemical properties: The phencyclidine derivative, ketamine hydrochloride, occurs as a white, crystalline powder. The commercially available solutions are slightly acidic (pH 3.5–5.5). Ketamine consists of two stereoisomers, S(+) ketamine and R(–) ketamine. The S(+) isomer has about 1.5–3-fold greater hypnotic potency and 3-fold greater analgesic potency than R(–) ketamine. Compared with the racemic mixture, S(+) ketamine is 1.5–2 times more potent. Racemic ketamine is a mixture of both enantiomers in equal amounts and comes as 1% (w/v), 5% (w/v) and 10% (w/v) preparations containing the preservative benzethonium chloride. In some countries S(+) ketamine is available as 0.5% (w/v) and 2.5% (w/v) solutions. Ketamine solutions are very stable, but should be protected from light and excessive heat. Ketamine can be administered by intramuscular, intravenous, subcutaneous or intraperitoneal injection. It is also effective when given orally or intranasally. Ketamine can be diluted with sterile water or physiological saline for injection. Because of illicit recreational use, in 1999 racemic ketamine became a Schedule III controlled drug in the USA.

Clinical properties: Ketamine penetrates the blood–brain barrier rapidly and has an onset of action after intravenous injection of 30–90 seconds in cats and dogs. After intramuscular injection it is distributed into body tissues rapidly and peak anaesthetic effects occur within 10–15 minutes.

Ketamine induces a dose-dependent CNS depression that leads to a dissociative state, characterized by profound analgesia and amnesia with maintained ocular, laryngeal, pharyngeal, pinnal and pedal reflexes. This catalepsy is caused (mainly) by inhibition of thalamocortical pathways and stimulation of the limbic system. The neuropharmacology of ketamine is complex and it interacts with multiple binding sites, including *N*-methyl-D-aspartate (NMDA) and non-NMDA glutamate receptors, nicotinic and muscarinic cholinergic, monoaminergic and opioid receptors. In addition, inhibition of voltage-dependent sodium and calcium channels has been described. It seems that the antagonism at the NMDA receptor accounts for the majority of the analgesic, amnesic and psychotomimetic effects.

After an intravenous bolus, racemic ketamine is distributed rapidly, followed by an elimination half-life of approximately 60 and 80 minutes in dogs and cats, respectively (see Figure 13.6). Recovery after a single dose occurs mainly by redistribution. Ketamine undergoes high hepatic extraction and is metabolized rapidly by the liver. The main metabolite, norketamine, has about 10–30% of the anaesthetic potency of ketamine. The cat also excretes ketamine as the active drug through the kidney. Accumulation of norketamine after repeated doses or ketamine infusions contributes to prolonged recovery and drowsiness. The parent compound and the metabolites undergo glucuronidation and are excreted via the kidney. Hepatic dysfunction impairs elimination of the drug and prolongs its action considerably.

The main pharmacokinetic difference between racemic ketamine and S(+) ketamine seems to be a higher elimination rate for the latter. Complete recovery after S(+) ketamine is faster and less likely to be associated with excitatory effects. However, racemic as well as S(+) ketamine anaesthesia is associated with increased muscle tone, muscle spasm and seizures and concurrent use of acepromazine, a benzodiazepine or an alpha-2 agonist is required to reduce these side effects and obtain a surgical state of anaesthesia. Therefore, in a clinical setting, the advantages of S(+) ketamine over racemic ketamine are influenced by the chosen premedication.

Ketamine has unique cardiovascular effects. Unlike other intravenous anaesthetics, it stimulates the cardiovascular system, resulting in increases in heart rate, blood pressure and cardiac output. This increase in haemodynamic variables is associated with increased myocardial work and oxygen consumption. A healthy heart can increase its oxygen supply by coronary vasodilation and increased cardiac output, but a compromised heart (hypertrophic, ischaemic heart) might not be able to mount such a response. Central stimulation of the sympathetic system is responsible for the cardiovascular stimulation. Concurrent use of sedatives will attenuate the stimulatory effects of ketamine. In contrast, ketamine also exerts direct myocardial depression (a negative inotropic effect). Normally the stimulatory effects predominate, but high intravenous ketamine doses can result in transient hypotension. In severely compromised animals or with concurrent use of other anaesthetics, ketamine may induce cardiovascular depression.

Ketamine has minimal effects on central respiratory drive. After bolus administration of an induction dose, initial respiratory depression occurs, often followed by a so-called 'apneustic' pattern of breathing, characterized by periodic breath holding on inspiration followed by short periods of hyperventilation. Generally, arterial and tissue oxygenation are well maintained. Potential respiratory problems can occur in cats and small dogs because of increased salivation, leading to upper airway obstruction or endotracheal tube occlusion. The swallow, sneeze and cough reflexes remain relatively intact after ketamine administration but 'silent' aspiration can still occur with ketamine anaesthesia.

Because of its excitatory effects on the CNS, ketamine increases cerebral metabolism, cerebral blood flow and ICP. Cerebrovascular responsiveness to carbon dioxide remains intact and therefore reducing P_aCO_2 attenuates the rise in ICP after ketamine. Ketamine has epileptogenic potential and should generally not be used in animals with known seizure disorders or in procedures known to possibly induce seizures (e.g. myelography). Ketamine also increases intraocular pressure and is therefore not suitable for intraocular surgery or open globe injuries. The eyes do not rotate with ketamine anaesthesia, making animals prone to corneal drying.

Recovery from ketamine anaesthesia can be associated with hyperexcitability, especially in cats, because animals become hypersensitive to noise, light and handling.

Ketamine is still licensed for use as the sole anaesthetic agent for cats and non-human primates. Because of the increased muscle tone, involuntary movements and the high incidence of excitation during recovery in cats, it should always be used in combination with a sedative or tranquillizer to offset these side effects (see Figures 13.7 and 13.8). Ketamine is a popular anaesthetic in cats because deep sedation or anaesthesia for short surgical procedures (e.g. castration) can be induced via the intramuscular route, a major advantage in uncooperative, fractious animals (Figure 13.10).

Drugs	Doses	Technique	Indication
Acepromazine Buprenorphine or Butorphanol Ketamine	0.02–0.05 mg/kg 0.01 mg/kg 0.2–0.4 mg/kg 20–30 mg/kg	Give acepromazine/opioid combination 15 minutes before ketamine	Short surgical procedures (30–40 minutes)
Xylazine Ketamine	1 mg/kg 5–10 mg/kg	Mixed in one syringe	Short surgical procedures (20–30 minutes)
Medetomidine Ketamine	0.04 mg/kg 5–7 mg/kg	Mixed in one syringe	Short surgical procedures (30–40 minutes)

13.10 Ketamine combinations for short surgical procedures in the cat given by the intramuscular route. Combinations with alpha-2 agonists can induce vomiting. (continues) ▶

Drugs	Doses	Technique	Indication
Medetomidine Butorphanol Ketamine	0.02 mg/kg 0.1 mg/kg 5 mg/kg	Medetomidine/opioid 15 minutes before ketamine	Short surgical procedures (30–40 minutes)
Romifidine Ketamine	0.05–0.1 mg/kg 10–20 mg/kg	Mixed in one syringe	Short surgical procedures (30–40 minutes)
Midazolam Ketamine	0.25 mg/kg 10–(20) mg/kg	Mixed in one syringe	Short minor procedures

13.10 (continued) Ketamine combinations for short surgical procedures in the cat given by the intramuscular route. Combinations with alpha-2 agonists can induce vomiting.

Ketamine readily crosses the placenta and neurological reflexes in puppies delivered by Caesarean section after ketamine–midazolam anaesthesia induction are reduced.

Its activity as a non-competitive antagonist at NMDA glutamate receptors and its ability to produce profound somatic analgesia have expanded the indications for ketamine. In subanaesthetic doses given in the perioperative period, ketamine may reduce the central 'wind-up' phenomenon, with a reduction in the requirement for postoperative analgesics. In addition, ketamine might be helpful in the treatment of chronic and neuropathic pain based on its interaction with NMDA receptors. Ketamine constant rate infusion (CRI) during inhalation anaesthesia provides preemptive analgesia and reduces the required concentration of the inhalation anaesthetic.

Practical use:

- Induction agent, sole anaesthetic for short surgical procedures (see Figures 13.7, 13.8 and 13.10).
- Effective after intravenous, intramuscular, subcutaneous, intranasal, oral or rectal administration.
- Pain can occur after intramuscular injection.
- Increased muscle tone and high incidence of convulsions (dogs) when used alone.
- Combine with benzodiazepine, alpha-2 agonist or acepromazine.
- Intact eye and laryngeal reflexes.
- Anaesthetic depths difficult to judge.
- Good somatic analgesia.
- Use eye ointment.
- Cardiovascular stimulation (heart rate, blood pressure, cardiac output increase).
- Do not use in patients with hypertrophic cardiomyopathy.
- Avoid in epileptics.
- Avoid in animals with increased ICP (trauma, tumours)
- Apneustic breathing (apnoea with high doses).
- Recover animal in a quiet, dimmed and heated room.

Tiletamine–zolazepam

Physicochemical properties: Tiletamine is chemically related to ketamine (phencyclidine derivative, cyclohexanone) with a longer duration of action. Zolazepam is a benzodiazepine (diazepinone minor tranquillizer) with muscle relaxant and anticonvulsant effects. Telazol® (USA) or Zoletil® (Europe) is a proprietary combination of zolazepam and tiletamine at a ratio of 1:1 (250 mg zolazepam, 250 mg tiletamine). The preparation comes as a lyophilized powder, which can be reconstituted with 5 ml saline, 5% dextrose or sterile water (50 mg/ml zolazepam, 50 mg/ml tiletamine). The clear solution is acidic (pH 2.0–3.5) and should be discarded if precipitation occurs. The prepared solution can be stored at room temperature for 4 days, and for 14 days when refrigerated. Telazol® is a controlled substance in the USA (Schedule III) and it is licensed in small animals for intramuscular injection, although intravenous injection is used frequently.

Clinical properties: Tiletamine alone produces a cataleptic, dissociative state similar to that produced by ketamine. High doses can produce unconsciousness and surgical anaesthesia in cats, but not in dogs, in which severe convulsions occur. Zolazepam has anticonvulsant and anxiolytic properties and produces muscle relaxation. Like the benzodiazepine group in general, its sedative effects are unreliable in healthy animals. Zolazepam alone causes only minimal CNS depression and has minimal cardiorespiratory effects.

The combination of tiletamine and zolazepam can produce sedation or general anaesthesia in dogs and cats. After intravenous injection, induction of anaesthesia is rapid (60–90 seconds). Onset of action after intramuscular injection varies between 1 and 7 minutes in cats, and 5 and 12 minutes in dogs. Intramuscular injection can be painful (due to the low pH of the solution). Duration of anaesthesia is dependent on the dose used (30–60 minutes).

In general, complete recovery from Telazol® anaesthesia can be long (4–5 hours) and is smoother in cats than in dogs. In cats, elimination half-life of zolazepam (4.5 hours) is longer than that of the tiletamine component (2–4 hours) and the recovery phase is still influenced by the tranquillizer. In dogs, zolazepam effects wane earlier (half-life 1 hour) than those of tiletamine (half-life 1.2 hours) and the recovery phase is characterized by muscle rigidity, excitation and seizure-like activity. High doses or repeated dosing will prolong and worsen recovery and therefore redosing is not recommended. Animals with renal disease have prolonged anaesthetic action and recovery periods.

Anaesthetic depth is difficult to judge because animals maintain ocular, laryngeal, pharyngeal and pedal reflexes.

Cardiovascular effects of Telazol® in cats and dogs are dose-dependent. In dogs, sinus tachycardia and premature ventricular complexes occur due to sympathetic stimulation, but Telazol® does not change the arrhythmogenic dose of adrenaline. In cats, heart rate responses are variable, but the cardiostimulatory effects of Telazol® should be avoided in cats with hyperthyroidism and hypertrophic cardiomyopathy. At lower doses, the overall haemodynamic state remains stable (blood pressure, cardiac output), whereas at higher doses cardiovascular depression occurs (reduced cardiac output, blood pressure and contractility).

Respiratory depression with hypoxaemia and hypercapnia occurs after intravenous injection and after high intramuscular doses of Telazol®. As with ketamine, hypersalivation is common and can be treated with atropine or glycopyrronium if necessary.

Like ketamine, tiletamine has excitatory effects on the CNS and increases cerebral metabolism, cerebral blood flow and ICP, and is therefore contraindicated in patients with head trauma or intracranial tumours. Tiletamine increases intraocular pressure and is therefore not suitable for intraocular surgery or open globe injuries. In cats a post-anaesthetic hyperthermic response can occur.

Practical use:

- Induction agent (intravenous).
- Sole anaesthetic agent only for diagnostic or minor surgical procedures.
- Induction agent for aggressive dogs and fractious cats (intramuscular).
- Dose recommendations refer to total drug.
- Effective after intravenous and intramuscular administration.
- Pain after intramuscular injection common.
- Intact eye and laryngeal reflexes.
- Anaesthetic depths difficult to judge.
- Do not redose.
- Use eye ointment.
- Do not use in patients with hypertrophic cardiomyopathy.
- Do not use in patients with pancreatic disease.
- Avoid in epileptics.
- Avoid in animals with increased ICP (trauma, tumours).
- Apneustic breathing (apnoea with high doses).
- Recover animal in a quiet, dimmed and heated room.
- Premedication with acepromazine, alpha-2 agonist or benzodiazepine reduces dose requirements and improves recovery.

Steroid anaesthetics

Alfaxalone

Physicochemical properties: The progesterone derivative alfaxalone is a neuroactive steroid. This molecule is insoluble in water and previously has been mixed with alfadolone acetate to increase its solubility. Alfadolone also has anaesthetic properties, with about half the potency of alfaxalone. The mixture of alfaxalone (9 mg/ml) and alfadolone acetate (3 mg/ml) in 20% (w/v) polyoxyethylated castor oil (Cremophor EL) is known as Saffan® (Schering Plough Animal Health). The viscid solution is isotonic and has a pH of about 7. Perivascular injection is not painful and does not produce tissue necrosis.

In veterinary anaesthesia, doses of Saffan® are expressed as mg per kg total steroid. The vehicle Cremophor EL induces non-specific mast cell degranulation and histamine release (true hypersensitivity and complement activation). In dogs and other canidae, prolonged hypotension, tachycardia, urticaria and oedema formation occur and Saffan® must not be used in these species. In cats, the response seems to be more localized to tissues with a high mast cell population. Transient facial (ear pinnae, nose) and paw oedema, scratching, sneezing and pawing of the face as manifestations of histamine release occur in about 25–69% of cats treated with Saffan®. However, pulmonary oedema and prolonged hypotension can also occur in cats.

Alfaxalone as the single anaesthetic steroid has recently been reformulated with the solubilizing agent 2-hydroxypropyl-beta cyclodextrin (Alfaxan®-CD RTU, Jurox Pty Ltd., Australia) and is registered for cats and dogs only in Australia, New Zealand and South Africa, but registration in the UK and other countries is currently under review. The Alfaxan® formulation exists as a sterile, colourless and clear solution with a neutral pH of approximately 7. Perivascular injection is not painful and does not produce tissue necrosis. This preparation is devoid of the adverse side effects related to Cremophor EL and can also be used in dogs.

Clinical properties: Neuroactive steroids produce hypnosis and muscle relaxation by enhancing the inhibitory effect of GABA on the $GABA_A$ receptor chloride channel complex. Anticonvulsive effects are low. Dependent on the dose, sedation or anaesthesia can be achieved. Intravenous injection leads to rapid relaxation and induction of anaesthesia (30–60 seconds) with dose-dependent duration. Intramuscular injection is effective, with onset of sedation/anaesthesia within 7–10 minutes, but with a very variable degree of effect. Subcutaneous injection is unsuitable for induction of anaesthesia.

Neither alfaxalone nor alfadolone acetate undergoes significant plasma protein binding. Glucuronidation processes play a major role in excretion of the drug and hepatic insufficiency will prolong anaesthetic time. Recovery depends more on drug metabolism than redistribution and cumulative effects are low. However, in one study in cats, anaesthetic time increased non-linearly with doses above 5 mg/kg (of both the Cremophor EL preparation and Alfaxan®).

In dogs, alfaxalone (Alfaxan®) is cleared from plasma very rapidly (see Figure 13.6). This is reflected by an average duration of anaesthesia (allowing endotracheal intubation) of 6 minutes and

26 minutes after 2 mg/kg and 10 mg/kg, respectively. In cats, dose-dependent disposition with a slower elimination than in dogs occurs. Doses of 5 mg/kg i.v. and 25 mg/kg i.v. resulted in mean anaesthesia times to complete recovery of 44 minutes and 68 minutes, respectively.

Saffan® alone produces a similar dose-dependent reduction in stroke volume, arterial pressure and central venous pressure to thiopental in cats. However, hypotension is not dose-related, can be profound and is accompanied by tachycardia, which is mainly the result of histamine release rather than the effects of the steroid anaesthetic itself. Saffan® produces excellent muscle relaxation and results in smooth anaesthesia induction. A bolus injection of Saffan® decreases cerebral metabolism, cerebral blood flow and ICP. Recovery from Saffan® anaesthesia can be excitable, although this can be alleviated by recovery in a quiet area.

Alfaxan® produces excellent anaesthesia induction and recovery, with dose-dependent changes in cardiovascular and respiratory variables and anaesthetic duration in dogs. At the recommended induction dose (see Figures 13.7 and 13.8) all cardiorespiratory parameters return to baseline within 15 minutes. Significant respiratory depression occurs only at between three and five times the recommended dose. Anaesthesia is characterized by excellent muscle relaxation and lack of response to electrical and mechanical noxious stimulation.

In cats, Alfaxan® at 5 mg/kg i.v. results in smooth anaesthesia induction with excellent muscle relaxation. Premedication with medetomidine, acepromazine, butorphanol or midazolam reduces the induction dose to 2–3 mg/kg i.v. (see Figure 13.8).

Practical use:

Saffan®:

- Do not use Saffan® in dogs
- Used as induction (and maintenance) agent in cats, but histamine release possible
- Dose recommendations refer to total steroid
- Best used intravenously; intramuscular administration less reliable
- Give to effect
- Facial and paw oedema, profound hypotension can occur in cats, treat with antihistamine
- Do not use in conjunction with barbiturates.

Alfaxan®:

- Induction agent; redosing possible
- Best used intravenously; intramuscular administration less reliable
- No accumulation and can be used as a maintenance agent
- Give to effect (see Figures 13.7 and 13.8):
  - Consider premedication (20–50% reduction in induction dose depending on premedication)
  - Consider physical status of the animal
  - Slow injection (60 seconds, one quarter of the dose every 15 seconds)
  - Maintenance: incremental dosing is *approximately* 0.1 mg/kg/minute (0.01 ml/kg/minute) in premedicated dogs and cats, although individual responses may vary. In practical terms, a 10 kg dog would require 10 mg or 1 ml for 10 additional minutes of anaesthesia, while a 5 kg cat would require 5 mg or 0.5 ml for 10 additional minutes of anaesthesia.

Neuroleptanalgesia

The concept of neuroleptanalgesia involves the combination of a neuroleptic agent (benzodiazepines, butyrophenones, phenothiazines) with a potent opioid analgesic. This technique can be used in two ways. At low doses, it is commonly used for sedation and premedication via the intramuscular route before general anaesthesia, which is described in detail in Chapter 12. At high doses, usually given by intravenous injection, the combinations can be used to produce sufficient CNS depression to allow endotracheal intubation and moderate surgical stimulation. The excitatory effects of high doses of opioids make this technique unsuitable for healthy cats, although it has been used in severely debilitated cats.

Neuroleptanalgesia is characterized by analgesia, suppression of motor activity, suppression of autonomic reflexes and behavioural indifference, but not 'true' unconsciousness. Neuroleptanalgesia combinations are not suitable for routine induction of anaesthesia in healthy, young animals, because a true anaesthetic state is not reached unless followed by another anaesthetic agent (nitrous oxide, volatile or injectable anaesthetic), or unduly high doses are used. However, in high-risk and debilitated patients, tranquillizer–opioid combinations can have a profound effect. The advantages of this technique are a wide safety margin and partial reversibility (by using opioid antagonists). The disadvantages are: possible occurrence of panting or marked respiratory depression (requiring artificial ventilation); occurrence of spontaneous movements; sensitivity to noise and light; and possible postoperative behavioural changes, especially when used as the sole anaesthetic agents. Bradycardia related to the high dose of an opioid can be treated with parasympatholytic agents (atropine, glycopyrronium).

The 'classic' neuroleptanalgesic mixtures contain phenothiazines or butyrophenones like acepromazine, proprionylpromazine, droperidol or fluanisone, which can lead to significant alpha-1 receptor blockade (hypotension unresponsive to adrenaline). Benzodiazepines (diazepam, midazolam) possess a wide safety margin with minimal cardiovascular depression and lack of alpha-1 effects. Therefore, combinations of an opioid with a benzodiazepine are well suited for induction of anaesthesia in severely debilitated high-risk patients (Figure 13.11). The time required to obtain conditions suitable for endotracheal intubation is longer than with other intravenous anaesthetics (>2–3 minutes) but haemodynamic stability is excellent.

Drugs	Dose	Maintenance	Comment
Midazolam/diazepam Hydromorphone or l-Methadone	0.2 mg/kg i.v. 0.1–0.2 mg/kg i.v. 0.5 mg/kg i.v.	Inhalant	Inject in alternate increments until desired effect (intubation) Give opioid first, wait few minutes, then administer benzodiazepine Do not mix in same syringe (excitement possible)
Midazolam Fentanyl	0.2 mg/kg i.v. 2–5 µg/kg i.v.	Inhalant	Give opioid first, wait few minutes, then administer benzodiazepine Do not mix in same syringe
Midazolam Sufentanil	0.9 mg/kg i.v. 3 µg/kg i.v.	Midazolam 0.9 mg/kg/h Sufentanil 3 µg/kg/h	Mixed in one syringe, give in increments until intubation possible Used in gastric dilatation–volvulus, endotoxaemic patients Requires intermittent positive pressure ventilation/oxygen Bradycardia possible Reverse midazolam with flumazenil if necessary at end (10–30 µg/kg i.v.)

13.11 Neuroleptanalgesia for induction of anaesthesia in debilitated and old dogs.

Total intravenous anaesthesia

TIVA refers to induction and maintenance of anaesthesia by intravenous drugs only. An intravenous anaesthetic (usually propofol) provides hypnosis, muscle relaxation and immobility, whereas analgesia is provided by an opioid, an alpha-2 agonist or ketamine. Both the analgesic and the anaesthetic can be given by the intravenous route as an infusion. Some anaesthetists prefer to provide the analgesic in the premedication by the intramuscular route and supplement it as required. Anaesthesia can be maintained by intermittent boluses, but continuous infusion produces a more stable plane of anaesthesia and is more economical in terms of total drug use. Drugs can be given as a CRI with or without manual adjustment (variable rate infusion, VRI). A better adjustment of anaesthetic depth can be achieved with target-controlled infusion (TCI) devices, which deliver a drug to a predicted blood concentration set by the veterinary surgeon.

Principles

Sedation or anaesthesia can be maintained by intermittent drug boluses. This technique is simple and does not require special equipment. The disadvantage of intermittent drug boluses is the large variation in plasma concentrations and subsequently excessive drug effect at the time of the bolus and inadequate effect before the next bolus. Continuous infusion results in less variation in plasma levels with fewer oscillations in haemodynamic, respiratory and central effects and thus is safer for the animal.

Pharmacokinetic models can be used to develop dosing regimes with intravenous anaesthetic infusions. Such models are a mathematical description of how the body 'disposes' a drug. For detailed accounts of pharmacokinetic principles and models, standard pharmacokinetic textbooks should be consulted (e.g. Riviere, 1999). The parameters describing the disposition process are usually estimated by administering a known dose of a drug and measuring the resulting plasma concentrations at various time points. Pharmacokinetic variables important for the basic description of intravenous drugs are the volume of distribution, total body clearance and elimination half-life (Figure 13.12).

Typically the drug concentration *versus* time curve is described as an exponential equation. Depending on the shape of the curve, the equation can have a single exponent (one-compartment model), two exponents (two-compartment model) or three exponents (three-compartment model), which reflect different rates of drug decay at different time points.

Parameter	Symbol	Description
Distribution half-life Elimination half-life	$T_{1/2\alpha}$ $T_{1/2\beta}$	Time required for an amount of drug in plasma to decrease by one half. The half-life is dependent on the extent of drug distribution in the body (volume of distribution) and excretion of drug from the body (clearance). About five times the elimination half-life is required to eliminate a drug from the body
Total body clearance	Cl_B	Volume of plasma (blood) cleared of a drug per unit time; total body clearance includes all elimination processes (liver, kidney, lung)
Volumes of distribution: Volume of the central compartment Volume of distribution at steady state Volume of distribution at pseudoequilibrium Apparent volume of distribution	 Vc Vd_{SS} Vd area Vd (B)	Theoretical or apparent degree of dilution of a drug within the body. A large volume of distribution implies extensive distribution of a drug to tissues. The lower limit is the plasma volume. The highly lipophilic anaesthetics have a very large volume of distribution. Disease states can alter the volume of distribution massively and thereby change dose requirements The volume of the different estimates varies, with $Vc < Vd_{SS} < Vd\ area < Vd\ (B)$ Vd_{SS} defines the extent of drug dilution at maximum distribution or when all compartments are in equilibrium; V_c is the volume from which clearance is determined and is used for target-controlled infusion calculations

13.12 Primary pharmacokinetic parameters describing drug disposition in the body.

Half-lives are derived from the rate of change in drug concentration; different half-lives are reported, depending on the model. In a one-compartment model, only the elimination half-life occurs; in a two-compartment model a distribution half-life and an elimination half-life are estimated; in a three-compartment model three half-lives exist. Intravenous anaesthetics are usually described by two- or three-compartment models: a rapid initial decrease in plasma drug concentration (distribution) is followed either by a second slower distribution phase or directly by the elimination phase. The description of drug disposition by different models for the same drug contributes to the often large variation in reported elimination half-lives (see Figure 13.6).

After infusion of an intravenous anaesthetic, the offset of effect (recovery) is not merely a function of the elimination half-life, but is affected by the rate of equilibration between plasma and effect site and by the duration of infusion. Therefore, the context-sensitive half-time has been introduced, which is defined as the time for the plasma concentration to decrease by 50% after termination of an intravenous infusion designed to maintain a constant plasma concentration. 'Context' refers to infusion duration. Considerable differences between the elimination half-life after a single intravenous bolus and context-sensitive half-times after different infusion times can be demonstrated for many drugs (thiopental, ketamine, fentanyl).

Dosing regimens for TIVA consist of a loading dose aimed to achieve an effective concentration of the drug in the plasma, or better at the effect site (brain), consistent with anaesthesia. In the case of anaesthesia, the loading dose of a drug is equivalent to an anaesthesia induction dose. With the knowledge of the volume of distribution of a drug and the effective plasma concentration, a loading dose can be calculated:

$$\text{Loading dose (LD)} = \text{desired plasma concentration (Cpt)} \times \text{volume of distribution } (Vd_{ss})$$

Many different volumes of distribution are reported in pharmacokinetic studies (see Figure 13.12) and there is considerable confusion about which one to use for estimation of a loading dose for a manual infusion regime. The volume of distribution at steady state (Vd_{SS}) seems to be a very robust estimate because it is independent of any elimination processes and constants, and avoids massive over- or underestimation of a loading dose as can occur with other distribution volumes.

Plasma concentrations and, thereby, anaesthesia are maintained by a maintenance infusion rate, which compensates for drug 'losses' (distribution, excretion, metabolism). Therefore, the maintenance dose can be derived from the knowledge of the total body clearance of a drug and the desired plasma concentration:

$$\text{Maintenance dose (MD)} = \text{Cpt} \times \text{total body clearance } (CL_B)$$

The ideal drug for TIVA does not accumulate and would allow infusion at a constant rate over prolonged periods of time. However, distribution processes over time, individual and breed differences in pharmacokinetics and sensitivity to a drug, and surgical stimulation make adjustments of the infusion rate necessary. Therefore, the infusion rate is rarely kept at a constant over the whole anaesthetic, but is adjusted to the animal's needs. A common approach is to keep either the analgesic or the propofol at a constant rate and infuse the other drug to effect (Figures 13.13 and 13.14).

Drugs	Induction/loading dose	Maintenance dose	Indication	Infusion
Propofol	4–6 mg/kg	0.2 mg/kg/minute or 2 mg/kg about every 5 minutes as required	Deep sedation, without endotracheal tube	CRI
Propofol	4–6 mg/kg	0.4–0.5 mg/kg/minute	Non-painful procedures	VRI
Propofol Fentanyl	2–4 mg/kg 5 µg/kg	0.1–0.2 mg/kg/minute 0.5 µg/kg/minute	Surgery	VRI CRI
Propofol Fentanyl	2–4 mg/kg 5 µg/kg	0.3 mg/kg/minute 0.16–0.3 µg/kg/minute	Surgery	CRI VRI
Propofol Alfentanil	2–4 mg/kg 5 µg/kg	0.3 mg/kg/minute 1 5 µg/kg/minute	Surgery	CRI VRI
Propofol Remifentanil	2–4 mg/kg No loading	0.3–0.5 mg/kg/minute 0.3–0.6 µg/kg/minute	Surgery	VRI CRI
Propofol Remifentanil	2–4 mg/kg No loading	Plasma target 3–3.5 µg/ml 0.2–0.5 µg/kg/minute	Surgery	TCI VRI

13.13 Infusion regimes for TIVA in the dog after premedication. CRI = Constant rate infusion; TCI = Target-controlled infusion; VRI = Variable rate infusion.

Drugs	Induction/loading dose	Maintenance dose	Indication	Infusion
Propofol	6–8 mg/kg	0.2 mg/kg/minute or 2 mg/kg every 5 minutes to effect	Deep sedation, without endotracheal tube	CRI
Propofol	6–8 mg/kg	0.4–0.5 mg/kg/minute	Non-painful procedures	VRI
Propofol Fentanyl	4–6 mg/kg 1 μg/kg	0.12–0.3 mg/kg/minute 0.1 μg/kg/minute	Surgery	VRI
Propofol Alfentanil	4–6 mg/kg 5 μg/kg	0.12–0.3 mg/kg/minute 0.5 μg/kg/minute	Surgery	CRI
Propofol Sufentanil	4–6 mg/kg 0.1 μg/kg	0.12–0.3 mg/kg/minute 0.01 μg/kg/minute	Surgery	CRI
Propofol Remifentanil	6–8 mg/kg No loading	0.3 mg/kg/minute 0.2–0.3 μg/kg/minute	Surgery	CRI VRI

13.14 Infusion regimes for TIVA in the cat after premedication and anaesthesia induction with propofol. CRI = Constant rate infusion; TCI = Target-controlled infusion; VRI = Variable rate infusion.

Target-controlled infusion

The idea of TCI systems is to aim at a specific drug plasma (effect site) concentration, which is known to produce a desired effect. Based on a mathematical (pharmacokinetic–pharmacodynamic) model, a microprocessor predicts changes in drug concentrations and controls an infusion device. Infusion rates are adjusted automatically by this system to obtain the targeted drug plasma concentration. With an open, model-based system, the anaesthetist sets the target concentration with the knowledge of drug effects. The plasma target is a calculated number based on a mathematical model and not a measured concentration. Therefore, the performance of TCI systems depends on the pharmacokinetic model used and requires careful evaluation. The next step in development of automated drug delivery systems is to feed the measured drug effect (i.e. blood pressure, EEG traces) back into the system. With such 'closed loop' systems the model is permanently updated based on actual drug effects rather than on drug concentration.

Infusion devices

Infusion devices are classified as either controllers or positive displacement pumps. Rate controllers simply control the flow produced by gravity. Infusion sets with regulating roller clamps come in different sizes labelled as number of drops producing 1 ml of fluid. They deliver fluids/drugs with an accuracy of ±10% depending on the height above ground.

Positive displacement pumps contain an active pumping mechanism. Volumetric infusion pumps (Figure 13.15) work with different delivery mechanisms (bellows, piston, peristaltic, shuttle) and can produce delivery rates of 0.1–1999 ml/h with an accuracy of ±5%. This type of pump often requires special tubing/infusion sets and cannot be used with regular infusion sets. Administration of anaesthetics or haemodynamic agents using a drip infusion via roller clamps or a volumetric infusion pump requires dilution of the very potent drugs to obtain dose rates (volume/time) suitable for administration by these systems. This can become a problem, particularly in very small animals.

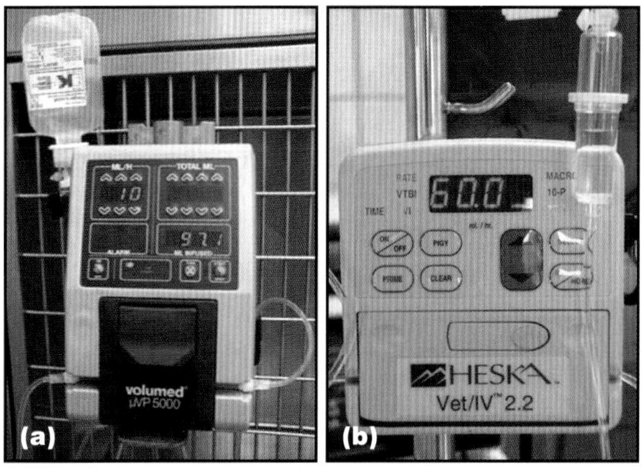

13.15 Volumetric infusion pumps.

Piston pumps also divide the millilitre dose into portions, which can produce a 'mini-bolus' effect within the patient, especially with diluted drugs with a very short half-life (e.g. vasopressors). Infusion by gravity with an infusion set is a simple way of administering an anaesthetic continuously, but is less accurate than with an infusion pump and requires careful calculation and adjustment of the drip rate.

Syringe pumps (Figure 13.16) that use a stepper motor with a drive screw (syringe drivers) are particularly suitable for the delivery of potent anaesthetics. Rates as low as 0.01 ml/h can be delivered with high accuracy (2–3%). Some syringe drivers include a calculator feature, which enables one to set the patient

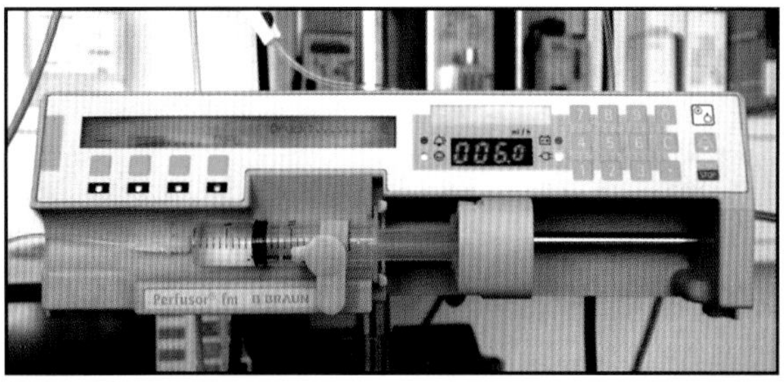

13.16 Syringe driver.

weight, the drug concentration and the infusion rate in dose/weight/time and the pump calculates the infusion in volume/unit time. Numerous pumps allow automatic recognition of syringe size and staged infusions, with a loading dose and a maintenance infusion being programmable. Special tubing is not required with syringe drivers. Syringe drivers can deliver drugs accurately, even to very small patients, and infusion of the anaesthetic can be adjusted independent of fluid administration.

Syringe drivers (e.g. Diprifusor® from Zeneca for propofol in humans) with inbuilt computer software and pharmacokinetic models to run TCIs, are not commercially available for dogs or cats at present. Syringe drivers (Graseby 3400, 3500), which can be controlled by a custom-built external computer and pharmacokinetic modelling software, have been used to target plasma concentrations of various drugs in experimental animal studies and for evaluation of a TCI protocol for propofol anaesthesia in dogs. Because of limited availability of infusion hardware and software, as well as evaluated population pharmacokinetics, the TCI idea is not yet ready to be used in veterinary practice.

TIVA protocols

Drugs used for maintenance of anaesthesia require a pharmacokinetic profile that allows adjustment of anaesthetic depth by changing the infusion rate over prolonged periods of time without significant accumulation and without significant prolongation of recovery (short context-sensitive half-time). This means rapid onset of effect, short duration of effect and high clearance rates with rapid metabolism to inactive substances and excretion.

Of the currently licensed drugs, propofol is the most suitable and most used for maintenance of anaesthesia by continuous infusion. Because propofol has poor analgesic properties it is often combined with fentanyl or one of its derivatives such as alfentanil, sufentanil or remifentanil. Medetomidine and ketamine can also given by infusion (see Chapter 9).

Diagnostic procedures, cast changes and surgical procedures with low invasiveness might be possible with low dose rates (low plasma concentrations) of propofol, which maintain spontaneous respiration. However, propofol is a respiratory depressant and causes hypoxaemia even when spontaneous respiration persists. Therefore, oxygen should be supplemented for all procedures lasting more than 15–20 minutes and equipment for intubation and basic artificial ventilation should be available. TIVA protocols for prolonged, invasive surgical procedures require concurrent administration of an effective opioid. With these combinations spontaneous respiration usually ceases and endotracheal intubation and mechanical ventilation are required.

Various propofol TIVA infusion regimes are used with excellent results in dogs for extended procedures (>2 hours), but prolonged recoveries have to be expected in Greyhounds (see Figure 13.13). In cats, it seems advisable to restrict duration of propofol infusions (30–60 minutes) because of cats' increased sensitivity to phenolic compounds and prolonged recoveries (see Figure 13.14).

Maintenance of anaesthesia with TIVA by means of an infusion pump or a syringe driver does not mean anaesthesia is automated without intervention. Anaesthesia monitoring and adjustment of anaesthetic depth by changing infusion rates should be as meticulous as during inhalation anaesthesia and by changing vaporizer settings.

Balanced anaesthesia

As with propofol TIVA, different analgesic compounds (opioids, medetomidine, ketamine, lidocaine) can be used as CRIs in conjunction with volatile agents, resulting in a type of balanced anaesthesia. The analgesic and anaesthetic-sparing properties of these drugs allow reduced concentrations of volatile agents and thereby less cardiovascular depression. Dose rates of CRIs for balanced anaesthesia techniques using various drugs are given in Figure 13.17. For descriptions of detailed pharmacology of the single drugs the reader is referred to Chapters 9 and 12.

Drugs	Induction/loading dose	Maintenance dose	Infusion	Comment
Fentanyl	3–5 μg/kg i.v.	0.08–0.3 μg/kg/minute	VRI to effect	IPPV Bradycardia
Alfentanil	2.5–5 μg/kg i.v.	0.5–5 μg/kg/minute	VRI	IPPV Bradycardia
Sufentanil	0.1–3 μg/kg i.v.	0.015–0.1 μg/kg/minute	VRI	IPPV Bradycardia
Remifentanil	No loading	0.2–0.6 μg/kg/minute	VRI	IPPV Bradycardia
Ketamine	0.3–0.5 mg/kg i.v.	2–20 μg/kg/minute (common 5 μg/kg/minute)	CRI	High doses lead to ketamine 'signs'
Medetomidine	No loading	1–1.5 μg/kg/h	CRI	Bradycardia

13.17 Constant rate infusions (CRIs) used in conjunction with inhalation anaesthesia in order to reduce anaesthetic requirements. Intermittent positive pressure ventilation (IPPV) becomes necessary. VRI = Variable rate infusion. (continues) ▶

Drugs	Induction/loading dose	Maintenance dose	Infusion	Comment
Dexmedetomidine	No loading	0.5–1 µg/kg/h	CRI	Bradycardia
Lidocaine	Dog: 2–4 mg/kg Cat: 0.25–0.75 mg/kg slow i.v.	25–80 µg/kg/minute 10–40 µg/kg/minute	CRI CRI	Care with lidocaine infusions in cats because of the potential for toxicity (seizures and severe bradycardia)
Morphine Lidocaine Ketamine (MLK)	Dog: 10 ml/kg Cat: no loading	3.3 µg/kg/minute 50 µg/kg/minute 10 µg/kg/minute infused at 10 ml/kg/h postoperative 2 ml/kg/h	CRI	5 mg morphine 75 mg lidocaine 15 mg ketamine in 250 ml NaCl

13.17 (continued) Constant rate infusions (CRIs) used in conjunction with inhalation anaesthesia in order to reduce anaesthetic requirements. Intermittent positive pressure ventilation (IPPV) becomes necessary. VRI = Variable rate infusion.

References and further reading

Adam H, Glen JB and Hoyle P (1980) Pharmacokinetics in laboratory animals of ICI 35 868, a new IV anaesthetic agent. *British Journal of Anaesthesia* **52**, 743–746

Beths T, Glen JB, Reid J, Monteiro A and Nolan A (2001) Evaluation and optimisation of target-controlled infusion systems for administering propofol to dogs as part of a total intravenous anaesthetic technique during dental surgery. *Veterinary Record* **148**, 198–203.

Boscan P, Pypendop B, Solano A and Ilkiw J (2005) Cardiovascular and respiratory effects of ketamine infusions in isoflurane-anesthetized dogs before and during noxious stimulation. *American Journal of Veterinary Research* **66**, 2122–2129

Ferré P, Pasloske K, Whittem T *et al.* (2006) Plasma pharmacokinetics of alfaxalone in dogs after an intravenous bolus of Alfaxan-CD RTU. *Veterinary Anaesthesia and Analgesia* **33(4)**, 229–236

Hall L, Clarke KW and Trim C (2001) *Veterinary Anaesthesia, 10th edn.* Saunders, Edinburgh

Hanna R, Borchard R and Schmidt S (1988) Pharmacokinetics of ketamine HCl and metabolite I in the cat: a comparison of i.v., i.m., and rectal administration. *Journal of Veterinary Pharmacology and Therapeutics* **11**, 84–93

Heit M, Pasloske K, Whittem T, Ranasinghe M and Li Q (2004) Plasma pharmacokinetics of alfaxalone in cats after administration at 5 and 25 mg/kg as an intravenous bolus of Alafaxan-CD RTU. In: *Proceedings of the American College of Veterinary Internal Medicine, Minneapolis*, pp. 849–850

Ilkiw J, Benthuysen J, Ebling W and McNeal D (1991) A comparative study of the pharmacokinetics of thiopental in the rabbit, sheep and dog. *Journal of Veterinary Pharmacology and Therapeutics* **14**, 134–140

Ilkiw J and Pascoe P (2003) Cardiovascular effects of propofol alone and in combination with ketamine for total intravenous anesthesia in cats. *American Journal of Veterinary Research* **64**, 913–917

Jackson A, Tobias K, Long C, Bartges J and Harvey R (2004) Effects of various anesthetic agents on laryngeal motion during laryngoscopy in normal dogs. *Veterinary Surgery* **33**, 102–106

Kaka J and Hayton W (1980) Pharmacokinetics of ketamine and two metabolites in the dog. *Journal of Pharmacokinetics and Biopharmaceutics* **8**, 193–202

Luna S, Cassu R, Castro G *et al.* (2004) Effects of four anaesthetic protocols on the neurological and cardiorespiratory variables of puppies born by caesarean section. *Veterinary Record* **154**, 387–389

McIntosh MP, Schwarting N and Rajewski RA (2004) *In vitro* and *in vivo* evaluation of a sulfobutyl ether beta-cyclodextrin enabled etomidate formulation. *Journal of Pharmaceutical Sciences* **93(10)**, 2585–2594

Mendes G and Selmi A (2003) Use of a combination of propofol and fentanyl, alfentanil, or sufentanil for total intravenous anesthesia in cats. *Journal of the American Veterinary Medical Association* **223**, 1608–1613

Muir W, Wiese AJ and March PA (2003) Effects of morphine, lidocaine, ketamine, and morphine-lidocaine-ketamine drug combination on minimum alveolar concentration in dogs anesthetized with isoflurane. *American Journal of Veterinary Research* **64**, 1155–1160

Murrell J, Notten RWV and Hellebrekers L (2005) Clinical investigation of remifentanil and propofol for the total intravenous anaesthesia of dogs. *Veterinary Record* **156**, 804–808

Musk G, Pang D, Beths T and Flaherty D (2006) Target controlled infusion of propofol – optimisation of induction target. *Veterinary Record* (in press)

Nolan A and Reid J (1993) Pharmacokinetics of propofol administered by infusion in dogs undergoing surgery. *British Journal of Anaesthesia* **70**, 546–551

Nolan A, Reid J and Grant S (1993) The effects of halothane and nitrous oxide on the pharmacokinetics of propofol in dogs. *Journal of Veterinary Pharmacology and Therapeutics* **16**, 335–342

Pascoe PJ, Ilkiw JE and Frischmeyer KJ (2006a) The effect of the duration of propofol administration on recovery from anesthesia in cats. *Veterinary Anaesthesia and Analgesia* **33(1)**, 2–7

Pascoe PJ, Raekallio M, Kuusela E, McKusick B and Granholm M (2006b) Changes in the minimum alveolar concentration of isoflurane and some cardiopulmonary measurements during three continuous infusion rates of dexmedetomidine in dogs. *Veterinary Anaesthesia and Analgesia* **33(2)**, 97–103

Pypendop B and Ilkiw J (2005) Pharmacokinetics of ketamine and its metabolite, norketamine, after intravenous administration of a bolus of ketamine to isoflurane-anesthetized dogs. *American Journal of Veterinary Research* **66**, 2034–2038

Riviere JE (1999) *Comparative Pharmacokinetics – Principles, Techniques and Applications.* Iowa State University Press, Ames, Iowa

Wortz E, Benson G, Thurmon J *et al.* (1990) Pharmacokinetics of etomidate in cats. *American Journal of Veterinary Research* **51**, 281–285

Wright M (1982) Pharmacologic effects of ketamine and its use in veterinary medicine. *Journal of the American Veterinary Medical Association* **180**, 1462–1471

Zhang J, Maland L, Hague B *et al.* (1998) Buccal absorption of etomidate from a solid formulation in dogs. *Anesthesia and Analgesia* **86**, 1116–1122

14

Inhalant anaesthetics

Nora S. Matthews

Introduction

Inhalant anaesthetics have specific advantages and disadvantages to the practising veterinary surgeon. For most patients, the advantages outweigh the disadvantages, which is why they have become a mainstay for most practices. Since methoxyflurane is no longer being manufactured on a large scale and has largely fallen out of use, the reader is referred to the previous edition of this manual or other texts for discussion of its use. Halothane is included for the sake of completeness, although its use and availability are also decreasing.

Advantages

All of the inhalants have the advantage that they are generally administered in oxygen and usually through an endotracheal tube (although a mask can be used). Both the addition of oxygen and a secured airway contribute to greater patient safety. The more modern inhalant anaesthetics (isoflurane, sevoflurane) act rapidly, produce less cardiac sensitivity to catecholamines and are minimally metabolized by the liver. Changes in depth of anaesthesia with modern inhalants can be produced more rapidly, compared with injectable or intravenous infusion techniques, with a rapid, complete recovery from anaesthesia. Their rapid elimination from the body, minimal metabolism by the liver or kidneys and decreased myocardial sensitization to catecholamines make the newer agents more appropriate for geriatric patients, patients with organ dysfunction and exotic species. Although it must be emphasized that there is no such thing as a completely safe anaesthetic, there are several reasons for the perception that isoflurane and sevoflurane are 'safer' than halothane, which are covered in the discussion of individual agents.

Disadvantages

The inhalant anaesthetics require the use of a costly anaesthetic machine, breathing system and vaporizer, which the user must understand and be able to trouble-shoot (see Chapters 4 and 5). For instance, the veterinary surgeon must be aware that carbon monoxide can be produced by the interaction of the volatile inhalants with soda lime. Pollution of the workplace is possible with inhalants and effective scavenging systems must be in place (covered later and in Chapter 5). Therefore, appropriate maintenance of the machine and use of fresh, moist soda lime is critical. In general, soda lime should be changed after every 6–8 hours of use and dry soda lime should be replaced, or the system flushed with oxygen to prevent the accumulation of carbon monoxide. Dose-dependent cardiopulmonary depression is produced by the inhalants and this must be carefully monitored.

Minimum alveolar concentration values

To use the inhalants effectively, the concepts of minimum alveolar concentration (MAC) values and solubility of the inhalant (usually blood/gas solubility, see later) must be understood. The minimum alveolar concentration is that concentration in the alveoli required to prevent 50% of a group of animals from responding with purposeful movement to a supramaximal noxious stimulus (Figure 14.1). It is a value obtained using reproducible laboratory techniques under stable conditions. This information then gives the veterinary surgeon an idea of the percentage concentration to set the vaporizer at to maintain an appropriate depth of anaesthesia. However, since the MAC value by definition only keeps 50% of animals anaesthetized, the

Physical properties and MAC	Halothane[a] ($CBrClH\text{-}CF_3$)	Isoflurane[b] ($CF_3\text{-}CHCl\text{-}O\text{-}CF_2H$)	Sevoflurane[b] ($CFH_2\text{-}O\text{-}(CF_3)_2$)	Nitrous oxide (N_2O)
MAC (dog/cat %)	0.87/1.14	1.28/1.63	2.35/2.58	222/255
Vapour pressure at 25°C	243	295	197	Gas
Blood/gas solubility (37°C)	2.0	1.43	0.63–0.69	0.47
ml of vapour/ml of liquid at 20°C	227	195	183	Not applicable

14.1 Physical characteristics and minimum alveolar concentration (MAC) of currently used inhalant anaesthetics. [a] = Halothane is a halogenated hydrocarbon. [b] = Isoflurane and sevoflurane are halogenated ethers.

actual alveolar concentration for clinical use needs to be 25–50% greater than the MAC value to achieve a light surgical plane of anaesthesia when volatile agents are used alone (see effects of drugs on MAC later). Higher concentrations (with the associated greater cardiopulmonary depression) will be needed for invasive procedures unless adjunctive analgesics are used. Certain situations, as well as drugs, can affect the minimum alveolar concentration.

Factors affecting MAC values

MAC values are generally measured in a limited population of healthy animals under controlled conditions. In clinical practice, these conditions are often not present; it is therefore important to recognize how other drugs and conditions will affect the MAC value.

Factors which decrease the MAC value of inhalant anaesthetics include:

- Pre-anaesthetic sedatives, injectable anaesthetics and many analgesics (Figure 14.2)
- High P_aCO_2 (above 90 mmHg (12 kPa))
- Hypoxaemia (P_aO_2 less than 40 mmHg (5.3 kPa))
- Haematocrit less than 10%
- Increasing age
- Hypothermia
- Pregnancy
- Concurrent illness.

Drug	Percentage decrease in MAC	Species studied	Reference
Buprenorphine	9–14 15–50	Cat Rat	Ilkiw *et al.*, 2002 Criado *et al.*, 2000
Butorphanol	8–19	Cat	Ilkiw *et al.*, 2002
Diazepam	53	Dog	Hellyer *et al.*, 2001
Electroacupuncture	15–21	Dog	Jeong and Nam, 2003
Fentanyl (transdermal)	18	Cat	Yackey *et al.*, 2004
Ketamine	25 Up to 75	Dog Cat	Muir *et al.*, 2003 Pascoe *et al.*, 2005
Lidocaine	19–43 3–52	Dog Cat	Valverde *et al.*, 2004 Pypendop and Ilkiw, 2005
Morphine	48	Dog	Muir *et al.*, 2003
MLK	45	Dog	Muir *et al.*, 2003
Epidural morphine	21–30	Cat	Golder *et al.*, 1998

14.2 Decrease in minimum alveolar concentration (MAC) of isoflurane associated with commonly used drugs or techniques. MLK = Morphine–lidocaine–ketamine combination.

The decrease in MAC may be significant; for instance, various lidocaine infusion rates have been found to decrease the MAC of isoflurane in dogs by 19–43% (see Figure 14.2). Clinically, this means the delivered concentration of inhalant should be decreased when a lidocaine infusion is used and close patient monitoring is essential to prevent overdosing the patient with anaesthetic. Conversely, when pre-anaesthetic or injectable induction drugs are not used, the amount of inhalant needed for maintenance will be increased.

Increases in MAC occur with elevation of body temperature and increased levels of catecholamines.

Factors which have little effect on MAC are:

- Duration of anaesthesia
- Circadian rhythms
- Hyper- or hypothyroidism
- Severe metabolic acidosis or alkalosis
- Hypertension
- Moderate hyper- or hypoventilation.

Anaesthetic breathing systems, gas flows and minimum alveolar concentration

It is important to understand that the vaporizer setting will only be reflective of patient alveolar inhalant concentration after the breathing system concentration is well equilibrated with inhalant under stable conditions. The concentration of inhalant in the system will depend on the choice of anaesthetic breathing system (non-rebreathing or rebreathing), and fresh gas flow rates used. Expensive monitors can measure inhaled (breathing system) concentrations of inhalant in fresh gas (see Chapter 7), and the alveolar concentration is measured in the exhaled breath. Rebreathing systems (circle or to-and-fro) tend to take longer to equilibrate with vaporizer settings during the early part of anaesthesia because these systems usually have a high internal volume, require lower fresh gas flow rates and attached patients are relatively larger compared to when non-rebreathing systems are used (e.g. Ayres T-piece, Bain, Lack; see also Chapter 5). Generally, alveolar concentrations more rapidly reflect vaporizer settings when non-rebreathing systems and high gas flow rates are used. Rebreathing systems can be more rapidly equilibrated with vaporizer output by temporarily using high fresh gas flows and increasing the vaporizer setting.

Uptake of inhaled anaesthetic gases into the body

Inspired anaesthetic gases are diluted by other gases (oxygen, nitrogen and carbon dioxide) in the patient's lung, so the rate of change of concentration of the volatile agent in the alveoli will depend on the size of the lung and the volume of gas which is being exchanged (i.e. minute ventilation). If the minute ventilation is small, the alveolar concentration will increase more slowly than if it is large. Once the anaesthetic gas reaches the alveoli, uptake by blood occurs; the rate of this uptake depends on the alveolar/blood anaesthetic concentration gradient (which is effectively 'pushing' the drug) and the blood/gas partition coefficient (which is effectively 'pulling' the drug). Agents with relatively low blood/gas solubility (such as isoflurane and sevoflurane) will have slower removal from the alveoli than agents with higher solubility (e.g. halothane) but this allows greater alveolar/blood anaesthetic concentration gradients to be established and therefore uptake is increased overall, leading to fast induction of anaesthesia. Anaesthetic agents with higher blood solubility (e.g. methoxyflurane or halothane) will produce slower inductions since gradients are not well established, and more of the agent will be retained in the blood and not transferred to the brain where the anaesthetic effect is produced. This is an oversimplification of a very complicated subject; for a detailed discussion see Eger (1974) or Sawyer (1982).

Cardiac output also influences anaesthetic uptake from the alveoli; generally, higher blood flow past the alveoli will promote greater anaesthetic uptake but large alveolar/blood anaesthetic concentration gradients are not established and, therefore, induction of anaesthesia is actually slowed during high cardiac output states. Sick animals with low cardiac output states have faster inductions.

Finally, uptake of anaesthetic agent by tissues must be considered. The vessel-rich group (brain, heart, intestines, kidneys, liver, spleen and endocrine organs) receive the majority of cardiac output, so the concentration of anaesthetic will equilibrate very quickly with the blood in these tissues.

Again, if we oversimplify the whole picture important factors in induction of anaesthesia are as follows:

- Ventilation must be sufficient to present anaesthetic molecules to the blood
- Inspired concentration of anaesthetic must be high enough to 'force' large numbers of molecules into blood and tissues
- Cardiac output as well as solubility in blood will interact to affect uptake and delivery of anaesthetic agents; the less soluble the agent, the smaller the influence of changes in blood flow on alveolar concentration
- Abnormalities in ventilation to perfusion ratio (V/Q mismatch; see Chapters 19, 20 and 21) will delay uptake of inhaled anaesthetics, and will slow induction.

Putting all of these conditions together can be demonstrated in the following potential clinical situation: a chamber induction (capacity 20 l) of an unpremedicated cat using isoflurane at a vaporizer setting of 2.0% (approx. 1.5 x MAC) with 2 l/minute oxygen flow rate. It will take a minimum of 10 minutes before the concentration in the box is close to 2.0% because of the low flow rates and high breathing system volume. It will be even longer before the alveolar concentration of inhalant in the cat stabilizes at this concentration. The unpremedicated cat is probably nervous, therefore its cardiac output may be increased, thereby slowing inhalant uptake by slowing build-up of alveolar concentration. This slower uptake may be offset by increased ventilation associated with the stressful situation. Therefore, it is normal to use higher oxygen flow rates and vaporizer settings to achieve anaesthesia more quickly. Premedication helps to relieve stress and may improve uptake of inhalant anaesthetic (by normalizing cardiac output) during mask or chamber induction of anaesthesia.

Anaesthetic index

The anaesthetic index (AI) is derived from the concentration of inhalant required to produce apnoea for 60 seconds (i.e. apnoeic concentration) divided by the MAC value for the inhalant. The lower the AI value, the greater the amount of respiratory depression produced by that inhalant. AI values for cats and dogs are presented in Figure 14.3.

Inhalational agent	Anaesthetic index	
	Cat	Dog
Halothane	N/A	2.9
Isoflurane	2.4	2.51
Sevoflurane	N/A	3.45

14.3 Anaesthetic index of commonly used inhalational agents in cats and dogs. N/A = Not available.

General characteristics of inhaled anaesthetics

To a large extent, the currently used volatile anaesthetics share the same characteristics; they all produce a dose-dependent decrease in cardiac output and blood pressure, depression of the central nervous system and have poor analgesic effects. None of the newer agents are particularly good analgesics when used alone (hence the common use of concurrent analgesics for very invasive procedures). Since the newer agents are all relatively insoluble and alveolar/blood gradients are rapidly established, depth of anaesthesia can be rapidly changed. The degree of respiratory depression varies slightly between each volatile agent, but generally they all produce dose-dependent depression.

Halothane

Halothane is a very potent (MAC value 0.9% in dogs) halogenated hydrocarbon which is falling out of favour due to decreased production (at least in the USA) and decreased cost of newer competing volatile anaesthetics. Halothane does require a preservative (0.01% thymol) and does not decompose in the presence of warm soda lime, but will attack aluminium, brass, lead, rubber and some plastics when moisture is present. It has a pleasant, non-irritating odour and is a respiratory depressant. Halothane reduces blood pressure, may result in bradycardia and will sensitize the myocardial conduction system to adrenaline, resulting in arrhythmias. It is licensed for both cats and dogs and, compared with methoxyflurane, induction and recovery are rapid. Significantly more halothane is metabolized by the liver (approximately 20–25%) than the other newer volatile anaesthetics (isoflurane and sevoflurane), making it inappropriate for patients with severe liver dysfunction and highlighting the importance of waste anaesthetic gas scavenging.

Isoflurane

Isoflurane is a fluorinated ether, which has been in use in small animal patients since the mid to late 1980s. Since it is very potent (MAC value for dogs is 1.28%) it is usually delivered using a precision, 'out-of-circuit' vaporizer. Isoflurane does not require a preservative and does not decompose in the presence of soda lime (at normal operating temperatures). It has a fairly strong, pungent odour and is a respiratory depressant, as well as producing dose-dependent cardiovascular depression. However, heart rhythm is stable. As it is much less soluble than halothane, induction, recovery and changes in depth of anaesthesia are rapid in comparison with halothane. Less than 1% of isoflurane is metabolized by the patient (since the majority is exhaled) making it a good choice of inhalant for patients with hepatic or renal dysfunction.

Sevoflurane

Sevoflurane is also a fluorinated ether, which has been more recently introduced into veterinary use (late 1990s). It is slightly less potent (MAC value for dogs is 2.36%) than isoflurane and requires a different vaporizer from that used for isoflurane (since the vapour pressure is different). Sevoflurane does not require a preservative, but can decompose in the presence of soda lime to produce compound A, which is nephrotoxic in rats. At normal oxygen flow rates (not <10 ml/kg/minute), production of compound A does not appear to be clinically relevant. Production of compound A is greater with Baralyme than with soda lime, and is greater at higher concentrations of sevoflurane and lower oxygen flow rates. Sevoflurane is metabolized to produce fluoride ions but no toxicity has been associated with this, even in patients with some renal dysfunction. However, since all anaesthetics can compromise renal function, the veterinary surgeon would be wise to administer intravenous fluids and monitor urine output. Sevoflurane is currently considerably more expensive than isoflurane, but, since it is less soluble than isoflurane, very rapid changes in the depth of anaesthesia are possible. One advantage of sevoflurane is that mask inductions are well tolerated (since it is not as pungent as isoflurane and does not induce coughing). The cardiovascular depression observed is similar to that observed with isoflurane, but the degree of respiratory depression (judged by anaesthetic index, see above) is less profound with sevoflurane. Approximately 3% of sevoflurane is metabolized by the patient, which means it is still a good choice for patients with hepatic or renal dysfunction.

Desflurane

Desflurane is also a fluorinated ether, which is only approved for use in humans. There has been some research into the use of desflurane in the veterinary field, but the main detractor has been the need for a very specialized vaporizer. Since desflurane has a very high vapour pressure (664 mmHg (88.5 kPa) at 20°C) it requires an expensive heated vaporizer to produce an accurate output. Although desflurane appears to have characteristics which make it attractive for use in animals (low blood/gas solubility of 0.42) with promising results in equine trials, it appears the cost of the vaporizer will prevent its popularity in veterinary anaesthesia at present. The MAC values of desflurane are 7.2% and 9.8% in the dog and cat, respectively.

Nitrous oxide

Nitrous oxide (N_2O) is a gaseous inhalant which has been widely used as an analgesic adjunct alongside the more potent inhalants. Due to its low solubility, it was widely used with halothane to speed anaesthetic uptake in the first few minutes of administration of N_2O (second gas effect). The second gas effect occurs when two anaesthetics are given together. Uptake of a large volume of N_2O (typically used at flow rates of several litres per minute) combined with the insolubility of N_2O augments uptake of volatile agent from the alveoli, thus increasing the delivery of the second gas (e.g. halothane, which is delivered in millilitres per minute) and concentrating the halothane 'left behind'. This second gas effect has been found not to be as advantageous with isoflurane or sevoflurane since they are already rapidly taken up from alveoli into the bloodstream.

Although true anaesthesia cannot be achieved in dogs or cats with N_2O alone (since the MAC value is so high), the use of N_2O at inspired levels of 50–65% facilitates appropriate anaesthetic depth without using higher concentrations of the more cardiopulmonary depressant volatile agents. Some have advocated using 75% N_2O with another volatile inhalant, but it is imperative that inspired oxygen concentrations are 33% or greater in anaesthetized patients. If 75% N_2O is used with 3% volatile inhalant, the amount of oxygen in the system is less than 22% (depending on how much carbon dioxide is in the system); in effect the inspired oxygen concentration in the system is now similar to room air. The maximum inspired N_2O can thus only be about 65% to allow adequate inspired oxygen levels. Fifty percent inspired N_2O (approximately 1 l/minute oxygen flow used with 1 l/minute N_2O) in a rebreathing system is still effective at lowering some volatile anaesthetic requirements and can be used. When using higher inspired concentrations of N_2O (50–65%) it is advisable to use a pulse oximeter to monitor oxygen saturation of haemoglobin. In a non-rebreathing system, setting the oxygen and N_2O flowmeters in a ratio of 1:2 (for example 1 l/minute oxygen and 2 l/minute N_2O) will still provide 33% inspired oxygen.

N_2O can be advantageous in that it produces mild sympathetic stimulation which tends to support the cardiovascular system. Caution should always be used with N_2O in patients where diffusion of the gas into currently existing closed gas pockets might be detrimental (e.g. a patient with gastric dilatation). The volume of the closed gas space will increase as N_2O crosses into the pocket faster than nitrogen leaves, and the volume increase can exacerbate problems further. The endotracheal tube cuff can also increase in volume, so patients receiving N_2O should also have the cuffs rechecked approximately half an hour after starting N_2O administration to avoid excess pressure on the tracheal mucosa. Adequate oxygen should also be provided during recovery to prevent diffusion hypoxia caused by the rapid outpouring of N_2O into the alveoli after its administration is discontinued. This rapid accumulation of N_2O can dilute oxygen levels within the alveoli and cause hypoxaemia. Supplemental oxygen should be continued for 5–10 minutes following termination of N_2O.

Calculation of inhalant volume used

Since the newer inhalants are more expensive, it is helpful to be able to approximate how much liquid inhalant will be used so that costs can be predicted (Figures 14.1 and 14.4). Cost per bottle divided by size of the bottle (in millilitres) equals cost per millilitre of liquid. Use of higher flow rates will result in more inhalant being used and greater expense; therefore, mask or chamber inductions and use of N_2O will increase the amount of volatile agents used. Other causes for greater use of volatile agents include leaks in the breathing system, e.g. leaking endotracheal tube cuffs or leaks around the soda lime canister.

3 x FGF (l/minute) x vol% = ml used/h

Example: if you are using 2 l/minute oxygen and sevoflurane is set at 4%, the estimate would be 24 ml/h. If the current cost of sevoflurane is £0.64 (US $1.00)/ml, it would cost the veterinary surgeon £15.36 (US $24)/h.

14.4 Calculation of liquid inhalant use. FGF = Fresh gas flow; Vol% = Vaporizer setting. (After Ehrenwerth and Eisenkraft, 1993).

Waste anaesthetic gases

It seems clear that exposure to waste anaesthetic gases should be minimized as much as possible to prevent associated health risks with this exposure. There is little evidence regarding risks of the newer agents, but in the USA, the National Institute for Occupational Safety and Health (NIOSH) (www.cdc.gov/niosh/hcwold.html), Occupational Safety and Health Administration (OSHA) (www.osha-slc.gov/dts/osta/anestheticgases/indexs.html#E) and American College of Veterinary Anesthesiologists (ACVA) all have recommendations for minimizing exposure. In the UK, such recommendations are contained in the 'Control of Substances Hazardous to Health' (COSHH) Regulations, available from the Health and Safety Executive (HSE). The ACVA recommendations acknowledge conflicting evidence but mention cancer, hepatic and renal disease, immunological effects and complications during pregnancy as being linked to trace gas exposure. Waste anaesthetic gas scavenging systems (see Chapter 5) should be routinely used on all equipment. Additional procedures related to case management can decrease exposure (Figure 14.5). Each country will have its own guidelines, but if pollution of the workspace is kept to a minimum through effective scavenging techniques the risks should be minimal (www.nohsc.gov.au/AboutNohsc/; www.ccohs.ca/oshanswers/chemicals/waste_anesthetic.html). In the UK, a list of approved workplace exposure limits is available from the HSE (www.hse.gov.uk).

Fill vaporizers in well ventilated areas and away from high traffic flow (fill vaporizers at the end of the working day)
Consider vaporizers with keyed filling systems to reduce exposure to liquid inhalant
Discard empty bottles with the tops attached and secured
Don't turn vaporizers on until the patient is attached to the breathing system
Scavenge gas from induction chambers (rather than leaving the top off)
Use endotracheal tubes with functional cuffs which have been inflated
Minimize mask inductions or maintenance with masks; use tightly fitting masks
Check anaesthetic machines and ventilators for leaks and fix them
Ensure anaesthetic equipment and vaporizers are regularly serviced
At finish of anaesthetic administration leave the patient attached to breathing system until extubation instead of letting the patient exhale into the room
Make sure recovery areas are well ventilated

14.5 Simple ways to minimize anaesthetic waste gas exposure.

Pollution of workspace and pregnant women

There is little reliable information available to provide answers regarding risks of exposure to anaesthetic gases for pregnant women. Pregnant women should consult their physicians regarding precautions that should be taken. Most institutions have the following precautions or guidelines for pregnant women if they need to continue working in environments where anaesthetic gases are used:

- Assign filling of vaporizers to other individuals
- Other individuals should fill vaporizers in areas with good ventilation
- Minimize or eliminate chamber and mask inductions
- Other individuals should empty induction chambers via scavenging systems, rather than opening the chamber into the room
- Consider wearing a facemask which filters organic vapours (e.g. 3M 7500 series half facepiece respirator with 6001 organic vapour chemical cartridges)
- Monitor concentrations of inhalant anaesthetics using exposure badges (see Chapter 5) to make sure that concentrations do not exceed COSHH/NIOSH guidelines
- In the recovery room it is important to leave the patient attached to the breathing system (with scavenging) after the vaporizer is turned off to scavenge as much exhaled agent as possible
- Avoid the use of N_2O unless scavenging is excellent. Chronic exposure to trace amounts of N_2O may be, although not proven, more serious to the unborn child than volatile agents. Note that activated charcoal scavengers do not adsorb N_2O, only volatile agents.

Summary

Overall, the use of inhalants contributes to safe and effective anaesthesia, but requires a good understanding of the agents and the equipment required. The author would also suggest that an inhalant used by itself, with no premedication or analgesics, is *not* necessarily the safest way to anaesthetize patients; the use of a more balanced technique (e.g. concurrent use of premedication and analgesics such as opioids, epidural anaesthesia or local techniques to provide analgesia) is recommended.

References and further reading

Burm AG (2003) Occupational hazards of inhalational anaesthetics. *Best Practice and Research. Clinical Anaesthesiology* **17**,147–161

Cornick-Seahorn J, Cuvelliez S, Gaynor J, McGrath C and Hartsfield S. (1996) Commentary and recommendations on control of waste anesthetic gases in the workplace. *Journal of the American Veterinary Medical Association* **209**, 75–77

Criado A, de Segura A, Tendillo F and Marsico F (2000) Reduction of isoflurane MAC with buprenorphine and morphine in rats. *Laboratory Animals* **34**, 252–259

Eger EI (1974) *Anesthetic Uptake and Action.* Williams and Wilkins Co, Baltimore

Ehrenwerth J (1993) Anesthesia vaporizers. In: *Anesthesia Equipment: Principles and Applications*, ed. J Ehrenwerth and JB Eisenkraft, pp. 57–88. Mosby Inc, St. Louis

Galloway D, Ko J, Reaugh H *et al.* (2004) Anesthetic indices of sevoflurane and isoflurane in unpremedicated dogs. *Journal of the American Veterinary Medical Association* **225**, 700–704

Golder F, Pascoe P, Bailery C, Ilkiw J and Tripp L (1998) The effect of epidural morphine on the minimum alveolar concentration of isoflurane in cats. *Journal of Veterinary Anaesthesia* **25**, 52–56

Hellyer P, Mama K, Shafford H, Wagner A and Kollias-Baker C (2001) Effects of diazepam and flumazenil on minimum alveolar concentrations for dogs anesthetized with isoflurane or a combination of isoflurane and fentanyl. *American Journal of Veterinary Research* **62**, 555–560

Ilkiw J, Pascoe P and Tripp L (2002) Effects of morphine, butorphanol, buprenorphine, and U50488H on the minimum alveolar concentration of isoflurane in cats. *American Journal of Veterinary Research* **63**, 1198–1202

Jeong SM and Nam TC (2003) Effect of electroacupuncture on minimum alveolar concentration of isoflurane in dogs. *Journal of Veterinary Medical Science* **65**, 145–147

Jones N, Clarke K and Clegg P (1995) Desflurane in equine anaesthesia: a preliminary trial. *Veterinary Record* **137**, 618–620

Muir W, Wiese A and March P (2003) Effects of morphine, lidocaine, ketamine, and morphine-lidocaine-ketamine drug combinations on minimum alveolar concentration in dogs anesthetized with isoflurane. *American Journal of Veterinary Research* **64**, 1155–1160

Mutoh T, Nishimura R and Sasaki N (2001) Effects of nitrous oxide on mask induction of anesthesia with sevoflurane or isoflurane in dogs. *American Journal of Veterinary Research* **62**, 1727–1733

Pascoe P, Ilkiw J, Craig C, Kollias-Baker C (2005) The effects of ketamine on the minimum alveolar concentration of isoflurane in cats. *Proceedings of the 30th Annual Meeting. American College of Veterinary Anesthesiologists*, Atlanta, GA, p. 77

Pypendop B and Ilkiw J (2005) Assessment of the hemodynamic effects of lidocaine administered IV in isoflurane-anesthetized cats. *American Journal of Veterinary Research* **66**, 661–668

Pypendop B, Ilkiw J, Imai A and Bolich J (2003) Hemodynamic effects of nitrous oxide in isoflurane-anesthetized cats. *American Journal of Veterinary Research* **64**, 273–278

Sawyer D (1982) The anesthetic period. In: *The Practice of Small Animal Anesthesia*, ed. D. Sawyer, pp. 45–120. WB Saunders Co, Philadelphia

Valverde A, Doherty T, Hernandez J and Davies W (2004) Effect of lidocaine on the minimum alveolar concentration of isoflurane in dogs. *Veterinary Anaesthesia and Analgesia* **31**, 264–271

Yackey M, Ilkiw J, Pascoe P and Tripp L (2004) Effect of transdermally administered fentanyl on the minimum alveolar concentration of isoflurane in cats. *Veterinary Anaesthesia and Analgesia* **31**, 183–189

15

Muscle relaxants

Derek Flaherty and Adam Auckburally

Introduction

Many drugs used for induction or maintenance of anaesthesia provide a degree of muscle relaxation, but in general this is only mild to moderate at conventional anaesthetic 'depths'. More profound muscle relaxation can be achieved in several ways:

- Provision of 'deep' anaesthesia. Although muscle relaxation will improve with increasing depth of anaesthesia, this is not recommended because of the associated increase in cardiopulmonary depression
- Local anaesthetic techniques. By paralysing the motor fibres responsible for maintenance of muscle tone, the use of local anaesthetics can provide profound muscle relaxation (see Chapter 10). However, local anaesthesia may not be applicable or achievable in all cases, and there is a steep learning curve associated with some of the commonly performed regional nerve blocks
- Centrally acting muscle relaxants. Benzodiazepines and alpha-2 adrenoceptor agonists both provide moderate to good muscle relaxation. However, because these agents achieve this through a centrally mediated action, they also have numerous other effects, many of which may be undesirable (see Chapter 12)
- Peripherally acting muscle relaxants. These are neuromuscular-blocking agents (NMBAs) that act at the neuromuscular junction (NMJ) to provide profound muscle relaxation ('paralysis') throughout the body. Although other agents can be considered as muscle relaxants due to the relaxation produced through their central effects (see above), in general the term 'muscle relaxant' is used specifically for NMBAs, and these form the focus of this chapter.

Microanatomy of the neuromuscular junction and physiology of normal neuromuscular transmission

An understanding of normal neuromuscular transmission is essential for appropriate use of muscle relaxant drugs.

Skeletal muscle cells are innervated by myelinated nerve branches of a motor neuron. As the nerve approaches the muscle cell, it loses its myelin sheath, and the region of contact between the nerve and muscle is known as the motor end-plate (Figure 15.1). Here, the muscle membrane becomes folded, and is separated from the nerve terminal by a distance of approximately 20 nm: this separation is known as the junctional (or synaptic) cleft. Within the nerve terminal are abundant vesicles containing the neurotransmitter acetylcholine (ACh), while on the crests of the folded muscle membrane lie postjunctional nicotinic ACh receptors.

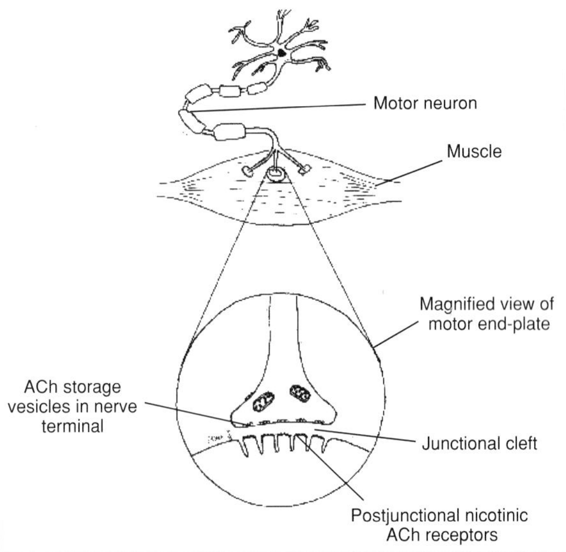

15.1 Microanatomy of the neuromuscular junction.

When an action potential reaches the nerve terminal, ACh storage vesicles fuse to the prejunctional membrane and release ACh into the junctional cleft by exocytosis. ACh then diffuses across the cleft to bind to the postjunctional receptors. The receptors comprise a pentameric protein structure, which, when stimulated, undergoes a conformational change, creating a transmembrane channel that allows movement of ions across the membrane. Two ACh molecules, binding to two distinct subunits of the pentameric structure, are required to activate opening of the ion channel. If one subunit remains unbound, or is occupied by another molecule, channel opening will not occur. The movement of ions generates an end-plate potential, and if enough ion channels are opened, the adjacent muscle membrane is depolarized and generates an action potential. Within the muscle membrane, this action potential traverses the T-tubule system and causes release of calcium ions from the sarcoplasmic reticulum, initiating excitation–contraction coupling and subsequent muscle contraction (Figure 15.2).

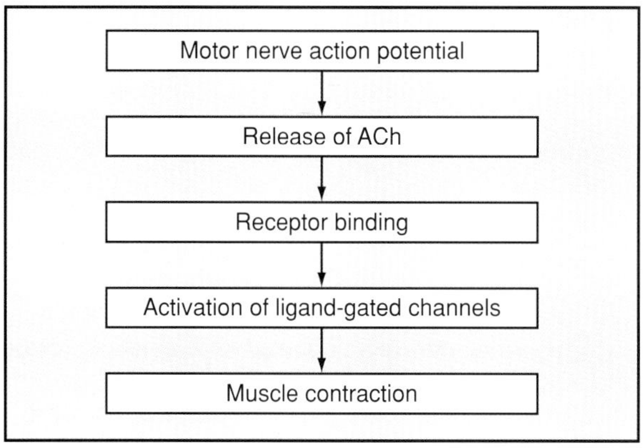

15.2 Summary of events leading to normal muscle contraction.

ACh remains bound to the postjunctional receptors for approximately 2 milliseconds, detaches, and is then rapidly hydrolysed into choline and acetate by the enzyme acetylcholinesterase, present in the junctional cleft. This terminates the action of ACh on the postjunctional nicotinic receptors, the transmembrane channel closes and muscle contraction terminates.

At physiological frequencies of nerve stimulation, neuromuscular transmission begins to fail only after a minimum of 75% of the postsynaptic ACh receptors have been blocked, with complete failure of transmission occurring with greater than 90% receptor blockade. This so-called neuromuscular 'margin of safety' implies that only 25% of ACh receptors need to be stimulated to induce normal neuromuscular transmission. The major implication from this is that during recovery from NMBAs, up to 75% of ACh receptors may still be blocked, with the patient exhibiting no detectable clinical signs, but with a reduced margin of safety.

Mechanism of action of muscle relaxants

Based on differences in their mechanisms of action, NMBAs can be classified as either depolarizing (non-competitive) or non-depolarizing (competitive).

The only depolarizing relaxant used clinically is suxamethonium (succinylcholine), which comprises two molecules of ACh joined together. Because of this structure, administration of suxamethonium causes the generation of an action potential through binding to postsynaptic ACh receptors. However, since suxamethonium is not metabolized by acetylcholinesterase, the drug remains bound to the receptors for a longer period of time, until blood concentration has declined sufficiently for the drug to diffuse down its concentration gradient from the neuromuscular junction into the plasma, allowing restoration of normal neuromuscular transmission. Plasma degradation of suxamethonium is mediated through the enzyme pseudocholinesterase (plasma cholinesterase), which is distinct from acetylcholinesterase. The prolonged binding of suxamethonium to the ACh receptor prevents normal neuromuscular transmission. The resultant clinical effect is one of initial muscle stimulation – due to the initial action potential (and manifested as widespread transient muscle fasciculations throughout the body) – followed by a longer period of muscle flaccidity. This normal pattern of suxamethonium-induced blockade is known as phase I block (phase II block is described later).

Non-depolarizing relaxants have a different chemical structure to that of suxamethonium, and although they also bind to the postsynaptic ACh receptors, they do not induce channel opening and consequent generation of an action potential. By preventing ACh reaching the receptors, they induce a competitive blockade, resulting in muscle paralysis. Thus, unlike suxamethonium, non-depolarizing relaxants do not produce initial muscle fasciculations prior to onset of muscle relaxation. Both subunit binding sites within the pentameric receptor structure do not need to be occupied by a non-depolarizing NMBA to produce paralysis; only one site can be occupied and the ion channel will still remain closed, even with one site occupied by an ACh molecule.

It is important to emphasize that muscle relaxant drugs are neither anaesthetic nor analgesic. It is therefore possible that if these agents are used inappropriately, a patient may be paralysed but fully conscious. This must be avoided at all costs by closely monitoring the adequacy of anaesthesia (see later).

Pattern of neuromuscular blockade

Because NMBAs paralyse all skeletal muscles within the body (including the respiratory musculature), it is essential that facilities for controlled ventilation are available whenever these drugs are used. Not all muscles are equally sensitive to relaxants, with the diaphragm in particular being relatively resistant: this is usually the last muscle to become paralysed, and the first to recover following administration of a relaxant. However, the musculature of the pharyngeal/laryngeal area is much more sensitive to the effects of NMBAs, and takes longer to return to normal function. Clinically, patients may appear to be ventilating adequately during recovery from a muscle relaxant, but may still succumb to upper airway obstruction once the endotracheal tube is removed. Because the diaphragm and intercostal muscles are less sensitive to NMBAs than other skeletal muscles in the body, attempts have been made to produce muscle relaxation without interference with respiratory function. An example is relaxation of the extraocular muscles (for intraocular surgery) by utilizing low doses of relaxant, while still maintaining spontaneous ventilation. This technique avoids the necessity for either a person devoted to manual ventilation of the lungs, or an expensive ventilator. Although some authorities have claimed success with this practice, it involves considerable risk of hypoventilation, and, in these authors' opinions, should be avoided. As inspired oxygen concentration is often at 100%, patients may be able to maintain oxygenation under these circumstances, but are often hypercapnic.

Monitoring the neuromuscular junction

Use of muscle relaxants should always be accompanied by assessment of the degree of neuromuscular blockade. This is most commonly performed by using a peripheral nerve stimulator (Figure 15.3a). This device delivers a small electrical current through a pair of electrodes attached to the skin overlying a peripheral nerve. The ulnar nerve on the medial aspect of the elbow (Figure 15.3b), the peroneal nerve at the lateral cranial tibia (Figure 15.3c), or the facial nerve on the lateral aspect of the face (Figure 15.3d) are most often used. The electrodes may be attached directly to the skin, or to subcutaneously placed needles. The response of the muscle groups innervated by these nerves is observed when the nerve stimulator is activated. It is important that the electrodes are attached over the nerve rather than the muscle body itself, otherwise direct electrical stimulation of the muscle may occur, resulting in a muscle response even in the presence of complete neuromuscular blockade. Although techniques such as mechanomyography and electromyography are commonly used to assess the muscle response for research purposes, they are too complex to be used clinically, and the veterinary surgeon has to rely on visual and tactile assessment of the evoked muscle response.

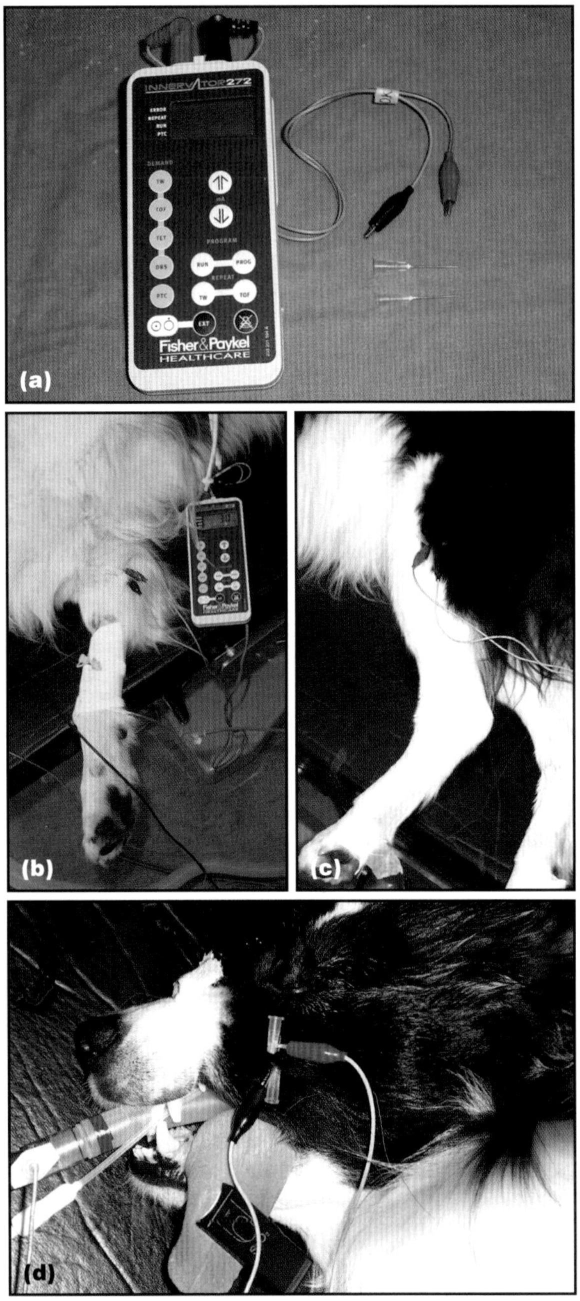

15.3 **(a)** Peripheral nerve stimulator with needle electrodes. **(b)** Placement of needle electrodes over the ulnar nerve on the medial aspect of the elbow. **(c)** Stimulation of the peroneal nerve can be achieved by electrode placement over the lateral head of the fibula. **(d)** Needle electrodes placed over the facial nerve as it exits the infraorbital foramen.

The nerve stimulator should be capable of producing a square wave pulse, with a current of at least 50 mA over a 1000 Ω load. The stimulus applied should be supramaximal to recruit all the nerve fibres: in the clinical setting, a supramaximal stimulus is usually achieved by increasing the nerve stimulator to the maximum current output.

Several different stimulation patterns are used to assess neuromuscular blockade.

Stimulation patterns

Single twitch

The single twitch is a stimulation pattern utilizing a single electrical pulse delivered at a rate between 1/sec and 1 per 10 seconds (1 Hz to 0.1 Hz). This pattern is principally used to assess onset of neuromuscular blockade, and has limited use in clinical anaesthesia.

Train-of-four

This is the commonest pattern of nerve stimulation used for assessing neuromuscular function. Four electrical pulses are applied to the nerve over a 2-second period (i.e. 2 Hz). In the absence of neuromuscular-blocking agents, four distinct muscle twitches will occur (T_1, T_2, T_3 and T_4), each of which are of identical strength (Figure 15.4a). If a non-depolarizing relaxant is then administered, the fourth twitch (T_4) in the train-of-four (TOF) will become weaker and eventually disappear, followed by the third twitch (T_3), then the second (T_2) and eventually the first (T_1) if sufficient relaxant is given (Figure 15.4bc). This phenomenon of a gradually decreasing muscle response to nerve stimulation during non-depolarizing NMBA-induced relaxation is known as *fade* (Figure 15.4b). Fade is thought to be due to a prejunctional effect of relaxants reducing the availability of ACh for release during nerve stimulation.

Since depolarizing relaxants only act postsynaptically, fade is observed solely with non-depolarizing agents, or in the presence of abnormal (phase II) suxamethonium blockade (see later). Although the TOF response to phase I suxamethonium blockade does not exhibit fade, all four twitches are reduced to an equal extent. With onset of non-depolarizing neuromuscular blockade, T_4 disappears when approximately 75% of ACh receptors are blocked; T_3 with approximately 80% blocked; T_2 with around 90% blocked; and loss of T_1 indicates essentially 100% blockade.

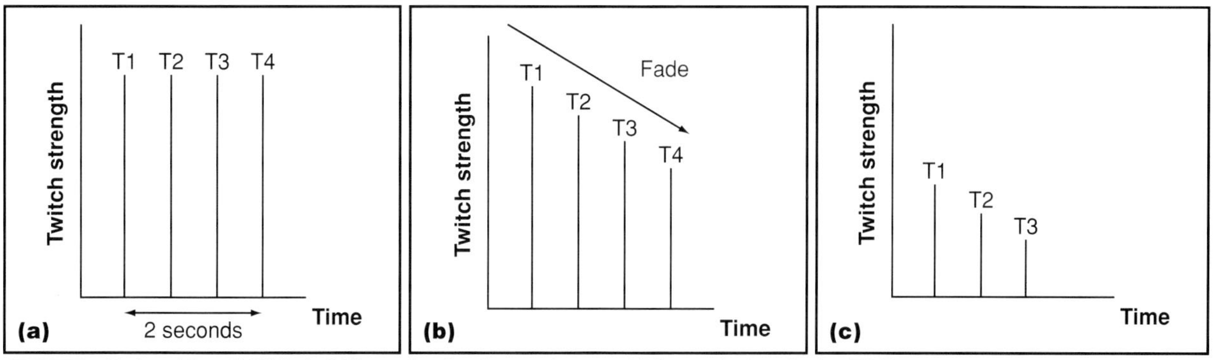

15.4 Train-of-four (TOF). **(a)** Normal animal, no relaxant. All four twitches in the TOF are present and of equal strength. **(b)** Onset of non-depolarizing blockade. Fade is present in TOF but all twitches are still visible. **(c)** Neuromuscular blockade is now more profound; the fourth twitch in the TOF has now disappeared and the remaining three twitches are weaker.

During recovery, the twitches reappear in reverse order (i.e. T_1 first). In addition to counting the number of muscle twitches in response to TOF (the 'TOF count') as a means of assessing the degree of neuromuscular blockade, attempts have been made (using mechanomyography in the research setting) to establish a TOF ratio (height of T_4/height of T_1) which is consistent with recovery of neuromuscular function to a degree that allows the patient adequate muscle strength for control of the airway. A TOF ratio of at least 0.9 in humans is considered optimal prior to endotracheal extubation.

It has been demonstrated in a number of studies that visual and tactile assessment of the TOF ratio is only able to detect fade when the TOF ratio is <0.4, implying that a significant degree of neuromuscular blockade may be missed by an observer in the clinical setting. This poor sensitivity of TOF in detecting residual neuromuscular blockade is probably related to the difficulty in comparing the strength of T_4 and T_1, while ignoring the two muscle twitches in between. TOF is used to assess both intraoperative muscle relaxation and recovery.

Tetanic stimulation

Tetanic stimulation ('tetanus') is defined as a sustained electrical stimulus of 50 Hz (occasionally 100 Hz) for a 5-second period. Because of the high frequency of stimulation, the muscle is unable to respond by producing 50 individual muscle contractions per second, and instead summates to produce one sustained muscle contraction. This pattern of stimulation is painful in the awake and minimally anaesthetized patient, but stresses the NMJ sufficiently that neuromuscular blockade can be detected by fade. Similar to TOF, tetanic fade can only be detected when significant degrees of neuromuscular blockade are present; the absence of obvious fade by visual and tactile assessment is not an indication of adequate neuromuscular transmission. Tetanic stimulation is principally used to assess recovery from neuromuscular blockade.

Double-burst stimulation

Double-burst stimulation (DBS) (Figure 15.5) comprises three short pulses at 50 Hz, a 750 millisecond pause followed by either three further 50 Hz pulses ($DBS_{3,3}$) or two 50 Hz pulses ($DBS_{3,2}$). The resultant muscle response is characterized by two individual muscle twitches (D_1 and D_2), which are stronger than those produced by TOF. The ratio of D_2:D_1 in DBS correlates closely with the TOF ratio T_4:T_1. However, it is easier to detect fade with DBS than TOF, since one is only comparing the strength of D_2 to D_1 in DBS, but T_4 to T_1 in TOF, whilst attempting to ignore T_2 and T_3. Visual and tactile assessment of DBS can detect fade at equivalent TOF ratios <0.6. Thus, although DBS may appear superior to TOF for detection of residual neuromuscular blockade, it does not completely rule out the presence of residual paralysis, since a TOF ratio >0.9 is required to ensure adequate neuromuscular recovery. DBS is used to assess recovery from neuromuscular blockade when there is no apparent fade to TOF (Figure 15.6).

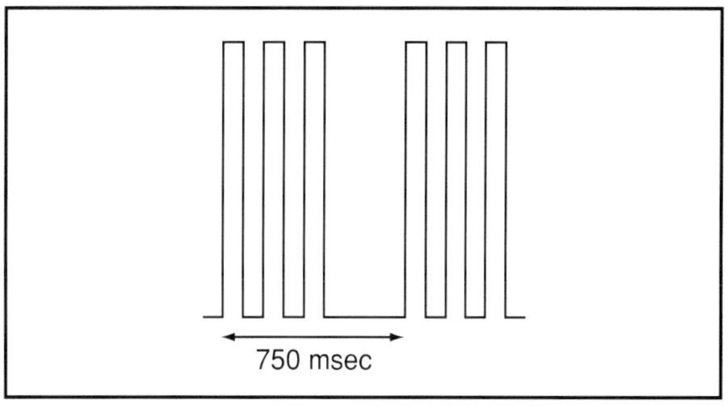

15.5 Double-burst stimulation ($DBS_{3,3}$). Each burst comprises three stimuli of 0.2 milliseconds duration with 20 milliseconds between each stimulus, the second burst following 750 milliseconds after the first. In the absence of neuromuscular blockade, this produces two distinct muscle twitches.

Pattern of nerve stimulation	Main use
Single twitch	Assessing onset of blockade
TOF	Assessing depth of block Assessing recovery from block
Tetanus	Assessing depth of block Assessing recovery from block
DBS	Assessing recovery from block

15.6 Main use of different peripheral nerve stimulation patterns. TOF is the most effective means of assessing depth of neuromuscular blockade. DBS is the most effective means of assessing recovery from neuromuscular blockade (i.e. the most reliable detector of fade).

Use of peripheral nerve stimulation

It is important to emphasize that peripheral nerve stimulation provides an indication *only* of the degree of neuromuscular blockade present – it gives no information on adequacy of anaesthesia. Therefore, a patient may have no response to nerve stimulation, but still be fully conscious.

Peripheral nerve stimulation serves two useful purposes. Firstly, it has been shown that ideal muscle relaxation for abdominal surgery is achieved when only one or two twitches remain in the TOF (80–90% of receptors blocked). This allows the veterinary surgeon to titrate the dose of neuromuscular-blocking drug to achieve suitable surgical conditions. Secondly, at the end of surgery, it permits an assessment of residual neuromuscular blockade. The TOF should have recovered to four equal-strength twitches again, with no fade detectable on DBS, before the animal is allowed to awaken and the endotracheal tube removed. It is important to recognize that, because individual muscle groups have differing sensitivities to relaxants, monitoring the response to ulnar nerve stimulation, for instance, gives limited information on the muscles of respiratory function. Consequently, even with apparently adequate recovery on nerve stimulation, the patient must be closely observed in recovery to ensure adequate airway control and ventilation.

Clinical assessment of recovery from muscle relaxants

Because none of the patterns of peripheral nerve stimulation described above can reliably assure adequate recovery of neuromuscular function (TOF ratio >0.9), clinical assessment of return of muscle strength should always be used in conjunction with nerve stimulation. Since the most serious consequence of residual paralysis (curarization) is inadequate ventilation and/or loss of airway control, many of these clinical tests of recovery have focused on assessing tidal volume or minute ventilation. However, diaphragmatic and intercostal muscle activity may have returned to normal even in the presence of significant degrees of weakness in other muscle groups, since the former are relatively resistant to the effects of NMBAs. Consequently, patients may have an entirely normal tidal volume, but have limited control of the upper airway musculature, and may be unable to maintain airway patency once extubated. Thus, the presence of a normal tidal volume during recovery from NMBAs gives very little information about the degree of residual curarization. Similarly, a normal end-tidal carbon dioxide value on capnography gives no indication of adequacy of upper airway muscle strength.

Other tests used in humans, such as assessment of vital capacity and maximum negative inspiratory pressure, are more difficult to utilize or interpret in animals. The ability to sustain a head lift for 5 seconds has been shown to correlate well with return of pharyngeal muscle strength in humans, and can probably be similarly interpreted in animals.

Monitoring adequacy of anaesthesia

Although some studies have suggested that anaesthetic requirements may be reduced by the administration of muscle relaxants (presumably through a reduction in afferent input to the CNS as a result of the loss of normal muscle tone), this is controversial. The animal must always be closely observed for signs of inadequate anaesthesia.

It is more difficult to assess the depth of anaesthesia in patients that have received NMBAs, since many of the signs and responses commonly monitored during 'conventional' anaesthesia will be absent or modified. For instance, while the eye will normally rotate ventrally at surgical planes of anaesthesia in the dog and cat, neuromuscular blockade of the extraocular muscles will cause the globe to remain centrally positioned. Similarly, although the presence or absence of the palpebral reflex is often used to quantify depth of anaesthesia, paralysis of the periocular muscles will obliterate this response, and no blinking will occur when the eyelids are stimulated. Paralysis of the respiratory musculature will also prevent any alteration in ventilatory pattern, regardless of whether the depth of anaesthesia is appropriate for the procedure being performed (bearing in mind that animals given NMBAs should be receiving intermittent positive pressure ventilation (IPPV) anyway). It goes without saying that the most classical sign of inadequate anaesthesia, gross movement, is impossible when muscle relaxants have been administered.

Assessment of anaesthetic depth in patients that have received NMBAs does, therefore, present some challenges, but alterations in sympathetic nervous system activity will usually provide a useful guide to the adequacy (or otherwise) of anaesthesia. In general, patients that are too lightly anaesthetized will be tachycardic and hypertensive, although some may demonstrate a form of vasovagal response, and become bradycardic and hypotensive. However, the latter appears to be much less common than the classical tachycardia/hypertension pattern. In addition, they may salivate excessively, demonstrate increased tear production and dilation of the pupils. End-tidal carbon dioxide values may also rise on the capnograph, and isolated muscle twitching may occur, particularly on the extremities, tongue or commissures of the mouth (Figure 15.7). This muscle twitching can occur even in patients who appear totally paralysed with TOF nerve stimulation, and although various theories have been proposed as to how this apparent anomaly may be possible, there is currently no universally accepted explanation.

Increase in pulse rate
Increase in arterial blood pressure
Salivation
Lacrimation
Increase in end-tidal carbon dioxide on capnograph
Muscle twitching, especially around head

15.7 Signs of inadequate anaesthesia during muscle relaxant use.

Patients that have received NMBAs and are excessively anaesthetized are likely to be hypotensive, and possibly bradycardic. Although it is potentially more difficult to detect excessive anaesthetic depth than it is to identify inadequate anaesthesia, every effort should be directed to ensuring the adequacy of anaesthesia in patients receiving NMBAs, since it is clearly unacceptable to have a patient aware but paralysed.

It is important to reiterate that monitoring of neuromuscular transmission with a peripheral nerve stimulator gives no information whatsoever on anaesthetic depth.

Indications for the use of muscle relaxants

Deep surgical dissection

Muscle relaxants are extremely useful to relax the abdominal musculature, particularly for dissection deep within the abdomen, e.g. nephrectomy and adrenalectomy. However, they will improve surgical conditions even for routine procedures, such as ovariohysterectomy. They are also of value during spinal surgery (e.g. laminectomies) in heavily muscled individuals.

Thoracic surgery

See Chapter 21. IPPV is mandatory during intrathoracic surgery. Although not required in every case, the use of muscle relaxants allows the veterinary surgeon a smooth 'take-over' of the patient's ventilation.

Dislocations and fractures

Muscle relaxants facilitate the replacement of dislocated joints. Although controversial, they may in addition also improve conditions during fracture reduction, especially in larger individuals: this depends on the degree of muscle fibrosis that has resulted from the initial trauma.

Intraocular procedures

See Chapter 17. By relaxing the extraocular muscles, NMBAs will produce a centrally positioned eye, which protrudes slightly. This facilitates intraocular surgery. In addition, paralysis of the respiratory musculature means that the patient can neither cough nor fight imposed ventilation, both of which would be detrimental: increased intrathoracic pressures significantly increase intraocular pressure. Muscle relaxants have no direct effect on pupillary size in dogs or cats because the iris is composed of smooth muscle, but they will cause pupillary dilation in birds, where the ciliary muscle is striated.

Endotracheal intubation

Because of the sensitivity of the feline larynx, it is routine practice to utilize local anaesthetic spray prior to attempting endotracheal intubation: this helps to avoid the development of laryngospasm. However, this technique imposes a time delay between induction of anaesthesia and establishment of a secure airway, because the local anaesthetic requires approximately 60 seconds to achieve its peak effect. While this is usually well tolerated in healthy cats, those with respiratory impairment (e.g. diaphragmatic rupture) may become severely hypoxaemic during this period.

Fortunately, relaxation of the larynx may also be achieved through the use of muscle relaxants. Although any NMBA may be used for this purpose, suxamethonium is the one most commonly chosen, because it has the fastest onset time of any muscle relaxant. Administration of suxamethonium immediately following the anaesthetic induction agent allows endotracheal intubation in a significantly shorter time than when local anaesthesia is used to desensitize the larynx. *This is the only situation where relaxants are administered prior to securing an airway by endotracheal intubation.*

Individual agents

Muscle relaxants are only administered once a patent airway has been established by endotracheal intubation (with the exception of suxamethonium for rapid intubation in cats as described above), a stable plane of anaesthesia has been achieved and facilities for controlled ventilation are immediately available. In addition, secure intravenous access should be available throughout the procedure because all muscle relaxants and antagonists are administered by this route.

Although many agents have been used to produce neuromuscular blockade over the years, only those currently used clinically will be considered here.

Depolarizing relaxants

Suxamethonium

Suxamethonium (succinylcholine) is the only depolarizing agent currently in use. It has the fastest onset time of any relaxant, and is generally relatively short acting. However, repeated or high doses can lead to a phase II block (as opposed to the phase I block usually produced), where the neuromuscular blockade assumes some characteristics of a nondepolarizing block and becomes relatively long acting. Phase II block can be detected by TOF monitoring because 'fade' develops, a characteristic not normally associated with suxamethonium-induced (phase I) blockade. Phase II block can develop in dogs following even a single dose of the drug, so it is seldom used in this species.

Suxamethonium has a number of other side effects which limit its usefulness. In particular, cardiovascular effects can be marked, with either bradycardia or tachycardia occurring, as well as arterial hypertension. Cardiac arrhythmias may also be seen. Because of the initial muscle fasciculations produced, suxamethonium is thought to cause actual muscle damage, and an increase in plasma potassium concentrations may be observed. This increase may be clinically significant in patients with pre-existing hyperkalaemia, e.g. cats with urinary obstruction. Suxamethonium can also increase intraocular pressure through sustained contraction of extraocular muscles, and can trigger malignant hyperthermia in the rare susceptible patient.

Since incremental doses of suxamethonium may induce a phase II block, the drug should only be administered as a single dose. No antagonist agent is available, and the duration of action is principally dictated by plasma cholinesterase levels, which vary widely between patients. As a result of these two factors, suxamethonium has limited use in veterinary anaesthesia, with the main indication being facilitation of endotracheal intubation in cats.

Dose:

- Dogs: 0.3 mg/kg i.v. provides approximately 25 minutes of relaxation. Not recommended (see above).
- Cats: 3–5 mg i.v. total dose for an adult cat provides approximately 5 minutes of relaxation.

Non-depolarizing relaxants

Non-depolarizing relaxants can be classified as either benzylisoquinoline (curariform) derivatives or aminosteroids, based on their chemical structure. With all these agents, potency is inversely related to onset time, i.e. the more potent the agent, the slower its onset. Increments may be given as required, using approximately one quarter to one third of the initial dose, and their effects can be antagonized with anticholinesterases (see below). Therefore, they offer much greater flexibility of use than suxamethonium. It is important to emphasize that the doses provided below for each drug are guides only, since patients vary widely in their requirements; use of a peripheral nerve stimulator is the only accurate method of determining the necessary dose and the need for additional increments.

Benzylisoquinolines

Atracurium: Atracurium is metabolized in the body both by non-specific esterases and by Hofmann degradation (a spontaneous breakdown at physiological pH and temperature), with <10% of the drug excreted unchanged by the liver and kidneys. Because of this unique method of metabolism, the action of atracurium is independent of renal and hepatic function, and it is generally the relaxant of choice for patients with hepatopathy or nephropathy. Laudanosine, one of the metabolites of atracurium, has been associated with precipitation of seizures; this is unlikely to occur in the clinical setting unless the animal has received massive doses of atracurium and additionally has hepatic impairment, because laudanosine is metabolized by the liver. Although atracurium has the potential to release histamine (particularly with high doses given rapidly), this appears to be uncommon in animals. However, the drug is probably best avoided in patients where histamine release may be detrimental, e.g. asthmatics.

Dose: In dogs and cats 0.25–0.5 mg/kg i.v. provides approximately 30–40 minutes of relaxation. The drug is also suitable for infusion: an initial bolus of 0.25 mg/kg being followed by an infusion of 0.4–0.5 mg/kg/h, started immediately after the bolus dose. The infusion should be prepared in 0.9% NaCl or 5% dextrose to minimize Hofmann degradation.

Cis*-atracurium:* *Cis*-atracurium is one of 10 stereoisomers of atracurium. It is metabolized in a similar way by Hofmann degradation, but non-specific esterases do not appear to play a part in its elimination. *Cis*-atracurium is more potent than atracurium, and has a reduced propensity to release histamine. Because of the greater potency, less *cis*-atracurium is required to produce an equivalent degree of neuromuscular blockade and consequently, less laudanosine is produced in comparison with atracurium.

Since histamine release is uncommon in animals following atracurium administration, and since the clinical significance of laudanosine production is limited, the precise advantages of *cis*-atracurium in veterinary anaesthesia are unclear. It may be the relaxant of choice in patients who are at risk from histamine release, and additionally have concurrent hepatic disease. The effects of *cis*-atracurium appear to be fairly unpredictable in animals.

Dose:

- Dogs: 0.15 mg/kg i.v. provides approximately 30 minutes of relaxation. Infusion rates of approximately 0.2–0.45 mg/kg/h following the initial bolus dose have also been used successfully.
- Cats: there are no published reports of the clinical use of *cis*-atracurium in cats.

Mivacurium: Mivacurium is unique amongst non-depolarizing relaxants in that it is metabolized by plasma cholinesterase at a rate of approximately 70–88% that of suxamethonium (in humans), and this produces a short duration of neuromuscular blockade. In addition (and unlike suxamethonium), mivacurium can be antagonized readily with anticholinesterases (see below). Although there is very limited information on its clinical use in animals, this agent has provided rapid onset, medium duration relaxation in cats. In dogs, however, mivacurium has a long duration of action unless administered at very low doses, although it does appear to be devoid of significant haemodynamic effects. It would seem, therefore, that mivacurium offers little benefit in animals over the more commonly used relaxants such as atracurium and vecuronium.

Dose:

- Dogs: 0.01 mg/kg, 0.02 mg/kg and 0.05 mg/kg i.v. provide relaxation for approximately 34, 65 and 151 minutes, respectively.
- Cats: 0.1 mg/kg i.v. provides approximately 25 minutes of relaxation.

Aminosteroids

Vecuronium: Vecuronium has negligible effects on the cardiovascular system, even at high doses. It undergoes only a minor degree of hepatic metabolism, and depends mainly on biliary excretion for termination of its effect. Duration of action may therefore be markedly prolonged in animals with hepatic disease. Vecuronium is supplied in a lyophilized form, which is then dissolved in water; the resultant solution is stable at room temperature for approximately 24 hours.

Dose: In dogs and cats, 0.1 mg/kg i.v. provides approximately 20–25 minutes of relaxation. Vecuronium can also be administered by intravenous infusion, an initial bolus dose of 0.1 mg/kg being followed immediately by infusion of 0.1 mg/kg/h.

Pancuronium: Pancuronium is a relatively long-acting relaxant. Although it generally has little effect on cardiovascular function, it can occasionally induce tachycardia and hypertension through a vagolytic and mild indirect sympathomimetic action.

Dose: In dogs and cats, 0.06 mg/kg provides approximately 45–60 minutes of relaxation.

Rocuronium: Rocuronium is an intermediate duration NMBA, with minimal cardiovascular side effects. It has the fastest onset of any non-depolarizing agent, being only slightly slower than suxamethonium, but this appears to be its only real advantage over other agents.

Dose:

- Dogs: 0.5 mg/kg i.v. provides approximately 30 minutes of relaxation. An infusion of 0.2 mg/kg/h started immediately after the initial bolus may be used to maintain relaxation.
- Cats: 0.6 mg/kg i.v. provides approximately 15 minutes of relaxation. There are no reports of the use of this drug by infusion in cats.

Short-acting and long-acting relaxants

It has been demonstrated in humans that shorter-acting relaxants are more easily antagonized than longer-acting ones. Therefore, for procedures where relaxation may be required for a relatively long period of time, it is now more common to administer short or intermediate duration agents, such as atracurium or vecuronium, and to provide incremental doses as required, rather than using longer-acting agents such as pancuronium.

Interactions between muscle relaxants and other drugs

A number of different agents may interact with muscle relaxants when administered concurrently:

- Volatile anaesthetic agents. These potentiate the effects of NMBAs both in terms of dose requirements and duration of action. Isoflurane appears more potent in this regard than halothane, while atracurium and vecuronium appear to be potentiated less than the longer-acting relaxants
- Injectable anaesthetic agents. At clinical doses, propofol appears to have minimal effect on the action of muscle relaxants. Ketamine potentiates all non-depolarizing relaxants in a dose-dependent manner in a primate model
- Antibiotics. Some antibiotics may prolong neuromuscular blockade by mechanisms that vary from agent to agent. Several sites at the NMJ may be affected. The most important antibiotics in this regard are the aminoglycosides, although the effect produced varies depending on the relaxant used, the concentration of the antibiotic achieved *in vivo*, and inter-patient variability. Close monitoring of the NMJ is certainly recommended if aminoglycosides and muscle relaxants are used concurrently during anaesthesia. Some authorities have suggested that administration of calcium salts may be useful to reverse any prolonged blockade that occurs when these agents are used together
- Anticonvulsants. Some anticonvulsants may shorten the duration of NMBAs, although this depends on the relaxant used and the anticonvulsant
- H_2 receptor antagonists. High-dose oral cimetidine prolongs vecuronium-induced blockade, while intravenous ranitidine has been shown to antagonize atracurium relaxation in rats, but not in humans. The clinical significance of the interaction between muscle relaxants and H_2 antagonists is unclear.

Use of muscle relaxants in the presence of concurrent disease

The presence of concurrent disease may influence the relaxant chosen, and may also require modification of the dose:

- Renal and hepatic disease. Atracurium (or *cis*-atracurium) is generally the relaxant of choice for patients with renal or hepatic disease because of the unique method of metabolism. Although renal elimination plays only a minor role in terminating the effects of vecuronium, studies in humans have demonstrated an increased duration of action in patients with renal failure
- Acid–base and electrolyte disturbances. The effects of acid–base disturbances on muscle relaxants are extremely complex and vary from agent to agent, but either potentiation or antagonism of relaxation may occur. Electrolyte disorders have similarly complex effects, but, generally, hypernatraemia and hypokalaemia will potentiate non-depolarizing agents, while hyponatraemia and hyperkalaemia will antagonize them
- Burn injuries. Patients with extensive burn injuries may develop resistance to non-depolarizing neuromuscular blockers, while administration of suxamethonium can produce severe hyperkalaemia and ventricular fibrillation
- Spinal cord injury. This may increase sensitivity to non-depolarizing agents, while administration of suxamethonium to these patients can induce hyperkalaemia
- Myasthenia gravis (MG). Patients with MG are extremely sensitive to the effects of non-depolarizing relaxants, and use of a nerve stimulator is mandatory if these agents are to be used in animals with this condition. An initial

dose of approximately one tenth of the normal dose of relaxant should be used, and small incremental doses administered as dictated by TOF monitoring.

Antagonism of neuromuscular blockade

Recovery from neuromuscular blockade may occur spontaneously, as the plasma concentration of relaxant diminishes (due to metabolism and elimination). This allows the drug to diffuse away from the NMJ, moving down its concentration gradient into the plasma. Alternatively, in the case of non-depolarizing relaxants, recovery may be hastened by administration of an anticholinesterase agent. These inhibit the effects of the enzyme acetylcholinesterase, which is responsible for the rapid degradation of ACh following its release. Consequently, anticholinesterases allow accumulation of ACh, which is then able to competitively displace the non-depolarizing relaxant from the postsynaptic ACh receptor and restore neuromuscular transmission. Anticholinesterase agents will not antagonize classic phase I suxamethonium blockade because the block induced is non-competitive (see earlier); there is some evidence, however, that they may facilitate reversal of a fully developed phase II suxamethonium block.

Anticholinesterases do not only allow a build up of ACh at the nicotinic receptors of the NMJ; ACh also accumulates at postganglionic parasympathetic muscarinic receptors throughout the body, and may produce a number of unwanted side effects, such as bradycardia and cardiac arrhythmias, bronchoconstriction and salivation. To prevent these muscarinic effects, anticholinesterases are usually administered in conjunction with antimuscarinic agents, such as atropine or glycopyrronium.

Two anticholinesterases are used clinically for antagonism of non-depolarizing induced relaxation: neostigmine and edrophonium. Neostigmine has a slow onset but long duration, whereas edrophonium has a more rapid onset but shorter duration. Atropine has rapid onset, short duration, and glycopyrronium slow onset, long duration. Therefore, the pharmacokinetic profile of atropine fits more closely with that of edrophonium, while that of glycopyrronium fits more closely with neostigmine. It is, therefore, most logical to use either an edrophonium–atropine or neostigmine–glycopyrronium combination for reversal of neuromuscular blockade. A neostigmine–glycopyrronium combination is commercially available (Robinul-Neostigmine, Anpharm). However, even though the pharmacokinetics of neostigmine–glycopyrronium and edrophonium–atropine are the most favourable, it is still not uncommon to see minor muscarinic effects when these combinations are used, particularly mild bradycardia or second-degree atrioventricular block. These effects are, however, usually transient. An edrophonium–atropine combination produces the fewest muscarinic side effects and is the combination of choice in patients where these may be detrimental, e.g. those with cardiac disease.

If a short-acting antagonist (edrophonium) is used with a long-acting relaxant (e.g. pancuronium), there is an increased risk of recurarization in the recovery period, i.e. the edrophonium may initially antagonize the blockade and restore normal neuromuscular transmission, but because edrophonium is shorter-acting than the relaxant, neuromuscular blockade may recur as edrophonium concentration at the NMJ declines. Thus, if longer-acting relaxants have been used, neostigmine is the anticholinesterase of choice. In addition, neostigmine will more reliably antagonize a more intense blockade than edrophonium. Neostigmine has, however, also been shown to possess neuromuscular-blocking capabilities, particularly if administered in high doses; consequently, the doses described below should not be exceeded.

The greater the TOF count prior to antagonism, the more likely the success in restoring neuromuscular transmission, and the less likely residual curarization or recurarization are to occur during recovery. Consequently, where time allows, it is preferable to allow restoration of all four twitches in the TOF prior to antagonism, although reversal can be achieved when only one twitch has reappeared. However, antagonism at this point will be more difficult, will require higher doses of anticholinesterase, and will also increase the risk of problems occurring in recovery. Inadequate antagonism of neuromuscular blockade at the end of anaesthesia risks residual curarization in the recovery period, which may incur serious consequences for the animal. Numerous studies in humans have demonstrated that patients commonly arrive at the recovery room with significant residual blockade still present, which is responsible for an increased incidence of complications, particularly involving the respiratory system.

Although antagonism is not always required following the use of muscle relaxants, it should certainly be considered when longer-acting NMBAs have been used, or when multiple boluses or infusions of these agents have been delivered. If in doubt as to the state of neuromuscular recovery, it is wise to err on the side of caution and administer an anticholinesterase.

Administration of anticholinesterases

Neostigmine and glycopyrronium are usually mixed in a ratio of 5:1 (2.5 mg neostigmine + 500 μg glycopyrronium/ml in the commercial preparation), with a total dose requirement of 0.01–0.1 mg/kg i.v. neostigmine, depending on the degree of blockade at the time of antagonism.

Edrophonium and atropine are usually mixed in a 25:1 ratio (1 mg/kg edrophonium + 40 μg/kg atropine) and given slowly intravenously to effect over several minutes.

In preference to mixing the antimuscarinic and anticholinesterase in the same syringe, some anaesthetists administer the antimuscarinic 1–2 minutes prior to the anticholinesterase to lessen the risk of muscarinic side effects occurring. However, cardiac instability may also occur with this approach because the antimuscarinic generally induces a transient tachycardia before the heart rate reduces once the anticholinesterase is administered.

It is vital that ventilatory support and a depth of anaesthesia adequate to prevent awareness are maintained until antagonism of neuromuscular blockade has been achieved. Failure to restore spontaneous ventilation may occur for several reasons (Figure 15.8).

Ongoing neuromuscular blockade (in absence of a peripheral nerve stimulator):
- Inadequate antagonism
- Hepatic/renal disease
- Acid–base/electrolyte disturbance

Excessive anaesthetic depth
Hypocapnia (over-ventilation)
Hypothermia

15.8 Common causes of failure to restore spontaneous ventilation following the use of muscle relaxants.

Non-depolarizing antagonist

Recently, a novel non-depolarizing antagonist has been described. This agent, Org 25969 (Sugammadex), is a modified cyclodextrin compound that works in a completely different way to anticholinesterases. Cyclodextrins have a ring structure with a hydrophilic surface, which makes them water soluble, but with the capability to encapsulate hydrophobic molecules within their central core. Org 25969 has principally been developed as a reversal agent for rocuronium, and it appears highly effective at rapidly 'mopping up' this molecule even during profound (or following prolonged) neuromuscular blockade. Once the rocuronium becomes encapsulated in the central core of the cyclodextrin molecule, it is no longer able to act at the NMJ. Org 25969 may also have some activity against vecuronium, but apparently to a much lesser extent than against rocuronium. Since Org 25969 produces antagonism without inhibition of acetylcholinesterase, muscarinic effects do not occur, and therefore the concurrent administration of antimuscarinic drugs is unnecessary. The ability rapidly to terminate even profound rocuronium-induced blockade without potential muscarinic side effects is a major benefit of Org 25969.

References and further reading

Auer U and Mosing M (2006) A clinical study of the effects of rocuronium in isoflurane-anaesthetized cats. *Veterinary Anaesthesia and Analgesia* **33(4)**, 224–228

Clutton RE (1994) Edrophonium for neuromuscular blockade antagonism in the dog. *Veterinary Record* **134**, 674–678

Corletto F and Brearley JC (2003) Clinical use of mivacurium in the cat. *Veterinary Anaesthesia and Analgesia* **30(2)**, 93–94

Dugdale AHA, Adams WA and Jones RS (2002) The clinical use of the neuromuscular blocking agent rocuronium in dogs. *Veterinary Anaesthesia and Analgesia* **29(1)**, 49–53

Shields M, Giovannelli M, Mirakhur RK *et al.* (2006) Org 25969 (sugammadex), a selective relaxant binding agent for antagonism of prolonged rocuronium-induced neuromuscular blockade. *British Journal of Anaesthesia* **96(1)**, 36–43

Smith LJ, Moon PF, Lukasik VM and Erb HN (1999) Duration of action and hemodynamic properties of mivacurium chloride in dogs anesthetized with halothane. *American Journal of Veterinary Research* **60(9)**, 1047–1050

16

Fluid therapy and blood transfusion

Paula F. Moon-Massat

General considerations

Introduction

Parenteral fluids are indicated for treatment or prevention of decreased oxygen delivery, hypotension and hypovolaemia, and electrolyte, metabolic and acid–base disorders. As a patient's physical condition deteriorates the importance of selecting the most compatible fluid increases. This chapter reviews the decision-making process for designing an appropriate fluid therapy plan for anaesthetized small animal patients.

Fluid dynamics

In emergency situations, fluids are often administered intravenously to restore vascular volume and cardiac output to levels that, at least, can sustain life until treatment is provided. Definitive fluid selection depends on matching the patient's individual needs with a fluid that has the composition and volume of distribution equivalent to the patient's deficit. Therefore, it is essential to know the composition of available solutions (Figure 16.1) and their equilibration within the fluid compartments of the patient (Figures 16.2 and 16.3). Equilibration of intravenous fluid is a balance of hydrostatic, osmotic and oncotic pressures and is also influenced by the permeability characteristics of the capillaries (Starling's law). Normal dog blood has a colloid osmotic (oncotic) pressure of 25–30 mmHg and an osmolarity of 280–310 mOsm/l. Normal vascular endothelium is permeable to small ions or electrolytes, but impermeable to large proteins. Hydrostatic pressure is rarely an important factor in determining a fluid type. Consequently, fluid osmotic and oncotic pressures are the most important criteria in patients without vascular permeability abnormalities.

Solution	COP (mmHg)	Osmolarity (mOsm/l)	pH	Na^+ (mmol/l)	Cl^- (mmol/l)	K^+ (mmol/l)	Ca^{2+} (mmol/l)	Mg^{2+} (mmol/l)	Buffer (mmol/l)
Isotonic crystalloids									
0.9% NaCl	0	308	5.0–5.7	154	154	0	0	0	0
D5W	0	252–278	4.0–6.5	0	0	0	0	0	0
Acetated Ringer's solution (Kendall-McGaw, Baxter)	0	294–310	7.4	141	98	5	0	1.5	27–29 acetate/ 23 gluconate
Lactated Ringer's solution (Baxter, Abbott, Animalcare)	0	273	6.5	130	109	4	1.5	0	28 lactate
Ringer's	0	310	5.8–6.1	147	156	4	2.25	0	0
Hypertonic crystalloids									
3% NaCl	0	1,026	5.0	513	513	0	0	0	0
7.5% NaCl	0	2,567	5.0–5.7	1,283	1,283	0	0	0	0
D5W/LRS	0	495–527	4–6	130	109	4	1.35	0	28 lactate
Iso-oncotic colloids									
3% Plasmagel	ND	310	ND	120	147	0	Some	0	Some
6% Albumin	30	310	5.5	154	154	0	0	0	0
6% Hetastarch (Du Pont, Fresenius Kabi)	30–35	310	5.5	154	154	0	0	0	0
6% Pentastarch (Du Pont Critical Care)	25	310	5.5	154	154	0	0	0	0
Haemaccel (Intervet)	25–29	ND	7.3	145	145	5.1	3.125	ND	ND

16.1 Electrolyte composition and physical properties of commonly available fluids. COP = Colloid osmotic pressure; D5W = 5% dextrose in water; HES = Hydroxyethyl starch; HS = Hypertonic saline; ND = No data. (continues) ▶

Solution	COP (mmHg)	Osmolarity (mOsm/l)	pH	Na^+ (mmol/l)	Cl^- (mmol/l)	K^+ (mmol/l)	Ca^{2+} (mmol/l)	Mg^{2+} (mmol/l)	Buffer (mmol/l)
Hyperoncotic colloids (in normal saline)									
Oxypolygelatin (Marshallton Veterinary Group)	45–47	200	7.4	145	100	0	1	0	30 carbonate
6% Dextran 70 (Baxter)	75	309	5.0	154	154	0	0	0	0
10% Dextran 40	>100	310	3.5–7.0	154	154	0	0	0	0
10% HES (Fresenius Kabi)	>100	308	Acidic	154	154	0	0	0	0
20% HES	>100	310	Acidic	154	154	0	0	0	0
Hypertonic-hyperoncotic									
7.5% NaCl-20% HES	>100	2,567	Acidic	1,283	1,283	0	0	0	0
7.5% NaCl-6% dextran 70	75	2,567	~4–5	1,283	1,283	0	0	0	0

16.1 (continued) Electrolyte composition and physical properties of commonly available fluids. COP = Colloid osmotic pressure; D5W = 5% dextrose in water; HES = Hydroxyethyl starch; HS = Hypertonic saline; ND = No data.

Fluid type	Examples	Volume needed to increase PV by one litre	Distribution	Examples of clinical indications
Colloid	Starch Gelatin Dextrans	1–1.5 litres	PV	Hypovolaemia, hypotension, normovolaemic haemodilution, hypoalbuminaemia
Hypertonic crystalloid	7.5% NaCl	300 ml	Immediate PV expansion causing ICFV reduction	Hypovolaemic shock, cerebral oedema
Hypotonic crystalloid	5% dextrose	14 litres	TBW	Free water deficit, hypernatraemia
Isotonic crystalloid	0.9% NaCl Lactated Ringer's	3–4 litres	ECFV (PV and ISFV expansion)	Dehydration, hypovolaemia, hypotension, normovolaemic haemodilution

16.2 Categories, distribution and clinical indications for commonly available fluids for intravenous fluid therapy. ECFV = Extracellular fluid volume; ICFV = Intracellular fluid volume; ISFV = Interstitial fluid volume; PV = Plasma volume; TBW = Total body water.

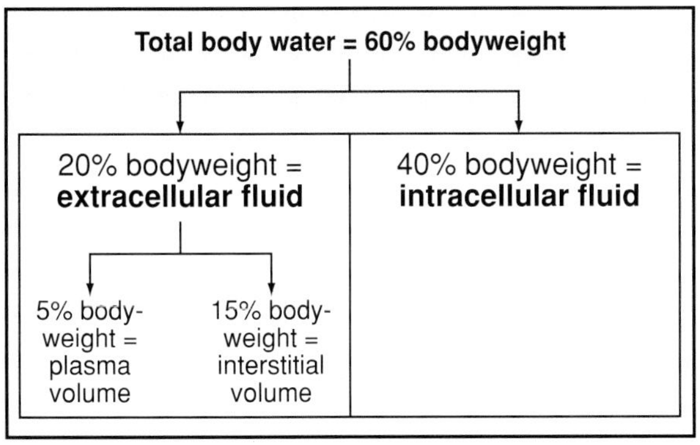

16.3 Distribution of fluid compartments. Intracellular fluid includes the fluid within red blood cells, as well as other cells. Interstitial fluid volume includes cerebrospinal and ocular fluids, and fluids in the pleural and peritoneal spaces.

Osmosis is the net movement of water across a semi-permeable membrane caused by the concentration differences of solutes across that membrane. *Osmotic pressure*, the pressure exerted by the particles within the solution, prevents the movement of water across the membrane. 'Tonicity' refers to the osmotic pressure of a fluid when compared with plasma. An 'isotonic' solution (approximately 300 mOsm/l) has the same proportion of particles and water as that found in plasma. Therefore, isotonic fluid administration produces no change in the osmotic pressure of plasma and no fluid shift between compartments. Sodium, the primary ion present in extracellular fluid, is also the main component of most electrolyte or 'crystalloid' solutions (see Figure 16.1). Sodium freely crosses capillary boundaries, taking water with it as it distributes throughout the entire extracellular fluid volume. Similarly, all isotonic electrolyte solutions will distribute themselves throughout the extracellular fluid volume.

A solution that is 'hypotonic' has fewer particles than the number present in plasma. Because the addition of a hypotonic solution decreases the plasma osmotic pressure, an osmotic pressure difference is established between intravascular and extravascular spaces. For equilibrium to be re-established, water moves out of the intravascular space (low osmotic pressure) and into the interstitial and intracellular spaces (high osmotic pressure). Conversely, when a 'hypertonic' solution is administered, water moves from the interstitial and intracellular spaces (low osmotic pressure) into the intravascular space (high osmotic pressure). The more hypertonic the solution, the larger the osmotic driving pressure and the more rapidly the water will move into and expand the plasma volume. This is the principal mechanism for the rapid plasma volume expansion after hypertonic saline administration and explains why a smaller volume of hypertonic saline causes a larger expansion of the plasma volume than an equivalent volume of isotonic saline. Eventually, the shifting water results in no pressure difference between compartments and the volume of administered electrolyte fluid redistributes evenly throughout the extracellular fluid compartment. Hence, hypertonic saline is transient in its effect.

Commercially available fluids provide the osmolarity of the fluid on the label and package insert. This information can be used to predict the degree and duration of plasma volume expansion after parenteral administration. There is one caveat to this, however, for crystalloid solutions containing glucose. Glucose molecules are unique because they only act as 'effective osmoles' initially (i.e. 5% dextrose in water is isotonic, 10% dextrose in water is hypertonic) and body water shifts as predicted based on osmotic pressures. However, through cellular transport and glucose metabolism, the tonicity of the final glucose-containing solution should be estimated assuming no glucose remains. Consequently, 5% dextrose in water, while isotonic in the container, is ultimately hypotonic in the body and should only be administered if the goal is to provide 'free water' to all fluid compartments. Such hypotonic solutions do not adequately replace standard fluid losses under conditions of anaesthesia and surgery and should not routinely be used for maintenance and volume replacement. Furthermore, they will cause intracellular and interstitial oedema more rapidly than if an isotonic fluid is used to maintain an equivalent degree of plasma volume expansion. The movement of free water into cells may either treat cellular dehydration or produce cellular oedema, depending on the situation of a given patient. Thus, it is imperative to consider the effects of a fluid's tonicity on the patient's fluid compartments.

In fluid selection, the second important property is *oncotic pressure* (*colloid osmotic pressure*, COP) and this is an extremely important component of transcapillary fluid dynamics. Oncotic pressure is the pressure exerted by large molecular weight molecules (molecular weight >30,000 Daltons) that normally do not cross the capillary membranes. Solutions containing these large molecules, either endogenous proteins (albumin) or synthetic molecules (e.g. starches), are considered 'colloid solutions'.

Normal oncotic pressure of plasma is 20–30 mmHg and, in most situations, it is assumed that plasma oncotic pressure is adequate if serum albumin is ≥25 g/l and total protein is ≥50 g/l. The contribution that plasma proteins (albumin, globulins) make to the total plasma *osmotic* pressure is small (approximately 4%) but they exert enough of a pressure difference to influence the vascular–interstitial distribution of water. It is primarily the plasma proteins that cause water to remain preferentially in the intravascular space. A normal capillary wall is relatively impermeable to such colloid molecules although the actual capillary permeability to colloids, endogenous or synthetic, depends upon the type of capillary as well as the nature of the colloid (size, shape and charge).

'Iso-oncotic' colloids have the same oncotic pressure as plasma and 'hyperoncotic' colloids have a higher oncotic pressure. Hyperoncotic fluid administration will increase plasma oncotic pressure and will draw water into the vascular compartment, similarly to hypertonic saline. However, unlike both isotonic and hypertonic crystalloids, colloid molecules cannot cross normal capillary membranes. Therefore, the plasma volume expansion after colloid fluid administration is maintained for a longer period of time than after administration of an equivalent volume of either isotonic or hypertonic crystalloid solutions.

Fluid types

Isotonic crystalloids

Isotonic crystalloids (lactated Ringer's, Isolyte) are inexpensive fluids used to expand both the vascular and the interstitial fluid compartments. They are commonly used to maintain plasma volume in anaesthetized uncomplicated patients; to replace deficits in dehydrated patients; to restore third-space losses; and to promote urinary flow. Within 30–45 minutes of administration, approximately 75–80% of the administered volume has left the intravascular compartment and redistributed primarily into the interstitial space. Therefore, the transient nature of crystalloids prevents sustained improvement in plasma volume and haemodynamic parameters unless they are administered as a continuous infusion. Large volumes of isotonic fluids, coupled with their large volume of redistribution, may promote peripheral and pulmonary oedema.

Another consideration is the acidity of the solution. The pH of common solutions varies greatly, some are acidifying, others alkalinizing, depending on whether or not buffers are added (see Figure 16.1). Chloride or lactate, the anions associated with the sodium and potassium cations in most fluids, can be used interchangeably for most patients. When there is concern for acidosis, the veterinary surgeon should select a fluid of the appropriate pH with the presence of a metabolizable buffer (acetate, gluconate or lactate).

Calcium-free solutions, such as saline (0.9% NaCl) and some commercial fluids (see Figure 16.1), can be administered simultaneously with blood products. Calcium-containing solutions, such as lactated Ringer's (Hartmann's), cannot be combined with blood products or microprecipitates may occur.

Hypertonic solutions

These rapidly expand the plasma volume, increase cardiac output and improve blood pressure. Hypertonic saline may directly increase myocardial contractility and decrease systemic vascular resistance. Hypertonic solutions also improve microcirculatory blood flow because of a reduction in endothelial cell size and a lower blood viscosity. For a more sustained effect, hypertonic crystalloids can be administered with a colloid.

Hypertonic solutions are useful in the initial treatment of hypovolaemic shock because of effective plasma volume expansion following rapid administration of a small volume. Replacement of only one quarter to one third of the lost volume of blood is needed to rapidly restore cardiovascular function compared with three to four times the lost volume necessary with isotonic crystalloids. Hypertonic solutions are a 'stop-gap' therapy and must be followed by administration of appropriate follow-up fluids (crystalloids, colloids or blood products). In addition to treatment of shock, slow infusions of hypertonic saline have been advocated for intraoperative use during cardiac surgery, to prevent tissue oedema from conventional fluid therapy. Three to five percent hypertonic saline also decreases intracranial pressure and total brain water in experimental traumatic brain injury models and may be useful in treating cerebral oedema.

Most of the adverse effects of hypertonic saline are transient but can be clinically relevant. The most important side effects are hypernatraemia, hyperchloraemia, hypokalaemia, hyperosmolarity and metabolic acidosis. For example, at the standard shock dose (4 ml/kg i.v. over 10 minutes), a hyperchloraemic metabolic acidosis can cause a transient decrease of 0.05 unit in pH that lasts approximately 10 minutes. Newer hypertonic solutions have attempted to prevent some of these side effects and both hypernatraemic–isochloraemic-acetate solutions and isonatraemic–hyperchloraemic solutions are being developed. Because of the hyperosmolarity, hypertonic saline administered through a small peripheral vein to a patient with poor perfusion may result in intravascular haemolysis and haemoglobinuria. Hypertonic saline also produces haemodilution of all blood components. Finally, ventricular arrhythmias can be observed occasionally during administration and their incidence may increase with the severity of the patient's condition.

The use of hypertonic saline in dehydrated patients or patients with ongoing, uncontrolled blood loss remains a controversial topic. With pre-existing cellular dehydration, hypertonic saline causes further decrease in cell size and it is important to administer an isotonic crystalloid promptly to replace this aggravated cellular fluid deficit. However, some evidence suggests that mild cellular dehydration does not compromise the efficacy of a single dose of hypertonic saline for treatment of hypovolaemia. Cardiovascular improvement is not sustained, however, with a second dose of hypertonic saline in these patients. In more severely dehydrated patients, mortality may actually increase with its use.

The other concern with hypertonic saline is that uncontrolled bleeding will worsen (due to the rapid increase in blood pressure) and mortality may increase. As with any fluid therapy, aggressive volume restoration to normotension can promote continued blood loss if the source of haemorrhage is not controlled. Therefore, it seems rational to provide only enough fluid to prevent tissue ischaemia and maintain life support as an initial measure. One must realize that striving for normal blood pressure in such situations may not be an appropriate end-point until bleeding has been controlled. 'Hypotensive resuscitation' (mean arterial blood pressure approximately 60 mmHg) is acceptable for short-term delays (<3 hours) until definitive treatment, regardless of the type of fluid used in initial resuscitation attempts.

Colloids

Clinical conditions of hypoalbuminaemia, blood loss, hypovolaemia, third-space fluid accumulation, sepsis and persistent hypotension are indications for colloid administration. The benefit of colloids is that they do not cross normal capillary walls and have a more sustained effect on plasma volume expansion than crystalloid solutions. Compared with plasma, synthetic colloids have a longer storage time, no risk of transmission of infectious diseases and no long-term sensitization effect. Although less expensive than plasma, they are more costly than crystalloids.

The volume of colloid administered is equal to or slightly greater than the lost volume of blood. Compared with isotonic crystalloids, this translates into less total fluid administered, less fluid distributed into extravascular spaces and less risk of peripheral oedema. However, both colloids and crystalloids have been associated with pulmonary oedema in patients with permeable capillaries. Diseased capillaries may leak both colloids and fluid into the interstitial space when 'gaps' become large enough, resulting in oedema. On the other hand, colloids that are larger than the 'gaps' may impede transport of water and small proteins through permeable capillaries. This property may have therapeutic benefit. Pentafraction (a derivative of starch for plasma substitution), in particular, may be useful in 'plugging' leaky capillaries in patients with sepsis, pulmonary dysfunction, burns and other diseases with increased capillary permeability.

Typically, colloids are categorized as a type of dextran, gelatin or starch (Figure 16.4). The plasma half-life is proportional to the size of the molecules. Molecules ≤50,000 Daltons are rapidly filtered unchanged by the kidneys while larger molecules are degraded, metabolized and excreted through renal and gastrointestinal pathways. Diseases that alter renal function or vascular permeability will alter the duration of plasma volume expansion. In addition, if high doses of smaller colloids are administered to a patient with renal dysfunction, renal tubular obstruction may occur, potentially causing acute renal failure.

Three potential disadvantages of all synthetic colloids are circulatory overload, anaphylactic reactions and coagulation disorders. Because of slow fluid redistribution, circulatory overload and haemodilution may occur if the patient is not properly monitored. As errors in fluid loading with colloids have a prolonged effect, the volume of colloid used should be carefully titrated. Central venous pressure, systemic blood pressure, capillary wedge pressure and urine output should be monitored in patients with pulmonary oedema, congestive heart failure or renal failure or other patients at risk for circulatory overload.

Historically, anaphylactic and anaphylactoid reactions have been reported in humans for all three classes of colloids and are estimated to be 0.33% overall. This incidence is small compared with the degree of reactions reported after administration of blood, penicillin, barbiturates or contrast media. The incidence in veterinary medicine is unknown although adverse reactions to dextrans have been reported in dogs (rarely) and rats (commonly). Reactions are usually immediate, even after administration of a small volume.

Colloid % solution Trade name	Albumin 5%	Polygeline 3.5%	Gelofusine	Dextran-40 10%	Dextran-70 6%	Hetastarch 6%	Pentastarch 10%	Tetrastarch 6%
Category	Protein	Gelatin		Dextran		Starch		
Substance		Polypeptide		Polysaccharide		Amylopectin (branched polysaccharide)		
Source	Blood			Bacteria		Maize or sorghum		
Mean (range) Weight ave. mol. wt (kD)	69	35 (5–50)	30	40 (15–75)	70 (20–175)	450 (10–1,000)	264 (150–350)	130
% Interstitial % Intravascular	20% 80%	50% 50%	50% 50%	0% 100%	0% 100%	0% 100%	0% 100%	0% 100%
Plasma $T_{1/2}$ (h)	>16	2–4	2–4	2–6	6–12	10–12	3–5	2–3
Total elimination		Very rapid	Very rapid	Very rapid	Rapid	Prolonged	Prolonged	
% adverse reactions (in humans, after 1980)	Fewest (0.001%)	Some (0.78%)		Few (0.2% if pretreat with dextran 1), common in rats		Extremely rare (0%)		
Coagulopathies		Rare			Reported	Reported		

16.4 Comparison of commonly available colloid solutions. The number average molecular weight of pentastarch is higher than hetastarch although the weight average molecular weight is lower, i.e. pentastarch has a narrower range of medium-weight molecules.

Therefore, initial, slow administration with careful monitoring is justified. Signs of an adverse reaction include hypotension, ischaemia, flushing, urticaria, respiratory compromise, pulmonary oedema and gastrointestinal disturbances. In a few extremely rare instances, administration of a colloid has been fatal.

Although all colloids affect coagulation, gelatins are the least detrimental, followed by starches and finally dextrans. For dextrans, the effects have been attributed to platelet coating, precipitation of coagulation factors, increased fibrinolytic activity and decreased functional von Willebrand factor. The effect on coagulation with dextrans appears to be dose-related. The manufacturer's recommended dose for 6% dextran 70 is up to 1.5 g/kg with the total dose not to exceed 20 ml/kg the first day, and half this dose on the following 2 days. Higher doses may increase blood viscosity, vascular resistance and afterload. A maximum rate of 2 ml/kg/h has not been associated with bleeding problems in people while large, rapid doses may cause haemorrhagic diathesis. There are no controlled data on the maximum safe dose for dextrans in veterinary medicine. Empirical doses of 5–10 ml/kg/h have been suggested for the treatment of hypoproteinaemia while doses from 5–15 ml/kg given as a rapid bolus, at a rate of 40–50 ml/kg/h, have been suggested for acute hypovolaemia. It has been reported that doses of 20 ml/kg, over 30 or 60 minutes, produced minimal haemostatic abnormalities in clinically normal dogs, but there were enough alterations to suggest dextrans may precipitate bleeding in dogs with marginal haemostatic function. The coagulation changes that can occur with hetastarch, although measurable, are not as pronounced. Hetastarch slightly prolongs partial thromboplastin and prothrombin bleeding times. Clotting factor VIII function is decreased 25–50%, and there is altered fibrin formation with hetastarch. Since both dextrans and starches have documented haematological effects that are due to more than simple haemodilution, one should consider avoiding them and using a gelatin or plasma in patients with coagulopathies or von Willebrand's disease, or blood products when massive blood loss is expected.

Albumin therapy

The administration of highly concentrated 25% human serum albumin (HSA) is becoming increasingly popular in veterinary medicine but with limited investigation regarding its safety and efficacy. HSA is an easily obtainable fluid that is extremely hyperoncotic (COP approximately 200 mmHg *versus* plasma approximately 25 mmHg). As described earlier, COP is important for maintaining intravascular volume and a hypertonic solution will draw extravascular fluids into the intravascular space. The slow redistribution of HSA decreases the likelihood of causing oedema and may assist in its treatment. Albumin also has other purported theoretical advantages over other synthetic colloids including, but not limited to, reducing microvascular permeability, decreasing platelet aggregation and antioxidant properties. At present, there are no commercially available species-specific albumin products. However, a study reported the use of 25% HSA in 64 dogs and 2 cats for treatment of severe hypoalbuminaemia (<15 g/l or <18 g/l, in the presence of hypovolaemia and dehydration) at a mean total dose of 5 ml/kg as either 2 ml/kg boluses or a 0.1–1.7 ml/kg/h infusion. The study concluded that administration of HSA was safe (two dogs developed facial oedema possibly associated with this treatment) and 25% HSA reliably increased blood pressure and albumin concentration. It was also suggested that HSA may be a good choice for critically ill patients with systemic inflammatory response syndrome (SIRS), gastric dilatation–volvulus, peritonitis and liver disease.

Despite use of albumin in human medicine since the 1940s, its use and risk:benefit ratio are still controversial. The 2004 'Saline *versus* Albumin Fluid Evaluation' (SAFE) study evaluated 6997 patients (ICU patients where fluid was indicated for intravascular volume depletion with the exception of liver transplantation, burn or cardiac surgery patients); it concluded that the 28-day mortality rate was the same with or without albumin therapy. There was no difference in other secondary outcomes (similar days in ICU, in hospital and need for mechanical ventilation). There was limited evidence that a subpopulation of patients with severe sepsis who received albumin had a more favourable outcome. On the other hand, the study also suggested that the subpopulation of patients with trauma (especially with brain injury) had a more favourable outcome if they did not receive albumin. The overall conclusion was that albumin, evaluated across the entire population, was safe without any clear efficacy advantage over saline.

Thus broad utilization of 25% HSA is not recommended at present. Absolute guidelines have not been determined and highly intensive monitoring of patients to prevent circulatory overload must occur if this potent colloid is used. Furthermore, the immunological effects of this human protein are not known in all species presented to the veterinariay surgeon.

Oxygen-carrying solutions

The inability to readily obtain blood products or perform a cross-match can have life-threatening consequences. Following over 60 years of research and development, only one blood substitute, Oxyglobin Solution, is commercially available. Oxyglobin Solution is a polymerized bovine haemoglobin (130 g/l) colloid in a balanced electrolyte solution (130 mmol/l Na^+, 4 mmol/l K^+ and 110 mmol/l Cl^-) with a pH of 7.8. It is stable at room temperature, has a 3-year shelf-life and there is no need for cross-matching, reconstitution, warming the solution or specialized transfusion administration sets. The potential for disease transmission is negligible. The plasma haemoglobin is able to carry oxygen to tissues and can temporarily replace the need for red blood cells (half-life is dose-dependent but ranges from 18–43 hours). Oxyglobin Solution has the same advantages as other colloids and a smaller volume than crystalloids can be used to maintain blood volume.

Oxyglobin is approved for use in dogs for treatment of anaemia and the recommended dose is 10–30 ml/kg bodyweight i.v. at a rate not to exceed 10 ml/kg/h, administered once. Blood loss, haemolysis and ineffective erythropoeisis are other common indications for its use. Controversy exists as to whether Oxyglobin is beneficial in dogs with immune-mediated haemolytic anaemia (IMHA). One report suggested an association with poor survival while a more recent report revealed that Oxyglobin had a positive effect on long-term survival. The difference in outcome may have been related to a difference in dosing strategy.

Oxyglobin has been administered (off-label) under experimental and clinical conditions to over two dozen different species, ranging from reptiles, birds and mammals to aquatic species. Regardless of the species or indication for its use, it is essential to respect Oxyglobin as a colloid. Because of its oncotic pressure (Figure 16.5), circulatory overload may occur, with development of pulmonary oedema and pleural effusion. As with all colloids, this can be prevented through careful monitoring of administration rate and minimizing the dose to the lowest effective dose. In fragile patients, invasive monitoring with a central venous pressure line is recommended. Signs of volume overload include pulmonary crepitations and crackles or diminished lung sounds (pleural effusion), decreased P_aO_2 or respiratory distress. Appropriate treatment involves slowing or discontinuing fluid administration, and providing diuretics and oxygen. Several reports indicate that cats may be especially sensitive to volume overload when Oxyglobin is administered at infusion rates and volumes approved for dogs, but such effects were not observed at lower rates (<2–5 ml/kg/h) and smaller volumes (≤10–15 ml/kg).

Parameter	Whole blood	Oxyglobin
Haemoglobin (g/l)	140–160	120–140
Osmolarity (mOsm/l)	280–310	280
Oncotic pressure (mmHg)	25–30	43
Viscosity (cp)	3.5	1.3
Half-life (h)	Varies	18–43 (dogs)
P_{50} (mmHg) [a]	26	34
Methaemoglobin (%)	<2	<3

16.5 Comparison of whole blood to a haemoglobin-based oxygen carrier, Oxyglobin Solution (HBOC-301). Note that the half-life of Oxyglobin is dose-dependent and values are based on doses ranging from 10 to 30 ml/kg. [a] P_{50} is the partial pressure at which 50% of haemoglobin is saturated with oxygen.

Results of a multicentre clinical trial using Oxyglobin in 64 anaemic dogs showed that the most commonly reported adverse reactions were transient discoloration of sclera and urine, vomiting and over-expanded vascular volume when Oxyglobin was administered at a higher than recommended rate. Less frequent adverse events that had an unknown relationship to the administration of Oxyglobin included diarrhoea, fever, cardiac arrhythmia and tachypnoea.

Priorities in fluid therapy

The initial goal in any fluid therapy plan is to maintain enough oxygen delivery to vital organs to sustain aerobic metabolism (Figure 16.6). Oxygen delivery (DO_2) is primarily based on cardiac output (CO), haemoglobin content (Hb) and arterial oxygen saturation of haemoglobin (S_aO_2):

$$DO_2 = CO \times C_aO_2$$

The arterial or mixed venous oxygen content (C_aO_2 or C_vO_2, respectively) is determined by the amount of oxygen bound to the haemoglobin plus the amount dissolved in the plasma. The full equation for oxygen delivery then becomes:

$$DO_2 = CO \times (1.36\,(Hb)(\%S_aO_2) + (0.003)(P_aO_2))$$

where the variable $0.003(P_aO_2)$ is the amount of oxygen dissolved in the plasma at that arterial oxygen tension (P_aO_2). The determinants of a patient's oxygen consumption ($\dot{V}O_2$) are dependent not only on the metabolic demands of the patient but also on adequacy of oxygen delivery. If oxygen delivery decreases, then more oxygen must be extracted from the blood to maintain the oxygen consumption of the patient. Estimates of adequate oxygen delivery can be made either by estimating the components of oxygen delivery itself or evaluating whether or not the oxygen extraction of the patient has increased, assuming an unchanged metabolic state. See 'Fluid therapy monitoring' for indirect methods of evaluating oxygen delivery and extraction.

Parameter	Normal range
Arterial haemoglobin saturation (S_aO_2) (%)	>95
Base deficit (mmol/l)	+2 to −2
Blood lactate (mmol/l)	<2
Cardiac index (ml/kg/minute)	100–150
Central venous pressure (cmH_20)	Awake: −3 to +4 Anaesthetized: 2–7
Gastric intramucosal pH	7.35–7.41
Heart rate (bpm)	Dog: 70–180 Cat: 145–200
Haematocrit (%)	Dog: 37–55 Cat: 25–45
Mean arterial blood pressure (mmHg)	80–110
Mixed venous haemoglobin saturation (S_vO_2) (%)	>65
Mixed venous oxygen tension (mmHg; kPa)	40; 5.3
Oxygen delivery (DO_2) (ml/minute)	500–800
Oxygen extraction (%)	20–30
Oxygen consumption (VO_2) (ml/minute/m^2)	110–160
Pulmonary artery wedge pressure (mmHg)	3–9
Urine output (ml/kg/h)	1–2

16.6 Normal values of cardiopulmonary parameters for monitoring of fluid therapy.

In situations such as acute haemorrhage, cardiac output and haemoglobin concentration will decline. Initially, the consequences of low cardiac output outweigh the consequences of low haemoglobin. Therefore, treating hypovolaemia is more important than treating anaemia and restoring *volume* is more important than maintaining haemoglobin concentration. The blood volume of a dog is 80–90 ml/kg and that of a cat is 60–70 ml/kg. A rough estimate for determining the fluid volume needed to restore blood volume can be calculated based on the final distribution of the chosen fluid type. When administering whole blood, give a volume equal to the volume deficit; when administering a colloid, give a volume equal to 1–1.5 times the volume deficit; and when administering an isotonic crystalloid give a volume equal to 3–4 times the volume deficit (see Figures 16.2 and 16.7).

Calculation of fluid volume needed:

1. Calculate the patient's normal blood volume (BV)
2. Estimate the percent blood loss, based on clinical signs and history
3. Calculate the volume deficit, VD = BV x % blood loss
4. Determine the resuscitation volume, based on:
   - Whole blood volume = VD
   - Colloid volume =1.5 x VD
   - Isotonic crystalloid volume = 4 x VD

Normal blood volume: Dog = 80–90 ml/kg; Cat = 60–70 ml/kg

Normal plasma volume: Dog = 36–57 ml/kg; Cat = 35–53 ml/kg

Shock fluid rates:

Isotonic crystalloid fluids: Dog = 80–90 ml/kg/h; Cat = 60–70 ml/kg/h

7.5% Hypertonic saline ± colloid: 4 ml/kg over 10 minutes

Blood replacement:

Volume (ml) of blood to administer =

$$\frac{(\text{desired Hb} - \text{existing Hb}) \times (\text{ml/kg BV} \times \text{recipient wt})}{\text{donor Hb}}$$

Plasma replacement:

Volume (ml) of plasma to administer =

$$\frac{(\text{desired TP} - \text{existing TP}) \times (\text{ml/kg PV} \times \text{recipient wt})}{\text{donor TP}}$$

Cryoprecipitate[a]:

Volume (ml) of cryoprecipitate to administer =

$$\frac{\text{recipient wt} \times \text{BV (l/kg)} \times [1 - \text{Hct(l/l)}] \times (\text{desired} - \text{current factor level (U/ml)})}{\text{factor level in plasma product (U/l)}}$$

Platelet-rich plasma[a]:

Expected 1-hour plt count ($\times 10^9$/l) =

$$\text{plt count before transfusion } (\times 10^9/\text{l}) + \frac{\text{unit plt count } (\times 10^9/\text{l}) \times \text{unit vol.} \times 0.51^b}{\text{recipient kg wt} \times \text{BV (l/kg)}}$$

16.7 Guidelines for calculating fluid and blood component replacement. BV = Blood volume; Hb = Haemoglobin concentration; Hct = Haematocrit; Plt = Platelet; PV = Plasma volume; TP = Total protein; wt = Weight in kg. [a] Reprinted from Mathews (1996) with permission of the publisher. [b] 0.51 corrects for splenic sequestration of transfused platelets.

Following volume restoration, the second priority is *haemoglobin* restoration. However, haematocrit values taken alone give no information about oxygen delivery or oxygen uptake by the tissues. If they did, elevated haematocrits in dehydrated patients would signify increased oxygen delivery, and fluid therapy would not be required. This rationale is obviously incorrect, implying that the common practice of transfusing red blood cells based on a specific haematocrit alone has little scientific basis. A more rational approach to determine if red cell transfusions are necessary is to evaluate oxygen delivery variables and look for evidence of inadequate oxygen consumption (see Figure 16.6). For example, with normovolaemic anaemia (following crystalloid fluid therapy or in chronic anaemia), red cell transfusion may not be necessary because blood volume is adequate and a compensatory increase in cardiac output may have occurred to meet oxygen delivery. However, red cell administration may be indicated if oxygen delivery is below normal and lactate is being produced in large amounts (suggesting anaerobic metabolism) or if oxygen extraction is greater than normal (suggesting tissue oxygen needs are greater than delivery). Normalization of these indicators of poor oxygen delivery and an increase in oxygen consumption after administration of blood or packed red cells should be considered a positive response. Transfusions should be continued until oxygen consumption is no longer dependent on haemoglobin content.

Other priorities in fluid therapy include correction or prevention of acid–base, electrolyte and metabolic disorders. Treatment is tailored to the individual patient and can be addressed either by selecting a fluid of appropriate pH and electrolyte composition (see Figure 16.1) or by adding a supplement to the fluid (Figure 16.8). Chronic abnormalities should be corrected slowly.

The pH of common solutions varies greatly: some are acidifying and others alkalinizing, depending on whether buffers have been added (see Figure 16.1). Chloride and lactate, the anions associated with sodium and potassium cations in most fluids, can be used interchangeably for most patients, but not for patients with acidaemia. When there is concern about acidosis, the clinician should select a fluid of the appropriate pH with a metabolizable buffer (acetate, gluconate or lactate) in preference to chloride, as chloride may promote a hyperchloraemic metabolic acidosis while the metabolizable anions can be converted to bicarbonate.

Perioperative considerations

Pre-anaesthetic considerations

A healthy adult's body is composed of 55–60% water, divided unequally into intracellular (40%) and extracellular (20%) volumes (see Figure 16.3). The extracellular fluid volume can be subdivided into the interstitial fluid volume and plasma volume. An estimate of the volume of fluids needed should be calculated to include pre-existing deficit, maintenance and ongoing losses (evaporative losses, surgical blood loss and third-space fluid loss).

Preoperatively, a minimum database of haematocrit, total protein, glucose, blood urea nitrogen and creatinine should be obtained and the patient should be evaluated for signs of dehydration or haemodynamic compromise. Clinical assessment includes evaluating skin elasticity, pulse rate and quality, mucous membrane colour, capillary refill time, respiratory rate and character, temperature of extremities, behaviour and mentation. The ability to assess extracellular fluid volume is important but often it must be estimated based on these non-specific clinical signs and abnormalities such as haemoconcentration, oliguria, azotaemia and acid–base or electrolyte alterations. A history suggestive of extracellular fluid deficits may include protracted gastrointestinal losses (vomiting, diarrhoea, bowel obstruction), sepsis, trauma or chronic diuretic administration. In some cases, additional information, such as mixed venous blood oxygen saturation or tension, buffer or base deficit calculations, blood lactate concentrations, urine output and urine specific gravity, will assist in determining adequacy of tissue perfusion and severity of metabolic abnormalities.

Whenever time permits, stabilization of oxygen delivery, pH and electrolyte balance should occur in the preoperative period to optimize the patient's ability to tolerate the subsequent cardiopulmonary depressant effects of general anaesthesia. In an emergency, however, while adequate oxygen delivery must still be restored, mild metabolic, electrolyte and acid–base disorders can be corrected during the intraoperative and postoperative periods. Treatment should always be initiated preoperatively for extreme hyperkalaemia (≥8 mmol/l), acidaemia (pH ≤7.2) or hypoglycaemia (<3.3 mmol/l). Fluids should be warmed prior to administration, because cold fluids will promote hypothermia and increase metabolic oxygen demands as the body attempts to maintain normothermia.

Supplement	Emergency dose	Osmolarity (mOsm/l)	pH	Composition (mmol/l)
Calcium chloride (10%)	0.05–0.1 ml/kg slowly	2,040	5.5–7.5	17 Ca^{2+} 68 Cl^-
Calcium gluconate (10%)	0.5–3 ml/kg slowly or 60–90 mg/kg/day	680	6–8.2	232.5 mmol/l Ca^{2+} ND gluconate
Dextrose (50%)	500 mg/kg diluted, for immediate bolus	2,530	4.2	ND
Magnesium sulphate (1 g/2 ml)	0.075–0.15 mmol/kg over 5 minutes	4,060	5.5–7.0	2.03 Mg^{2+} ND SO_4^{2-}
Mannitol (25%)	0.25–3 g/kg diluted and given slowly over 30 minutes	1,373	4.5–7.0	ND
Potassium chloride (2 mmol/ml)	0.5 mmol/kg/h	4,000	4–8	2,000 K^+ 2,000 Cl^-
Sodium bicarbonate (8.4%), (1 mmol/ml)	0.3 x bodyweight in kg x base deficit (mmol/l) Give one third over 20 minutes and rest over 4 hrs or 1 mmol/l immediately	2,000	7.8	1,000 Na^+ 1,000 HCO_3^-

16.8 Intravenous fluid supplements. ND = No data.

Choice of fluid will depend upon the condition of the patient:

- For most routine surgical patients, a balanced, isotonic crystalloid solution is an appropriate choice administered at 5–10 ml/kg/h
- *Dehydration* will decrease the intracellular, interstitial and plasma fluid volumes and these patients need volume expansion of all fluid compartments. Practically, however, one relies on the patient's own physiological mechanisms to control intracellular fluid deficits. Therefore, a balanced isotonic crystalloid is an acceptable fluid choice
- If massive *acute blood loss* or severe hypotension occurs, a crystalloid is an acceptable initial fluid choice, provided that colloids and blood products are immediately available to maintain blood volume as soon as indicated during the procedure
- In more *chronic, progressive types of hypovolaemia*, the patient needs restoration of both blood volume and interstitial fluid volume and will benefit from combination of an isotonic crystalloid (to replace interstitial fluid deficit and maintain urine output) and colloid (to maintain plasma volume)
- *Septicaemic conditions* or *severe ischaemic episodes*, from any cause, can decrease blood volume but increase intracellular and interstitial volumes because of changes in capillary and cell membrane permeability and secondary fluid shifts. Such patients need fluids to support oxygen delivery but fluids should be chosen that will minimize further tissue or organ oedema
- With a pre-existing *metabolic acidosis* or when there is concern for future acidosis, the pH of the initial fluid should be near that of plasma (see Figure 16.1), and acetate or gluconate (easier to metabolize than lactate) may be a better buffer choice in severely ill patients. In mild to moderate metabolic acidosis, efforts should be made to improve circulating blood volume and oxygen delivery either by increasing the volume of fluid being administered or by erythrocyte restoration to improve oxygen content. Stored blood and packed red cells are extremely acidotic and fresh whole blood is preferred to prevent worsening acidaemia in critical patients. With severe acidaemia (pH <7.2), administration of an alkalinizing solution may be of temporary benefit while the underlying cause is treated. A buffer should not be administered through the same catheter as either a calcium-containing solution (lactated Ringer's) or any type of blood product.

Intraoperative considerations

Two concerns for intraoperative maintenance fluid choices are whether to administer glucose, and how much water, sodium and potassium are necessary to replace losses. Glucose has, in the past, been given perioperatively to decrease protein catabolism and prevent hypoglycaemia. This may be of special concern for diabetic patients, patients with liver disease or paediatric patients. However, the stress response that results from anaesthesia and surgery produces an 'anti-insulin' effect, making it difficult to predict the glucose requirements for an individual patient. Except where hypoglycaemia is likely, routine administration of glucose has two disadvantages. Firstly, hyperglycaemia may cause an osmotic diuresis and dehydration. Secondly, studies have indicated that hyperglycaemia may worsen neurological ischaemia and outcome after traumatic brain injury. This latter finding may also have clinical relevance for other critically ill patients. To prevent hypoglycaemia, one can formulate a 2.5% dextrose infusion by adding 5 ml of 50% dextrose to 100 ml of an isotonic crystalloid solution. This allows additional dextrose to be administered without the concern of also administering free water. Blood glucose should then be re-evaluated periodically and additional glucose added to the solution if necessary (blood glucose <4.5–6.0 mmol/l).

The electrolytes sodium and potassium must be replaced in the perioperative period. Slight variations in the fluid concentrations are generally well compensated by the kidneys. The average maintenance sodium requirements are approximately 30 mmol/l and potassium requirements approximately 20 mmol/l. There are no other short-term requirements for other electrolytes except in instances where severe derangements have occurred (see Figure 16.8). Water requirements include the need to replace gastrointestinal, renal and insensible losses (e.g. respiratory, cutaneous). Additional fluids are required to replace blood and third-space fluid losses and to prevent general anaesthesia-induced hypotension from vasodilation and myocardial depression.

Even awake animals are intolerant of acute blood loss and rapid intervention is essential. With hypovolaemic shock, the mortality rate is directly related to the magnitude and duration of the ischaemic insult. Since life-saving compensatory reflexes are obtunded or removed in patients under general anaesthesia, these patients are even more sensitive to acute blood loss and hypovolaemia. Furthermore, seemingly small volumes of blood loss may not be tolerated in sick, debilitated or traumatized patients.

The first priority after blood loss is to restore blood volume (and red cells, if needed) and secondarily to replenish interstitial fluid deficits that may have occurred due to compensatory 'transcapillary refill'. In emergency situations, blood volume and cardiac output restoration will occur with any fluid that re-expands plasma volume (crystalloids, colloids or blood products). However, less viscous colloids and crystalloids flow faster through intravenous tubing than more viscous blood products. Hence, any acellular solution will flow faster than whole blood and whole blood will flow faster than undiluted packed red cells. Therefore, cardiac output is most rapidly restored with colloids and least rapidly restored with packed red cells. Due to differences in compartment distribution, the volume of crystalloids must be at least three times greater than the volume of colloid infused to have an equivalent effect on cardiac output. With mild to moderate haemorrhage, crystalloids are still beneficial because this type of fluid also replaces the interstitial fluid deficit.

In severe haemorrhage, administering a colloid followed by a crystalloid will restore the blood volume and interstitial fluid volume rapidly. In addition, acellular solutions will decrease haemoglobin concentration through haemodilution, and decrease blood viscosity. This decrease may improve microcirculatory blood flow without detrimental effects on oxygen delivery. Conventional shock doses of an isotonic crystalloid fluid are 90 ml/kg/h for dogs and 60 ml/kg/h for cats (one blood volume in an hour). The fluid rate should be slowed as soon as favourable responses are observed. If the patient remains unstable, or initial blood loss is severe, fluids such as colloids and blood may be necessary to maintain intravascular volume during the critical period, with fluid rates dictated by the patient's clinical condition. The standard 'shock' colloid dose is 5–20 ml/kg over 15–30 minutes. For emergency blood volume expansion, hypertonic saline plus a colloid can be life-saving. The standard emergency hypertonic saline/dextran dose is 4 ml/kg i.v. of 7.5% hypertonic saline with 1–2 ml/kg + 6% dextran 70 over a 10-minute period followed by conventional fluid therapy. If hypertonic saline is given more rapidly, paradoxical hypotension due to direct vascular relaxation and vasodilation may occur. This hypotension, in the face of a life-threatening hypovolaemia, can be detrimental and even fatal. If hypertonic saline is administered more slowly than the above rate, fluid shifting will still occur but the onset may be slower and maximum effect may be obtunded. Lower hypertonic saline doses or rates may be necessary in patients with cardiac disease to prevent circulatory overload and cardiac failure.

It should be noted that the crystalloid and colloid 'shock' doses are only approximate starting doses. The safe maximum rate or volume that can be administered is undetermined for any fluid. In one study, 8–14% dehydrated but otherwise healthy dogs received intravenous lactated Ringer's for 1 hour at doses of: 90 ml/kg/h (A); 225 ml/kg/h (B); or 360 ml/kg/h (C). Clinical signs of circulatory overload were absent or mild in groups A and B while dogs in group C showed marked serous nasal discharge, coughing and dyspnoea within 20 minutes of fluid administration. One may conclude that isotonic crystalloid fluids probably can be administered faster than 90 ml/kg/h but slower than 360 ml/kg/h in otherwise healthy dogs (with no pulmonary oedema, sepsis or heart disease). The rule of thumb is to infuse fluids as slowly as possible but as fast as necessary to produce haemodynamic stability. While 'shock' doses should be decreased as soon as the clinical condition permits, it is equally important to be aggressive during initial resuscitation because duration of tissue ischaemia affects outcome. Cellular oedema and injury to major organs can continue after apparently successful resuscitation due to the no-reflow phenomenon and reperfusion injury from sustained ischaemia.

Third spacing is the abnormal accumulation of fluid in normal extracellular locations. It is caused by expansion of the interstitial fluid space, ascites, hydrothorax or fluid accumulation around traumatized tissues (including excessive surgical manipulation of the gastrointestinal tract). Loss of fluid into these spaces needs to be considered when calculating fluid replacement. This fluid movement may lead to hypovolaemia (if the fluid came from the vasculature), dehydration (if the fluid came from the extracellular space) and/or hypoproteinaemia (if the third-space fluid has high protein content). The third-space fluid can accumulate in regions that may further compromise circulation to an organ or within an organ and produce poor tissue perfusion. In human patients, guidelines for third-space fluid losses are calculated based on degree of expected tissue trauma; these losses are corrected in addition to the fluids calculated to replace blood loss. The more the tissue damage, the more the third spacing of fluids. Estimated fluid rates for an anaesthetized patient are approximately 4 ml/kg/h for procedures with minimal trauma, 6 ml/kg/h for moderate trauma and 8 ml/kg/h for extreme tissue trauma. For all patients, clinical monitoring will determine if the rate is adequate or should be adjusted.

Postoperative fluid considerations

Most patients receive a high fluid rate preoperatively and intraoperatively in order to maintain intravascular blood volume. In the postoperative phase, this fluid may redistribute to extravascular spaces thus causing a decrease in intravascular volume. At the same time, the patient is awakening from anaesthesia and the return to normal blood pressure increases glomerular filtration and diuresis. Patients may need additional fluids for several hours after the anaesthetic period to compensate for this inappropriate diuresis. The diuresis may mask signs of hypovolaemia, as it appears that the patient has adequate urine production. Furthermore, patients that were not hydrated prior to anaesthesia may continue to be dehydrated following the anaesthetic procedure and will require additional fluid volume. On the other hand, interstitial overexpansion may develop after administration of isotonic crystalloids. Once haemodynamic stability has returned, this sequestered fluid is mobilized, returned to the plasma volume and eventually removed from the body. Mobilization of accumulated fluids tends to occur maximally around the third postoperative day, with continued fluid shifting for up to 10 days, depending on the circumstances and severity of surgical trauma.

Special conditions

Cardiac function

Patients with decreased cardiac function do not tolerate excessive fluid administration. Large sodium loads should be avoided. Colloids are an acceptable alternative but must be titrated carefully because overexpansion of the plasma volume with colloids cannot be corrected very quickly.

Oliguria

Patients with acute oliguria also need to be monitored carefully. An acceptable plan would be to infuse an isotonic crystalloid while monitoring urine output, central venous pressure, blood pressure and heart rate. The patient's response to a small fluid challenge may help differentiate the origin of the oliguria. Signs of urine output greater than 0.5 ml/kg/h indicate prerenal oliguria. If fluid challenge causes neither signs of improvement nor toxicity and there is concern that further fluids may result in unacceptable risk, fluid rates should be decreased. In these patients, concurrent therapy may include dopamine or diuretic administration. If colloids are chosen, careful titration and monitoring are essential because many colloids are cleared by the kidneys and may have a prolonged effect or worsen renal disease.

Central nervous system

Patients with traumatic brain injury and/or elevated intracranial pressure are very fragile and react quickly to insufficient or excessive fluid administration. Unfortunately, no single fluid is superior in this situation and extreme care must be taken in evaluating the patient's response. The volume and type of fluid depend on whether or not the patient is haemodynamically stable and if the blood–brain barrier is thought to be intact. The goal is to provide a systolic blood pressure greater than 90 mmHg without detrimentally affecting cerebral perfusion pressure. Paradoxically, cerebral perfusion pressure can decrease with fluid therapy due to redistribution of water into the cerebral interstitial and intracellular spaces, increasing cerebral oedema and causing secondary brain injury. The normal blood–brain barrier is relatively impermeable to both protein and sodium, causing water normally to move in or out of brain cells and the interstitium based on primarily capillary osmotic pressure and secondarily on oncotic pressure. Sodium changes are, therefore, more important than protein changes. Thus, even a slightly hypotonic solution, such as lactated Ringer's (although classified as an isotonic solution in Figure 16.1) may promote cerebral oedema. Isotonic saline, with supplemental potassium, may be a more appropriate fluid. However, prolonged saline use is not advisable because the patient may become hypernatraemic or hyperchloraemic and the fluid is devoid of other important electrolytes. Three to five percent hypertonic saline solution lowers intracranial pressure and may decrease cerebral oedema as well as provide rapid haemodynamic stability. Resuscitation with colloid-containing solutions also has been associated with lower intracranial pressure than resuscitation with isotonic crystalloid solutions. Specifically, pentafraction is composed of very large molecules and may 'plug' leaks in the blood–brain barrier.

Solutions containing glucose should be avoided in patients with any type of neurological disease. It is thought that patients with increased intracranial pressure with elevated plasma glucose have a worse neurological outcome because glucose promotes cellular metabolism leading to anaerobic conditions and intracellular lactic acidosis. Pure dextrose-containing solutions will also cause cerebral oedema due to the addition of free water. If dextrose must be administered to treat hypoglycaemia, it is imperative to add the dextrose to an isotonic solution and not use dextrose in water.

Fluid therapy monitoring

The goal of monitoring is to evaluate for adequate tissue oxygen delivery (see Figure 16.6), assess the effect of any changes to fluid administration and rule out deleterious consequences of fluid therapy. It has been found that in high-risk surgical patients, survivors frequently have supranormal oxygen delivery indices compared with those who later die. Thus, intensive monitoring is necessary in critically ill patients, even if there are no outward clinical signs of hypoperfusion. The challenge, however, is that there is no practical way directly and repeatedly to measure oxygen delivery, blood volume, extracellular fluid volume, etc. One must rely on both subjective and objective information. Subjective signs of adequate tissue perfusion include mentation, mucous membrane colour, capillary refill time, temperature of extremities and other signs of perfusion. Useful objective data include heart rate, direct or indirect arterial pressure, pulse quality, central venous pressure, temperature, pulse oximetry, blood pH and gas tensions, electrolytes, haematocrit, total protein, blood urea nitrogen, urine output and response to fluid challenges as well as calculation of oxygen indices (see Figure 16.6).

Many of the common cardiovascular monitoring techniques have limitations. For example, changes in blood pressure and heart rate are important but non-specific, insensitive markers of hypovolaemia due to blood loss. Hypotension may just as easily be due to excessive anaesthetic depth, the type of anaesthetic used, cardiac dysfunction or decreases in systemic vascular resistance. Non-invasive blood pressure measurements can yield equally low values in both hypovolaemic and hypothermic patients and it is difficult to differentiate between these two conditions, since they often co-exist. Cardiac filling pressures, such as central venous pressures and pulmonary artery wedge pressures, show a poor correlation to the presence and extent of blood loss until the blood loss is severe (>30%). Cardiac filling pressures are normally low (central venous pressure is 0–7 cmH_2O), and many types of monitors are insensitive to small changes in pressure. These measurements may not be practically useful because changes are not easily or accurately measured (see also Chapter 7).

Periodic assessment of the patient's packed cell volume (PCV) or haematocrit will detect acute anaemia and its direct effect on oxygen delivery. The haematocrit is often measured in patients with acute blood loss and during fluid therapy but it should be remembered that the haematocrit, by itself, is not an appropriate method of evaluating blood loss. Since whole blood is lost during haemorrhage, the haematocrit will not change acutely, only the total volume of blood will decrease. After several hours, with transcapillary refill and conservation of sodium and water by the kidneys, the haematocrit will decrease. This decrease may not be maximal for up to 24 hours. If, simultaneously, the patient is treated with asanguinous intravenous fluids to promote normovolaemia, the haematocrit will decrease further as a result of haemodilution of remaining red cells. Neither of these decreases in haematocrit is an indication of ongoing blood loss. However, a decrease in haematocrit *plus* dependency on continued fluid therapy to maintain haemodynamic stability is more suggestive of ongoing blood loss.

Indirect indicators of oxygen delivery

Even after apparently adequate intravenous fluid resuscitation following a hypovolaemic or hypotensive incident, unrecognized tissue hypoperfusion may be present. This unseen hypoperfusion is the most likely cause of many postoperative complications that develop in critical patients, such as acute renal failure, hepatic failure or systemic inflammatory response syndrome. Monitoring oxygen indices (e.g. oxygen extraction, mixed venous partial pressure of oxygen) is one method of evaluating global oxygen delivery and tissue perfusion. In most situations where tissue oxygen delivery falls, tissue *oxygen extraction* will increase as a method of obtaining more oxygen. The normal S_aO_2 is >95% and the $S_{\bar{v}}O_2$ >65%, giving a normal extraction of 20–30%. When the patient is breathing room air, this corresponds to an arterial oxygen tension of approximately 100 mmHg (13.3 kPa) and a mixed venous oxygen tension of approximately 40 mmHg (5.3 kPa).

The oxygen extraction will increase, and $S_{\bar{v}}O_2$ (and corresponding mixed venous oxygen tension) will decrease, as tissues take out more and more oxygen from the inadequate amount of delivered blood. At the point where extraction can no longer increase, tissue oxygen consumption becomes dependent on oxygen delivery (the critical oxygen delivery threshold). Experience suggests that the transition from compensated hypovolaemia to uncompensated hypovolaemic shock takes place when $S_{\bar{v}}O_2$ falls below 50% and oxygen extraction approaches 50–60%. Thus, oxygen extraction >30% is a marker of profound tissue hypoperfusion and oxygen extraction >50% indicates hypovolaemic shock. Other possible differential diagnoses for increased oxygen extraction are anaemia, hypermetabolism or use of a solution containing a haemoglobin-based oxygen carrier (HBOC).

A rough estimate of oxygen extraction can be performed using a pulse oximeter (in lieu of an arterial blood gas analyser or arterial haemoximeter) and a mixed venous blood gas measurement in which oxygen saturation values are provided. Arterial oxygen saturation minus venous oxygen saturation ($S_aO_2 - S_{\bar{v}}O_2$) roughly describes the percentage extraction and this technique is known as 'dual oximetry'. The extraction ratio can also be calculated using the formula:

$$(C_aO_2 - C_vO_2)/C_aO_2$$

where C_aO_2 and C_vO_2 are arterial and venous oxygen content (described earlier). Monitoring blood lactate concentrations or the base deficit from a central vein or mixed venous blood gas sample will provide additional information on the development of lactic acidosis from hypoperfusion. A lactate concentration >4 mmol/l or a base deficit lower than –10 mmol/l suggests profound oxygen debt.

Blood transfusion

The classical indications for blood product transfusions are treatment or prevention of decreased oxygen delivery, hypoproteinaemia, hypovolaemia and coagulation disorders. Commercial animal blood banks now make specific blood component therapy possible in some areas (Figure 16.9).

Blood volume is critical for homeostasis. Clearly, blood volume will decrease during haemorrhage but it can also decrease with diseases associated with hypoproteinaemia (due to decreased intravascular oncotic pressure). Initially, blood volume can be restored with either crystalloid or colloid therapy. However, two points need to be considered in deciding whether blood therapy is indicated: the haemoglobin content of the patient's blood and the rate of blood loss.

Absolute minima in haemoglobin content are controversial for both awake and anaesthetized patients and should be evaluated in conjunction with the other determinants of oxygen delivery. Cardiac output and blood flow may increase to compensate for a decrease in haematocrit, but when they are maximized, correcting a low haematocrit becomes critical. Conventional wisdom suggests that a patient can tolerate a low haematocrit when awake or if the anaemia is of chronic duration. For these patients, a haematocrit of 18–20% is often well tolerated. However, when anaesthesia is required, blood products are necessary sooner because of increased fluid needs during surgery, depressed compensatory reflexes, myocardial depression and vasodilation from the anaesthetic drugs. Haematocrits below 25–27% may limit oxygen delivery and delay wound healing.

Disorder	Fresh whole blood	Stored whole blood	Packed red cells	Platelet-rich plasma	Fresh frozen plasma	Cryoprecipitate	Stored or frozen plasma
Acute haemorrhage	**x**	x	x (plus colloid)		x (plus red cells)		x (plus red cells)
Anaemia	x	x	**x**				
Coagulopathy	x			x	**x**	x	
Hypoproteinaemia				x	x		**x**
Platelet function abnormality				**x**	x		
Replace specific clotting factors					x	**x**	
Thrombocytopenia	x			**x**			
von Willebrand's disease				x	x	**x**	

16.9 Indications for blood component therapy. Bold type indicates best choice of blood component for that disorder.

Therefore, depending on the length of anaesthesia and the invasiveness of the surgical procedure, the pre-anaesthetic haematocrit is recommended to be at least 30–34% in dogs and 25–29% in cats.

The most common indications for administration of a blood product during anaesthesia are acute blood loss or normovolaemic anaemia from acellular fluid administration. Signs of blood loss, such as tachycardia and hypotension, are inconsistent, imprecise and unreliable in anaesthetized patients; therapy should *not* be withheld until these signs are observed. Even in awake, healthy patients, an acute blood loss of 30–40% may cause reflex tachycardia and vasoconstriction to be limited, with sudden and profound onset of hypotension and hypovolaemic shock. In awake, previously healthy patients, an acute blood loss of >40% is usually fatal unless immediate intravascular volume and haemoglobin restoration occur. Under anaesthesia, the amount of permissible blood loss is much lower. An anaesthetized patient with an acute blood loss of ≥10% may require a blood transfusion, especially if the patient becomes haemodynamically unstable, prolonged anaesthesia time is predicted, or additional blood loss is likely.

The actual blood volume of a patient should be calculated to determine the significance of lost fluids in the perioperative period and to predict the necessary volume of fluid replacement. Calculating the exact blood volume in larger animals is often overlooked but it is important to have an estimate. Blood volume is generally calculated as 8–9% bodyweight (80–90 ml/kg) in dogs (45% cells and 55% plasma), and approximately 6% bodyweight (60 ml/kg) in cats (36% cells and 64% plasma). Therefore, for an equivalent bodyweight and equivalent volume of lost blood, the loss is a greater percentage of a cat's blood volume compared with that of a dog. Obviously, the same volume of blood loss in different-sized animals will clearly affect the smaller animal more profoundly. For small patients, counting and weighing Q-tips and gauzes may become essential to assess accurately blood or fluid loss, while measuring the PCV of and estimating the volume of fluid in the suction canister may be necessary in larger patients.

Blood types and incompatibility reactions

Cross-matching

Cross-matching tests evaluate for serological incompatibility between donor and recipient blood. They are useful for determining the likelihood of a transfusion reaction under the patient's current medical conditions. Cross-matching tests check for the presence of haemolysing or haemagglutinating antibodies in plasma (or serum) that are directed against red blood cell antigens. When red blood cells are to be administered to a patient, a *major cross-match* should be performed (washed donor red cells and serum of recipient), while a *minor cross-match* (washed recipient red cells and serum of donor) is recommended when plasma products are to be administered.

Cross-matching is performed in both dogs and cats not only to decrease the risk of transfusion reactions but also to decrease the risk of sensitizing the recipient if future transfusions become necessary. Transfusion reactions may occur in previously sensitized animals, animals with naturally occurring isoantibodies or those with neonatal isoerythrolysis.

Blood typing

Blood typing reveals blood group antigens on the red blood cell surface. Blood typing is recommended whenever red blood cells are to be administered. A blood typing card to classify dogs as DEA 1.1 positive or negative and cats as type A, type B or type AB is available for convenient in-house use (see Appendix of manufacturers, below). These tests require only a small volume of whole blood (approximately 50 µl for dogs and 150 µl for cats) to perform the assay. Although the canine card allows for rapid and reliable identification of DEA 1.1, it has been reported that weak reactions may also occur to DEA 1.2-positive dogs. Likewise, the feline card has been reported to have weak reactions to type AB blood. In the case of such reactions, dog and cat blood types should be verified at a qualified laboratory using another typing method (e.g. tube or gel).

Canine blood types: There are approximately 12 different canine blood types (Figure 16.10). The most antigenic is DEA 1.1, followed by DEA 1.2 and DEA 7. In contrast to cats, dogs do not appear to have any clinically important naturally occurring antibodies to other canine blood types. The low incidence of DEA 1.1, 1.2 and 7 and the lack of naturally occurring antibodies have two important clinical implications. Firstly, if neither donor nor recipient has ever received a transfusion before, a cross-match will not detect any alloantibodies even if the individual blood samples are of two different blood types. Secondly, a random, first-time transfusion is unlikely to cause an immediate incompatibility reaction because 4–14 days are required for the recipient to produce antibodies to donor cells.

	Canine blood types (DEA)							
	1.1	1.2	3	4	5	6	7	8
USA	33–45	7–24	5–10	87–98	12–25	67–99	8–45	40
Netherlands	38	4	5	56	8	74	31	17
Japan	44	22	24	ND	ND	60	ND	ND

16.10 Population incidences (percentages) of canine blood types. Adapted from Giger *et al.* (1995).

For canine blood transfusions, it is recommended that all blood donors be blood typed and, ideally, DEA 1.1-, 1.2- and 7-negative (with DEA 1.1 the most important). Approximately 40% of all dogs are DEA 1.1-positive. However certain breeds, such as the Greyhound, have a low frequency of DEA 1.1, 1.2 and 7 antigens, and are especially suitable donors. These dogs can be considered 'universal donors' because the other blood types cause minimal antigenic stimulation in unsensitized dogs. It is preferable to blood type the recipient as well, to prevent a delayed haemolytic reaction and to prevent sensitization (see below) but, in emergency situations, this can be foregone. However, a blood type and cross-match should *always* be performed if either the donor or recipient has previously received a blood transfusion.

Canine incompatibility reactions: An immediate or delayed reaction can occur with incompatible blood types. If a cross-match is not available and the dogs are of different blood types, the recipient dog may destroy the donor red cells as antibodies develop. This *delayed haemolytic transfusion reaction* can be observed as a rapid decline in the haematocrit over 1–2 weeks after the transfusion and is easily overlooked or misdiagnosed on follow-up blood work. The dog also is now sensitized to that blood type, and all future transfusions with blood of that type may cause an *acute haemolytic reaction.*

An acute haemolytic reaction occurs when mismatched blood is administered to a previously sensitized recipient. The most severe reaction will occur when a previously DEA 1.1-sensitized dog receives another DEA 1.1 blood transfusion. The signs of an acute transfusion reaction are variable and can develop within minutes to hours after the transfusion has begun. The severity of signs is roughly proportional to the amount of incompatible blood received and degree of incompatibility. Common signs include fever, vomiting, urticaria, haemoglobinaemia and haemoglobinuria. The reaction can be fatal, with initial signs of severe hypotension, bradycardia and dyspnoea. If the animal survives this phase, a second phase may occur in which the patient becomes tachypnoeic, hypertensive and tachycardic, and may develop other cardiac arrhythmias. Stabilization, if it is to occur, generally follows within 30 minutes.

Feline blood types: Cats have an AB blood group system; the most common blood type is type A (Figure 16.11). A and B are alleles, with A being dominant. The third cat blood type, type AB, is inherited separately as a third allele that is recessive to A and co-dominant with B. In certain breeds, type B can be very common compared with the general population (Figure 16.11) and historical information from owners or breeders may be important. Thirty five percent of type A cats and 70% of type B cats have natural isoagglutinins against the opposite red blood cell antigens. Type AB cats do not have any alloantibodies against either type A or B red blood cells. There is no 'universal' donor.

For feline blood transfusions, it is recommended that both donor and recipient cats are blood typed. Blood typing prevents acute or delayed transfusion reactions and avoids sensitizing a cat that may not have naturally occurring alloantibodies. If blood typing is not available, a major and minor cross-match should be performed. Small 'test doses' of blood to recipient should never be administered. Type A donors are preferred because of their common blood type but access

Domestic Shorthair		Type A (%)	Type B (%)
USA	Northeast	99.7	0.3
	North central	99.6	0.4
	Southeast	98.5	1.5
	Southwest	97.5	2.5
	West coast	95.3	4.7
Other countries	Australia (Brisbane)	73.7	26.3
	Argentina	97.3	2.7
Europe	Austria	97.0	3.0
	England	97.1	2.9
	Finland	100	0
	France	85.1	14.9
	Germany	94.0	6.0
	Italy	88.8	11.2
	Netherlands	96.1	3.9
	Scotland	97.1	2.9
	Switzerland	99.6	0.4
Purebred cats ([a]breeds with isolated type AB cats)		**Type A (%)**	**Type B (%)**
Abyssinian		84	16
American Shorthair		100	0
Birman [a]		82	18
British Shorthair [a]		64	36
Burmese		100	0
Cornish Rex		67	33
Exotic Shorthair		73	27
Japanese Bobtail		84	16
Maine Coon		97	3
Norwegian Forest		93	7
Oriental Shorthair		100	0
Persian		86	14
Scottish Fold [a]		81	19
Siamese		100	0
Somali [a]		82	18
Sphinx [a]		83	17
Tonkinese		100	0

16.11 Blood type A and B frequencies in cats. Reprinted from Giger and Oakley (1988) with permission from the publisher.

to a type B cat is advisable. Cats with type AB blood are best transfused with type AB blood or, at the very least, type A blood. There are two reasons for not using type B donor blood:

- More type B cats have isoagglutinins than type A cats
- Any anti-A alloantibodies in type B donor blood will recognize A antigens in the recipient type AB blood, causing a more severe haemolytic reaction than if type A donor blood is used.

Feline incompatibility reactions: Naturally occurring alloantibodies are much more common in cats than in dogs, so a random, first-time blood transfusion will have a higher likelihood of a reaction (approximately 36%). The mean half-life of feline red cells is approximately 30 days in cats that receive a matched blood type. Type A cats with anti-B serum that receive mismatched blood will have decreased red cell survival (half-life of approximately 2 days) and a modest, sometimes clinically inapparent, transfusion reaction. However, type B cats with anti-A serum that receive type A blood will have tremendously decreased red cell survival (half-life of approximately 1 hour) and will exhibit marked systemic reactions consistent with an acute intravascular haemolytic transfusion reaction. In such situations, as little as 1 ml of blood can be fatal.

Calculating the transfusion volume needed

Formulae have been devised to estimate the volume of whole blood or blood component to administer to a patient (see Figure 16.7). Alternatively, some less precise 'rules-of-thumb' are available:

- For whole blood, administer 10–40 ml/kg for a dog or 5–20 ml/kg for a cat and remeasure the patient's haematocrit
- Use 2 ml/kg whole blood for every 1% desired increase in haematocrit.

All of these 'rules-of-thumb' are rough estimates, because they do not take into account the haematocrit of the donor or that cats and dogs have a different ratio of red cell mass to plasma volume. A pre-calculated chart is also available for cats (Figure 16.12).

For *plasma albumin*, approximately 22 ml/kg of plasma will be necessary to increase albumin by 5 g/l. A relatively large volume of plasma is required for very little effect and using plasma for treatment of hypoalbuminaemia is not ideal.

Using *fresh frozen plasma* for coagulopathies, the dose is 10–20 ml/kg bodyweight. This dose may be repeated several times to obtain the desired effect.

If *cryoprecipitate* is needed, the 'rule-of-thumb' dose is approximately 1 ml/kg, or 1 unit/10 kg.

Transfusion administration and complications

Route of administration

Jugular, cephalic or saphenous veins and intraosseous femoral or humeral sites are all acceptable routes for blood administration. Intraperitoneal transfusion is not advisable since rate of peritoneal absorption is slow (40% absorbed after 24 hours).

Preparation

Refrigerated blood and blood products should be warmed gently to body temperature before transfusing (not to exceed 37°C). Packed red cells should only be diluted with 0.9% saline. Frozen bags of plasma must be handled carefully to prevent cracking during the thawing process. Thawing of frozen plasma, conducted with a circulating warm water bath with the temperature between 30 and 37°C, generally takes about 30 minutes. Frozen plasma can be microwaved and ready to administer after approximately 3–5 minutes. To microwave frozen plasma, the plasma bag is placed in a container of water, without its sides touching the container, and the container placed in the

		PCV of donated blood (including anticoagulant)										
		30%	32%	34%	36%	38%	40%	42%	44%	46%	48%	50%
PCV of recipient	4%	35.9	33.7	31.7	29.9	28.4	27.1	25.8	24.4	23.3	22.4	21.6
	6%	30.8	28.8	27.3	25.7	24.4	23.1	22.0	20.9	20.2	19.4	18.5
	8%	25.7	24.0	22.7	21.3	20.2	19.4	18.3	17.6	16.7	16.1	15.4
	10%	20.5	19.4	18.0	17.2	16.3	15.4	14.7	14.1	13.4	12.8	12.3
	12%	15.4	14.5	13.6	12.8	12.1	11.7	11.0	10.6	10.1	9.7	9.2
	14%	10.3	9.5	9.0	8.6	8.1	7.7	7.3	7.0	6.6	6.4	6.2

Example:	PCV of recipient	6%
	PCV of donated blood	46%
	Weight of recipient	3.2 kg
	Volume of blood required per kg body weight *(see above table)*	20 ml
	Multiplied by weight of the recipient	20 ml x 3.2 kg
	Total volume of blood required	64 ml

16.12 Volume of blood (ml) needed for transfusion per kilogram (kg) of recipient cat. (Note: to convert kilograms (kg) into pounds (lbs) divide by the conversion factor of 2.2.) Adapted from Norsworthy (1977).

centre of a microwave oven (700 W setting). The plasma unit is microwaved for 5–10-second periods and is agitated for 3–5 seconds by hand between exposures (to prevent localized overheating). Microwave thawing of canine fresh frozen plasma does not alter the one-stage prothrombin time, factor VIII coagulant activity and von Willebrand factor antigen. Thawed plasma should be used within 6–8 hours and should never be refrozen. Whole blood and other blood components should never be 'warmed' in a microwave.

Stored blood and packed red cells quickly become acidotic and have higher ammonia levels than fresh whole blood. Citrate-phosphate-dextrose, the anticoagulant solution in most blood collection bags, has a pH of 5.5. Thus, the pH of even a freshly drawn bag of blood will decrease to approximately 7.0 or 7.1. With additional storage, lactic and pyruvic acids produced by red cell metabolism and glycolysis will accumulate and the pH may decrease to 6.9 after 3 weeks of storage. A contributing factor to acidosis of stored blood is hypercapnia. However, excess carbon dioxide is rapidly removed if the patient has adequate ventilatory function. Stored blood alterations should be considered and addressed in patients with pre-existing acidosis, those with hepatic encephalopathy or in critically ill patients.

Autotransfusion

The best method of autotransfusion is to estimate the volume of blood loss preoperatively, harvest this amount from the patient and store it several days to a week prior to the surgery. Alternatively, blood can be withdrawn from the patient immediately prior to the procedure and replaced with appropriate crystalloids or colloids, a technique called 'normovolaemic haemodilution'. This blood can then be given intraoperatively when needed without concern about incompatible transfusion reactions. Intraoperative salvage techniques for autotransfusion have some definite drawbacks but can be performed. Intraoperative salvage is preferably done with some type of automated cell saver or blood salvage system. The blood is aspirated from the surgical field, mixed with anticoagulant and transferred to a reservoir unit. In the reservoir, it is filtered, centrifuged, washed and resuspended. Complications include haemolysis, coagulopathies, decreased calcium and air embolism. Salvaged blood should not be reinfused if the blood may contain tumour cells, urine, bile, faecal matter or other contaminants.

Desmopressin acetate

DDAVP (Rhinyle, Octim, Vasopressin) is used to release factor VIII and von Willebrand factor transiently from endothelial stores. It is administered to human patients with selected types of von Willebrand's disease prior to surgery. The recommended dose is 0.1–0.3 mg/kg i.v., using the human intranasal drops diluted with sterile saline and administered over 10 minutes. The peak effect is obtained 30–50 minutes after administration and the duration of response is transient (approximately 6 hours). In dogs, a dose of 1–5 μg/kg s.c. has been used empirically as an alternative to transfusion therapy for some patients with von Willebrand's disease, or to increase factor VIII levels in the blood donor dog 30 minutes prior to collection. Limitations to DDAVP include the transient effect, failure of some dogs to respond (presumably because some dogs have minimal von Willebrand factor, even in storage) and patients who become refractory after repeated treatments. Thus, DDAVP can only be considered an adjunct therapy in some specific patients and should not be considered a reliable substitute to transfusion therapy.

Administration and rate

A blood filter must always be used to remove microthrombi. A human adult filter is generally acceptable but, when small volumes of blood are being administered, an 18 micron micropore filter can also be used safely with less blood being trapped in the filter apparatus (see Appendix of manufacturers below).

Blood products should always be administered through a separate intravenous line with no latex, or, at least, with compatible fluids that do not contain calcium or bicarbonate (e.g. 0.9% NaCl). Do not administer drugs through the blood intravenous line and do not add any medication to the blood bags. Gently oscillate the bag to mix the contents periodically during administration.

An extremely slow rate of administration is initially indicated to allow observation for signs of an acute transfusion reaction. Even with appropriate serological screening, non-immunological transfusion reactions can occur due to improper storage or transfusion technique, or contamination with infectious organisms. As already mentioned, a transfusion reaction can have a wide variety of clinical signs and, should any occur, the transfusion must be immediately aborted. If no transfusion reaction develops, the rate can be increased to the desired rate. If possible, the final rate should be as slow as possible to obtain the desired result over 4–8 hours, unless the patient is severely hypovolaemic. A standard rate of approximately 4–5 ml/kg/h is generally adequate for conditions of mild hypovolaemia. If the patient is normovolaemic, the rate should be slower (2.5–5 ml/kg/h) to prevent circulatory overload. In patients with pre-existing cardiac disease, the rate may need to be further decreased to 0.5–1 ml/kg/h. At the other extreme, 5–15 ml/kg/h is recommended to treat acutely hypovolaemic animals and, in a life-threatening emergency, rates up to 40–60 ml/kg/h may be required (bolus technique).

Monitoring of the patient receiving transfusions

In this instance, monitoring means evaluating the response to therapy and looking for signs of *acute transfusion reactions* such as change in attitude, vomiting, pruritis, altered capillary refill time, fever, tachycardia, dyspnoea or erratic respiration, peripheral oedema, disseminated intravascular coagulation, urticaria, hypotension, icterus or haemoglobinaemia. Blood pressure, heart rate, body temperature, urine output and haematocrit measurements, evaluation of serum colour and electrocardiography are recommended to monitor patients receiving a blood transfusion during anaesthesia. Acute haemolysis is indicative of direct incompatibility. If hyperthermia occurs, even mild, up to 4–5 hours post-transfusion, the most likely cause is incompatibility between donor white blood cells and recipient antigens.

For any reaction, treatment involves stopping the blood transfusion immediately and providing supportive care. If the reaction is mild, the transfusion can be reinitiated at a slower rate. Corticosteroids (dexamethasone sodium phosphate at 2 mg/kg i.v. or methyl prednisolone at 10 mg/kg i.v.) and diphenhydramine (0.5 mg/kg i.m.) are often used to prevent or lessen the signs of an acute haemolytic transfusion reaction. There is, however, no current objective evidence to support use of these drugs. Donor antibodies reacting to recipient white blood cell antigens may cause white blood cell aggregates or emboli to lodge in the recipient's lungs. This may result in pulmonary oedema and has been termed 'transfusion-induced acute lung injury'. Serial arterial blood gas analyses and pulse oximetry may detect this complication in an anaesthetized and conscious patient.

Some adverse reactions may not be due to incompatible blood types, but to improper handling or administration of blood:

- Units containing dark brown or black blood should be discarded, because they may be colonized by bacteria and can lead to sepsis
- Bleeding can occur if large volumes of factor-free blood components are administered
- In patients affected with coagulopathies, monitoring platelet number, activated clotting time, partial thromboplastin time, prothrombin time and buccal mucosal bleeding time may be beneficial
- Lung microemboli can cause respiratory insufficiency if the blood product is not filtered properly
- Circulatory overload can occur if blood is administered in excess or too rapidly, particularly in patients with pre-existing cardiac or renal disease. These patients should be monitored for classical signs of vascular overload, such as an increase in central venous pressure, dyspnoea, vomiting, chemosis or pulmonary oedema
- Citrate toxicity can occur if large volumes of blood are rapidly administered and the ability of the liver to metabolize citrate is transiently overwhelmed. Citrate binds calcium, causing signs of transient hypocalcaemia with hypotension, a narrow pulse pressure, and, rarely, cardiac arrhythmias. Usually this complication is self-limiting but calcium supplementation may be necessary in some cases (see Figure 16.8). Ionized calcium concentrations in critically ill patients should be measured during transfusions and whenever massive transfusions are rapidly administered.

Appendix of manufacturers

Abbott Laboratories, Abbott Park, IL

Animalcare, York, UK

Baxter Healthcare Corp, Deerfield, IL; Baxter Healthcare, Newbury, UK

Du Pont Pharmaceuticals, Wilmington, DE; Du Pont Critical Care, Waukegan, IL; Du Pont, Stevenage, UK

Fresenius Kabi UK, Runcorn, UK

Intervet, Milton Keynes, UK

Kendall-McGaw, Inc., Irvine, CA

Marshallton Veterinary Group, West Chester, PA, 1-800-833-3090

HEMO-NATE neonatal filter: Gesco International, PO Box 690188, San Antonio, Texas, USA 78269; Utah Medical Products, Garrycastle Industrial Est., Athlone, County Westmeath, Ireland

Oxyglobin Solution: Biopure Corp., Cambridge, Massachusetts, USA; European Union Arnolds Veterinary Products Ltd, UK; +44 (0) 17 43 44 1632

RapidVet-H (Canine 1.1), RapidVet-H (feline): Catalog #HC105, DMS Laboratories, Flemington, NJ; 1-800-567-4367; UK: Woodley Equipment Company; +44 (0) 12 04 66 9034

References and further reading

Callan MB and Rentko VT (2003) Clinical application of a hemoglobin-based oxygen-carrying solution. *Veterinary Clinics of North America Small Animal Practice (Hematology edition)* **33(6)**, 1277–1293

Conroy JM, Fishman RL, Reeves ST, Pinosky ML and Lazarchick J (1996) The effects of desmopressin and 6% hydroxyethyl starch on Factor VIII-C. *Anesthesia and Analgesia* **83**, 804–807

Cornelius LM, Finco DR and Culver EH (1978) Physiologic effects of rapid infusion of Ringer's lactate solution into dogs. *American Journal of Veterinary Research* **39**, 1185–1190

Giger U, Gelens CJ, Callan MB and Oakley DA (1995) An acute hemolytic transfusion reaction caused by dog erythrocyte antigen 1.1 incompatibility in a previously sensitized dog. *Journal of the American Veterinary Medical Association* **206(9)** 1358–1362

Giger U, Kilrain CG, Filippich LJ and Bell K (1989) Frequency of feline blood groups in the United States. *Journal of the American Veterinary Medical Association* **195,** 1230–1232

Giger U and Oakley D (1988) Current feline transfusion therapy: unique issues in cats. In: *Proceedings of the VI International Veterinary Emergency and Critical Care Symposium*, pp. 207–210

Giger U, Stieger K and Palos H (2005) Comparison of various canine blood-typing methods. *American Journal of Veterinary Research* **66(8)**, 1386–1392

Grundy SA and Barton C (2001) Influence of drug treatment on survival of dogs with immune-mediated hemolytic anemia: 88 cases (1989–1999). *Journal of the American Veterinary Medical Association* **218**, 543–546

Lundy EF, Kuhn JE, Kwon JM, Zelenock GB and D'Alecy LG (1987) Infusion of five percent dextrose increases mortality and morbidity following six minutes of cardiac arrest in resuscitated dogs. *Journal of Critical Care* **2**, 4–14

Marino PL (1997) *The ICU Book, 2nd edn.* Williams & Wilkins, Baltimore

Mathews KA (1996) Blood/Plasma transfusion. In: *Veterinary Emergency and Critical Care Manual*, pp. 10–11. Life Learn Inc., Guelph, Ontario

Matthew CB (1994) Treatment of hyperthermia and dehydration with hypertonic saline in dextran. *Shock* **2(3)**, 216–221

Moon PF and Kramer GC (1995) Hypertonic saline-dextran resuscitation from hemorrhagic shock induces transient mixed acidosis. *Critical Care Medicine* **23(2)**, 323–331

Moon PF, Gabor L, Gleed RD and Erb HN (1997) Acid-base, metabolic and hemodynamic effects of sodium bicarbonate or tromethamine administration in anesthetized dogs with experimentally induced metabolic acidosis. *American Journal of Veterinary Research* **58(7)**, 771–776

Moon PF, Hollyfield-Gilbert MA, Myers TL, Uchida T and Kramer GC (1996) Fluid compartments in hemorrhaged rats after hyperosmotic crystalloid and hyperoncotic colloid resuscitation. *American Journal of Physiology* **207**, F1–F8

Norsworthy GD (1977) Blood transfusion in the cat. *Feline Practice* **7,** 29–31

SAFE Study Investigators (2004) A comparison of albumin and saline for fluid resuscitation in the intensive care unit. *New England Journal of Medicine* **350**, 2247–2256

Stieger K, Palos H and Giger U (2005) Comparison of various blood-typing methods for the feline AB blood group system. *American Journal of Veterinary Research* **66(8)**, 1393–1399

Turrentine MA, Kraus KH and Johnson GS (1988) Plasma from donor dogs, pretreated with DDAVP, transfused into a German Shorthair Pointer with type II von Willebrand's disease. *Veterinary Clinics of North America* **18**, 275

Weinkle TK, Center SA, Randolph JF *et al.* (2005) Evaluation of prognostic factors, survival rates, and treatment protocols for immune-mediated hemolytic anemia in dogs: 151 cases (1993–2002) *Journal of the American Veterinary Medical Association* **226(11)**, 1869–1880

17

Ophthalmic surgery

Sarah Thomson

Introduction

Anaesthesia for ophthalmic surgery presents several challenges. The type of surgery being performed and the condition of the eye have implications for patient handling, as well as for the analgesic and anaesthetic protocols. Many patients presenting for ocular surgery are geriatric or have concurrent disease, such as diabetes mellitus. Brachycephalic breeds are predisposed to corneal ulceration and general anaesthesia may be complicated by brachycephalic obstructive airway syndrome. Positioning and draping for ophthalmic surgery often restricts access to the head and forelimbs with subsequent effects for monitoring techniques. Specialized equipment, such as ventilators and nerve stimulators, is valuable for many intraocular and corneal surgeries. This chapter considers ocular physiology, ocular pain and analgesia, the systemic effects of ocular drugs and the management of patients requiring different types of ophthalmic surgery.

Physiology relevant to anaesthesia

Intraocular pressure

Anaesthetic management should minimize changes, principally increases, in intraocular pressure (IOP) over the entire anaesthetic period. Preoperatively, this is important with deep corneal lesions as an increase in IOP can cause the globe to rupture. Intraoperative rises in IOP during intraocular surgery can cause vitreous prolapse and retinal detachment. Postoperative intraocular haemorrhage and wound breakdown may occur with serious consequences.

IOP is maintained by the interaction of several factors (Figure 17.1). Aqueous humour originates from the ciliary processes of the ciliary body, resulting from active secretion (catalysed by the enzyme carbonic anhydrase), diffusion and ultrafiltration of plasma. Aqueous humour flows into the posterior chamber, through the pupil into the anterior chamber and exits the eye via the iridocorneal drainage angle, ultimately reaching the venous circulation (Figure 17.2). Clinically, IOP is influenced by central venous pressure (CVP), arterial carbon dioxide tension, arterial oxygen tension, extraocular muscle tone, head position, external pressure on the globe, drugs and arterial blood pressure (Figure 17.3).

Rate of production of aqueous humour
Facility of outflow of aqueous humour
Choroidal blood volume
Vitreous volume
Rigidity and compliance of sclera
Tone of extraocular muscles
External pressure

17.1 Factors that maintain intraocular pressure (from Almeida *et al*., 2004).

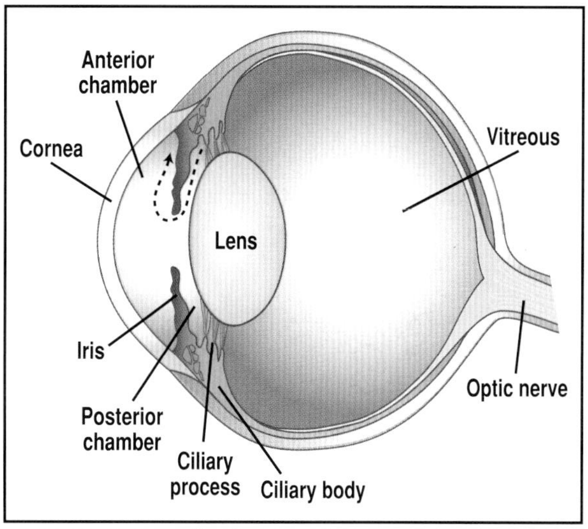

17.2 Schematic diagram of the cross-section of a globe. Arrow shows direction of flow of aqueous humour from the site of production into the anterior chamber.

Central venous pressure

Raised CVP can increase IOP by reducing venous drainage and aqueous humour outflow. Vomiting, gagging and coughing are all possible causes, so potentially emetic drugs, such as morphine, hydromorphone and medetomidine, should be avoided. Laryngeal and pharyngeal reflexes can be minimized during intubation of the trachea by attaining an adequate degree of unconsciousness before attempting to intubate. Topical lidocaine is commonly applied to the larynx of cats, and intravenous lidocaine (1 mg/kg i.v.) or fentanyl (1–2 µg/kg i.v.) may be used in dogs to minimize the response to intubation. In humans, intravenous lidocaine has been shown to prevent increases in IOP associated with endotracheal intubation when administered

Factor increasing IOP	Common causes	Action to reduce risk
↑ Central venous pressure	Vomiting	Avoid morphine, medetomidine
	Gagging, coughing at intubation and extubation	Adequate plane of anaesthesia prior to intubation Extubate slightly early to avoid coughing Drugs to reduce response: fentanyl (1–2 µg/kg i.v.), lidocaine (topical spray in cats or 1 mg/kg i.v. in dogs)
	Barking, crying	Sedation, analgesia
	Pressure on jugular veins	Use cross leads or harness Avoid neck bandages Positioning in surgery to avoid pressure on neck area and a slight elevation of the head Care with jugular blood sampling
	↑ Intrathoracic or intra-abdominal pressure	Care with maximum inflation pressures during IPPV Avoid pressure on abdomen when lifting Avoid responses to intubation/extubation
↑ External pressure	Accidental pressure on globe	Care when handling/moving/positioning for surgery Care with facemasks
	Self-trauma	Analgesia Sedation Elizabethan collar Bandage feet
	Stay sutures in sclera	Use muscle relaxants
↑ Arterial CO_2 tension	Hypoventilation	IPPV
↑ Hydrostatic pressure	Positioning during surgery	Slight elevation of head compared with body
Drugs	Suxamethonium increases extraocular muscle tone	Do not use when ↑ IOP to be avoided
	Ketamine increases extraocular muscle tone	Do not use when ↑ IOP to be avoided
↑ Arterial blood pressure	Sympathetic stimulation	Ensure adequate plane of anaesthesia Ensure good analgesia Sedate as appropriate

17.3 Factors influencing intraocular pressure.

1–3 minutes prior to intubation. Fentanyl usually has an onset time of 2–3 minutes. If protective airway reflexes are diminished, care must be taken to protect the airway to avoid aspiration of gastric contents. Removing the endotracheal tube before normal reflexes return may also avoid coughing and gagging, but may not be appropriate in all patients, such as brachycephalic breeds where upper airway collapse may occur. Pressure around the neck due to leads, bandages, jugular blood sampling and poor positioning under anaesthesia can raise CVP by compressing the jugular veins. A slight elevation of the head reduces venous pressure and therefore IOP.

Arterial carbon dioxide concentration

Hypoventilation may occur during anaesthesia, resulting in increased blood carbon dioxide tension (P_aCO_2) and subsequent vasodilation of ocular vessels and elevation of IOP. Hyperventilation can reduce IOP by causing vasoconstriction. However a recent study showed that hyperventilation to achieve hypocapnia had no effect on IOP in dogs, probably due to the intermittent positive pressure ventilation (IPPV) increasing intrathoracic pressure and therefore CVP, with resultant effects on IOP. Ventilation, either spontaneous or manual, should aim to maintain the end-tidal carbon dioxide concentration within normal limits (35–45 mmHg (4.7–6.0 kPa)).

External pressure

External pressure on the globe is a particular risk during handling and restraint of the patient, which is particularly important at induction. Non-depolarizing neuromuscular-blocking agents, which may be used to produce a centrally positioned globe to facilitate ocular surgery, can lower IOP by relaxing the extraocular muscles. Alternative positioning methods such as stay sutures may increase the IOP, as well as poor patient and head positioning and heavy drapes. Preoperative measures such as good analgesia and sedation are helpful, as are bandaged paws and Elizabethan collars postoperatively to minimize self-trauma.

Drug effects

Most general anaesthetic and analgesic drugs will lower or maintain IOP within normal limits, due to some depression of the cardiovascular system. Volatile inhalational agents reduce or produce no significant effects on IOP in dogs. Due to the interaction of various drugs and factors during the perioperative period it is difficult to predict the effect of an individual drug on IOP in a particular case. However certain drugs are known to significantly increase IOP and are generally avoided in ocular procedures when an increase in IOP could be detrimental. For example, drugs that increase muscle tone, such as suxamethonium and ketamine, increase IOP due to contraction of the extraocular muscles. Ketamine also increases IOP in dogs when used in combination with diazepam. Morphine, hydromorphone and medetomidine can induce retching and vomiting, which may increase IOP. However a sedative drug combination including a low dose of medetomidine may be preferable to sedate fractious or aggressive patients, where high levels of restraint are more likely to increase IOP. Although pre- and intraoperative administration of parenteral anticholinergic drugs has not been associated with raised IOP in dogs, these drugs are usually avoided in patients with pre-existing glaucoma.

Arterial blood pressure

Arterial blood pressure has some influence on IOP by affecting choroidal blood volume. Common causes of hypertension under general anaesthesia (mean arterial blood pressure >110 mmHg) include inadequate analgesia or depth of anaesthesia, which may be rapidly controlled by potent opioids such as fentanyl (1–5 μg/kg i.v.).

Cataract surgery

Postoperative hypertension (POH) is the term to describe a temporary increase in IOP shortly after cataract surgery. POH is common in the postoperative period. Studies have shown that this occurs 3–5 hours postoperatively in 18–48.9% of dogs undergoing cataract surgery. Any further increase in IOP due to non-ocular factors should therefore be avoided.

Oculocardiac reflex

The oculocardiac reflex is infrequently reported in dogs and cats, but may be initiated during ocular surgery and can cause bradycardia, arrhythmia or cardiac arrest. Application of pressure on the globe, manipulation or traction of the globe and extraocular tissues during surgery (e.g. enucleation) and retrobulbar nerve blocks can elicit the reflex. The afferent sensory component of the reflex is transmitted via the ciliary nerves of the ophthalmic branch of the trigeminal nerve to the trigeminal sensory nucleus. The efferent arm originates from the visceral motor nucleus of the vagus nerve and so the impulse continues through the vagus nerve to exert motor effects on the heart. Suggested ways to reduce the likelihood of the reflex occurring are aimed at minimizing globe manipulation during surgery. These include maintaining an adequate plane of anaesthesia, careful surgical technique, relaxation of extraocular muscles by the use of muscle relaxants and moderate hypocapnia to reduce IOP.

The pre-emptive use of anticholinergic drugs (atropine and glycopyrronium) to prevent the reflex is now thought to be unnecessary for several reasons. The incidence of the reflex is low; in one study only one out of 72 dogs undergoing ocular surgery where muscle relaxants were used showed cardiac signs that could be attributed to the reflex. The incidence is likely to be greater in young animals, due to a higher vagal tone in this age group. Anticholinergic drugs have adverse effects on the heart such as tachycardia (which increases myocardial oxygen consumption) and arrhythmias. If anticholinergic drugs are administered as part of the premedication, their effect will be variable and may be negligible during surgery. Retrobulbar nerve blocks may reduce the incidence or degree of the reflex, but are associated with complications and the retrobulbar injection itself can induce the response.

It is important to be aware that the oculocardiac reflex may occur, particularly in young animals, to monitor the patient carefully and use a good balanced anaesthetic technique. If the reflex occurs, the surgical stimulation should be immediately stopped, and the depth of anaesthesia assessed and adjusted if appropriate. If a bradycardia or bradyarrhythmia continues, an anticholinergic should be administered intravenously.

Position of globe

Under a surgical plane of anaesthesia the globe of cats and dogs usually rotates ventromedially. Corneal or intraocular surgery may be facilitated by an immobile and centrally positioned globe (Figure 17.4). This is usually achieved by the use of muscle relaxants, which paralyse the extraocular muscles, or by using stay sutures in the sclera. Other techniques, which are not advised due to the risk of associated complications, are a retrobulbar nerve block or a deep plane of anaesthesia (Figure 17.5). Commonly used non-depolarizing muscle relaxants include atracurium, vecuronium and pancuronium (see Chapter 15). IPPV is required during muscle paralysis. Extraocular muscles are sensitive to the effects of muscle relaxants; they are more quickly paralysed and remain paralysed longer than many other muscle groups, e.g. diaphragm and intercostal muscles. In this way, the globe can be centrally positioned even if chest movements are detectable or several twitches are visible using a train-of-four stimulation on the peroneal or ulnar nerve. The selection of drug and dose will depend on the expected length of the surgery, the cost of the drug, any concurrent disease and the anaesthetic regime.

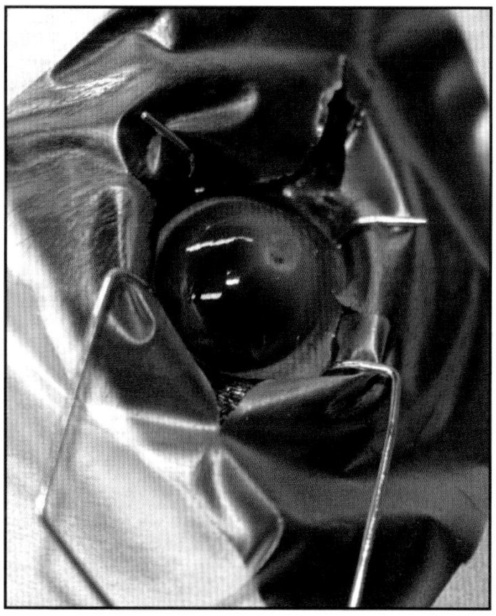

17.4 A centrally positioned and immobile globe.

Techniques	Method	Advantages	Disadvantages
Currently used	Muscle relaxants	Monitor degree of paralysis with nerve stimulator Reversible Short acting Predictable response Reduces IOP	Lose normal signs of anaesthesia and pain Requires IPPV Need to ensure no residual effect/fully reversed before allowing spontaneous ventilation
	Stay sutures	No requirement for drugs No requirement for IPPV	Increases surgical difficulty Increases surgical and anaesthetic time Increases IOP
Not advised	Deep plane of anaesthesia	No need for additional drugs	Cardiovascular and respiratory depression Unpredictable effects on globe
	Nerve block	Avoid use of systemic drugs	Complications: haemorrhage, globe rupture, optic nerve damage

17.5 Methods to produce a centrally positioned globe.

Tear production

It is widely accepted that sedation and general anaesthesia are associated with reduced tear production. General anaesthesia significantly lowers tear production in dogs for up to 24 hours following anaesthesia. The reduction in tear production was found to be related to the length of the general anaesthetic, with anaesthetic durations over 2 hours producing a longer effect. Various drugs have been associated with reduced tear production in dogs, e.g. acepromazine, medetomidine, atropine, hydromorphone, diazepam, butorphanol, xylazine, buprenorphine, fentanyl and pethidine (meperidine). The drug combination of xylazine and butorphanol appears to be synergistic in its reduction of tear production. Reduced tear production can lead to corneal drying and, therefore, corneal ulceration. Tear substitutes are therefore beneficial for patients undergoing sedation or general anaesthesia. Application every 90 minutes during the anaesthetic and at appropriate intervals postoperatively has been advocated. This is particularly important in brachycephalic breeds, during prolonged general anaesthesia and following the administration of muscle relaxants or ketamine.

Ocular pain

Analgesia for ocular surgery should aim to be pre-emptive (before the noxious stimulus) and multimodal (using different classes of drugs) as much as possible. When planning an analgesic regime for an animal with ocular pain or undergoing ophthalmic surgery, several considerations are important (Figure 17.6).

Consideration	Examples of clinical situation	Drug selection
Intraocular pressure (IOP)	Glaucoma Eye at risk of rupture, e.g. deep corneal ulcer After intraocular surgery	Avoid drugs which cause vomiting (morphine, medetomidine)
Corneal healing	Corneal ulcer, corneal trauma After corneal or intraocular surgery	Topical local anaesthetics are epitheliotoxic and delay corneal healing NSAIDs may delay healing
Age of animal	Geriatric cataract surgery	Caution with NSAIDs if impaired renal/hepatic function
Concurrent disease	Diabetic patients	Avoid steroids
Pupil size	Mydriasis required for: • Phacoemulsification (cataract surgery) • Lendectomy	Opioids may produce miosis (dogs), mydriasis (cats)
Concurrent medication	Long-term use of topical steroids	Topical drugs may have systemic effects
Degree of pain	Stages of intraocular or corneal surgery associated with most pain are: • Corneal incision • Corneal sutures	Topical local anaesthetic prior to incision and intraoperatively Short-acting potent opioids (e.g. fentanyl) provide additional analgesia
Type of pain	Intraocular (glaucoma, uveitis)	Systemic NSAIDs and opioids Atropine for uveitis
	Corneal surface, e.g. corneal ulceration, corneal foreign body	Additionally local anaesthetics for initial investigations or very short-term analgesia. Avoid self-trauma (foot bandage, Elizabethan collar)
Corneal sensitivity	Brachycephalic breeds have reduced corneal sensitivity	Other breeds may have higher analgesic requirements

17.6 Considerations in determining an analgesic regime for ocular pain.

Type of pain

The sensory nerve supply to the eye originates from the ophthalmic division of the trigeminal nerve. Nerves enter the corneal stroma at the limbus, and branch repeatedly, providing a rich innervation to the anterior stroma and epithelium. The central cornea has the greatest density of nerve endings and is therefore the most sensitive part of the cornea. The corneal epithelium and anterior stroma are more densely populated with sensory neurons and pain receptors than the deeper corneal layers (Figure 17.7). In clinical terms this means that a superficial ulcer is often more painful than a deeper ulcer, although the latter is more serious. There are breed-associated variations in the sensitivity of the cornea to painful stimuli. Brachycephalic breeds of dogs and cats have the least sensitive corneas and may display minimal signs of ocular pain, in contrast to dolichocephalic breeds, which may have higher analgesic requirements. In addition to pain receptors, the cornea has pressure receptors within the deeper stroma; these are associated with pain in glaucoma.

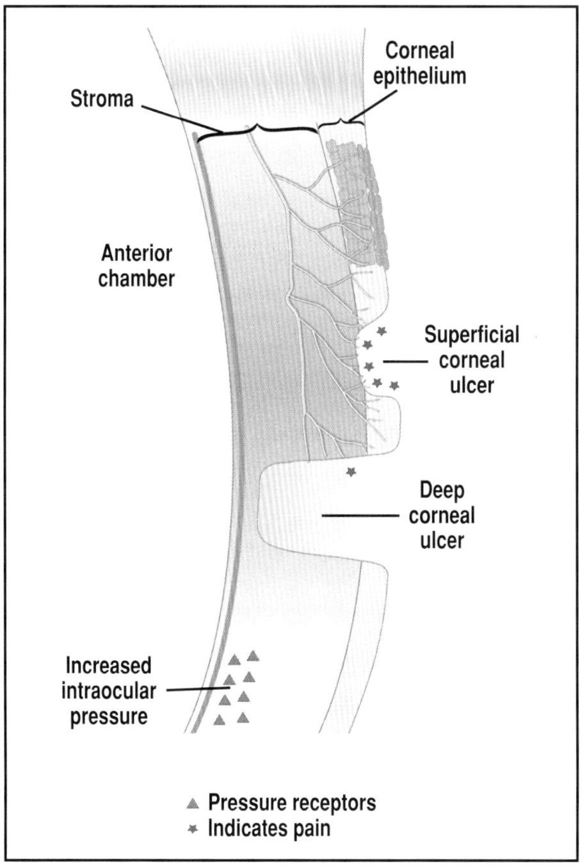

17.7 Schematic diagram of a cross-section of the canine cornea, showing the sensory nerve supply and how this affects the degree of pain associated with deep and superficial corneal ulcers.

Ocular pain can be considered simply as surface pain (cornea and conjunctiva) and intraocular pain. The classic clinical signs of ocular pain include blepharospasm, increased lacrimation and photophobia. Self-trauma is also a very common sign of ocular discomfort. These signs are non-specific and are seen with either surface or intraocular pain. Signs of pain will depend on the patient, the severity of the disease process and the condition itself. Surface pain, e.g. a corneal ulcer, is typically acute and intense. It is temporarily alleviated by topical local anaesthesia (see below) for diagnostic purposes or for very short-term analgesia (Figure 17.8).

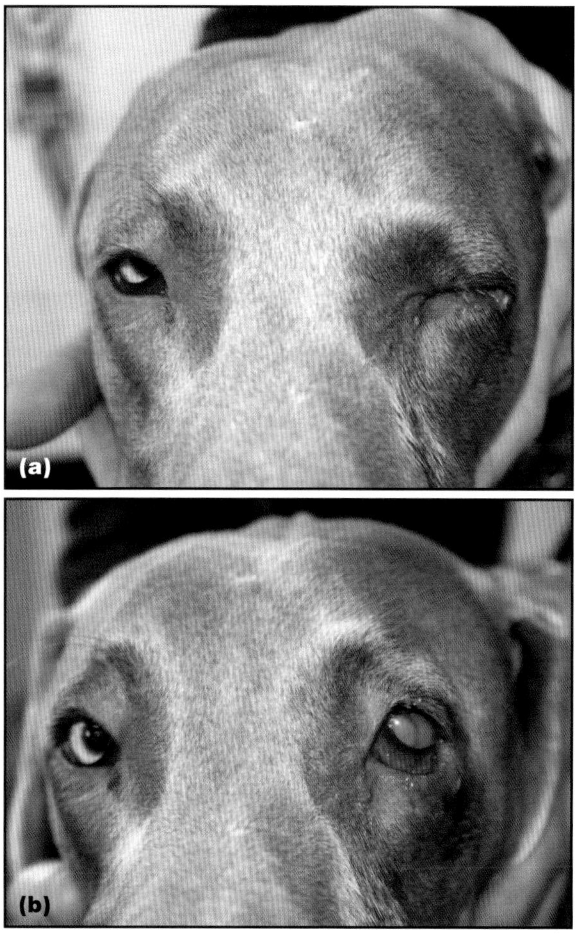

17.8 **(a)** Ocular surface pain before topical local anaesthetic. **(b)** Ocular surface pain after local anaesthetic.

Intraocular pain occurs with glaucoma or uveitis. In contrast to surface pain, intraocular pain is not alleviated by topical anaesthesia. Intraocular pain is characterized by dullness and depression, as well as blepharospasm, lacrimation and photophobia. A patient may present with both ocular surface and intraocular pain, e.g. a corneal insult and secondary uveitis (reflex or axonal uveitis). Systemic non-steroidal anti-inflammatory drugs (NSAIDs) and opioids are widely used to provide ocular analgesia but it is also important to address the ocular condition, for example by reducing IOP in glaucoma, and by relieving painful uveal muscular spasm (associated with miosis in uveitis) with topical atropine.

The degree of pain is predictable in some instances. An example is cataract surgery (phacoemulsification) in which most pain is anticipated at the beginning and end of the surgery, during the corneal incision and suturing, respectively.

Drugs

Local anaesthetics

Although topical local anaesthetics are very effective in providing short-term analgesia for ocular surface pain, they are epitheliotoxic and impede corneal healing, and are therefore contraindicated for the treatment of pain associated with corneal ulcers. Their use should be limited to diagnostic purposes and for analgesia during corneal or conjunctival surgery. Commonly used topical local anaesthetics include proxymetacaine (proparacaine) and amethocaine (tetracaine). Side effects such as pain on application and chemosis are more common with amethocaine than with proxymetacaine. Both drugs have a rapid onset of action (less than 15 seconds). The serial application of topical anaesthetic eye drops has been reported to increase both the duration and depth of surface anaesthesia. Retrobulbar injection of lidocaine or bupivacaine can provide analgesia prior to enucleation, but may be associated with complications and is uncommonly performed.

The safety of intraocular lidocaine for use following intraocular surgery has recently been studied. Intracameral (into the anterior chamber) injection of preservative-free 1% and 2% lidocaine caused no adverse effects in dogs. Another study evaluated the analgesic effects of intravenous lidocaine during intraocular surgery in dogs, administered preemptively as a bolus of 1 mg/kg, followed by a continuous rate infusion of 1.5 mg/kg/h. This provided analgesia equivalent to that attained with an intravenous infusion of morphine (bolus of 0.15 mg/kg followed by 0.1 mg/kg/h). No adverse effects on heart rate or blood pressure were detected.

Non-steroidal anti-inflammatory drugs

NSAIDs can be administered systemically or topically. NSAIDs exhibit analgesic and anti-inflammatory effects by preventing and reducing the production of prostaglandins (see Chapter 9). The release of prostaglandins into the eye can result in various changes (Figure 17.9). Ocular inflammation should be minimized to prevent serious sequelae such as cataract formation, retinal degeneration and glaucoma. Prostaglandins are also thought to be involved in the axonal reflex in dogs, in which an insult to the cornea, conjunctiva or eyelid can cause anterior uveitis.

Systemic NSAIDs such as carprofen and meloxicam are used preoperatively primarily for analgesia and to prevent ocular inflammation during intraocular surgery. Commencing NSAID therapy several hours preoperatively, or the day before if possible, appears to have beneficial ocular effects.

Vascular permeability changes
Vasodilation
Breakdown of blood–aqueous barrier
Miosis
Intraocular pressure changes
Photophobia
Reduction of ocular pain threshold

17.9 Effects of prostaglandins and subsequent inflammation on the eye (Giuliano, 2004).

Topical NSAIDs are used perioperatively and also in the management of ocular inflammatory conditions such as keratitis and uveitis. Flurbiprofen is most commonly used preoperatively for intraocular surgery, in contrast to ketorolac, which is more often used for keratitis and uveitis. The mechanism of action is primarily by the inhibition of prostaglandin production, although a direct analgesic effect of topical NSAIDs on corneal nerve endings has also been postulated. NSAIDs may also reduce aqueous outflow and so should be used cautiously in patients with severe intraocular inflammation when secondary glaucoma is a concern. Topical NSAIDs may adversely affect corneal healing and their use should be minimized or avoided with corneal ulceration.

Opioids

Methadone is a pure mu opioid receptor agonist that produces excellent analgesia, mild sedation and, when compared with morphine, has the advantage of not inducing vomiting. Hydromorphone can be used postoperatively without inducing vomiting, or can be given intravenously for intraoperative analgesia after induction of anaesthesia. Doses can be repeated and more potent opioids, such as fentanyl or alfentanil, administered intraoperatively to achieve the required analgesic effect. Buprenorphine is a partial mu opioid receptor agonist and so may not provide adequate analgesia for ocular surgery associated with a high degree of pain. Furthermore, the intraoperative use of potent mu opioid agonists is restricted as their analgesic effects may be antagonized by buprenorphine. Opioids also affect pupil size and this is discussed later.

Opioid receptors (delta and mu) have been found in the corneal anterior stroma and epithelium of dogs. The use of a topical 1% morphine solution in dogs with corneal ulcers has been shown to provide ocular analgesia with no adverse effect on corneal healing. However topical morphine is rarely, if ever, used in clinical practice.

Ophthalmic drugs relevant to anaesthesia

Figure 17.10 summarizes the potential systemic effects of drugs used in ophthalmology.

Carbonic anhydrase inhibitors

Carbonic anhydrase inhibitors may be used for the long-term treatment of glaucoma. IOP is reduced by the inhibition of carbonic anhydrase, which is involved in aqueous humour production. Systemic carbonic anhydrase inhibitors (e.g. acetazolamide) can produce significant side effects due to reduced bicarbonate ion reabsorption in the proximal renal tubules. Hyperchloraemic metabolic acidosis and hypokalaemia may result, particularly if the animal has a reduced appetite. Clinical signs include vomiting, diarrhoea, polyuria, polydipsia, panting, weakness and anorexia. Topical formulations of carbonic anhydrase inhibitors (e.g. dorzolamide) have now largely replaced their systemic counterparts due to a minimal risk of side effects.

Timing of drug use	Drug	Type of drug	Route of application	Use of drug	Possible systemic effects
Preoperative medication	Acetazolamide	Carbonic anhydrase inhibitor	Systemic – intravenous, oral	Reduce IOP	Metabolic acidosis, hypokalaemia, hyperchloraemia, hypocalcaemia Vomiting, diarrhoea, anorexia, weakness
	Brinzolamide Dorzolamide	Carbonic anhydrase inhibitor	Topical	Reduce IOP	Minimal
	Timolol Betaxolol	Beta-1 selective beta-blocker	Topical	Reduce IOP	Bradycardia
	Apraclonidine	Alpha-2 adrenoceptor agonist	Topical	Reduce IOP Mydriasis (dog) Miosis (cat)	Bradycardia Toxicity in cats
	Pilocarpine	Parasympathomimetic	Topical	Miosis	Vomiting, diarrhoea, arrhythmia, bronchospasm
	Mannitol	Osmotic diuretic	Systemic – intravenous	Reduce IOP	Dehydration, electrolyte disturbances, hyponatraemia, plasma hyperosmolarity Volume expansion When renal failure: risk of hypervolaemia, pulmonary oedema, cardiac failure
	Glycerol	Osmotic diuretic	Systemic – oral	Reduce IOP	Vomiting, diarrhoea, dehydration, risk of renal failure
	Prednisolone	Steroid	Topical	Reduce inflammation	Iatrogenic hyperadrenocorticism
	Flurbiprofen Ketorolac	NSAIDs	Topical	Reduce inflammation	Minimal (generally safe to use with concurrent systemic steroids)
Intraoperative use	Phenylephrine	Alpha-1 adrenergic agonist	Topical	Mydriasis	Hypertension Reflex bradycardia
	Atropine	Anticholinergic	Topical	Mydriasis Cycloplegia (raised IOP)	Tachycardia Cardiac arrhythmias Constipation Hypersalivation (atropine is an anti-sialogogue but is bitter, so topical eyedrops may cause paradoxical hyperptyalism in cats and some dogs) Bronchodilation
	Acetylcholine	Neurotransmitter	Intracameral	Miosis	Bradycardia Hypotension
	Adrenaline	Alpha and beta adrenoreceptor agonist	Intracameral	Mydriasis	Tachycardia Hypertension Arrhythmias

17.10 Systemic effects of drugs used in ophthalmology.

Osmotic diuretics

Osmotic diuretics such as mannitol or glycerol are sometimes used prior to anaesthesia to reduce IOP in acute situations, e.g. lens luxation and glaucoma. Mannitol causes an initial increase in cardiac preload, which may precede dehydration and hyponatraemia caused by diuresis. These drugs should therefore be avoided in cases of renal insufficiency or cardiac failure.

Topical ocular drugs

Topical ocular drugs may have systemic effects due to uptake across the cornea, ocular blood vessels, nasolacrimal and pharyngeal mucosa and by ingestion. Systemic effects are variable and depend on factors such as the dose and volume applied, contact time with the ocular surface and bodyweight. Topical beta-blockers, used in glaucoma, could potentially produce systemic effects of bradycardia and bronchospasm. Pilocarpine, used in the management of glaucoma and keratoconjunctivitis sicca, may cause vomiting. The long-term use of topical prednisolone may produce changes associated with hyperadrenocorticism, e.g. polyuria, polydipsia and increased alkaline phosphatase.

Phenylephrine

Phenylephrine is sometimes used perioperatively for haemostasis due to its vasoconstrictive effect and to produce mydriasis. Hypertension with reflex bradycardia in conscious and anaesthetized dogs due to the topical application of 2.5% and 10% solutions of phenylephrine has been reported. In these cases, very low dose acepromazine (1–5 μg/kg i.v.) was sufficient to treat phenylephrine-induced hypertension. Phenylephrine should be avoided in patients with conditions that are associated with systemic hypertension, such as diabetes mellitus, hyperadrenocorticism and renal disease.

Adrenaline

Intracameral adrenaline (epinephrine) is frequently used during intraocular surgery to produce mydriasis. It is administered either as a single injection or as a component of the intraocular irrigating solution. Tachycardia, hypertension or arrhythmias are occasionally observed after intracameral injection of adrenaline. Petersen-Jones and Clutton (1994) found that by using a balanced anaesthetic technique and maintaining monitored parameters within normal limits, intraocular adrenaline (100 μg injection and irrigating solution containing 2 μg/ml) was not associated with cardiac effects, even in patients anaesthetized with halothane. However, halothane can potentiate catecholamine-induced arrhythmias and is probably best avoided in this situation.

Acetylcholine

Intracameral acetylcholine is sometimes used to achieve miosis after phacoemulsification and has been associated with hypotension and bradycardia in a small number of geriatric humans.

Effects of anaesthetic and analgesic drugs on the eye

Pupil size is a consideration in certain intraocular procedures, such as cataract extraction and lendectomy, when mydriasis is required to enable surgical access. Topical mydriatics, such as tropicamide and atropine, and intracameral adrenaline are examples of drugs frequently administered to produce mydriasis. Over the perioperative period many drugs can potentially affect pupil size, in addition to factors such as anaesthetic depth and the species involved. In the clinical setting where several topical and systemic drugs are used to prepare the animal for ocular surgery, the effects of individual drugs become confusing and unimportant. Different studies have shown different effects for the same drugs but there are some well described examples. Opioids can produce varying effects dependent on the type of opioid and the species. Parenteral morphine and hydromorphone result in miosis in dogs (direct stimulation of the oculomotor nucleus), whereas they cause mydriasis in cats (catecholamine release from the adrenal glands). Ketamine causes a marked mydriasis. Clinical experience has shown methadone to be an excellent choice of opioid for intraocular surgery. Being pure mu agonists, methadone or hydromorphone provide good analgesia and mydriasis appears to be readily achieved with standard topical and intracameral agents. The effects of anaesthetic and analgesic drugs on IOP have been discussed.

Anaesthetic management

Preoperative assessment

A full clinical examination and detailed history from the owner are particularly important as many animals presenting for ocular surgery are geriatric and may have concurrent disease. Diabetic patients should ideally be stabilized prior to general anaesthesia (see Chapter 25). The anaesthetic regime will depend on several factors, and animals can broadly be divided into those requiring intraocular surgery, ocular surface surgery and adnexal surgery (Figures 17.11 and 17.12).

An important consideration is whether preoperative increases in IOP will be detrimental to the eye. Examples include deep corneal ulcer, full thickness corneal laceration, iris prolapse and anterior lens luxation. In these cases preoperative rises in IOP should be avoided by using harnesses rather than neck leads, by using gentle restraint during examination and intravenous catheter placement and by using sedation as appropriate, particularly to reduce barking. Premedication producing a moderate to marked degree of sedation has the advantage of reducing the amount of restraint needed to handle fractious or boisterous animals with fragile globes. Acepromazine and methadone (or buprenorphine or hydromorphone) are good choices for routine cases; low doses of medetomidine or midazolam (in cats) can improve sedation. As medetomidine and hydromorphone can induce vomiting, each case should be assessed individually to determine the greatest risk to the eye. Blind or partially sighted animals may be particularly nervous in a new environment and so verbal reassurance, gentle handling and careful leading when walking are important.

Age
Concurrent disease
Diabetes mellitus Hyperadrenocorticism Brachycephalic obstructive airway syndrome Cardiac disease Systemic hypertension Renal disease Hypothyroidism
Current medication
NSAIDs Steroids Carbonic anhydrase inhibitors
Renal and hepatic function
Affects drug selection, e.g. muscle relaxants – vecuronium avoided in hepatic disease, pancuronium avoided in renal disease Avoid osmotic diuretics in renal disease or cardiac failure
Temperament of patient
Sedation may be required in aggressive, boisterous animals
Analgesia requirements
E.g. intraocular and corneal surgery – local anaesthetics reduce response to corneal incision and suturing
When increases in IOP should be minimized
Pre- and intraoperative most important for deep corneal ulcers Intra- and postoperative important during phacoemulsification or for cataract surgery
Requirement for muscle relaxants
Often needed for corneal and intraocular surgery Must provide IPPV, monitor degree of neuromuscular block, reversal agents

17.11 Considerations in formulating an anaesthetic plan for ocular surgery.

Site of ocular surgery	Surgical procedure	Considerations	Muscle relaxants required
Intraocular	Phacoemulsification for cataracts	• May be diabetic • May be blind • Avoid ↑ IOP intra- and postoperatively • Corneal incision and sutures likely to produce most response to surgery	Yes
	Lendectomy for lens luxation	• Avoid ↑ IOP perioperatively • May be glaucomatous and painful	Yes
	Intraocular tumour excision or biopsy	• Avoid ↑ IOP intra- and postoperatively • Haemorrhage risk	Yes
	Ocular trauma, intraocular foreign body	• May involve any intraocular structures • Assess for and treat other injuries, e.g. head trauma • Analgesia • Avoid ↑ IOP • May require preoperative stabilization if haemorrhage or shock	Yes
Corneal surface	Keratectomy	• Analgesia – topical local anaesthetics • Minimize frequency of treatment with drugs that delay corneal healing, e.g. topical anaesthetics, topical NSAIDs	Yes, but not essential
	Conjunctival or corneal grafts, corneal trauma, iris prolapse	• Avoid ↑ IOP as risk of globe rupture • Pain with superficial ulcers, corneal surgery – topical local anaesthetics • Caution with drugs that delay corneal healing	Yes
	Corneal foreign body removal	• Avoid ↑ IOP as risk of globe rupture • Pain – topical local anaesthetics • Caution with drugs that delay corneal healing	Yes, but not essential
Adnexal	Eyelid and eyelash surgery	• Soft tissue pain and inflammation – analgesia with NSAIDs and opioids • Risk of self-trauma postoperatively	No
	Nictitans gland surgery		
	Parotid duct transposition		
	Tumour resection		
	Biopsy		
Globe	Enucleation	• Risk of haemorrhage • Avoid ↑ IOP if risk of globe rupture • Monitor for oculocardiac reflex • Retrobulbar anaesthesia	No

17.12 Considerations relevant to different types of ocular surgeries.

An intravenous catheter placed in the saphenous vein, as opposed to the cephalic vein, improves venous access during ocular surgery. Intravenous induction, with combinations of propofol or thiopental with diazepam (0.1–0.2 mg/kg i.v.) and/or fentanyl (2 μg/kg i.v.), has several advantages over a mask induction with inhalational agents for patients with fragile globes. The mask itself can exert external pressure on the globe and the slower induction with inhalational agents may result in more struggling and stress, all potential causes of raised IOP. Brachycephalic breeds are predisposed to corneal ulcers, which may require surgical intervention. Preoxygenation and a rapid induction sequence are particularly important in these breeds to allow endotracheal intubation and control of ventilation. Hypoventilation should be avoided during induction to prevent hypercapnia and an increase in IOP.

A cuffed or tight-fitting (in cats) endotracheal tube is important, particularly as IPPV will be needed when muscle relaxants are administered. Armoured endotracheal tubes are more resilient to kinking, and right-angled connectors are also useful but increase dead space. Securing the tube to the mandible avoids interference with the surgical site. As space may be restricted near the patient's head by surgical equipment, elongated anaesthetic breathing systems may be needed (Figure 17.13). Tubing with a smooth

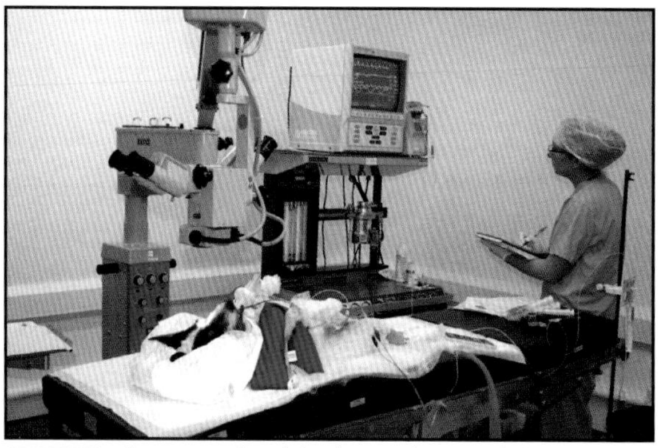

17.13 An example of the layout in an ophthalmology theatre.

internal surface will help to reduce resistance in long breathing systems, but IPPV may be needed to prevent hypoventilation.

Maintenance

Isoflurane and sevoflurane vaporized in oxygen and nitrous oxide are excellent choices for maintaining anaesthesia. Halothane may potentiate arrhythmias associated with intraocular adrenaline. Isoflurane and sevoflurane are associated with rapid recoveries from anaesthesia, an advantage in diabetic patients. An isotonic crystalloid such as lactated Ringer's solution is usually infused intravenously at 10 ml/kg/h during anaesthesia. Glucose-containing intravenous fluids may be required in hypoglycaemic diabetic animals, e.g. 5% glucose in either 0.9% saline solution or lactated Ringer's solution.

Attention should be paid to maintaining the animal's body temperature, particularly as some ocular surgeries are time consuming and hypothermia can affect the duration of action of drugs, e.g. the degradation of atracurium is temperature dependent. During phacoemulsification the irrigating solution can leak on to the patient's head, further cooling the patient. Heat and moisture exchangers, low-flow anaesthesia (using a circle system or mini Lack where possible), insulation, air warmers and water-beds are all ways to prevent hypothermia.

Instrumentation of the patient must be completed before the surgeon drapes the surgical site, as access is then very limited (Figure 17.14). Capnography is extremely useful to ensure that end-tidal carbon dioxide levels are maintained within normal limits during IPPV. Disconnection of the endotracheal tube or connector from the anaesthetic breathing system can occur and is more difficult to detect immediately without a capnograph trace. Pulse oximetry probes can be placed on the tongue, or on more accessible sites such as the vulva, prepuce, digits or tail. Monitoring of heart rate and blood pressure is important for several reasons but especially because there are potential systemic effects associated with topical and intracameral drugs (see above). Also there is limited access to the head to monitor depth of anaesthesia, and pain and a light plane of anaesthesia during neuromuscular blockade can produce tachycardia and hypertension. Direct monitoring using an arterial catheter (e.g. placed in the dorsal pedal artery) is the most accurate way to measure blood pressure and allows collection of arterial blood samples to measure serial glucose levels in diabetic patients. Doppler and oscillometric non-invasive blood pressure measurements are easy to perform, but can be inaccurate in certain circumstances (see Chapter 7).

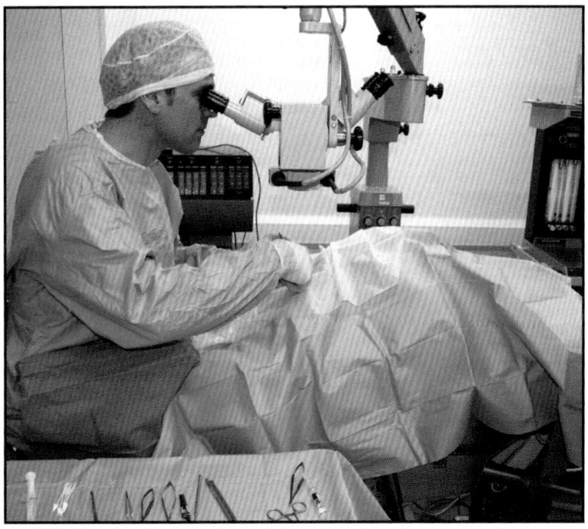

17.14 An illustration of the restricted access for the anaesthetist.

The peroneal nerve of the hindlimb is the most readily accessible site to attach a nerve stimulator and this should not interfere with the surgeon (Figure 17.15).

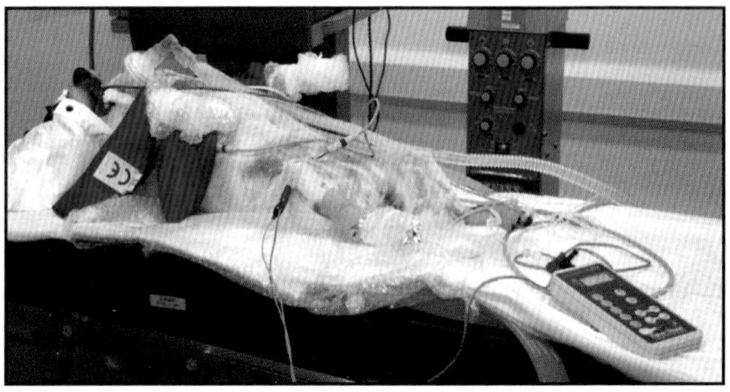

17.15 Photograph showing the positioning of electrodes for stimulation of the peroneal nerve.

Recovery

Adequate reversal of neuromuscular blockade should be monitored using a nerve stimulator. The nerve stimulator may be used to ensure that there are four equal twitches on the train-of-four mode, and two equal twitches on a double-burst stimulation mode before allowing the patient to attempt to ventilate spontaneously. This is achieved either by allowing the neuromuscular-blocking agent to wear off, or by administering an anticholinesterase and anticholinergic combination (see Chapter 15). The adequacy of spontaneous ventilation can be assessed by observing the patient's chest movements and by ensuring normal end-tidal carbon dioxide concentrations (35–45 mmHg) and pulse oximetry readings (over 95%) before extubation. Tidal volume can be measured with a Wright's respirometer attached to the endotracheal tube, but these delicate devices can be expensive to purchase. Alternatively, to ensure there is enough respiratory muscle tone, the rebreathing bag can be detached (do this in a well ventilated room) and a hand temporarily placed under the bag attachment pipe to seal the circuit. When the dog breathes, the lack of gas reservoir will cause the circuit pressure to become negative. A dog should be able to produce -10 to -15 cmH_2O circuit pressure. Ensure the bag is replaced as soon as the test has been performed.

The eye may be more fragile on recovery than induction, e.g. phacoemulsification, or less fragile, e.g. conjunctival graft. However, in all cases action should be taken to prevent rises in IOP. Extubation should avoid eliciting a cough, and so may be performed earlier than normal in appropriate animals. The recovery from anaesthesia and the postoperative period should be as calm as possible to minimize the risk of intraocular haemorrhage or ocular trauma. Gentle, quiet handling and good analgesia are essential. Sedation is important in excited and disorientated animals and those who are barking or crying despite analgesia. Physical trauma to the eye can occur while the patient is moved, during a poor recovery or by scratching or rubbing the ocular region. Applying bandages to distal limbs and the use of Elizabethan collars can help prevent self-trauma. Opioids can be repeated after surgery while the patient is hospitalized and systemic NSAIDs are often continued longer into the postoperative period. Acepromazine (20 μg/kg i.v.) is also useful in the postoperative period to lessen dysphoria and restlessness.

Acknowledgements

The author would like to thank Heidi Featherstone BVetMed DVOphthal Dip ECVO MRCVS, Davies Veterinary Specialists, UK for reviewing this chapter and for ophthalmology advice and Dr David Gould BSc(Hons) BVM&S PhD DVOphthal Dip ECVO MRCVS, Davies Veterinary Specialists, UK for ophthalmology advice.

References and further reading

Almeida DE, Rezende ML, Nunes N and Laus JL (2004) Evaluation of intraocular pressure in association with cardiovascular parameters in normocapnic dogs anaesthetised with sevoflurane and desflurane. *Veterinary Ophthalmology* **7(4)**, 265–269

Barrett PM, Scagliotti RH, Merideth RE, Jackson PA and Alarcon FL (1991) Absolute corneal sensitivity and corneal trigeminal nerve anatomy in normal dogs. *Progress in Veterinary and Comparative Ophthalmology* **1(4)**, 245–254

Bartfield JM, Holmes TJ and Raccio-Robak N (1994) A comparison of proparacaine and tetracaine eye anaesthetics. *Academic Emergency Medicine* **1(4)**, 364–367

Biricik HS, Ceylan C, Sakar M (2004) Effects of pethidine on tear production in dogs. *Veterinary Record* **155(18)**, 564–565

Blocker T and van der Woerdt A (2001) A comparison of corneal sensitivity between Brachycephalic and Domestic Short-haired cats. *Veterinary Ophthalmology* **4(2)**, 127–130

Brinkley Jr JR and Henrick A (1984) Vascular hypotension and bradycardia following intraocular injection of acetylcholine during cataract surgery. *American Journal of Ophthalmology* **97(1)**, 40–42

Chahory S, Clerc B, Guez J and Sanaa M (2003) Intraocular pressure development after cataract surgery: a prospective study in 50 dogs (1998–2000). *Veterinary Ophthalmology* **6(2)**, 105–112

Chen X, Gallar J and Belmonte C (1997) Reduction by anti-inflammatory drugs of the response of corneal sensory nerve fibres to chemical irritation. *Investigative Ophthalmology and Visual Science* **38(10)**, 1944–1953

Clutton RE, Boyd C, Richards DLS and Schwink K (1988) Significance of the oculocardiac reflex during ophthalmic surgery in the dog. *Journal of Small Animal Practice* **29**, 573–579

DiBartola SP (2000) Metabolic acid–base disorders. In: *Fluid therapy in Small Animal Practice, 2nd edn*, ed. SP DiBartola, pp. 211–240. WB Saunders, Philadelphia

Dodam JR, Branson KR and Martin DD (1998) Effects of intramuscular sedative and opioid combinations on tear production in dogs. *Veterinary Ophthalmology* **1(1)**, 57–59

Erickson SR and Yousuf MJ (1991) Hypotension and bradycardia possibly associated with intraocular injection of acetylcholine. *DICP: the Annals of Pharmacotherapy* **25(11)**, 1178–1180

Frischmeyer KJ, Miller PE, Bellay Y, Smedes SL and Brunson DB (1993) Parenteral anticholinergics in dogs with normal and elevated intraocular pressure. *Veterinary Surgery* **22(3)**, 230–234

Gerding PA, Turner TL, Hamor RE and Schaeffer DJ (2004) Effects of intracameral injection of preservative-free lidocaine on the anterior segment of the eyes in dogs. *American Journal of Veterinary Research* **65(10)**, 1325–1330

Giuliano EA (2004) Nonsteroidal anti-inflammatory drugs in veterinary ophthalmology. *Veterinary Clinics of North America: Small Animal Practice* **34(3)**, 707–723

Gum GG, Gelatt KN and Ofri R (1999) Physiology of the eye. In: *Veterinary Ophthalmology, 3rd edn*, ed. KN Gelatt, p. 154. Lippincott, Williams and Wilkins, Philadelphia

Hendrix DVH, Ward DA and Barnhill MA (2002) Effects of anti-inflammatory drugs and preservatives on morphologic characteristics and migration of canine corneal epithelial cells in tissue culture. *Veterinary Ophthalmology* **5(2)**, 127–135

Herring IP, Bobofchak MA, Landry MP and Ward DL (2005) Duration of effect and effect of multiple doses of topical ophthalmic 0.5% proparacaine hydrochloride in clinically normal dogs. *American Journal of Veterinary Research* **66(1)**, 77–80

Herring IP, Jacobson JD and Pickett JP (2004) Cardiovascular effects of topical ophthalmic 10% phenylephrine in dogs. *Veterinary Ophthalmology* **7(1)**, 41–46

Herring IP, Pickett JP, Champagne ES and Marini M (2000) Evaluation of aqueous tear production in dogs following general anaesthesia. *Journal of the American Animal Hospital Association* **36(5)**, 427–430

Hofmeister EH, Mosunic CB, Torres BT *et al.* (2005) Effects of diazepam, ketamine, and their combination on intraocular pressure in normal dogs (Abstract). *Veterinary Anaesthesia and Analgesia* **32(4)**, 237

Krohne SG, Blair MJ, Bingaman D and Gionfriddo JR (1998) Carprofen inhibition of flare in the dog measured by laser flare photometry. *Veterinary Ophthalmology* **1(2–3)**, 81–84

McMurphy RM, Davidson HJ and Hodgson DS (2004) Effects of atracurium on intraocular pressure, eye position, and blood pressure in eucapnic and hypocapnic isoflurane-anaesthetised dogs. *American Journal of Veterinary Research* **65(2)**, 179–182

Millichamp NJ, Dziezyc J and Olsen JW (1991) Effect of flurbiprofen on facility of aqueous outflow in the eyes of dogs. *American Journal of Veterinary Research* **52(9)**, 1448–1451

Pascoe PJ, Ilkiw JE, Stiles J and Smith EM (1994) Arterial hypertension associated with topical ocular phenylephrine in dogs. *Journal of the American Veterinary Medical Association* **205(11)**, 1562–1564

Petersen-Jones SM and Clutton RE (1994) Use of intraocular adrenaline during cataract extractions in dogs. *Veterinary Record* **135(13)**, 306–307

Samuelson DA (1999) Ophthalmic anatomy. In: *Veterinary Ophthalmology, 3rd edn*, ed. KN Gelatt, p. 46. Lippincott, Williams and Wilkins, Philadelphia

Smith LJ, Bentley E, Shih A and Miller PE (2004) Systemic lidocaine infusion as an analgesic for intraocular surgery in dogs: a pilot study. *Veterinary Anaesthesia and Analgesia* **31(1)**, 53–63

Smith PJ, Brooks DE, Lazarus JA, Kubilis PS and Gelatt KN (1996) Ocular hypertension following cataract surgery in dogs: 139 cases (1992–1993). *Journal of the American Veterinary Medical Association* **209(1)**, 105–111

Stephan DD, Vestre WA, Stiles J and Krohne S (2003) Changes in intraocular pressure and pupil size following intramuscular administration of hydromorphone hydrochloride and acepromazine in clinically normal dogs. *Veterinary Ophthalmology* **6(1)**, 73–76

Stiles J, Honda CN, Krohne SG and Kazacos EA (2003) Effect of topical administration of 1% morphine sulphate solution on signs of pain and corneal wound healing in dogs. *American Journal of Veterinary Research* **64(7)**, 813–818

Sullivan TC, Hellyer PW, Lee DD and Davidson MG (1998) Respiratory function and extraocular muscle paralysis following administration of pancuronium bromide in dogs. *Veterinary Ophthalmology* **1(2-3)**, 125–128

Wang YM, Chung KC, Lu HF *et al.* (2003) Lidocaine: the optimal timing of intravenous administration in attenuation of increase of intraocular pressure during tracheal intubation. *Acta Anaesthesiologica Sinica* **41(2)**, 71–75

Ward DA (1999) Clinical pharmacology and therapeutics. In: *Veterinary Ophthalmology, 3rd edn*, ed. KN Gelatt, pp. 339–340. Lippincott, Williams and Wilkins, Philadelphia

Ward DA, Ferguson DC, Ward SL, Green K and Kaswan RL (1992) Comparison of the blood-aqueous barrier stabilising effects of steroidal and non steroidal anti-inflammatory agents in the dog. *Progress in Veterinary and Comparative Ophthalmology* **2(3)**, 117–124

Wilkie DA (1990) Control of ocular inflammation. *Veterinary Clinics of North America: Small Animal Practice* **20(3)**, 693–713

18

Dental and oral surgery

Tanya Duke-Novakovski

Introduction

The patient population presented for dental or maxillofacial surgery can be varied, but many patients will pose a greater anaesthetic risk because of their age, brachycephalic anatomy or due to airway problems caused by trauma or cancer. Procedures involving the head and neck can pose airway security concerns, risk of haemorrhage and difficult monitoring conditions if access to the head is denied. This chapter addresses some of the concerns regarding administration of an anaesthetic to a patient presented for dental or oral surgery.

Principles and potential problems

Airway security

The airway should be adequately secured using endotracheal intubation, as debris, blood and irrigation fluids in the oral cavity will enter unprotected airways and cause aspiration pneumonia. This potentially fatal condition is easier to prevent than cure. Endotracheal tubes should be checked prior to use for defective cuffs and obstructed lumens. The length should be cut to fit the patient from mid neck to the level of the incisor teeth. A properly positioned endotracheal tube will reduce apparatus dead space and the risk of endobronchial intubation. Excessively long endotracheal tubes protruding from the oral cavity are prone to kinking and are difficult to secure to the jaw with gauze bandage. Knots placed around the endotracheal tube itself can become loose in the presence of irrigation fluids and saliva, and increase the risk of accidental extubation. Knots should be tied around the endotracheal tube connector for greater security and not tied around the endotracheal tube. Pharyngeal packing can be used for greater airway security, but it is imperative that it is removed before extubation. A length of damp gauze bandage is superior to individual surgical swabs since bandage can be packed tightly around the endotracheal tube, and is less likely to be forgotten if the free end is left visible.

During manipulations of the head, kinking of the endotracheal tube, extubation and circuit disconnections are possible. These problems are common during diagnostic imaging as the patient is positioned for radiographs in a darkened room. Flexion of the neck has the potential to move the caudal tip of the endotracheal tube into a bronchus, which can cause problems such as hypercapnia and potential hypoxaemia. The inflated cuff can cause damage to the mucosal lining of the trachea, and should be deflated and reinflated after extreme position changes. Overinflation of the cuff, and/or rotating patient position through 180 degrees without temporarily disconnecting the endotracheal tube from the circuit can cause tracheal damage or rupture, especially in cats. Inspiration against an obstructed airway caused by a kinked endotracheal tube may lead to dyspnoea, cyanosis and pulmonary oedema. If extreme flexion of the head is necessary, a guarded endotracheal tube can be used. These tubes have a stiff, spiral wire running through the endotracheal tube wall and are less prone to kinking. In spontaneously breathing patients, inadvertent disconnection allows air breathing, reduced inspired anaesthetic concentrations and decreased depth of anaesthesia. Surgical drapes conceal accidental circuit disconnection unless sudden emptying of the rebreathing bag is observed. Apnoea alarms and capnographs are useful for detecting accidental disconnection.

Long anaesthetic periods

Lengthy procedures require close attention to life support. Oxygen should be delivered at an inspired concentration of at least 33% to compensate for the anaesthesia-induced deterioration in pulmonary function, even in healthy, young patients (hypoventilation, reduced functional residual capacity, atelectasis and ventilation/perfusion mismatch).

Reduced cardiac output and arterial blood pressure produced by the administration of anaesthetic drugs should be offset by fluid therapy via an intravenous catheter. Intravenous Hartmann's (lactated Ringer's) solution should be administered at a rate of 10 ml/kg/h. Catheters are best removed when the patient is fully conscious following recovery from anaesthesia.

Hypothermia results from lengthy anaesthesia time and the use of cool irrigation fluids. Hypothermia can cause anticholinergic-resistant bradycardia, reduced cardiac output and haemoconcentration. Cardiac fibrillation can occur at a body temperature of about 28°C. Requirements for anaesthetic agents are reduced due to hypothermia and care should be taken not to administer a relative overdose of anaesthetic agent. External heat can be supplied with heating blankets, warmed intravenous and irrigation fluids, and commercial forced warm air heating devices. Thermal injuries due to 'hot spots' are rarely produced by circulating warm water blankets, but may occur when using electrical heating mats. Patient insulation can be provided with towels, bubble packing or aluminium foil. Hyperthermia can occasionally occur in large, heavy-coated dogs connected to rebreathing circuits for long periods. Active cooling should be initiated before damage occurs to vital organs. Body temperature should be monitored during long procedures in order to avoid hypo- or hyperthermia.

Haemorrhage

Blood loss and hypovolaemia may occur in some procedures. Loss should be estimated either by weighing blood-soaked swabs or measuring the amount of blood in a suction jar. Intravenous fluid rates should be increased to 30–40 ml/kg/h to compensate for hypotension. As blood loss approaches 20% of circulating volume, fluid replacement therapy with whole blood or packed red blood cells should begin. Colloids such as gelatins, dextrans or starches can be used at a dose of up to 20 ml/kg, but while they support tissue perfusion, they are not a replacement for red blood cells. If haemorrhage is anticipated during the procedure, cats and dogs should be cross-matched with a healthy donor or blood-typed beforehand.

An alternative to cross-matching with a donor is autologous transfusion. A few days prior to surgery, 10% of the patient's blood volume is removed and replaced with intravenous fluids. The blood is stored at 4°C in acid-citrate-dextrose transfusion packs until required. Before potentially haemorrhagic procedures, the patient should have a full haemotological examination and clotting profile performed. See Chapter 16 for further information.

If haemorrhage is anticipated, it might be prudent to avoid vasodilating drugs such as acepromazine in the premedication. Some veterinary surgeons might argue, however, that moderate hypotension would decrease blood loss.

Haemostasis

Vasoconstrictors such as adrenaline should not be used for haemostasis if the patient is anaesthetized with halothane. A few drops can be used with caution in a 1:20,000 dilution if the patient is anaesthetized with isoflurane, and monitored with an electrocardiogram. Phenylephrine at the same dilution is less arrhythmogenic, but even with a few drops, this drug can be absorbed and increase systemic vascular resistance through alpha-adrenergic receptor stimulation.

Analgesia

The head and neck are sensitive areas of the body, and some procedures produce strong surgical stimulation, resulting in a variable plane of anaesthesia. A widely varying plane is often the result of poor analgesia. Opioids should be provided at the time of premedication, and local nerve blocks considered prior to surgery (details of nerve blocks are provided in Chapter 10). Further increments of injectable opioids can be provided intraoperatively during lengthy procedures and/or nitrous oxide can be administered. Analgesics should be continued into the recovery period.

Patients requiring dental procedures

Geriatric patients

Dental procedures range from simple deciduous teeth extractions in young, healthy patients to lengthy, complicated procedures in older, systemically compromised patients. Most patients requiring anaesthesia for dental procedures are considered to be geriatric (75–80% of the animal's anticipated lifespan is completed). Even clinically healthy geriatric patients have physiological changes that can influence the course of anaesthesia. Older patients are distressed and confused by a change in routine and require constant reassurance. Age-related changes in the cardiopulmonary system include:

- Decreased ability to compensate for blood pressure and circulating volume changes
- 30% decrease in cardiac output
- Decreased lung compliance
- High small-airway closing volume
- Decreased partial pressure of oxygen in arterial blood (P_aO_2).

A noticeable increase in circulation time is seen during induction, and further increments of injectable anaesthetic agents should not be given too soon. Chapter 28 contains further information on geriatric anaesthesia.

Brachycephalic patients

Many brachycephalic patients will require dental or maxillofacial procedures, and these patients pose an anaesthetic challenge. Upper airway obstruction from stenotic nares, elongated soft palate, laryngeal saccule eversion, laryngeal collapse, laryngeal oedema and hypoplastic trachea should be anticipated. The degree of obstruction may be assessed from the clinical history and pre-anaesthetic physical examination. Upper airway problems may benefit from surgical correction at the time of planned dental procedures. Cor pulmonale may result from severe chronic upper airway obstruction and any clinical signs thereof should be investigated further. Induction of anaesthesia causes relaxation of pharyngeal musculature and upper airway obstruction is increased until endotracheal intubation is performed, and the obstruction bypassed with the endotracheal tube. Xylazine and medetomidine should be avoided during premedication as these drugs exacerbate upper airway obstruction through their muscle relaxation properties.

Mild sedation using a low dose of acepromazine with either buprenorphine or pethidine (meperidine) or butorphanol is usually adequate in dogs. Boxers can be prone to vasovagal syncope with acepromazine, and either they should concurrently receive an anticholinergic or the phenothiazine should be avoided. Fractious dogs should not be muzzled, but an Elizabethan collar can be useful to prevent handlers from being injured. Preoxygenation by mask for 5 minutes will help prevent hypoxaemia during induction, but mask induction using an inhalational agent should be avoided where possible. Mask induction takes longer and the dog is prone to further airway obstruction until conditions are suitable for intubation. A rapid, reliable induction technique should be used with such drugs as thiopental, propofol, alfaxalone or ketamine/benzodiazepine, and endotracheal intubation rapidly performed. Alfaxalone/alfadolone can be used in brachycephalic cats.

The best way to avoid problems with upper airway obstruction following extubation is to use anaesthetic drugs with rapid elimination. Induction drugs with relatively short plasma half-lives, such as propofol or a ketamine/benzodiazepine combination, ensure a rapid recovery, and return of the patient's ability to maintain its own airway. Isoflurane and sevoflurane provide more rapid recoveries than halothane.

Even by taking these precautions, once the endotracheal tube is removed, there is still a risk of obstruction until the patient is fully awake. Obstruction can be alleviated by pulling the patient's tongue forwards and keeping its mouth open to encourage mouth breathing. Hypoxia can be alleviated by administering oxygen. Placing the patient in sternal recumbency allows more uniform expansion of the lungs, and may promote more rapid return to consciousness.

If dyspnoea is observed because the extubated patient has been administered a potent mu opioid agonist, such as morphine, methadone or hydromorphone, for postoperative analgesia, an alternative to reintubation may be to reverse the agonist. Low doses of naloxone can be used to reverse sedation, although some analgesia may also be reversed. Butorphanol (0.2 mg/kg i.v. over 1 minute) can also be used for reversal and to provide analgesia.

Anaesthesia for routine dental procedures

Pre-anaesthetic preparation

It is important to ensure that a thorough clinical examination has been performed on the patient prior to administration of an anaesthetic. Many procedures are considered to be routine, and clients may believe that anaesthetizing their pet will be straightforward. In older patients there is increasing likelihood of systemic disease, which may have gone unnoticed by the client. A thorough examination will help to eliminate unforeseen problems in the perioperative period. Elective procedures can be delayed until the patient is stable, and urgent procedures can be undertaken with the veterinary surgeon (and client) cognizant of problems that may occur. Further information regarding systemic disease and anaesthesia may be found in other chapters on anaesthetic management.

Premedication

Many geriatric patients are likely to be distressed by the upheaval in their routine and association with strangers in unfamiliar surroundings. Premedication provides a calming effect and makes the patient more manageable. Important considerations for dental anaesthesia include the provision of intraoperative analgesia with an opioid, the ability to reduce the amount of major depressant anaesthetic agents and the reduction of their undesirable side effects. Combinations of acepromazine and opioid are suitable in most cases. Alpha-2 adrenoceptor agonists should only be used in young, healthy patients, and only when there is a full appreciation of the side effects. Oxygen and ventilatory support must be available when these drugs are used.

Anticholinergics can reduce undesirable parasympathetic effects, such as salivation and bradycardia. The duration of action of glycopyrronium is 2–3 hours and it is a more potent antisialogogue than atropine. Further information can be found in Chapter 12.

Induction

The passage from consciousness to unconsciousness should be smooth and excitement-free. In healthy dogs and cats, thiopental, propofol, ketamine/benzodiazepine and steroid-based anaesthetics (alfaxalone or alfaxalone/alfadolone) are recommended as they produce a reliable, rapid induction. In patients with cardiopulmonary compromise or severe hepatic or renal disease, they should be used with caution (see Chapters 19, 20 and 22). Xylazine/ketamine or medetomidine/ketamine combinations for induction of anaesthesia should not be used in geriatric or debilitated patients. See Chapter 13 for further details regarding injectable drugs.

Maintenance

For short procedures of less than 15 minutes, incremental boluses of short-acting injectable anaesthetics, such as thiopental, propofol, benzodiazepine/ketamine and alfaxalone or alfaxalone/alfadolone, can be used. Barbiturates and propofol, however, do not provide effective analgesia for invasive procedures. Dental procedures can be lengthy and this will increase risks of deterioration in physiological status, especially in older, compromised patients, and anaesthesia is best maintained with an inhalational technique. The technique involves the administration of oxygen and greatly improves oxygen delivery at tissue levels.

Anaesthetic management for trauma and elective oral surgery

Patients requiring elective procedures, such as hemimandibulectomy, can be thoroughly examined, and any concurrent disease stabilized before anaesthesia is induced. Any consequences of the surgical procedure, such as haemorrhage, should be anticipated. The upper airway should be examined for potential difficulties with intubation. Patients with traumatic injuries must be stabilized, and other potential injuries addressed before anaesthesia. Most procedures can be managed with conventional orotracheal intubation, but occasionally passing the endotracheal tube through a pharyngotomy site, or a tracheotomy, may be necessary (see below).

Preoxygenation should be performed in case there are difficulties with intubation. Once the patient is stable, rapid-sequence induction techniques after light premedication (if used at all) can be used to establish an airway. Maintenance of anaesthesia can be provided by inhalational techniques. Positioning for surgery is important and the endotracheal tube must be securely tied to prevent accidental disconnections. Right-angled adaptors can be attached to the endotracheal tube adaptor to enable breathing systems to be diverted away from the surgical site. Breathing systems with heavy valves at the patient end (Magill) should be avoided since they could place drag on the endotracheal tube.

Surgical drapes may make examination of eye position impossible and monitors measuring end-tidal anaesthetic agent concentration are expensive, although very useful for this type of procedure. Less expensive pulse oximeters and capnographs can aid decisions regarding anaesthetic depth. It should be ensured that any monitoring probes (for example pulse oximeter probes) placed on the head area are secured, otherwise they may become dislodged during the procedure and can be difficult to replace. Alternative sites should be used if possible.

Recovery and analgesia

Good nursing, analgesics, warmth, fluids and continuous observation will help to eliminate postoperative problems. Before extubation the pharyngeal area should be inspected for fluids, blood clots and foreign objects so they can be removed. Suction apparatus is useful to ensure that the pharynx is dry. Cats should be closely watched during recovery, as they are prone to upper airway obstruction if the nasal passages are occluded with blood and debris. Until cats are fully recovered from the effects of the anaesthetic, they appear reluctant to mouth breathe after extubation. Anaesthetic agents providing rapid recovery are useful to decrease the time from extubation until the cat is fully aware of its surroundings.

Delirious recoveries may be the result of pain, excitatory anaesthetic agents or hypoxia.

Patients recovering from oral surgery often try to rub their faces, and sedatives, analgesics or an Elizabethan collar may help prevent self-inflicted trauma. For restless patients, acepromazine can be administered at a low dose (0.02 mg/kg i.v.). Some patients will greatly benefit from oxygen administration by mask or nasal catheter during recovery.

Analgesics should be provided perioperatively (see Chapters 9 and 10). Opioids are the analgesics of choice for the perioperative period and can be administered systemically. Continuous infusions of morphine, lidocaine and/or ketamine can be used during the procedure and may be continued into the recovery period when pain is anticipated to be severe (see Chapter 13). Regional nerve blockade can be performed before or after surgery using mandibular and infraorbital blocks with local anaesthetics. Placing the local anaesthetic before surgery can decrease the amount of other anaesthetic drugs needed and lower the postoperative requirement for analgesics. Fentanyl patches and newer non-steroidal anti-inflammatory drugs, such as meloxicam or carprofen, are also useful.

Special techniques

The difficult airway

Occasionally, alternative techniques are required to secure an airway. Conventional laryngoscopy and intubation techniques may be impossible to perform in traumatized patients, patients with cancer and patients who are unable to open their jaws wide enough for visualization. The following techniques can be attempted if necessary. A wide range of endotracheal tube diameters should be selected for all techniques. An emergency tracheotomy kit should also be available in case the patient gets into difficulties during the intubation process. Anaesthesia can be maintained using incremental doses of short-acting injectable anaesthetic drugs until inhalational techniques can be used. Preoxygenation for a measured 5 minutes is necessary for all patients with anticipated intubation difficulties. A feeding tube attached to an oxygen line may be slid into the trachea temporarily to insufflate oxygen if the patient becomes hypoxaemic during the intubation procedure.

Placing an endotracheal tube using a guide stylet

A fairly stiff feeding tube or equivalent plastic tubing can be used as a guide over which an endotracheal tube can be placed into the trachea. The guide is twice the length of the endotracheal tube and should be carefully inserted into the trachea using a laryngoscope. The laryngoscope is then removed and the chosen endotracheal tube threaded over the stylet. The stylet will guide the endotracheal tube into the correct position.

Placing an endotracheal tube using a bronchoscope

The endotracheal tube can be placed over a narrow bronchoscope and the distal end of the bronchoscope directed into the trachea. Once the bronchoscope is in the trachea the endotracheal tube can be slid off the bronchoscope and secured. This technique has limitations in small dogs and cats as the narrowest diameter of bronchoscope available may not be small enough.

Retrograde placement of an endotracheal tube

A long guide wire, such as a stiff feeding tube, is inserted into the trachea via a small tracheotomy and passed into the mouth. An endotracheal tube is then passed over the end within the mouth and inserted into the trachea. The guide is then removed.

Pharyngotomy for diversion of the endotracheal tube

Occasionally, the endotracheal tube may be required to pass from the trachea through a temporary pharyngotomy to connect with the breathing circuit. This allows the surgeon access to the oral cavity without the hindrance of an endotracheal tube. Once the endotracheal tube is in place, a pharyngotomy can be performed and the proximal end of the endotracheal tube removed from its adaptor and passed mediolaterally through the pharyngotomy site, and the adaptor reconnected allowing anaesthesia to continue with an inhalational technique. Injectable anaesthetic drugs (propofol, thiopental) may be required to maintain anaesthesia during movement of the endotracheal tube.

After surgical preparation of the cervical area and angle of the mandible, an index finger is introduced into the oral cavity. The finger locates the pyriform sinus rostral to the epihyoid bone (Figure 18.1). The tissues are incised and dissected through to the oral cavity. The forceps may need to be thrust through the mucosa, and their end grasps the proximal end of the endotracheal tube to pull the tube laterally. The incision can be closed in a routine manner once it is not required.

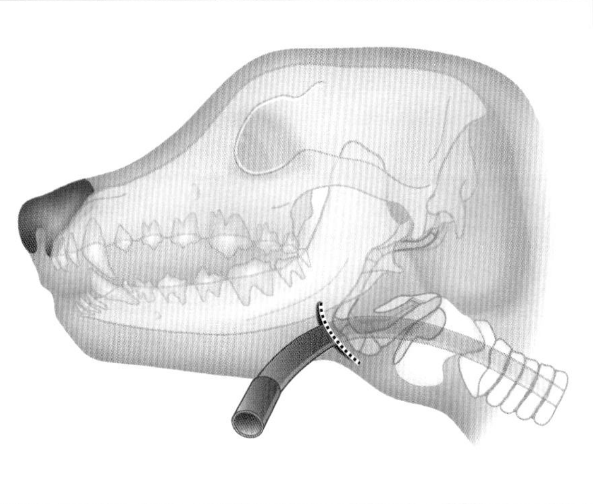

18.1 Placement of an endotracheal tube through a pharyngotomy site.

Elective tracheotomy

A patient that can otherwise breathe normally, but cannot open its mouth, should have anaesthesia induced and maintained with incremental boluses of an injectable anaesthetic agent until the jaws are opened or a tracheotomy is performed.

Elective tracheotomies can be performed under aseptic conditions while there is an orotracheal tube in place. The ventral surface of the trachea at the level of the second, third or fourth tracheal rings is exposed by a midline incision and the sternohyoideus muscles retracted. Two stabilizing sutures are placed around tracheal rings at the site of tracheal incision to facilitate apposition later. A transverse incision between rings is made through the annular ligament and mucosa up to 65% of the circumference of the trachea. Alternatively, a U-shaped ventral tracheal flap is created based on the second tracheal ring and extending two rings distally. The flap is raised as a hinge to allow placement of the tracheotomy tube. This flap is used for long-term intubation as it prevents excessive pressure of the tube on the surrounding tissue. Postoperatively the incision should be left to granulate, but this does require intensive care to allow cleaning of the tracheotomy site and constant observation of the patient. Some veterinary surgeons prefer to close the incision postoperatively, but there may be a risk of subcutaneous emphysema, localized swelling and subsequent risk of airway obstruction.

Feeding tubes

In patients that cannot feed and drink normally, a nasogastric, pharyngostomy, oesophagostomy or gastrostomy tube offers an alternative method of providing nutrition and fluids (see *BSAVA Manual of Canine and Feline Emergency and Critical Care*; Crowe, 1986). Basic information is presented here regarding the first three tube positions.

Indwelling nasogastric intubation

After desensitizing the nasal mucosa, a lubricated 5 or 6 French polyvinyl infant feeding tube is passed into the ventral nasal meatus. Placement into the oesophagus is easy in the anaesthetized patient with an endotracheal tube. In conscious patients the head should be held with the nose pointing down while the tube is advanced as this helps prevent accidental insertion into the trachea. The tube should be advanced until the distal end is positioned in the distal oesophagus (preferred location) or in the stomach. The stylet, if used, should then be removed. Placement should be verified, by radiography or by auscultation of bubbles when air or sterile saline is instilled through the tube. The tube should then be capped and sutured in place with butterflies made from sticky tape. An Elizabethan collar will be necessary in some patients to prevent them from removing the tube. Although easy to perform, this technique is limited to short periods of feeding with liquidized foods.

Pharyngostomy tube

This tube is placed by a technique similar to that described for a pharyngotomy endotracheal tube, but long-term maintenance can result in dysfunction of the larynx and aspiration. The technique of placement is therefore modified slightly in order that the tube exits as caudodorsally as possible, close to the entrance to the oesophagus. In the modified technique, the incision is made in the lateral wall of the pharynx, caudodorsal to the hyoid apparatus.

Oesophagostomy tube

This site is currently the preferred position for placement of a feeding tube. It avoids the complications of peritonitis from gastrotomy tubes, and the risks of aspiration and damage to mucosa from the previously described sites. Under anaesthesia, the lateral cervical region is clipped and prepared for surgery; the left side is commonly used, but the right side can be used if necessary. Curved forceps are inserted into the proximal cervical oesophagus via the pharynx. The tips of the forceps are then turned laterally and pressure applied so the instrument can be palpated. A skin incision large enough to accommodate the feeding tube is made over the tips of the forceps. The forceps can be pushed through the oesophagus, or an incision can be made in larger dogs. The feeding tube is premeasured and marked from stomach or distal oesophagus to incision site. The distal end is grasped by the forceps and pulled through the oesophagus out of the mouth. With the aid of the forceps the distal end is then turned on itself to pass back into the oesophagus until the loop disappears. The distal tip is correctly positioned using the mark on the tube. This method helps to straighten the tube, and limit kinks (Crowe and Devey, 1997). An alternative technique is to place a van Noort oesophagotomy tube using the appropriate introducer.

References and further reading

Crowe DT (1986) Enteral nutrition for critically ill or injured patients. Part I, II, III. *The Compendium on Continuing Education for the Practicing Veterinarian* **8**, 603–826

Crowe DT and Devey JJ (1997) Esophagotomy tubes for feeding and decompression: clinical experience in 29 small animal patients. *Journal of the American Animal Hospital Association* **33**, 393–403

Hardie EM, Spodnick GJ, Gilson SD, Benson JA and Hawkins EC (1999) Tracheal rupture in cats: 16 cases. *Journal of the American Veterinary Medical Association* **214**, 508–512

Hartsfield SM (1990) Anesthetic problems of the geriatric dental patient. *Problems in Veterinary Medicine* **2**, 24–45

Hobson HP (1995) Brachycephalic syndrome. *Seminars in Veterinary Medicine and Surgery (Small Animal)* **10**, 109–114

King L and Hammond R (1999) *Manual of Canine and Feline Emergency and Critical Care.* BSAVA Publications, Cheltenham

Mitchell SL, McCarthy R, Rudloff E and Pernell RT (2000) Tracheal rupture associated with intubation in cats: 20 cases. *Journal of the American Veterinary Medical Association* **216**, 1592–1595

Muir WW III and Hubbell JAE (1995) *Handbook of Veterinary Anaesthesia, 2nd edn.* Mosby, St Louis

Rochette J (2005) Regional anesthesia and analgesia for oral and dental procedures. *Veterinary Clinics of North America: Small Animal Practice* **35**, 1041–1058

Quandt JE, Robinson EP, Walter PA and Raffe MR (1993) Endotracheal tube displacement during cervical manipulation in the dog. *Veterinary Surgery* **22**, 235–239

19

Cardiovascular disease

R. Eddie Clutton

Introduction

The cardiovascular system consists of the heart, blood vessels and controlling elements of the autonomic nervous system. It is functionally divided into the right and left circulations: the right delivers venous blood to the lungs for oxygenation, whilst the left maintains blood pressure and drives tissue perfusion, i.e. maintains delivery of adequate volumes of oxygenated blood (DO_2) to peripheral tissue per unit time so that whole body oxygen requirements ($\dot{V}O_2$) are met. Thus, 'cardiovascular disease' refers to any pathology limiting peripheral blood flow, including:

- Diseases of the heart, i.e. myocardium, valves and the cardiac conducting system
- Arterial disease
- Impaired autonomic nervous control of cardiovascular function
- Abnormal blood flow characteristics
- Hypovolaemia.

Cardiovascular disease is frequently encountered in companion animal practice: congenital cardiac anomalies are common, while cardiopulmonary function deteriorates with age. Acquired cardiac disease is common in dogs and cats. Animals with cardiovascular disease may require an anaesthetic for diagnostic tests, for the surgical correction of anomalies or for operations unrelated to the condition. Cardiovascular disease increases risk from anaesthesia because:

- Cardiovascular depression is the most important side effect of most anaesthetics; anaesthesia increases the likelihood of cardiovascular failure and death
- Cardiovascular disease affects other organ systems in ways that increase anaesthetic risk. The most important affect the heart itself, e.g. chronic hypertension causes ventricular hypertrophy
- Cardiovascular diseases alter drug disposition (Figure 19.1)
- Cardiovascular therapy involves drugs (Figures 19.2, 19.3 and 19.4) which may interact with anaesthetics or produce adverse effects during anaesthesia.

Risks from anaesthesia are reduced if:

- An accurate diagnosis is established. Management depends on identifying and understanding the condition's primary (haemodynamic) and secondary effects
- Reversible risk factors are identified and treated preoperatively
- Cardiovascular reserve is recruited by preoperative preparation
- The anaesthetics used offset, rather than aggravate, the haemodynamic effects of the condition
- The adverse haemodynamic effects of surgery are understood and minimized
- Problems of secondary complications, altered drug behaviour and drug interactions are recognized
- A range of autonomic nervous and cardiovascular (adjunct) drugs is available
- Perioperative physiological monitoring is adequate.

Effect	Consequences
Reduced drug volume of distribution	Greater sensitivity to injectable anaesthetics; reduced doses and/or infusion rates required. This is greatest with drugs given by intravenous rather than intramuscular or subcutaneous injection
Slower circulation time	Slower response after intravenous injection; longer delay required between incremental injections
Poor peripheral perfusion	Lower drug bioavailability after intramuscular, subcutaneous or oral drug administration
Reduced cardiac output	Increased rate of inhalation anaesthetic uptake. More rapid induction rate and a more rapid response to altered vaporizer settings. Greater attention required to vaporizer settings
Reduced renal perfusion	Reduced renal clearance of drugs. Metabolic acidosis increases sensitivity to weak acidic drugs, e.g. thiopental, non-steroidal anti-inflammatory drugs (NSAIDs). Hypoalbuminaemia increases unbound:bound drug fraction, increasing sensitivity to albumin-bound compounds
Reduced hepatic blood flow	Diminished extraction of drugs undergoing extensive hepatic metabolism; prolonged effect
Increased pulmonary ventilation/ perfusion inequality	Slower onset and response to altered concentrations of inhalation anaesthetics

19.1 Pharmacokinetic effects of cardiovascular disease.

Drug	Indications	Dose	Side effects
Digoxin	Heart failure Atrial premature complexes Atrial tachycardia Atrial fibrillation Sinus tachycardia due to heart failure	Rapid intravenous: using 250 µg/kg injectable solution, prepare 10–20 µg/kg. Inject 50% i.v. and wait 30–60 minutes. Give 25% dose i.v. and wait another 30–60 minutes before giving the final aliquot, if necessary Rapid oral: Using tablets, 10–30 µg/kg is given at presentation and again at 12 hours Maintenance: 10–20 µg/kg divided q12h	Perioperative arrhythmias: sinus block, atrioventricular (AV) block, AV junctional rhythm, atrial and ventricular ectopic beats, ventricular tachycardia Anorexia; vomiting; diarrhoea; lethargy; ataxia. Toxic signs occur at lower concentrations in presence of hypokalaemia. Toxicity enhanced by hyperkalaemia, alkalosis, hypoxaemia, hypercalcaemia, hypomagnesaemia Monitor ECG throughout rapid digitalization. Any possibility that preoperative bradycardia/bradyarrhythmias result from digoxin toxicity should prompt administration of a test dose of atropine 20 µg/kg to ensure intraoperative heart rate increases are possible
Diuretics			
Loop	Rapid elimination of excessive fluid	Furosemide: 2–5 mg/kg every hour i.v., rapid onset and effective in dogs and cats Then 1–4 mg/kg i.m. or orally q8–24h thereafter	Should be used only with vasodilators, i.e. ACE inhibitors Hypovolaemia; hypotension Hypokalaemia aggravates digoxin toxicity Metabolic alkalosis; hypochloraemia Use carefully in conditions in which cardiac output relies on ventricular filling pressures Monitor effect by weight loss
Thiazides	Slow elimination of excessive fluid	Hydrochlorothiazide: 2–4 mg/kg orally q12h	As above
Potassium-sparing	Slow elimination of excessive fluid	Spironolactone: 1–2 mg/kg orally q12–24h Amiloride: 0.125 mg/kg orally q24h	Plasma potassium levels unchanged
Phosphodiesterase inhibitors	See below		
Potassium	Hypokalaemia following prolonged diuretic therapy and/or cachexia	Cats 2–6 mmol/day orally Dogs 0.2–0.5 mmol/kg orally q8h	Hyperkalaemia and arrythmias when plasma levels exceed 7 mmol/l. Potassium-sparing diuretics (spironolactone, amiloride and triamterene) do not warrant K^+ supplementation

19.2 Drugs for preoperative preparation of animals in heart failure. Sodium intake should be restricted to 10–40 mg/kg/day (0.1–0.4% diet dry matter). If possible, cases should receive a formulated low-sodium diet or a prescription diet, e.g. Hill's k/d or h/d.

Drug	Indications	Dose	Side effects
Glyceryl trinitrate	Emergency venodilation/ afterload reduction, e.g. pulmonary oedema	Ointment applied q6–12h to medial pinna: Dogs 6–50 mm Cats 3–6 mm	Hypotension, tachycardia, azotaemia
Nitroprusside	Rapid afterload reduction	Infusion: 1–15 µg/kg/minute (dogs)	Hypotension, tachycardia, azotaemia Rapid effects; monitor blood pressure
Hydralazine	Reduce afterload (arteriolar dilation), e.g. acute mitral valve regurgitation	0.5–3.0 mg/kg orally q12h (dogs)	Acute: hypotension, tachycardia Chronic: hypernatraemia, hypokalaemia
Alpha-1 antagonists	Reduce afterload	Prazosin: Dogs <15 kg 1 mg orally q8–12h Dogs >15kg 2 mg orally q8–12h Cats 0.25–1 mg orally q8–12h Phenoxybenzamine: Dogs 0.2–1.5 mg/kg orally q12h Cats 0.5–1 mg/kg orally q12h	Hypotension, tachycardia, depression, weakness Effects wane with constant use
ACE inhibitors	Non-emergency afterload control	Enalapril: Dogs 0.25–1 mg/kg orally q12–24h Cats 0.25 mg/kg orally q12–24h Benazepril: Dogs 0.25–0.5 mg/kg orally q24h Cats 0.5–1.0 mg/kg orally q24h Imidapril: Dogs and cats 0.25 mg/kg orally q24h Ramipril: Dogs 0.125 mg/kg orally q24h	Hypovolaemia, hypotension, tachycardia, hyperkalaemia. May aggravate hypotensive effects of acepromazine (use lower acepromazine dose and prepare for crystalloid infusion)

19.3 Vasodilators for preoperative preparation of animals in heart failure. (continues) ▶

Drug	Indications	Dose	Side effects
Phosphodiesterase inhibitors	Mixed effects: inotropy, chronotropy, diuresis, vasodilation	Pimobendan: Dogs 0.2–0.6 mg/kg orally q24h Propentophylline: Dogs 2.5–3 mg/kg orally q12h	
Calcium channel blockers	Vasodilation and weak negative chronotropic and inotropic effects	Amlodipine: Dogs 0.05–0.1 mg/kg orally q12–24h Cats 0.625–1.25 mg orally q24h	

19.3 (continued) Vasodilators for preoperative preparation of animals in heart failure.

Drug	Indications	Dose	Side effects
Type 1a	Ventricular arrhythmias and ventricular tachycardia	Procainamide 4–8 mg/kg over 5 minutes then 25–50 µg/kg/minute	Procainamide causes myocardial depression, hypotension and ECG abnormalities if given rapidly
	Malignant ventricular arrhythmias, refractory supraventricular tachycardia (SVT), acute atrial fibrillation	Quinidine 6–10 mg/kg i.m. or 6–20 mg/kg orally q6–8h (dogs)	Hypotension, arrhythmias
Type 1b	Malignant ventricular arrhythmias	Lidocaine 2–4 mg/kg i.v. then 25–75 µg/kg/minute	
Type 2	Tachyarrhythmias	Propranolol: 50 µg/kg i.v. every 2 minutes to effect maintenance 0.25–1 mg/kg orally q8h (dogs & cats) Atenolol: Dogs 0.5–2.0 mg/kg orally q12h Cats 6.25–12.5 mg/cat orally q24h	Hypotension, bradycardia, bronchospasm, obtunded sympathetic responses to hypovolaemia, hypercapnia, hypoxaemia etc. Acute aggravation of congestive failure
Type 3	Ventricular arrhythmias	Amiodarone: Dogs 10–15 mg/kg orally q12h for 1 week then 5–7.5 mg/kg q12h for 2 weeks, thereafter 7.5 mg/kg q24h	Bradycardia, atrioventricular blockade, hypotension
Type 4 Calcium channel blockers	SVT, ventricular tachycardia, atrial fibrillation	Diltiazem: Dogs 0.5–1.5 mg/kg orally q8h Cats 1.75–2.5 mg/kg orally q8–12h Verapamil: Dogs and cats 0.5–1.0 mg/kg orally q8h	Bradycardia, other arrhythmias, hypotension, acute aggravation of congestive failure
Antimuscarinics	Bradyarrhythmias	Atropine 20–40 µg/kg i.m. or s.c. Glycopyrronium 5–10 µg/kg i.m. or s.c. Isopropamide 2.5–5 mg/kg orally q8–12h Propantheline: Dogs 1–2 mg/kg orally q8–12h Cats 7.5 mg/kg orally q8–12h	Tachycardia
Beta-1 agonists	Bradyarrhythmias	Isoprenaline 5–10 mg orally q6–8h (dogs) Terbutaline: Dogs 1.25–5 mg/dog orally q8–12h Cats 300 µg–1.25 mg/cat orally q8–12h	Severe tachycardia
Magnesium	Refractory ventricular arrhythmias	Dogs and cats 0.5 mmol/kg/day by infusion	

19.4 Anti-arrhythmic drugs for preoperative preparation of animals in heart failure.

Cardiovascular disease: management

Preoperative examination

Preoperative examination establishes the diagnosis and predicts the capacity of the cardiovascular system to withstand anaesthesia and surgery. It forms the basis of preoperative preparation and anaesthetic technique selection. While the most important indicators of severe cardiovascular disease are diminished exercise tolerance, dyspnoea, syncopal episodes and 'fits' (seizures), no *single* sign or test predicts an animal's capacity to tolerate anaesthesia and surgery. Overall status must accommodate both the haemodynamic derangement and the effect of secondary changes. However, the most useful and practical index of cardiopulmonary 'fitness', at least in dogs, is exercise tolerance.

A thorough medical history review and physical examination may establish a diagnosis, although more complex studies, such as radiography, electrocardiography, arterial blood gas analysis, ultrasonography and cardiac catheterization, are often required. The stress associated with such investigations in conscious animals may produce spurious test results, or worse, may precipitate deterioration. Veterinary cardiologists should be recruited to establish the diagnosis if necessary.

Thoracic radiographs provide information on cardiac chamber enlargement and assist in identifying pulmonary changes. Animals in extremis should be examined in the lateral decubital position while being supplied with oxygen.

Electrocardiography should be performed on most cases (certainly all dogs) with cardiovascular disease, especially when pulse irregularities are detected. A cursory examination suffices for risk assessment because arrhythmias are more important in anaesthesia than chamber enlargement or axis deviation. A single lead electrocardiogram (ECG) can be taken from the standing or resting orthopnoeic animal. Many sedatives, e.g. alpha-2 agonists, are arrhythmogenic while some, e.g. acepromazine, are anti-arrhythmic.

Arterial blood gas analysis quantifies the lungs' ability to oxygenate blood and may be useful for risk assessment in cases with cor pulmonale. Arterial puncture may be stressful, which will affect results by lowering carbon dioxide and increasing or decreasing oxygen tension.

Venous blood samples should be taken to determine hepatic and renal function when tricuspid valve disease, low cardiac output or passive venous congestion are present. The haematocrit, plasma haemoglobin concentration, serum protein and plasma electrolyte levels (sodium, potassium and chloride) should also be examined.

Sedation/anaesthesia for diagnostic tests

Sedation or anaesthesia may be required for some tests. Sedation may *seem* safer and more convenient than general anaesthesia. However, sedative effects may be unpredictable, provide an inadequate duration of effect, cause adverse physiological changes and fail to provide the conditions required for invasive physiological measurement and tracheal intubation (should ventilatory support become necessary). In contrast, general anaesthesia allows tracheal intubation and intermittent positive pressure ventilation (IPPV). The depth of anaesthesia can be adjusted during the investigation, according to the degree of stimulation. General anaesthesia with volatile agents provides rapid recoveries after prolonged investigations because their elimination is independent of hepatic and renal function.

Preoperative preparation

Preoperative preparation aims to reduce risk by reversing the effects of pre-existing disease; adequate preoperative preparation can reduce the risk of anaesthesia in most cases, and depends on the extent of dysfunction present and the intended operation. The need for adequate preparation must be balanced against the pressing needs for surgery. Elective operations should be postponed until therapy has achieved its maximum effect, and undesirable drug effects are controlled. The primary condition must be treated first, as most secondary complications resolve spontaneously with improved cardiovascular function.

Primary condition

Uncontrolled cardiac failure is a contraindication to general anaesthesia and must be treated. Cardiac function can be improved by the following steps:

1. Eliminating retained fluids with diuretics, sodium-free diets and interventions such as pericardiocentesis.
2. Improving myocardial contraction with pimobendan, digoxin, beta-1 agonist drugs or phosphodiesterase inhibitors.
3. Reducing cardiac work with vasodilators, cage rest and anxiolytic drugs.
4. Controlling arrhythmias persisting after steps 1–3.

General details are given in Figures 19.2 and 19.3. Specific details, which vary according to the condition, are described below. Some arrhythmias, e.g. third-degree atrioventricular (AV) block, arise *de novo* (are not secondary to cardiovascular disease), and are solely responsible for inadequate cardiac output. These are treated with suitable anti-arrhythmic drugs or by pacemaker implantation.

Cardiac failure may result from non-cardiac disease, e.g. hyperthyroidism and phaeochromocytoma, in which case treatment must address the inciting condition.

Secondary complications

Secondary effects of cardiopulmonary disease which are life-threatening, e.g. ventricular arrhythmias, warrant immediate therapy. Other secondary effects may persist after the primary condition is treated because of irreversible pathology. In all cases, the effect of any cardiovascular condition on vital tissue perfusion should be assessed.

Arrhythmias: These are the most important secondary complication because:

- Some reduce cardiac output and cause hypotension. The haemodynamic significance of benign arrhythmias may increase in cardiac disease
- Untreated, benign arrhythmias may degenerate into lethal rhythms such as ventricular fibrillation, asystole or electromechanical dissociation during surgery. Veterinary surgeons must be able to differentiate malignant and benign arrhythmias from artefacts and be able to rapidly treat the former
- Spontaneously arising intraoperative arrhythmias indicate a deterioration in the myocardial environment as a result of poor management, e.g hypoxia, hypercapnia and changes in pH, temperature and electrolyte values.

Some arrhythmias resolve as cardiac function improves. If they do not, an alternative cause must be investigated and/or non-specific anti-arrhythmic therapy instituted (see Figure 19.4). For simplicity, preoperative arrhythmias are categorized here as bradyarrhythmias and tachyarrhythmias.

Bradyarrhythmias: Preoperative bradycardia may be secondary to hypoglycaemia (insulinoma), hyperkalaemia (hypoadrenocorticism), hypertension (polycythaemia) or hypothyroidism. It may be iatrogenic (digoxin and beta-1 antagonists) or idiopathic, e.g.

canine sick sinus syndrome. Bradycardia (or bradyarrhythmia) requires investigation because further slowing is likely during anaesthesia. At very low heart rates, reduced cardiac output and coronary arterial flow may lead to cardiac arrest.

When emergency surgery is needed in animals with bradyarrhythmias, the heart's ability to increase rate is tested first with atropine (Figure 19.5) and then isoprenaline (Figure 19.6). A positive response indicates the appropriate therapy for controlling intraoperative bradyarrhythmias. If neither increase heart rate, surgery should be postponed, conducted at the subject's peril, or artificial ventricular pacing should be instituted.

Drug class	Indications	Drug	Precautions
Type 1a	Ventricular arrhythmias and ventricular tachycardia	Procainamide 4–8 mg/kg over 5 minutes then 25–50 µg/kg/minute	Procainamide causes myocardial depression, hypotension and ECG abnormalities if given rapidly
Type 1b	Malignant ventricular arrhythmias	Lidocaine 2–4 mg/kg i.v. then 25–75 µg/kg/minute	
Type 2	Tachyarrhythmias	Propranolol 50 µg/kg i.v. every 2 minutes to effect, maintenance 0.25–1 mg/kg orally q8h (dogs and cats) Esmolol 50–100 µg/kg every 5 minutes to effect, then infuse 50–200 µg/kg/minute (dogs and cats)	Hypotension, bradycardia, bronchospasm, obtunded sympathetic responses to hypovolaemia, hypercapnia, hypoxaemia, etc., acute aggravation of congestive failure
Type 4	Supraventricular arrhythmias	Verapamil: Dogs 50 µg/kg i.v. over 10 minutes, repeat four times 25 µg/kg doses at 5 minute intervals Cats 20 µg/kg i.v. over 3 minutes, repeat eight times at 5 minute intervals	
	Refractory ventricular arrhythmias	Magnesium sulphate 0.5 mmol/kg/day by infusion (cats and dogs)	
Antimuscarinics	Hypotension due to slow heart rate, bradycardia, bradyarrhythmias	Atropine 20–40 µg/kg i.v. Glycopyrronium 5–10 µg/kg i.v.	
Negative chronotropes	Idiopathic tachycardia, tachyarrhythmias	Morphine 0.25–0.5 mg/kg i.v. Alfentanil 1–5 µg/kg every 5 minutes i.v. Fentanyl 1–2.5 µg/kg i.v. repeated every 20 minutes or so Digoxin 5–10 µg/kg i.v. Neostigmine 25–50 µg/kg i.v. Edrophonium 1 mg/kg i.v.	Monitor heart rate and ECG; severe bradycardia and hypotension in overdose

19.5 Anti-arrhythmic drugs used for rapid control of haemodynamic variables during anaesthesia.

Drug class	Indications	Drug	Precautions
Beta-1 agonists	Hypotension due to poor myocardial contractility and/or bradycardia	Dobutamine 1–20 µg/kg/minute Dopamine 1–20 µg/kg/minute Isoprenaline 10–100 µg/kg/minute Adrenaline 22–33 µg/kg i.v. then 0.01–0.1 µg/kg/minute	Monitor heart rate (HR) and ECG; severe tachycardia, hypertension and ventricular arrhythmias in overdose
Beta-1 antagonists	Tachycardia, tachyarrhythmias, arrhythmias associated with myocardial hypoxia Hypotension due to reduced cardiac output in hypertrophic cardiomyopathy Hypotension due to excessive heart rate	Propranolol 50 µg/kg every 2 minutes Esmolol 50–100 µg/kg every 5 minutes to effect, then infuse 50–200 µg/kg/minute (dogs and cats)	Monitor HR and ECG; severe bradycardia and hypotension in overdose
Alpha-1 agonists	Hypotension due to alpha-1 antagonists and/or inadequate systemic vascular resistance	Phenylephrine 10 µg/kg every 5–15 minutes i.v. Noradrenaline 0.01–0.05 µg/kg/minute i.v.	Monitor HR and urine output; bradycardia and oliguria in overdose
Alpha-1 antagonists	Hypertension due to excessive alpha-1 agonist activity, myocardial hypoxia due to high afterload	Phentolamine 25–100 µg/kg i.v.	Monitor HR and blood pressure (BP); hypotension in overdose
Vasodilators	Severe hypertension/rapid afterload reduction	Sodium nitroprusside infusion: 1–15 µg/kg/minute i.v. (dogs)	Hypotension, tachycardia, azotaemia Rapid effects; monitor BP
	Emergency venodilation/afterload reduction (pulmonary oedema)	Glyceryl trinitrate ointment 0.6–5 cm (dogs) 0.6–1.25 cm (cats) q6–12h to medial pinna	Hypotension, tachycardia, azotaemia Rapid effects; monitor BP

19.6 Adjunct drugs used for rapid control of haemodynamic variables during anaesthesia.

Tachyarrhythmias: Preoperative tachycardia or tachyarrhythmia should be investigated because they may jeopardize myocardial oxygen balance (m(D–V)O_2) (Figure 19.7). Myocardial hypoxia may result in ventricular arrhythmias and eventually cardiac arrest. This is likely when catecholamines are released (Figure 19.8). Vagal manoeuvres, e.g. carotid sinus massage and ocular pressure, may convert atrial tachycardia to sinus rhythm, but rarely do, in which case digoxin, beta-1 antagonists or calcium channel blockers are required.

Factors reducing myocardial oxygen delivery (mDO_2)
Low blood oxygen tension (P_aO_2)
Low haemoglobin concentration
Coronary vasospasm (severe hypocapnia)
Low arterial blood pressure
Increased heart rate
Factors increasing myocardial oxygen demand (mVO_2)
Increased heart rate
Systolic wall tension, afterload
Contractility
Basal metabolic rate

19.7 Factors affecting myocardial oxygen balance (m(D–V)O_2). Note that tachycardia is particularly dangerous as it simultaneously increases oxygen demand while reducing oxygen delivery.

Conditions increasing plasma catecholamine levels
Noxious surgical stimulation ± inadequate anaesthesia/analgesia
Endotracheal intubation under 'light' anaesthesia
Hypotension
Hypoxaemia
Hypercapnia
Hypoglycaemia
Hyperthermia
Severe hypothermia
Postoperative pain
Endocrine disease
Hyperthyroidism
Phaeochromocytoma
Drugs
Antimuscarinic drugs
Beta agonist drugs
Thyroxine
Phosphodiesterase inhibitors

19.8 Factors increasing perioperative sympathetic nervous activity.

Pulmonary oedema: Pulmonary oedema indicates left heart failure and occurs in mitral valve incompetence, mitral stenosis and aortic stenosis (Figure 19.9). It must be treated preoperatively because it decreases lung compliance (increases lung 'stiffness'), increases work of breathing and impairs oxygenation. The management of congestive cardiac failure will resolve pulmonary oedema in chronic cases. In acute episodes, diuretics (e.g. furosemide) and vasodilators (e.g. hydralazine) may be required.

Blood pH changes: Blood gas abnormalities caused by cardiopulmonary disease may aggravate the primary condition and create self-reinforcing cycles. For example, low cardiac output causes tissue hypoperfusion and metabolic acidosis. The latter further depresses cardiac contractility. Treatment should be directed at the primary lesion whether it be hypoperfusion, renal failure or inadequate pulmonary perfusion.

Polycythaemia: Polycythaemia (haematocrit >0.55) results from any condition causing hypoxia, e.g. right-to-left intrapulmonary (neoplasm, bronchitis) or extrapulmonary (ventricular septal defect) shunts. It increases blood viscosity and mimics elevated systemic vascular resistance. The latter increases ventricular wall tension during systole, which increases oxygen demand and eventually leads to ventricular failure. In peripheral tissue, viscous blood 'sludges' in capillaries and limits delivery of oxygenated blood. High haematocrit values are lowered preoperatively by normovolaemic haemodilution: the simultaneous removal of blood and infusion of plasma, colloids or crystalloid solutions.

Right heart failure: Right ventricular failure raises central venous pressure (CVP) and favours capillary transudation throughout the body, resulting in pleural and/or pericardial effusion, ascites, hepato- and splenomegaly and/or peripheral oedema. Pleural and pericardial effusions may restrict ventilation while pericardial fluid accumulation impedes cardiac filling (cardiac tamponade).

Renal dysfunction: *Hyperkalaemia* associated with renal dysfunction is arrhythmogenic and must be lowered with sodium bicarbonate, insulin–glucose solutions or cation-exchange resins, or its effects countered with calcium gluconate (see Chapter 23). In extreme cases, peritoneal dialysis may be required.

Azotaemia (as well as hyperkalaemia and acidaemia) can cause bradyarrhythmias and increase myocardial sensitivity to anaesthetics. The nature of treatment depends on whether failure is predominantly renal or prerenal.

Hypoalbuminaemia renders animals sensitive to albumin-bound drugs like thiopental, while lowered plasma oncotic pressure facilitates pulmonary oedema formation. In conjunction with high CVP, hypoalbuminaemia contributes to peritoneal, pleural and pericardial effusions.

Liver dysfunction: Preoperative coagulation tests are mandatory if there is any suspicion of impaired clotting. Coagulopathies are treated using preoperative fresh blood infusion, even before minor operations such as dentistry.

Adequate blood glucose concentrations (4.1–14.8 mmol/l) must be maintained perioperatively with intravenous dextrose solutions. Impaired cerebral glucose delivery, which is more likely with cardiovascular disease, will result in severe neuronal damage.

Severe hepatic dysfunction may also impair the rate of elimination of long-acting drugs like pentobarbital and acepromazine.

Category			Example	Problems	Management goals
Low cardiac output	Fixed	Obstructive (valvular)	Mitral and aortic regurgitation and stenosis, pulmonary hypertension	HR unable to increase output in response to challenge. Intolerant of **any** changes affecting cardiac output Increased systemic vascular resistance (SVR) causes hypertension; more importantly, reduced SVR, venomotor tone or heart rate causes marked hypotension	Maintain or increase HR (not >20% resting) Maintain sinus rhythm
		Cardiac tamponade			Avoid falls in SVR
		Fixed heart rate (HR)	Canine sick sinus syndrome		Avoid myocardial depression/maintain contractility
		Ventricular	Cardiomyopathy 'End-stage' heart disease		Avoid myocardial ischaemia Maintain preload
	Variable	Inefficient HR	Ventricular tachycardia	Myocardial hypoxia, hypotension	Reduce HR and variables decreasing myocardial oxygen balance
			Hypothyroidism	Myocardial hypoxia, hypotension	Increase HR
		Inadequate contractility	Cardiomyopathy 'End-stage' heart disease	Myocardial hypoxia, hypotension	Maintain contractility Minimize variables decreasing myocardial oxygen balance
		Inadequate preload	Hypovolaemia, septicaemia	Hypotension	Maintain preload Increase SVR Avoid high inflation pressures during IPPV
		Excessive afterload	Polycythaemia, hypertension, cor pulmonale	Myocardial hypoxia, arrhythmias, end-organ damage in brain, eyes, heart, kidneys and peripheral vessels	Reduce SVR or pulmonary vascular resistance
High cardiac output			Secondary to hypermetabolic conditions: hyperthyroidism, phaeochromocytoma, hypercapnia	Slow induction of anaesthesia with volatile agents Increased risk of myocardial hypoxia, arrhythmias High output failure in response to catecholamines	Avoid increases in HR Suppress myocardial contractility Suppress afterload Avoid catecholamine release

19.9 Classification of cardiac failure.

Other considerations in preoperative preparation

Effective circulating blood volume: Preoperative fluid deficits must be resolved and the overzealous use of diuretics avoided in those conditions in which cardiac output depends on preload.

Anaemia: A haemoglobin concentration of 120–150 g/l is required to produce a normal arterial blood oxygen content of 16.1–20.1 ml/dl. In anaemia, maintaining delivery of adequate volumes of oxygenated blood depends on commensurate rises in cardiac output. This increases myocardial work which, in the face of reduced arterial blood oxygen content, may lead to myocardial hypoxia. Anaemia should be resolved preoperatively by blood transfusion with fresh whole blood in acute (haemorrhagic) losses, or packed cells (haematocrit >0.65) in chronic (normovolaemic) anaemia. Stored blood should be transfused 24 hours preoperatively to allow *in vitro* storage lesions to resolve. Over-transfusion must be avoided as it increases ventricular afterload and promotes pulmonary oedema, whilst also excessively increasing preload.

Hypokalaemia caused by loop diuretics: This should be treated preoperatively because hypokalaemia prevents anti-arrhythmic drugs converting ventricular tachycardia to sinus rhythm. The treatment of choice is oral potassium supplementation, although crystalloid infusions with added potassium chloride may be required in collapsed animals. The infusion rate should ensure that potassium administration does not exceed 0.5 mmol/kg/h and the ECG should be monitored (see Figure 19.2 and Chapter 22).

Pyrexia: This stimulates cardiovascular activity by increasing the metabolic rate and raising oxygen and glucose consumption and carbon dioxide production. Beyond this there is little problem with mild hypermetabolism *per se*, although the cause must be identified; there is considerable risk when pyrexia results from endocarditis or meningitis. Some antibiotics, e.g. aminoglycosides and chloramphenicol, may interact adversely with anaesthetic drugs.

Drugs in preoperative preparation: Many drugs used to treat heart failure (see Figures 19.2, 19.3 and 19.4) produce undesirable side effects and complicate anaesthesia. For example, digoxin causes arrhythmias, and opinions differ over its preoperative use. Some recommend that animals in cardiac failure facing elective operations should be digitalized but have the morning dose withheld on the day of operation. However, digitalized animals facing emergency operations should not have the drug withdrawn. In non-digitalized animals facing emergency operations, the infusion of inotropes such as dobutamine may be as effective, and less hazardous than rapid intravenous digitalization. It is felt that antimuscarinic drugs should not be used in digitalized animals as their action negates digoxin's positive effects.

As a rule, attempting to limit potential interactions by withdrawing drugs before anaesthesia is likely to cause more problems than are solved. The fear of interactions should not be used as an excuse for inadequate preparation. Ideally, surgery is postponed until therapy has achieved a maximal effect, and drug side effects have been minimized.

Anaesthetic techniques

Major surgery can be performed in sedated animals using local anaesthesia, providing the surgical site is amenable to local anaesthetic techniques. This option is made more feasible when nerve locators are used. However, high sedative doses may cause greater physiological disturbance than a properly administered general anaesthetic, and local anaesthetic injected into the spinal or epidural space can cause severe hypotension under certain circumstances.

Pre-anaesthetic medication with a neuroleptanalgesic combination (e.g. acepromazine and buprenorphine), induction with an ultra short-acting injectable anaesthetic (e.g. propofol) and 'light' general anaesthesia produced with a volatile anaesthetic (and possibly nitrous oxide) provides adequate conditions for minor operations in animals with modest disease, providing attention is paid to ventilation, temperature, circulating blood volume and perioperative analgesia. However, this approach would be inadequate in cases with advanced disease undergoing major operations because it would not prevent the autonomic nervous responses to noxious (surgical) stimulation, which adversely affect cardiovascular function. In these cases, a balanced anaesthetic technique is more appropriate. This involves using the lowest dose of anaesthetic capable of producing unconsciousness (which minimizes myocardial depression) with a potent analgesic (to obtund reflex responses to surgery) and a muscle relaxant (to improve surgical conditions). Nitrous oxide is frequently included because it has few cardiovascular effects and reduces the delivered concentration of volatile agent required to produce a given depth of anaesthesia. Balanced anaesthesia is not without complications: neuromuscular-blocking agents eliminate both spontaneous respiration and the most obvious sign of inadequate anaesthesia: movement. Pre-emptive and polymodal analgesic techniques should be used in major operations with the objective of minimizing, if not eliminating, postoperative pain.

Drug selection

The goals of anaesthesia in animals with cardiovascular disease are to:

- Provide analgesia and muscle relaxation for surgery
- Optimize myocardial and tissue oxygenation by ensuring adequate blood oxygenation
- Maintain cardiac output at levels that meet tissue perfusion
- Maintain systemic arterial blood pressure at levels that sustain major organ (cerebral, coronary, renal and hepatic) blood flow
- Preserve a positive myocardial oxygen balance.

The chosen anaesthetic should:

- Reverse the haemodynamic disorder by mimicking the effects of medical therapy. This requires a knowledge of drug effects (summarized in Figure 19.10)
- Be compatible with drugs used perioperatively to improve cardiovascular function
- Be suitable in the presence of secondary cerebral, myocardial, hepatic or renal complications
- Be minimally affected by altered pharmacokinetics.

As a rule, the drugs chosen should have minimal effects on myocardial contractility and peripheral venous tone. Selecting the most appropriate anaesthetic for a given case is simplified by categorizing acquired cardiovascular diseases (see Figure 19.9). However, selection is made difficult by the virtual absence of data on anaesthetic drug behaviour in companion animals with cardiovascular disease. The information summarized in Figure 19.6 is simplified and erroneously implies that drug behaviour is predictable. However, it is frequently changed by diseases and/or co-administered medication. A preoccupation with drug suitability based on theoretical haemodynamic effects diverts attention from the fact that other perioperative factors, e.g. hypovolaemia, hypothermia and pain, may critically exacerbate cardiovascular dysfunction. In any case, the adverse haemodynamic effect of an anaesthetic can often be negated: the myocardial depressant effect of halothane is reversed to some degree by infusing fluids and inotropes.

The assumption that newer anaesthetics are safer for animals with cardiovascular disease is misconceived and dangerous. Drugs often behave differently in animals with cardiovascular disease and so, when using unfamiliar drugs, it is difficult to determine if an undesirable effect is normal, or reflects deteriorating conditions. Anaesthetics perceived as 'safer' might provide a temptation to anaesthetize cases which would previously have been regarded as unacceptable risks. Under these circumstances, the use of unfamiliar drugs (which are unlikely to be safer) in susceptible subjects may have dire consequences. Ultimately, anaesthetic risk depends as much on the veterinary surgeon's experience with a drug as it does on the drug's known adverse cardiovascular effects. It is better to choose any fundamentally safe (and familiar) technique over one which may in theory be more appropriate, but which

Drug	Cardiac output	Inotropy	Heart rate	Systemic vascular resistance	Mean arterial blood pressure	Pulmonary vascular resistance	Central venous pressure	Electrocardiogram
Acepromazine	↔↓	↔	↔↓	↓↓	↓	?	↓	Type 1b anti-arrhythmic effect, may cause some slowing, primary atrioventricular block
Diazepam	↔	↔	↔	↔↓	↔	?	↔	
Midazolam	↔↓	↔↓	↔↑	?	↔↓	?	?	
Morphine	↔	↔	↓	↓	↔	?	↓↓	Bradycardia, bradyarrhythmias, though tachycardia/hypotension (histamine release) may follow rapid intravenous injection of *any* opioid
Pethidine (meperidine)	↔↓	↔↓	↑	↔↓	↓	?	↑	
Butorphanol	↔	↔	↔↓	↔	↔↓	?	?	
Buprenorphine	↔	↔	↔↓	↔	↔↓	?	?	
Atropine	↑	↔	↑↑↑	↔	↔↑	?	?	Tachycardia, ventricular arrhythmias
Xylazine Medetomidine	↓	↔	↓↓↓	↑-↓	↑-↓	?	?	Bradycardia, primary and secondary AV blockade. Xylazine may 'sensitize' myocardium to catecholamines
Thiopental	↓	↔↓	↑↑	↔↓	↓	?	↓	Occasionally causes transient ventricular arrhythmias
Saffan® (alfaxalone/ alfadolone)	↓	↓	↑↑	↓	↓	↑	↓	
Ketamine	↑↑	↑↑	↑	↑	↑↑	?	?	
Propofol	↓	↓	↔↓	?	↓	?	?	
Etomidate	↔	↔	↔	↔	↔	?	?	
Halothane	↓↓	↓↓	↔↓	↔	↓	↔↓	↑	Sensitizes myocardium to catecholamines
Isoflurane	↔↑	↔↓	↑	↓↓	↓↓	↔↓	↑	
N_2O	↔↑	↓	↑	↔	↔↑	↑	↔	
Desflurane	↑	↔↓	↑	↓↓	↓↓	↔↓	↑	
Sevoflurane	↔↑	↔↓	↔	↓	↓	↓	?	
Fentanyl	↔↓	↔	↓↓	↔	↔↓	?	↔	Bradycardia, bradyarrhythmias (negated by co-injection of atropine)
Alfentanil	↔↓	↔	↓↓	↔	↔↓	?	↔	Bradycardia, bradyarrhythmias (negated by co-injection of atropine)

19.10 Summary of the haemodynamic effects of sedatives and anaesthetics. Data have been derived from several species and sources. Drug effects will be influenced by physiological, pathological and pharmacological factors unique to individual patients, so under certain conditions, minimal or even opposite changes to those described may be seen. Non-steroidal anti-inflammatory drugs (e.g. carprofen and ketoprofen) have not been included in this list because of *minimal* direct haemodynamic effects. ↑ = Increased; ↓ = Decreased; ↔ = No change; ↔↑ = No or slightly increased effect; ↔↓ = No or slightly decreased effect; ↑-↓ = Biphasic effect; ? = No information found.

is unfamiliar. However, this recommendation should not be taken as one of support for familiar, yet fundamentally unsafe, techniques.

Pre-anaesthetic medication

Neuroleptanalgesic combinations based on low dose acepromazine and opioids are useful in dogs and cats. The opioid chosen depends on several factors, including its haemodynamic effects. The author favours morphine, except when increases in heart rate are desired, when pethidine (meperidine) is used instead. Neuroleptanalgesic combinations are safe in cats: morphine (0.1–0.25 mg/kg) does not produce undesirable neurological effects providing it is injected intramuscularly with acepromazine (0.05–0.1 mg/kg).

Diazepam- or midazolam-based combinations offer theoretical benefits because benzodiazepines are largely devoid of cardiovascular effect. However, they are unreliable sedatives and often cause stimulation, even in depressed animals. They are useful in cats combined with ketamine and/or acepromazine.

Medetomidine should not be used for pre-anaesthetic medication in sick animals. The availability of an antagonist (atipamezole) does not justify its use, or that of other alpha-2 agonists, in high-risk cases because of the cardiovascular changes they produce (see Chapter 12).

Antimuscarinic drugs (atropine and glycopyrronium) may be used to increase heart rate, or to prevent bradycardia if this is likely to develop. However, they should not be used routinely as they cause arrhythmias in animals whose myocardial oxygen balance is precarious. There appears to be little evidence for the widespread conviction that glycopyrronium is safer than atropine.

Once pre-anaesthetic medication has been given, severely debilitated and/or deeply sedated animals should be monitored closely, though unobtrusively. There are advantages in applying the ECG and other physiological monitors at this time, providing they do not upset the subject. In very sick animals, central venous and/or arterial catheters may be placed under local anaesthesia, while enriching inspired air with oxygen will rarely do harm at this stage and can be achieved in several ways, e.g. nasal or transtracheal catheterization if the direct application of a mask is resented.

Induction

Induction of anaesthesia must be stress-free and not unduly compromise haemodynamic function. The objective is to provide conditions *just* sufficient for atraumatic tracheal intubation using a minimum effective dose of anaesthetic. However, anaesthesia must be adequate for tracheal intubation otherwise ventricular arrhythmias may arise, at least in dogs. 'Bucking' against the endotracheal tube also promotes lung collapse. Neglecting to intubate the airway of animals with cardiovascular disease is indefensible.

There are no ideal induction techniques. Some veterinary surgeons favour either drug combinations, or a series of drugs given in sequence for their minimal cardiovascular effects: benzodiazepines and opioids feature predominately in these techniques. However, most have their own specific disadvantages and offer few advantages over properly administered thiopental or propofol. Etomidate is popular in the USA because of its minimal effects on cardiovascular function. Problems with intravenous anaesthetics usually arise from a failure to appreciate abnormal pharmacokinetics (see Figure 19.1) rather than from drug effects *per se*. Any ultra short-acting injectable anaesthetic is suitable, providing the minimum effective dose is given carefully, i.e. a normal dose is prepared, but a lower than normal dose given initially, and at a slower rate. A longer interval must be left between deciding that intubation conditions are inadequate, and making further injections.

In severely compromised, sedated animals, the author uses halothane or sevoflurane delivered in a 1:2 oxygen:nitrous oxide mixture by facemask. At the first sign of resistance to the mask, a hypnotic dose of thiopental (1–3 mg/kg) or propofol (1 mg/kg) is injected intravenously. These doses eliminate reaction to the facemask but do not cause apnoea, so induction with the volatile agent continues. Despite atmospheric pollution, the technique allows for rapid recovery when problems arise.

Induction by facemask, or by the combination of facemask with subanaesthetic doses of intravenous agents, is feasible in well sedated cats. Chamber induction is another option in well sedated animals because it obviates the need for stressful restraint and ensures continuous oxygen delivery.

Transient ventricular arrhythmias are not uncommon during induction. The incidence seems to be reduced if intravenous anaesthetic solutions are diluted, e.g. 1.25% thiopental, and injected more slowly. Nevertheless, syringes pre-filled with rapidly acting antiarrhythmic drugs (e.g. lidocaine and atropine) should be available and the ECG monitored throughout.

Post-induction apnoea is normal with intravenous anaesthetics, especially propofol, and may cause haemoglobin desaturation. However, apnoea following normal doses is inconsequential providing the trachea is intubated briskly and the lungs inflated with oxygen-enriched gas, at a rate of two to three breaths per minute.

Maintenance

Ideally, the drugs used to provide surgical conditions should be non-cumulative and preserve cardiovascular function. Volatile anaesthetics profoundly depress haemodynamic function and so the minimum effective dose, i.e. the dose *just* preventing autonomic nervous responses to surgery, must always be used. The minimum effective dose is lowered (and haemodynamic function preserved) by other drugs, notably nitrous oxide, opioid analgesics, lidocaine, ketamine and benzodiazepines (see Chapter 13). The infusion of combinations of drugs to reduce volatile anaesthetic requirements also exerts desirable polymodal and pre-emptive analgesic effects. The author favours an alfentanil–ketamine combination, infused at doses of 1 and 10 μg/kg/minute, respectively. Similar objectives have been met elsewhere using a morphine, lidocaine and ketamine combination (Muir *et al.*, 2003).

By relieving volatile anaesthetics from the task of relaxing skeletal muscle, neuromuscular-blocking agents also lower anaesthetic requirements. In veterinary anaesthesia, inhalant anaesthesia still offers considerable advantages over total intravenous techniques.

Body position

Extreme body positions must be avoided: head-up body positions reduce venous return while severe head-down positions impair breathing, reduce functional residual capacity and lower cerebral perfusion pressure. Excessive thoracic limb fixation with ties may lower chest wall compliance and increase the work of breathing in spontaneously breathing animals.

Depth of anaesthesia

Anaesthetic overdose and inadequate anaesthesia are equally undesirable in animals with unstable cardiovascular function. Stress responses to surgery involving catecholamine release increase whole-body oxygen demand, heart rate, cardiac contractility and afterload and so threaten myocardial oxygen balance. Inadequate anaesthesia produced with theoretically appropriate drugs is probably more hazardous than adequate conditions provided by inappropriate agents. In one study, increasing the inspired concentration of halothane, a notorious arrhythmogenic drug, was effective at suppressing ventricular arrhythmias in both dogs and cats (Muir *et al.*, 1988). Pre-emptive and polymodal pain therapy are very desirable in cases with cardiovascular disease.

Anaesthetic overdose depresses cardiovascular function and so the depth of anaesthesia must be closely monitored. Depth should be altered to meet variations in surgical stimulation and maintained using minimum effective doses. Autonomic nervous responses to surgery are best controlled with potent analgesics, e.g. intravenous alfentanil or fentanyl, rather than intravenous or inhalational anaesthetics.

Surgical manipulation

During operations involving thoracic viscera, unavoidable manipulation of the heart and great vessels may limit cardiac output. Rotating the heart kinks the great veins and impairs ventricular filling. Accidental epicardial stimulation with surgical instruments produces ventricular ectopic beats while the use of cold irrigation fluids impairs contractility.

Ventilatory mode

Cardiovascular disease frequently affects pulmonary function. The end result(s) of ventilatory inadequacy (hypoxia, hypercapnia or both) are poorly tolerated by animals with cardiovascular disease. Hypoxia and hypercapnia are arrhythmogenic because they simultaneously promote sympathetic nervous activity (and solicit an increase in cardiac work) while impairing myocardial contractility.

Anaesthetized, spontaneously breathing animals normally hypoventilate and retain carbon dioxide. However, the thoracic pump is preserved and providing respiratory depression is not severe, cardiac output is not unduly depressed. Severe hypoventilation may occur in animals with chest wall and neural lesions (see Chapter 20). Controlled ventilation is required whenever spontaneous breathing fails to maintain normal arterial blood gas values. However, by raising the mean intrathoracic pressure, it inhibits the thoracolumbar pump and causes systemic hypotension. Pulmonary vascular impedance increases during inspiration and momentarily lowers right ventricular stroke volume. This may be hazardous when pulmonary blood flow is reduced, i.e. in pulmonary embolism, severe pulmonary valve stenosis or pulmonary hypertension, when injudicious IPPV may critically lower pulmonary blood flow.

Careful IPPV, which is usually advantageous in animals with cardiovascular disease, achieves an adequate minute ventilation volume with minimal elevation of the mean intrathoracic pressure. This requires that the inspiratory:expiratory (I:E) time ratio is short (about 1:3), that airway pressures are kept at a minimum (ideally 15–20 cmH_2O) and that there is no positive end-expiratory pressure (PEEP). High inflation pressures may be beneficial in conditions characterized by left-to-right shunts, e.g. patent ductus arteriosus, because they limit volume-loading of the left ventricle. Positive inflation pressures also oppose pulmonary transudative forces and should be used if pulmonary oedema is likely.

Fluid balance

Fluid loss, haemorrhage or venodilation are poorly tolerated whenever ventricular filling pressures are needed to maintain cardiac output, e.g. cardiac tamponade. In such cases, a large-bore catheter should be dedicated to fluid administration. Ideally, fluids are replaced as they are lost, and on a 'like-for-like' basis. Body fluids are lost as blood (haemorrhage), urine, water vapour, by evaporation from the respiratory tract and surgical site, and as transudate into a 'third-space' created by surgery (third-space losses). Only haemorrhage and urinary loss are easily quantified. Blood loss is measured by weighing swabs (1 ml blood weighs 1.3 g) and for each 1 ml blood shed, 1 ml blood or colloid solution or 3 ml of crystalloid solution are given. Third-space losses into damaged tissue are impossible to quantify but many accept that crystalloid solution infusions of 5, 10 or 15 ml/kg/h in dogs, or 3, 6 or 9 ml/kg/h in cats compensate for the effects of mild, moderate and major operations, respectively. Concessions are necessary when 'ideal' fluids are unavailable. The common statement that sodium-containing solutions should not be used in animals with cardiac disease is a counsel of perfection and when critical perioperative hypovolaemia arises, the rapid administration of *any* isotonic fluid will be life-saving (a sodium load can be dealt with later using loop diuretics).

Increased ventricular pre- and afterload and reduced pulmonary compliance result from over-transfusion with blood and colloid, and to a lesser extent crystalloid solutions, and must be avoided in cases with left heart failure as it may lead to pulmonary oedema. Haemorrhage during corrective cardiovascular surgery is usually not excessive but the aorta or pulmonary artery can be inadvertently damaged, with critical results. The means of rapidly transfusing large volumes of blood or colloid, i.e. adequate fluid stocks and a pressurizing device, should be available.

Body temperature

Hypothermia is a common complication in young animals undergoing surgery for the correction of cardiac anomalies in which viscera are exposed for prolonged periods. This is undesirable as hypothermia depresses ventilation, increases blood viscosity and shifts the oxyhaemoglobin dissociation curve to the left. Arrhythmias arise spontaneously in the chilled heart, with ventricular fibrillation becoming increasingly likely as temperatures approach 28°C. In recovery, hypothermia initiates shivering, which increases whole body oxygen requirements four-fold. The core temperature should be preserved throughout the perioperative period using prophylactic, rather than active, measures. Irrigation fluids should be warmed to 37°C before use.

Deliberate hypothermia involves actively cooling cerebral and myocardial tissue to 16–20°C in order to reduce oxygen requirements during periods of deliberate circulatory arrest. At these temperatures, the artificial support of both pulmonary and cardiovascular function (cardiopulmonary bypass) is mandatory.

Monitoring

There is no single measure of adequate cardiovascular function during anaesthesia and so an overall picture is gained by measuring and interpreting many variables. In cases with modest cardiovascular disease undergoing minor surgery, a minimum acceptable level of monitoring would include the continuous surveillance of unconsciousness, pulse rate and quality (by palpation), mucous membrane colour, capillary refill time, respiratory rate, depth and rhythm, core (oesophageal) temperatures, absolute blood loss, the *rate* of bleeding and blood colour at the surgical site. If skin temperature is measured simultaneously, the core–peripheral temperature gradient, which may reflect tissue perfusion, can be calculated. Heart and lung sounds are most easily monitored using an oesophageal stethoscope. The high prevalence of cardiac arrhythmias in companion animal anaesthesia justifies ECG monitoring, while simplicity and the value of information supports the measurement of urine output. Measuring CVP is useful in cases where cardiac output depends on ventricular preload. Pulse oximetry is easy to perform and gives vital information, providing the probe permits accurate measurement. Devices with a 'bouncing' plethysmograph are useful because they display pulsatile blood flow and indicate mechanical cardiac activity. In high-risk cases, arterial blood pressure should be monitored directly. Capnography is useful as a guide to effective IPPV, and to give early warning of critical haemodynamic events. The major advantages of capnography and pulse oximetry over serial arterial blood-gas analysis in general practice is that they are economically feasible. However, the inexperienced are advised against the indiscriminate use of complicated electronic monitors in high-risk cases as these may, in producing excessive information of varying quality, detract from the appraisal of vital signs. In any case, monitoring a given variable can only be fully justified if the veterinary surgeon can interpret its significance and make an appropriate response.

Neuromuscular blockade

Neuromuscular-blocking agents are useful in animals with severe cardiovascular disease when administered by individuals trained in their use. The penalty for misuse by the inexperienced is high. Atracurium, vecuronium and rocuronium are devoid of significant cardiovascular effects and may be used to improve surgical conditions and facilitate IPPV (see Chapter 15). Overdose, which may prolong recovery, is avoided if drug administration is based on continuous monitoring of neuromuscular transmission. Postoperative hypoventilation is prevented if neuromuscular block is antagonized; an edrophonium (1 mg/kg) and atropine (40 µg/kg) mixture injected over 2 minutes does not produce autonomic nervous or ECG changes in dogs.

Cardiovascular adjunct drugs

Rapid- and short-acting formulations of drugs used for preoperative preparation can be used during surgery to offset adverse haemodynamic events, providing they are safe when given intravenously. Haemodynamic problems encountered during anaesthesia in animals with cardiovascular disease, and their treatment, are examined in Figure 19.6. The control of intraoperative arrythmias is detailed in Figure 19.5.

Recovery

Problems during recovery are most common in cases which have not undergone corrective surgery, because the cardiovascular system has now to contend with pain, hypoventilation and hypothermia. Intraoperative monitoring and medications should continue until urine output is adequate, the ECG is stable and the extremities are warm and perfused. Pain must be aggressively managed, preferably with a polymodal approach; after cranial laparotomy or thoracotomy, pain from the incision site discourages deep breathing and promotes lung collapse. Periodic repositioning may be necessary in animals which do not inspire deeply. Inspired gas should be enriched with oxygen until the animal can maintain adequately saturated haemoglobin (saturation of haemoglobin with oxygen measured by pulse oximeter (S_pO_2) >90%) while breathing room air. This is especially important in the shivering animal.

Acquired cardiovascular conditions

In veterinary practice, it is common for acquired cardiovascular diseases to complicate anaesthesia in older animals presented for straightforward operations. The following sections describe the anaesthetic management for common examples of cardiovascular conditions listed in Figure 19.9.

Mitral valve incompetence

Mitral valvular incompetence resulting from endocardiosis begins as a fixed, low cardiac output condition. During systole, a proportion of the stroke volume flows back into the left atrium (Figure 19.11). Later, ventricular failure supervenes, with atrial fibrillation and pulmonary oedema complicating the clinical picture. In time, high back pressure from the pulmonary veins leads to right ventricular and congestive failure.

Preoperative preparation aims to enhance aortic flow, reduce the regurgitant fraction of stroke volume and control pulmonary oedema. This is achieved with angiotensin converting enzyme (ACE) inhibitors, diuretics, beta-1 agonists, pimobendan, cage rest and low-sodium diets. Atrial fibrillation, if present, should be converted to sinus rhythm preoperatively because the atrial contribution to ventricular filling becomes more important when cardiac output is reduced by disease. This often occurs incidentally with afterload-reducing therapy: reducing the regurgitant fraction volume reduces left atrial dilation.

Anaesthesia is managed as for fixed, low-output conditions. However, in unprepared animals facing emergency operations, the problem is one of low cardiac output and poor contractility (see Dilated cardiomyopathy, below). In addition to the haemodynamic objectives listed in Figure 19.10, anaesthesia in animals with leaking mitral valves should aim to:

- Produce mild reductions in systemic vascular resistance (promotes forward flow)
- Produce modest increases (<10% preoperative values) in heart rate (reduces regurgitant fraction and prevents falls in diastolic pressure and hence coronary perfusion)
- Avoid bradycardia and hypertension (which increases valvular regurgitation).

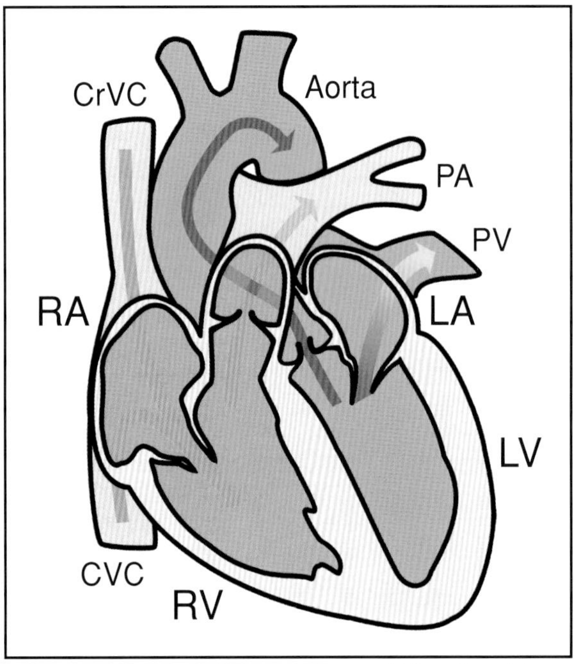

19.11 Mitral valve incompetence. CrVC = Cranial vena cava; CVC = Caudal vena cava; LA = Left atrium; LV = Left ventricle; PA = Pulmonary artery; PV = Pulmonary vein; RA = Right atrium; RV = Right ventricle.

Pre-anaesthetic medication with low dose acepromazine combined with an opioid agonist drug with chronotropic activities, e.g. pethidine (meperidine), usually provides adequate sedation whilst fulfilling haemodynamic objectives. High dose acepromazine may cause hypotension, particularly if ACE inhibitors have been given. Of the ultra short-acting intravenous anaesthetics suitable for induction in animals with mild to moderate disease, etomidate has the least depressant effects. A venous catheter should be placed before induction so that fluids can be infused in case venodilation (as occurs with thiopental) reduces ventricular filling. In severely affected animals, a combined mask/intravenous technique is suitable. Isoflurane has several advantages over halothane in these cases. Nitrous oxide mildly increases systemic vascular resistance but the benefits of inclusion usually outweigh the disadvantages. Ventricular preload should be maintained using intravenous fluids, while IPPV is of value when there are signs of pulmonary oedema.

Mitral valve stenosis

Managing mitral valve stenosis, which fixes cardiac output by limiting left ventricular filling during diastole, is a considerably greater challenge than mitral valve regurgitation. In this condition, cardiac output depends on blood transfer across the stenotic valve (Figure 19.12). This is greatest at slow heart rates (increases diastolic filling time) and when sinus rhythm, rather than atrial fibrillation, is present. However, the small left ventricle limits stroke volume and heart rate slowing may cause hypotension. Coincidental increases in left atrial and pulmonary venous pressures lead to atrial fibrillation and pulmonary oedema, respectively. As in any fixed low-output condition, anaesthesia must:

- Maintain cardiac output
- Maintain, or produce modest increases in, heart rate
- Maintain systemic vascular resistance
- Maintain sinus rhythm
- Avoid injudicious IPPV.

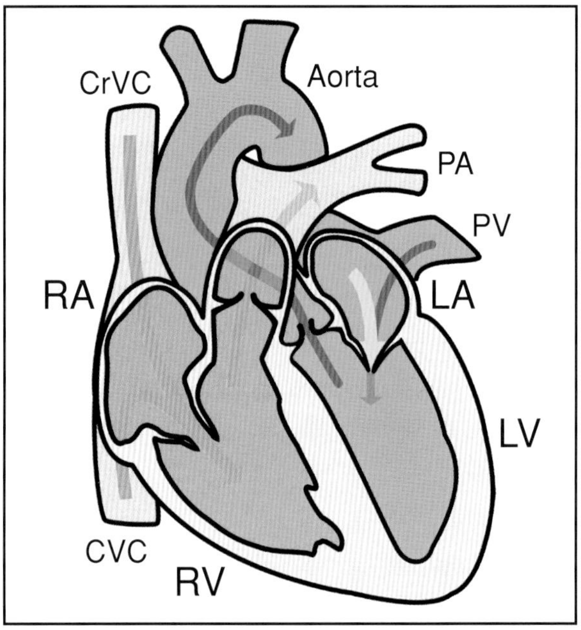

19.12 Mitral valve stenosis. CrVC = Cranial vena cava; CVC = Caudal vena cava; LA = Left atrium; LV = Left ventricle; PA = Pulmonary artery; PV = Pulmonary vein; RA = Right atrium; RV = Right ventricle.

The challenge here is in maintaining cardiac output whilst avoiding pulmonary oedema by overtransfusion or by increasing right ventricular output. Fluids must be given on a strict 'as needed' basis, while inotropes should only be used when signs of right ventricular failure are present. Cardiac output relies on the maintenance of heart rate and systemic vascular resistance. The latter should be maintained with alpha-1 agonist drugs; peripheral vasodilators will cause severe hypotension. While IPPV restricts pulmonary fluid transudation, it increases right ventricular afterload and so must be imposed judiciously. Furthermore, the lungs may have limited compliance (being engorged with extra blood) and require higher pressures for inflation.

Cardiac tamponade

The pericardium is only slightly distensible and so space-occupying masses or effusions within the pericardial sac readily raise intrapericardial pressure and restrict atrial and right ventricular filling. This reduces left ventricular stroke volume and renders cardiac output dependent upon heart rate, while arterial and venular constriction maintain blood pressure. When the elastic limits of the pericardial sac are reached, a small volume increment causes disproportionate rises in intrapericardial pressure and a critical reduction in cardiac output.

Some causes of cardiac tamponade, e.g. congenital peritoneopericardial diaphragmatic hernia, are amenable to surgical treatment. Preoperatively, pericardial effusions must be relieved (pericardiocentesis). Diuretics must be used carefully in animals with signs of oedema: over-use may reduce right-sided filling pressure. Anaesthesia should aim to:

- Avoid *any* reduction in heart rate
- Avoid *any* reduction in systemic vascular resistance.

Bradycardia will critically reduce cardiac output; positive chronotropes must be available and ready for use. Adequate cardiac output also depends on adequate ventricular filling pressure; hypovolaemia and other factors limiting venous return must be avoided. If IPPV is necessary, a low tidal volume/high frequency pattern will achieve alveolar ventilation with minimum effects on mean intrathoracic pressure. CVP should be monitored because it reflects right ventricular filling pressures. (It should also fall dramatically after pericardectomy.) Drugs causing marked arteriolar or venular dilation must be avoided where possible.

Canine sick sinus syndrome

Artificial pacemaker implantation is required when spontaneous cardiac pacemaker activity fails to initiate adequate cardiac output, e.g. in dogs with high-grade second-degree heart block, third-degree heart block, persistent atrial standstill and canine 'sick sinus syndrome'. Slow preoperative heart rates may respond to drugs such as isopropamide, propantheline, isoprenaline or terbutaline. This indicates drugs which may prove effective for controlling critical pre-implantation bradycardia, e.g. atropine, glycopyrronium or isoprenaline, and which should be made available before anaesthesia begins.

The operation usually takes place in two stages. A temporary pacing wire is passed via the external jugular vein into the right ventricle, often under neuroleptanalgesia and the infiltration of overlying tissue with local anaesthetic. Once the electrode tip of the pacemaker wire is located at the right ventricular apex (under fluoroscopy) and the heart is 'captured' (i.e. responds to the pacemaker unit), then general anaesthesia can be induced with little risk, and the permanent pacemaker implanted in the soft tissue of the neck or abdomen. The latter approach involves thoracotomy; the pacing wire is passed through the diaphragm before its insertion into the ventricular epicardium.

It may occasionally be more convenient to position the temporary pacing wire under general anaesthesia, when there is a real risk of cardiac arrest. The risk is reduced in the following ways:

- Choosing pre-anaesthetic medication that does not reduce heart rate or increase systemic vascular resistance
- Making available intravenous drugs which have proven chronotropic effect in the subject
- Monitoring the ECG as soon as pre-anaesthetic medication is given
- Attempting endotracheal intubation only once the animal is adequately anaesthetized (any ultra short-acting intravenous anaesthetic is suitable)
- Making provisions for emergency transvenous pacing and direct current (DC) defibrillation.

Dilated (congestive) cardiomyopathy

Large-breed male dogs are predisposed to dilated (congestive) cardiomyopathy (DCM), which is characterized by severe left ventricular systolic dysfunction. The left ventricle is thin-walled, flabby and dilated. Both atrial and ventricular arrhythmias are common and most dogs eventually develop both left and right heart failure, with pulmonary oedema. While some dogs respond to therapy, others die suddenly. In cats, DCM results from taurine deficiency, produces characteristic signs of right, not left, failure, and responds to dietary taurine supplementation (250 mg q12h).

Animals with DCM can die suddenly under anaesthesia and so adequate preoperative preparation is mandatory. Therapy involves management of pleural effusions (by thoracocentesis), pulmonary oedema (with furosemide) and heart failure (with pimobendan, digoxin, furosemide and vasodilators such as ACE inhibitors, prazosin or hydralazine). This is particularly important when atrial fibrillation is present. The haemodynamic goals of anaesthesia are to:

- Maintain cardiac output
- Avoid factors reducing myocardial oxygen balance.

Preoperative heart rate should be preserved and arrhythmias treated as they arise. Isoflurane offers advantages over halothane although inotropes and chronotropes may still be required. Venous return must be maintained using fluids.

Traumatic myocarditis (myocardial contusions)

Blunt thoracic trauma of sufficient force to contuse the epicardium (and fracture a thoracic limb) frequently results in ventricular arrhythmias which develop 24–48 hours later. These, combined with other effects of injury, e.g. pain, anxiety and hypovolaemia, produce an inefficiently high heart rate which threatens myocardial oxygen balance and makes ventricular fibrillation more likely. Other consequences of trauma, e.g. electrolyte and acid–base disturbances, also promote arrhythmias. Road traffic accident cases with thoracic limb fractures and/or thoracic injury should undergo ECG examination preoperatively. The treatment of arrhythmias is aimed at reducing plasma catecholamine levels and involves anxiolysis and analgesia, cage rest, the administration of oxygen and the restoration of effective circulating blood volume. Low dose acepromazine with morphine given intramuscularly eliminates arrhythmias in many cases. In others, lidocaine infusion may be necessary, given as an intravenous bolus and followed by a constant rate infusion. Procainamide may be necessary on the rare occasions that lidocaine fails. In animals with traumatic myocarditis, the haemodynamic effects of anaesthesia should:

- Reduce heart rate
- Avoid factors reducing myocardial oxygen balance
- Suppress arrhythmias.

Neuroleptanalgesic combinations are suitable for pre-anaesthetic medication. Preoperative anti-arrhythmic therapy, i.e. lidocaine infusion, should be maintained throughout the operative period and into recovery if necessary. Anaesthetics slowing or reducing myocardial oxygen demand, e.g. halothane, may be more suitable than those which maintain cardiac output, e.g. isoflurane and sevoflurane.

Hypovolaemia: absolute and relative

When intravascular volume losses exceed gains, e.g. haemorrhage, polyuria, vomiting and diarrhoea, effective circulating blood volume falls and limits ventricular preload, causing a low, variable cardiac output state. This also occurs when a normal volume circulates within an expanded vascular bed, e.g. in vasodilation caused by Gram-negative septicaemia. Restoring effective circulating blood volume obviates the problems associated with absolute or relative hypovolaemia and so elective surgery should be postponed until this is achieved. A greater challenge arises in cases requiring anaesthesia before fluid resuscitation is complete, e.g. when post-traumatic emergency surgery is required to locate and control internal haemorrhage. In these cases, anaesthesia must:

- Maintain ventricular filling pressures
- Maintain systemic vascular resistance
- Avoid high lung inflation pressures.

Ventricular filling pressures are maintained with intravenous fluids. Fluid balance should be monitored critically by accurately recording gains (i.e. infused volume) against losses (e.g. haemorrhage and urine). CVP is the preferred indicator of volume adequacy although the rate and degree of jugular venous distension after digital occlusion at the thoracic inlet provides an estimate. Systemic vascular resistance is preserved by avoiding vasodilatory drugs and/or giving alpha-1 agonists. Acepromazine should not be used at doses >12.5 μg/kg, if at all. Great care is required in giving all injectable drugs because the volume of distribution is smaller (see Figure 19.1). Surgical anaesthesia should rely more on high doses of analgesics rather than inhaled anaesthetics. High intrathoracic pressures must be avoided if IPPV is imposed, as these reduce venous return.

Cor pulmonale

Risks from anaesthesia are high in cor pulmonale because problems with lung pathology and right ventricular failure are combined. Right ventricular pathology secondary to pulmonary hypertension results from lung diseases like chronic bronchitis and bronchiectasis. Chronic hypoxia arising from lung disease causes pulmonary vasoconstriction and aggravates the condition. Pulmonary hypertension eventually leads to right-sided congestive heart failure.

Elective operations are postponed until all reversible elements of pulmonary disease have been treated and pulmonary arterial pressure lowered. The latter is achieved most simply with oxygen, which reverses pulmonary hypoxic vasoconstriction. In chronic conditions, bronchodilators and antibiotics may be beneficial (see Chapter 20). If right-sided failure is present, cage rest, low-salt diets and short-term diuretic therapy should be imposed. Positive inotropes (e.g. pimobendan and digoxin) should only be used if signs of congestive failure are obvious. Polycythaemia may necessitate normovolaemic haemodilution. In treating pulmonary hypertension, vasodilators may cause more problems than they solve so should be used carefully, if at all. Anaesthesia should aim to:

- Maintain or reduce pulmonary vascular resistance
- Avoid excessive lung inflation pressures.

Nitrous oxide increases pulmonary vascular resistance and this has led many to condemn its use in cases with pulmonary hypertension. However, volatile anaesthetics reduce pulmonary vascular resistance to a greater extent and so compensate for this. If IPPV is required, the airway pressures imposed must be the lowest required for adequate lung inflation.

Canine hypertension

Anaesthesia in dogs with hypertension is complicated in at least four ways:

- Increased left ventricular afterload and mass jeopardizes myocardial oxygen balance
- Hypertension occurs in diseases which elevate risk, e.g. polycythaemia and primary renal disease
- Chronic hypertension damages the brain, eyes, heart, kidneys and peripheral vessels
- Chronic hypertension shifts the autoregulation curve for renal and cerebral perfusion to the right. Blood flow in these organs becomes pressure-dependent at relatively high values. Blood pressure values that would ensure adequate perfusion in normotensive animals are inadequate in hypertensive cases.

Anaesthesia should be delayed, if possible, until normal arterial pressure is restored with low-sodium diets, diuretics, high doses of ACE inhibitors, beta-1 antagonists, alpha-1 antagonists or calcium channel blockers such as amlodipine. This may take several weeks. When faced with non-elective operations, anaesthesia must:

- Maintain or modestly increase blood pressure
- Maintain or modestly reduce systemic vascular resistance
- Avoid factors reducing myocardial oxygen balance.

Management depends on extensive monitoring and the judicious use of both inotropes and vasoactive adjunct drugs because it is not possible to achieve these haemodynamic goals simultaneously. Preoperative heart rate should be preserved and arrhythmias treated if they arise. Isoflurane offers some advantages over halothane, although inotropes and chronotropes may still be required. Venous return must be maintained with intravenous fluid administration.

Feline hyperthyroidism

See also Chapter 25. Thyroidectomy is the treatment of choice for hyperthyroidism. However, the preoperative restoration of euthyroidism and normal cardiac output using methimazole (2.5 mg orally q12h) for 2–3 weeks is necessary, otherwise anaesthesia is complicated by the presence of high-output cardiac failure and ventricular arrhythmias. Occasionally, emergency (non-thyroid) surgery may be necessary in unprepared animals. In these patients, pre-induction stress (caused by excessive restraint, an unsympathetic environment, pain, etc.) must be minimized. Consequently, oxygen, which may be needed to alleviate dyspnoea, should be given by chamber, rather than mask. Pre- and intraoperative cardiac hyperactivity and arrhythmias must be managed with beta-1 antagonist drugs, such as propranolol or esmolol. The goals of anaesthesia are to:

- Avoid all factors reducing myocardial oxygen balance
- Suppress ventricular arrhythmias.

Acepromazine exerts useful anti-arrhythmic effects and should be included in pre-anaesthetic medication. If subsequent sedation is inadequate, a chamber induction using sevoflurane (over isoflurane) may prove less stressful than an intravenous technique. Anaesthetics increasing or maintaining heart rate and contractility (e.g. ketamine, isoflurane) are probably less safe than those with a depressant effect (e.g. halothane). Drugs increasing afterload and ventricular wall tension, e.g. alpha-2 agonists, should not be used, while the factors listed in Figure 19.8 must be avoided. The other effects of elevated metabolic rate (increased oxygen consumption and carbon dioxide production) should be considered when setting flows to breathing systems and when IPPV is imposed.

Hypertrophic cardiomyopathy

Hypertrophic cardiomyopathy (HCM) is rare in dogs but is not uncommon in young to middle-aged male cats. It may occur secondary to hyperthyroidism. In some cases of HCM, a muscular subaortic stenosis forms during systole, which momentarily restricts left ventricular outflow and promotes mitral regurgitation. The effects of obstruction are greater when heart rate and myocardial contractility are increased and when left ventricular diastolic volume and ventricular afterload are decreased, all of which lower cardiac output when HCM is present. Often asymptomatic, its first signs may be pulmonary oedema or sudden death during anaesthesia.

Cats with HCM must not be stressed preoperatively (see Feline hyperthyroidism, above) but should receive supplemental oxygen. Heart failure, if present, is controlled with furosemide and vasodilators (glyceryl trinitrate ointment, benazepril or enalapril). Calcium channel blockers, such as diltiazem, exert a useful anti-arrhythmic and a positive lusitropic effect. Tachycardia may respond to atenolol. Pulmonary oedema, if present, is treated using oxygen, furosemide, cage rest and glyceryl trinitrate ointment, while pleural effusions are relieved by thoracocentesis. The goals of anaesthesia are to:

- Prevent heart rate increases
- Suppress contractility
- Suppress ventricular arrhythmias
- Maintain filling pressures
- Maintain or increase systemic vascular resistance
- Avoid all factors reducing myocardial oxygen balance.

Halothane may have advantages over isoflurane in this condition. Intraoperative hypotension should be treated with alpha-1 agonists such as phenylephrine, rather than beta-1 agonists, while hypertension should be controlled by increasing the delivered concentration of volatile agent; vasodilators are unsuitable. High perioperative heart rates arising from surgical stimulation should be controlled with analgesics such as alfentanil; beta-1 antagonists may be used if the cause is non-physiological.

Congenital cardiovascular conditions

Cardiac anomalies may be asymptomatic in young animals requiring incidental operations, and present little challenge beyond the haemodynamic effects of the lesion itself. However, some anomalies are associated with rapid cardiovascular deterioration. In these, limited cardiovascular reserve may be critically eroded when invasive operations are performed on immature animals. The small size of very young animals makes anaesthesia and surgery technically difficult, while physiological immaturity creates further problems. However, the advantages of postponing surgery are less significant than the disadvantage of a disproportionately increasing anaesthetic risk. It is nearly always safer to perform surgery on young, small animals rather than wait until the subject is larger and in advanced cardiac failure.

Accidental hypothermia is almost inevitable during surgical correction of cardiac anomalies:

- Small subjects have a high surface area:volume ratio
- The subjects are physiologically immature
- Operations are long
- A large visceral surface is exposed

- Animals are 'deeply' anaesthetized
- The lungs are ventilated with cold medical gases
- Irrigation fluids, which are extensively used, may be inadequately warmed.

Advanced techniques often required during cardiovascular surgery, e.g. thoracotomy, cardiopulmonary bypass and induced hypothermia, complicate anaesthesia, influence drug disposition and, when performed improperly, increase morbidity and mortality.

Congenital conditions can be classified in the same way as acquired disorders (see Figure 19.9) but further description is frequently necessary. Many anomalies are characterized by abnormal left-to-right or right-to-left conduits, through which blood shunts between the left (systemic) and right (pulmonary) circulation. Shunts are frequently of major clinical significance.

Left-to-right shunts are found in the more common form of patent ductus arteriosus (PDA), atrial septal defects (ASDs) and ventricular septal defects (VSDs) and are associated with massive increases in pulmonary blood flow and volume overload of either the left (PDA), right (ASD) or both (VSD) ventricles.

Right-to-left shunts are characterized by oxygen-resistant cyanosis and polycythaemia and are more dangerous. They are present in PDAs complicated by persistent pulmonary hypertension (see below). In all types, pulmonary flow is reduced so response to inhaled anaesthetics is sluggish while thoracic limb–brain circulation time is more rapid.

Patent ductus arteriosus

In the most common type of PDA, a proportion of left ventricular output enters the pulmonary artery and recirculates through the lung, i.e. there is a left-to-right shunt (Figure 19.13a). The reduced ejection fraction entering the descending aorta leads to hypotension in the absence of compensation. Diastolic blood pressure is typically low as the low resistance pulmonary vessels provide 'run-off'. In time, the increased left ventricular volume load and right ventricular pressure load lead to biventricular hypertrophy. Treatment involves surgical ligation of the ductus arteriosus.

Postparturient pulmonary vascular resistance remains high in some cases, and the resulting pulmonary hypertension causes ductal blood to flow in a right-to-left direction (Figure 19.13b). This is characterized by cyanotic mucous membranes in the rear half of the body, e.g. the penis, and normal mucous membranes in cranial structures. This occurs because oxygenated blood still flows down the brachiocephalic trunk and left subclavian artery which arise from the aorta proximal to the ductus. Surgery is inadvisable in these cases because the ductus arteriosus functions as a relief valve; ligation precipitates right heart failure.

Beyond the challenges of thoracotomy, anaesthesia and surgery in young, asymptomatic dogs carry few problems. Risk increases if surgery is delayed and decompensation occurs; left atrial dilation may precede fibrillation. When signs of heart failure are present, the animal should be stabilized and treatment continued until radiographic evidence of cardiomegaly, pulmonary congestion and pulmonary oedema is minimal. During surgery, the haemodynamic objectives are to minimize, and yet maintain, a left-to-right pressure gradient. This is achieved by anaesthetics which:

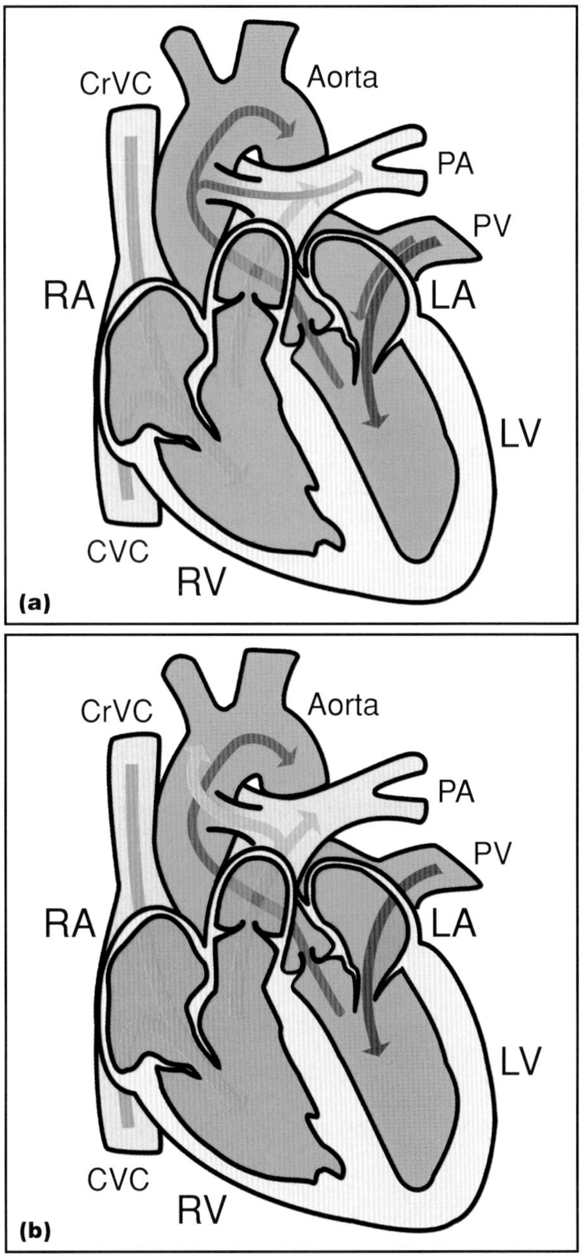

19.13 **(a)** Left-to-right patent ductus arteriosus. **(b)** Right-to-left patent ductus arteriosus. CrVC = Cranial vena cava; CVC = Caudal vena cava; LA = Left atrium; LV = Left ventricle; PA = Pulmonary artery; PV = Pulmonary vein; RA = Right atrium; RV = Right ventricle.

- Maintain cardiac output
- Avoid profound decreases in systemic vascular resistance
- Avoid marked increases in pulmonary vascular resistance.

Cardiac output is maintained with fluids and inotropes given to maintain, or produce slight increases in, heart rate. A modest reduction in systemic vascular resistance is desirable, as this increases systemic blood flow, reduces right ventricular afterload and may reduce left-to-right blood flow before ligation.

These effects are likely to be achieved with isoflurane or sevoflurane. Excessive lung inflation pressures are undesirable; increasing pulmonary over systemic vascular resistance could cause right-to-left shunting during parts of the cardiac cycle and lower S_pO_2. Increased pulmonary blood flow means the level of unconsciousness changes sluggishly after vaporizer settings are changed.

Ductal ligation is often associated with a transient reflex bradycardia (Bramham's sign) arising in response to raised diastolic pressure. If this occurs, the ligature should be slackened and re-tightened more slowly. There is no justification for atropine in this situation.

Ligation of a right-to-left shunting PDA is rarely performed, although occasionally it may be necessary to anaesthetize affected animals for incidental operations. These patients are at considerable risk from anaesthesia because they are usually hypoxic (P_aO_2 <60 mmHg (<7.9 kPa)) and polycythaemic. Attempts should be made to reverse the shunt, by the judicious use of alpha-1 agonists such as phenylephrine, which increase systemic vascular resistance, and alpha-2 antagonists, such as tolazoline, which lower pulmonary vascular resistance.

Pulmonic stenosis

In limiting right ventricular outflow, stenotic pulmonary valves raise right ventricular systolic pressures, which may render the tricuspid valve incompetent and cause right atrial enlargement (Figure 19.14). In time, the right ventricle hypertrophies and then fails. The condition is corrected by surgery or balloon valvuloplasty. The latter involves passing a balloon-tipped catheter via the jugular vein, the right atrium and the right ventricle up the pulmonary outflow tract and into the stenosis. The balloon is then inflated with the intent of physically dilating the stenosis.

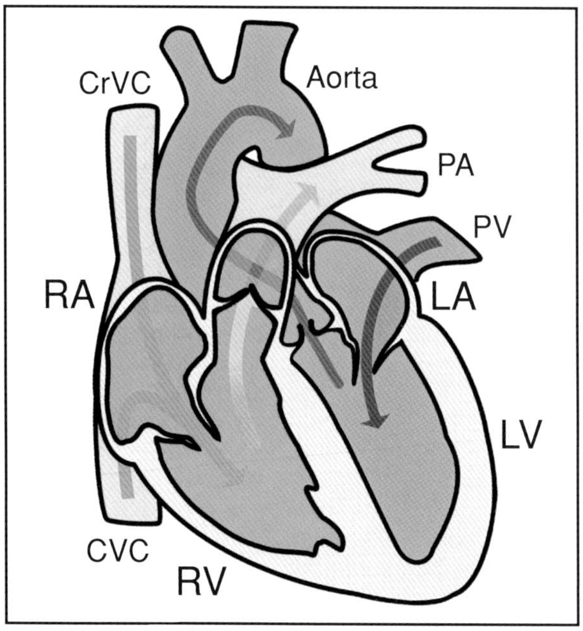

19.14 Pulmonic stenosis. CrVC = Cranial vena cava; CVC = Caudal vena cava; LA = Left atrium; LV = Left ventricle; PA = Pulmonary artery; PV = Pulmonary vein; RA = Right atrium; RV = Right ventricle.

Signs of right ventricular failure must be treated before an operation because the ventricle will be sensitive to the depressant effects of anaesthetics and IPPV. The haemodynamic goals of anaesthesia are to:

- Maintain myocardial contractility
- Maintain or modestly reduce heart rate
- Maintain right ventricular preload
- Avoid excessive lung inflation pressures.

Any volatile anaesthetic is suitable for this operation; isoflurane and sevoflurane maintain contractility but halothane reduces heart rate and so improves right ventricular filling. Dobutamine may be used to increase right ventricular contractility providing it does not increase heart rate. Adequate preload should be maintained by infusing fluids.

Aortic stenosis

Stenotic aortic valves (Figure 19.15) restrict left ventricular output and initiate hypertrophy and greater contractility, which in turn threatens myocardial oxygen balance. This is particularly hazardous because reduced diastolic arterial pressure, which is characteristic of aortic stenosis, leads to a critical reduction in coronary blood flow and sudden death (the coronary arteries arise from the aorta downstream from the stenotic valves). The condition can be treated by valvotomy (which necessitates cardiopulmonary bypass) or balloon valvuloplasty (which does not). Animals with this condition may require incidental operations.

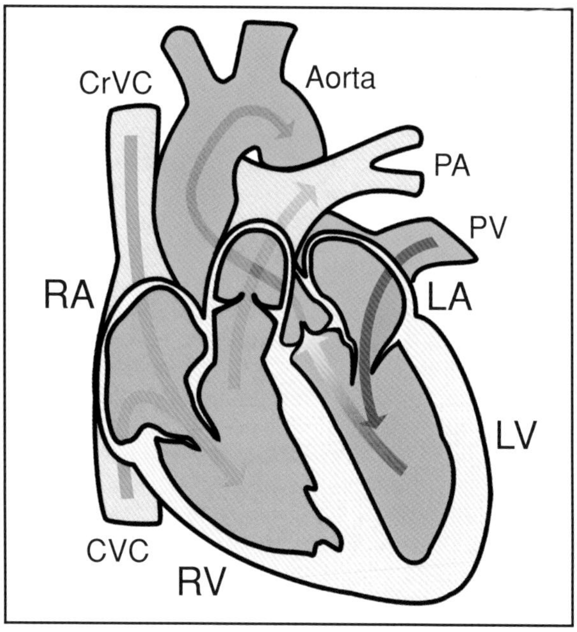

19.15 Aortic stenosis. CrVC = Cranial vena cava; CVC = Caudal vena cava; LA = Left atrium; LV = Left ventricle; PA = Pulmonary artery; PV = Pulmonary vein; RA = Right atrium; RV = Right ventricle.

Advanced cases with congestive failure respond poorly to diuretics, low-salt diets and rest, although beta adrenergic antagonists may be beneficial in long-term management of increased intraventricular pressures and hypertrophy. The haemodynamic goals of anaesthesia are to:

- Avoid hypotension by maintaining systemic vascular resistance, not increasing cardiac output
- Maintain heart rate within 20% of preoperative values
- Avoid factors reducing myocardial oxygen balance.

Arrhythmias are common in this condition and cause severe reductions in cardiac output. Bradycardia lowers cardiac output because the stroke volume is fixed, while tachycardia decreases the time for cardiac filling. In these cases, slight reductions in blood pressure cause disproportionately large reductions in coronary arterial filling pressure and delivery of oxygenated blood to the myocardium. Maintaining sinus rhythm is important as the left ventricle depends on synchronized atrial contractions to assure left ventricular filling (junctional or escape rhythms must be controlled as they arise). Intravascular fluid volume must be maintained. Providing heart rate and rhythm are maintained, the myocardium is not overly depressed and effective circulating blood volume is maintained, the most likely cause of intraoperative hypotension is drug-induced vasodilation. This must be remedied promptly with alpha-1 agonists.

Ventricular septal defect

The consequences of a ventricular septal defect (VSD) depend on its size and the shunt direction. The latter depends on the right-to-left ventricular pressure differential which in turn depends on pulmonary and systemic vascular resistance, respectively. Normally, blood flows left to right, because left ventricular pressures exceed those in the right. However, chronic hypoxia causes pulmonary hypertension, which may increase pulmonary vascular resistance to the point where shunt flow ceases or changes direction.

Anaesthesia for surgical correction requires cardiotomy and cardiopulmonary bypass. However, dogs with VSD may require anaesthesia for other operations. Cardiac failure must be treated if present. The haemodynamic goal of anaesthesia is to maintain a left-to-right shunt. This occurs if anaesthetics maintain systemic vascular resistance above pulmonary vascular resistance.

Blood pressure should be maintained with alpha-1 agonists, while high lung inflation pressures should be avoided.

Management of intraoperative arrhythmias

In general, intraoperative arrhythmias are more likely and of greater consequence in animals with cardiovascular disease. For simplicity, they have been divided here into brady- and tachyarrhythmias.

Bradyarrhythmias

Any factor listed in Figure 19.16 may slow heart rate during anaesthesia and cause significant hypotension and coronary hypoperfusion.

Cause	Treatment
Inadequately treated/ recurring preoperative causes	See Figures 19.2, 19.5 and 19.6
Anaesthetics	Establish causative agent; consider positive chronotropes
Anaesthetic overdose	Reduce delivered concentration of inhaled drug and ventilate lungs
Hypothermia	End surgery and re-warm; consider gastric or colonic lavage
Hypertension	Consider vasodilators and/or beta-1 antagonists
Vagal stimulation	Check surgery
Hyperkalaemia	Hyperventilate, with oxygen, give bicarbonate (1 mmol/kg over 10 minutes)
Severe acidosis	Hyperventilate lungs with oxygen and give bicarbonate (as above)
Severe hypoglycaemia	50% dextrose
Severe hypoxia	Ventilate lungs with 100% oxygen
Terminal myocardial hypoxia	Initiate cerebral-cardiopulmonary resuscitation (CCPR)

19.16 Causes of intraoperative bradyarrhythmias and suggested treatment. Note that 'lightening' anaesthesia or beginning surgery, if it has not already started, are the simplest treatments for drug-induced bradycardia. Antimuscarinic drugs safely reverse opioid-induced bradycardia but their use with alpha-2 agonists is controversial. When bradycardia, bradyarrhythmias or atrioventricular conduction blocks can be linked with specific surgical manipulations, surgery must be suspended and the level of anaesthesia assessed. 'Light' animals should have anaesthesia and surgery continued more gently. If the problem persists then atropine, glycopyrronium or isoprenaline should be given.

Tachyarrhythmias

Severe tachycardia reduces cardiac output and threatens myocardial oxygen balance; both are particularly undesirable in animals with myocardial disease. Unexpectedly high heart rates may disclose an undetected hypovolaemia or another physiological derangement (Figure 19.17). The rate of change of heart rate may indicate aetiology, e.g. sudden heart rate increases suggest inadequate anaesthesia or surgical stimulation, while insidious changes indicate progressively deteriorating blood gas values or hypovolaemia. The following responses are appropriate whenever tachycardia or tachyarrhythmias arise:

- The level of unconsciousness is evaluated, and any possible link between surgery and rhythm disturbance examined. If one exists, anaesthesia is deepened and surgery continued with gentler manipulation. If this is unsuccessful, short acting vagomimetic opioids such as alfentanil or morphine should be given
- Several lung inflations with oxygen-rich gas are imposed. These often suppress arrhythmias resulting from hypercapnia and/or hypoxaemia

Cause	Response
Inadequate anaesthesia or analgesia	Increase inspired concentration of volatile agent, low dose of intravenous anaesthetic, alfentanil or fentanyl (see Figure 19.5)
Hypercapnia	IPPV
Hypoxaemia	Provide 100% oxygen and IPPV
Hypotension, shock, septicaemia	Rapid intravenous fluids
Drugs	Discontinue beta-1 agonists, if given (see Figure 19.5)
Hyperthermia	Consider abdominal lavage with ice-cold fluids
Hypokalaemia	Give KCl (0.05 mmol/kg over 1 minute, repeat if necessary)
'Idiopathic' tachycardia	See Figure 19.5, non-specific negative chronotropes
Hyperthyroidism	See Figure 19.5, non-specific negative chronotropes

19.17 Causes of intraoperative tachycardia and suggested treatment.

- Fluid infusion rate is increased. This often slows heart rates elevated by hypovolaemia or hypotension, although the response may be slow and modest.

Intraoperative ventricular arrhythmias

Untreated tachyarrhythmias may degenerate into more dangerous rhythms: over time, multifocal ventricular premature complexes can convert to a ventricular tachycardia, which in turn can lead to ventricular fibrillation and cardiac arrest. Tachyarrhythmias must be treated aggressively, initially using the three responses described above. Lidocaine is used whenever these fail or are only partly effective. However, its beneficial effects are often short-lived and, although repeated injections can be given, it is preferable to give lidocaine (mixed with normal saline) as a constant rate infusion (see Figure 19.4). If lidocaine is ineffective, intravenous procainamide may be used. Alternatively, magnesium sulphate may prove effective. When ventricular premature complexes persist and deteriorate into ventricular tachycardia, cardioversion with an externally synchronized DC non-phasic defibrillator in conjunction with lidocaine should be attempted. If lethal rhythms arise, then cerebral-cardiopulmonary resuscitation (CCPR) must be initiated.

Note that intraoperative ventricular premature complexes arising in digitalized animals may indicate a relative digoxin overdose caused by hypokalaemia. The commonest cause of this is respiratory alkalosis, i.e. excessive mechanical ventilation. In minor cases, a reduction in alveolar ventilation may effect a cure, otherwise potassium chloride (up to 0.05 mmol/kg) should be given intravenously over 1 minute. A repeated dose may be necessary.

References and further reading

Atlee JL (1990) *Perioperative Cardiac Dysrhythmias: Mechanisms, Recognition, Management.* Year Book Medical Publishers, Chicago

Muir WW, Hubbell JAE and Flaherty S (1988) Increasing halothane concentration abolishes anesthesia-associated arrhythmias in cats and dogs. *Journal of the American Veterinary Medical Association* **192**, 1730–1735

Muir WW, Wiese AJ and March PA (2003) Effects of morphine, lidocaine, ketamine, and morphine-lidocaine-ketamine drug combinations on minimum alveolar concentration in dogs anesthetized with isoflurane. *American Journal of Veterinary Research* **64**, 1155–1160

20

Respiratory disease

R. Eddie Clutton

Introduction

Respiratory disease is often encountered in companion animals presented for non-pulmonary surgery. Infectious respiratory diseases are common and the lungs of older animals living in urban environments may suffer from the effects of air pollution. Pulmonary function deteriorates with age, and the lungs are a common target for metastatic disease. Conditions characterized by chronic vomiting are associated with aspiration pneumonia.

The principal function of the pulmonary system is gas exchange, i.e. to replenish venous blood with oxygen and to remove carbon dioxide. This depends on ventilation: the bulk flow of fresh gas into the alveoli. In turn, ventilation depends on an unobstructed airway and an effective respiratory muscle effort, and is controlled by medullary respiratory centres. The latter increase ventilation in response to high plasma carbon dioxide levels (>40 mmHg (>5.3 kPa)) and/or low oxygen tensions. Efficient gas exchange also depends on processes within the lung that match alveolar ventilation (V) with alveolar perfusion (Q). On this basis, pulmonary disease can be defined broadly as any process threatening gas exchange, i.e. any condition:

- Obstructing the airway
- Impairing respiratory muscle effort
- Depressing the neural control of breathing
- Impairing ventilation/perfusion (V/Q) ratios.

In this chapter, respiratory disease has been categorized as:

- Difficult orotracheal intubation
- Upper airway obstruction
- Hypoventilation caused by abnormal chest wall and neural function
- Impaired oxygenation caused by V/Q discrepancies (chronic obstructive pulmonary disease, asthma/bronchoconstriction).

Pulmonary disease increases risk from anaesthesia because:

- Anaesthetics suppress protective upper airway reflexes, impair mucociliary function, depress ventilation and derange processes ensuring V/Q matching
- Pulmonary disease affects other organ systems in ways that increase risk, e.g. blood gas derangements cause arrhythmias, whilst chronic hypoxia leads to polycythaemia
- The management of pulmonary diseases may involve drugs affecting anaesthesia
- Pulmonary disease alters the uptake of inhalation anaesthetics
- Conditions preventing gas movement into the alveolar space are life-threatening and demand immediate treatment.

The risk from anaesthesia in animals with pulmonary disease is reduced if:

- An accurate diagnosis is established
- The underlying pathophysiological processes are understood
- Pulmonary function is improved preoperatively
- The anaesthetic offsets, rather than aggravates, the effects of underlying pathophysiological processes
- Perioperative physiological monitoring is adequate.

Difficult orotracheal intubation

Conditions preventing mouth opening and orotracheal intubation are seldom associated with other respiratory disease, so affected animals breathe normally when conscious. However, it may be impossible to secure the airway after induction, so it is then at risk from soft tissue obstruction and/or the aspiration of nasopharyngeal material, e.g. saliva or regurgitated stomach contents. Conditions complicating orotracheal intubation include:

- Eosinophilic myositis
- Movement-limiting temporomandibular joint (TMJ) pathology
- Jaw fractures
- Painful or space-occupying orbital pathology.

Identifying these problems preoperatively allows their circumvention by performing tracheotomy under deep sedation and local anaesthesia. However, in many cases the condition's significance may not be recognized until the animal is unconscious and attempted intubation proves difficult or impossible.

If tracheotomy under sedation is not possible, the animal must be rendered unconscious, the mouth forcibly opened and the trachea intubated as rapidly as possible. A means of transtracheal oxygenation and intermittent positive pressure ventilation (IPPV) (i.e. tracheotomy) must be available in case this is impossible. Steps must be taken to lower the risk of regurgitation and aspiration (adequate fasting and avoidance of morphine and alpha-2 agonists) and of excessive salivation (alpha-2 agonists, high dose ketamine, etomidate). Before induction, oxygen by mask may prove advantageous.

The ideal induction technique, i.e. that which would provide analgesia yet preserve breathing, does not exist, but diazepam–ketamine combinations are preferred over thiopental, propofol or alfaxalone. Once the animal is unconscious (and in sternal recumbency) strong gauze straps are passed over the mandible and maxilla and sufficient force exerted until the mouth can be opened and the glottis identified. When painful TMJ pathology is present, profound analgesia or deep general anaesthesia is required to prevent reactions to TMJ articulation. If the mouth cannot be opened, so direct laryngoscopy is impossible, a blind intubation technique must be attempted, as in the horse. Non-steroidal anti-inflammatory drugs (NSAIDs) should be given before the animal recovers from anaesthesia, when many show signs of severe discomfort.

Upper airway obstruction

Upper airway obstruction can range in severity from cases with mildly stertorious breathing to life-threatening emergencies, necessitating immediate endotracheal intubation or tracheotomy. It may result from the anatomical peculiarities of brachycephalic breeds or be acquired, for example:

- Laryngeal hemiparalysis
- Subepiglottic cysts
- Intermandibular masses
- Laryngospasm
- Pharyngeal and retropharyngeal:
  - Neoplasia (Figure 20.1)
  - Abscessation
  - Oedema
  - Haemorrhage
  - Air (pneumomediastinum)
- Collapsing trachea
- Iatrogenic:
  - Laryngeal surgery
  - Tracheal surgery.

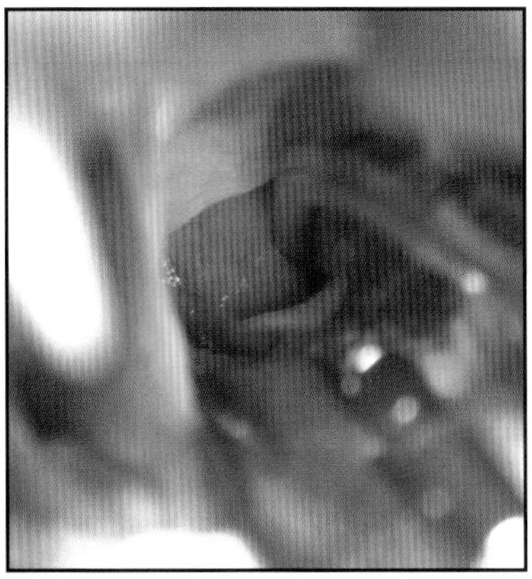

20.1 Retropharyngeal mass causing obstruction of the airway.

Management of life-threatening upper airway obstruction

Animals with near-complete upper airway obstruction present in extremis, i.e. collapsed and cyanotic. These patients must be preoxygenated (during the brisk preparation for tracheotomy) using a large-bore (14 gauge) needle introduced into the tracheal lumen downstream from the obstruction, or as close to the thoracic inlet as possible. An emergency tracheotomy is then performed with or without local anaesthetic and/or sedation produced with rapidly acting drug combinations, e.g. intravenous acepromazine (0.025–0.05 mg/kg) and alfentanil (2.5–5 μg/kg). Later, a more permanent tracheostomy is performed under general anaesthesia.

Management of less severe obstruction

With less critical cases, the problem is diagnosed and temporarily alleviated at presentation, with corrective surgery being performed either immediately or at a later date. The clinical signs of upper airway obstruction (stridor, stertor, dyspnoea, increased inspiratory effort) are aggravated by hyperventilation, which is brought about by physical exertion, anxiety, excitement or hyperthermia. This occurs because of the Bernoulli effect: an increase in gas velocity, which occurs when gases traverse a constriction, lowers the pressure at that point and promotes collapse (Figure 20.2). Consequently, the initial treatment of upper airway obstruction aims to calm the animal by using sedatives and respiratory depressant drugs if necessary. Low dose acepromazine (0.025–0.05 mg/kg), combined with a non-emetic opioid, e.g. methadone or butorphanol, is suitable for this purpose. Body temperature, if elevated, should be reduced in a stress-free manner using cold wet towels and fans. Enriching inspired gas with oxygen is beneficial if achieved in a non-stressful way. Intravenous access, attempted once the animal is calm, facilitates the administration of further sedatives if required. It also allows intravenous anaesthetics to be given for the purpose of performing upper airway examination, emergency tracheotomy (in cases where the aforementioned measures fail to relieve dyspnoea) and the surgical correction of the precipitating condition.

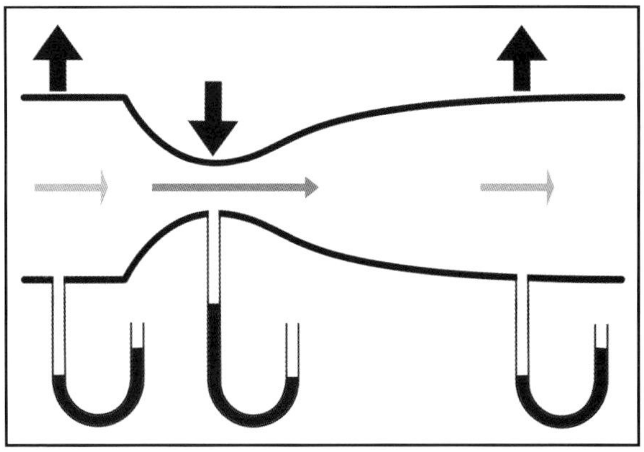

20.2 The Bernoulli effect. Gas flowing through a conduit accelerates across a constriction, e.g. a collapsing trachea, which creates a fall in pressure in the conduit and promotes its collapse.

Once a suitable degree of either sedation or anaesthesia and jaw relaxation are present, the oropharynx and upper respiratory tract are examined under direct vision, using a bright light source and a long-bladed laryngoscope. The retropharyngeal area and trachea are palpated for unusual structures, which may compress the airway. The effects of obstructive lesions are relieved by passing an adequately sized endotracheal tube beyond the obstruction site because this allows oxygen to be delivered and the lungs to be inflated (and protected) until a normal airway is restored. However, tracheal intubation may not be possible if space-occupying pharyngeal lesions obstruct the view of the rima glottidis and make blind intubation impossible. For these reasons, facilities for emergency tracheotomy should always be available. In cases where the obstruction cannot be bypassed by endotracheal tubes, e.g. cases of distal cervical/intrathoracic tracheal collapse, endotracheal intubation is still required as it allows the imposition of controlled hyperventilation: overcoming the animal's spontaneous breathing efforts with IPPV overcomes all forces promoting airway collapse.

Laryngeal paralysis

Disturbed motor innervation of laryngeal muscles results in varying degrees of laryngeal paralysis. Idiopathic acquired laryngeal paralysis occurs most commonly in older, large-breed dogs, while a hereditary form is less frequently encountered in puppies. In its mildest form, affected dogs present with exercise intolerance, a chronic honking cough, inspiratory stridor and a change in the bark. Diagnosis is made under anaesthesia by visual examination of the vocal folds and treatment involves a laryngeal tie-back operation. Both procedures are commonly performed during the same anaesthetic although surgery may sometimes be postponed to allow inflammation and oedema to subside.

Anaesthesia for the diagnosis of laryngeal paralysis requires attention because anaesthetics affect laryngeal activity and can complicate diagnosis. Pre-anaesthetic medication should produce a calm and anxiety-free animal, but high opioid doses are best avoided because breathing must continue throughout induction. After pre-anaesthetic medication with neuroleptanalgesic combinations, anaesthesia is best induced using sevoflurane delivered by mask until adequate jaw relaxation allows direct laryngoscopy. The mask is then removed and laryngeal function assessed until jaw tone and/or head movement precludes further investigation, when the mask is re-applied. The cycle of deepening anaesthesia by mask application and lightening anaesthesia during laryngeal examination can be repeated until a diagnosis is established. When no pre-anaesthetic medication is given, minimum effective doses of thiopental have been recommended for laryngeal examination because it has the least effect on arytenoid function.

Diagnosis involves examining the vocal folds to ensure they abduct symmetrically and adequately on inspiration, and is facilitated by an observer announcing inspiration and expiration when the chest wall moves. This helps the veterinary surgeon link barely perceptible arytenoid movements with the respiratory cycle. Another strategy involves doxapram, which if injected intravenously at 0.5–1.1 mg/kg in lightly anaesthetized animals (as indicated by jaw relaxation in the presence of positive palpebral and toe-pinch withdrawals) produces passive, paradoxical arytenoid motion in dogs with laryngeal paralysis; i.e. the arytenoid cartilages are drawn inward by negative airway pressure on inhalation, and are forced apart by exhaled air. Respiratory effort and depth are also greatly increased in dogs with laryngeal paralysis because of complete glottic constriction during inspiration.

During prolonged laryngeal examination, blood oxygen levels can be maintained by directing an oxygen stream from a narrow bore tube towards the rima glottidis at rates of 1–5 l/minute. Once a diagnosis is made, the animal may be allowed to recover although most cases will proceed to surgery. In this case, anaesthesia is deepened using volatile agents delivered by mask, or by intravenous anaesthetic, until conditions for endotracheal intubation are present.

Maintaining anaesthesia for laryngeal tie-back surgery presents no extraordinary challenges providing that the endotracheal tube tip lies distal to the glottis. Airway discontinuity is rarely a problem as surgery does not broach the airway. Postoperative complications are minimized by keeping the animal calm (sedated) and preventing vocalization and coughing. Morphine (or butorphanol) given after laryngeal examination but before surgery begins may achieve this. Postoperative swelling may be reduced by the presurgical administration of NSAIDs.

Brachycephalic obstructive airway syndrome

In brachycephalic breeds, upper airway gas flow is restricted by the combination of stenotic nares, soft palate dislodgement and the entrainment of superfluous pharyngeal tissue into the hypoplastic tracheal airway. The prolonged imposition of abnormally high negative inspiratory pressures eventually causes laryngeal saccule eversion, nasopharyngeal inflammation and arytenoid cartilage collapse.

The management of severely dyspnoeic, brachycephalic dogs is similar to that for cases with laryngeal paralysis, with one exception. While sedative–anxiolytic drugs improve ventilation by slowing inspiratory flows, they also relax naso- and oropharyngeal smooth muscle, which might aggravate obstruction. For this reason, any animal with signs of brachycephalic obstructive airway syndrome (BOAS) must remain under continuous surveillance from the time sedatives are given until either anaesthesia is induced and the trachea intubated (or a tracheotomy performed) or all signs of sedation have waned. In conjunction with the brachycephalic state, BOAS increases anaesthetic risk in dogs facing corrective or incidental (non-airway) surgery:

- Sedative pre-anaesthetic medication may exacerbate dyspnoea (see above). Very low dose acepromazine (12.5 μg/kg) combined with butorphanol (before minor superficial surgery) or stronger analgesics, e.g. pethidine (meperidine), in all other cases, is satisfactory

- At induction, the loss of protective airway reflexes may result in total airway obstruction. Therefore, preparation for rapid endotracheal intubation (or tracheotomy) must be complete. The ideal induction agent does not exist. Thiopental produces a rapid loss of consciousness and allows brisk intubation, but in recovery contributes to residual sedation and obstruction when returning pharyngolaryngeal reflexes necessitate tracheal extubation (which is most likely after short procedures). Propofol given over 45–60 seconds (in an attempt to avoid hypotension and apnoea) does not allow rapid airway control, although it provides a rapid and complete recovery, which means that protective airway reflexes are strong when returning pharyngeal activity prompts extubation. The use of anti-tussive drugs, e.g. butorphanol, may prolong tolerance of endotracheal tubes. This is desirable because it prolongs the time available for effective oxygenation, volatile anaesthetic elimination and injected drug clearance
- Redundant facial skin complicates head presentation for endotracheal intubation. Bandage strips passed behind the canine teeth (under the maxilla and over the mandible), in a way that everts labial skin from the oral cavity, circumvent these problems
- Abnormal canine teeth and jaw development render traditional mouth gags insecure. This is less important when tapes are used, as above
- Redundant pharyngeal soft tissue may obscure the rima glottidis and hamper intubation. The use of tapes, an experienced assistant and a laryngoscope greatly facilitates intubation. An assistant elevates the head at about 45° by lifting the two ends of the maxillary strip, while the anaesthetist opens the mouth by pulling downwards on both mandibular strips
- The glottis and trachea are commonly much smaller than anticipated. Therefore, a range of tube sizes (from 5.0 mm) should be made available
- The risk of airway obstruction persists during recovery, after tracheal extubation. After corrective airway surgery, blood clots, haemorrhage and swelling may counter the benefits of a surgically corrected airway. In contrast, dogs not undergoing airway surgery are likely to obstruct if sedation persists after endotracheal extubation. For this reason, insoluble inhalant anaesthetics, e.g. nitrous oxide with either sevoflurane or isoflurane, should be used in preference to halothane. Postoperative pain causes panting and will promote obstruction. Pre-emptive NSAIDs and butorphanol may provide adequate analgesia for minor procedures but the use of local anaesthetics should be considered after major surgery.

Tracheal surgery

Anaesthetic challenges during tracheal surgery are: competition for space, unintended tracheotomy and postoperative airway obstruction. The former can lead to breathing system disconnection, endotracheal tube obstruction and cuff damage or deflation.

Tracheal surgery *per se* presents no problems, providing the endotracheal tube tip and cuff lie distal to the point of surgery, as this will allow IPPV to be imposed whilst preventing environmental contamination with anaesthetic. Postoperative airway obstruction may result from haemorrhage, postoperative swelling and/or laryngeal paralysis resulting from iatrogenic recurrent laryngeal nerve trauma. Pre-emptive glucocorticoids or NSAIDs will reduce postoperative swelling, while tracheobronchial suction applied before endotracheal extubation should clear the airway and reduce the risk of distal airway collapse and/or postoperative coughing.

Chest wall/neural and pulmonary conditions

Conditions affecting the lower airway, chest wall and the control of breathing are seldom emergencies and so preoperative preparation is possible. Anaesthesia in animals with pulmonary disease is straightforward, providing the underlying pathophysiology is understood and reversed.

Preoperative examination

A thorough review of the medical history and physical examination may establish a diagnosis, although more complex procedures, such as radiography, electrocardiography (ECG), arterial blood gas analysis, ultrasonography, primitive lung function tests and bronchoscopy, may be required. It should be appreciated that many investigations are stressful, and may affect results or precipitate severe dyspnoea.

Haematology

An elevated haematocrit provides supporting evidence for significant cardiopulmonary disease because chronic hypoxia causes secondary polycythaemia. It should be appreciated that a polycythaemic animal may appear cyanotic even when oxygen saturation is normal.

Arterial blood gas analysis

Arterial blood gas analysis provides useful quantitative information on the lungs' ability to oxygenate blood, eliminate carbon dioxide and influence acid–base status. Venous samples are less useful as they do not reflect pulmonary function.

Thoracocentesis

Aspiration through an 18–21 gauge needle or a 14–16 gauge intravenous cannula inserted through the seventh or eighth intercostal space can relieve dyspnoea and assist diagnosis when accumulated air or liquid prevent adequate lung expansion. Needles or cannulae are normally inserted at the lateral point of the thorax, although more dorsal (air) or ventral (liquid) sites are used if the nature of the fluid is known (see Chapter 21 for further details).

Radiography

Radiographs are valuable for examining intrathoracic lesions. For animals with respiratory embarrassment, inappropriate positioning in the lateral and/or dorsal position may cause distress and struggling, and is potentially hazardous. Dyspnoea related to body position (orthopnoea) is avoided by using the lateral decubitus and dorsoventral projections.

Pulse oximetry

Pulse oximetry is well tolerated and may be applied in the conscious animal breathing air. It should be appreciated that low oxygen saturation of haemoglobin (S_pO_2 values <90%) may be due to factors other than pulmonary disease.

Bronchoscopy

The introduction of flexible bronchoscopes that can be passed through gas-tight grommets of suitable endotracheal swivel connectors has greatly facilitated bronchoscopy, although, in very small animals, effective ventilation ceases if the endoscope obstructs the airway.

Anaesthesia of animals with chest wall and neural disorders

Figure 20.3 lists conditions in which bulk gas flow into the alveoli is inadequate for maintaining normal carbon dioxide levels (oxygenation may not be impaired). Animals with these conditions develop severe hypercapnia, respiratory acidosis and possibly hypoxaemia when sedated or anaesthetized unless the lungs are periodically inflated with at least 20% oxygen.

Before surgery, an attempt should be made to address the cause (Figure 20.3), as in many cases this will limit the adverse haemodynamic effects of IPPV. Pre-anaesthetic medication must not impair spontaneous breathing and the animal should not be left unattended until anaesthesia is induced. During this interval, inspired gas should be enriched with oxygen. Anaesthesia can be induced with any ultra short-acting intravenous agent providing the trachea is intubated without unnecessary delay. When restrictive chest wall changes and/or impaired neural control are the only contributors to respiratory depression, the risk of anaesthesia effectively disappears once the trachea is intubated and periodic lung inflation begun. However, some conditions also involve pulmonary pathology compromising blood oxygenation, in which case additional measures are required.

When painful chest wall lesions (e.g. pleurisy) prevent adequate ventilation, the administration of analgesics, even those with respiratory depressant effects, improves breathing.

Aetiology	Location	Response
Neural factors	Overdose with depressant drugs	Antagonism
	Intracranial tumours	Methods reducing intracranial pressure
	Severe hypothermia or hyperthermia	Restore normal temperature
	Infection: meningitis or encephalitis	Antibiotics
	Head trauma	Methods reducing intracranial pressure
	Status epilepticus	Anticonvulsant therapy
Pleural resistance	Pleuropericardial herniation	No immediate treatment; head-up position
	Diaphragmatic herniation	No immediate treatment; head-up position
	Pleuritis (pain)	Analgesics
	Hydro-, pyo-, pneumo-, chylothorax	Thoracocentesis; drain
	Haemothorax	Thoracocentesis; drain, autotransfuse
Abdominal resistance	Pancreatitis (pain)	Analgesics
	Tympany	Gastric decompression
	Haemoperitoneum	Abdominal paracentesis; autotransfusion
	Pregnancy	Impose head-up position
	Pyometra	Impose head-up position
	Ascites	Abdominal paracentesis; slow drainage

20.3 Causes and preoperative treatment of chest wall/neural conditions. Note that hypoventilation caused by pain may disappear once consciousness is lost. There is risk of vasculogenic shock if large volumes of fluid are withdrawn rapidly from either the thoracic or the abdominal cavity, so haemodynamic variables should be monitored during aspiration and preparations made for the rapid administration of crystalloid solution, plasma substitute solution or whole blood. (continues) ▶

Aetiology	Location	Response
Thoracic wall resistance	Obesity	Weight reduction programme if possible
	Restrictive bandaging	Remove if possible
	Flail chest	Apply bandages; analgesics
	Injury (pain)	Analgesics
	Skeletal abnormalities, e.g. kyphosis, lordosis, pectus excavatum	No treatment
	Myasthenia gravis	Physostigmine, corticosteroids
Lower airway obstruction	Collapsing trachea	Sedation, endotracheal intubation
	Foreign body	Bronchoscopy
	Neoplasia	None
	Oedema	See Chapter 19
	Cardiomegaly	Diuretics, see Chapter 19
Pulmonary resistance	Pulmonary oedema	See Chapter 19
	Extensive fibrosis	No treatment
	Pulmonary hypertension	Oxygen

20.3 (continued) Causes and preoperative treatment of chest wall/neural conditions. Note that hypoventilation caused by pain may disappear once consciousness is lost. There is risk of vasculogenic shock if large volumes of fluid are withdrawn rapidly from either the thoracic or the abdominal cavity, so haemodynamic variables should be monitored during aspiration and preparations made for the rapid administration of crystalloid solution, plasma substitute solution or whole blood.

Pulmonary conditions

In some conditions, blood oxygenation improves by simply enriching inspired gas with oxygen. In others, endotracheal intubation and periodic lung inflation with oxygen (rather than air) are necessary. Specific therapies are required when chronic obstructive pulmonary disease (COPD) or bronchospasm are present.

Inadequate oxygenation

Many conditions altering V/Q ratios and/or retarding gas diffusion across the alveolar–capillary membrane are associated with a diminished ability to oxygenate blood. These include:

- Neoplasia
- Pneumonia
- Pulmonary contusion
- Embolism
- Chronic bronchitis
- Chronic emphysema
- Heart–lung anomalies
- Pulmonary oedema.

Preoperative preparation with drugs that produce a 'wide, dry and clean' airway (Figure 20.4) aims to relieve reversible pathology and optimize pulmonary function. Attempts to improve ventricular function may be appropriate in conditions characterized by chronic pulmonary hypertension (see Chapter 19). When disease is severe, the option of using local anaesthetic techniques and sedation should be considered.

Drugs	Indication	Dose	Side effects
Antibiotics	Bacterial infection of the respiratory tree Increased airway secretions	For Gram-negative, a fluoroquinolone is generally used (e.g. enrofloxacin 5 mg/kg orally q24h) For Gram-positive, amoxicillin–clavulanate (11–22 mg/kg orally q12h), or ampicillin (10–20 mg/kg orally q12h) plus β-lactam to extend spectrum for anaerobes Doxycycline (10 mg/kg orally q24h) or a fluoroquinolone for suspected *Bordetella* pneumonia Inhalation of gentamicin in nebulized saline may be useful for Gram-negative pneumonia (including *Bordetella*) Conduct Gram stain to guide initial therapy; final antibiotic choice based on culture and sensitivity results: many Gram-negative pathogens have unpredictable sensitivities	Potential for adverse interactions with anaesthetics

20.4 Drugs used for preoperative preparation of animals with pulmonary diseases. (continues) ▶

Drugs	Indication	Dose	Side effects
Diuretics	Pulmonary oedema and viral pneumonias (these have obstructive and restrictive components and enhance V/Q discrepancies) Conditions with increased lung water	See Chapter 19	May aggravate purulent conditions by increasing the viscosity of airway secretions
Bronchodilators	May produce intrapulmonary 'steal' when gas flow is restricted by external airway compression. Airway dilation in healthy lung diverts inspired gas from affected region whose V/Q ratio is then further lowered		
Antimuscarinics	Bronchoconstriction	Atropine 40 μg/kg i.v.	Airway secretions made more viscid
Beta-2 agonists	Bronchoconstriction	Terbutaline: Dog 1.25–5 mg/dog orally q8–12h Cat 0.3–1.25 mg/cat orally q8–12h	
Phosphodiesterase inhibitors	Bronchoconstriction	Aminophylline: Dogs 10 mg/kg i.v. q6–8h Cats 6.6 mg/kg orally q12h or 2–5 mg/kg slow i.v. Etamiphylline: Cats and dogs <10 kg 70–140 mg i.m., s.c. or 100 mg orally q8h Dogs 10–30 kg 140–420 mg i.m., s.c. or 100–300 mg orally q8h Dogs >30 kg 420–700 mg i.m., s.c. or 300–400 mg orally q8h Theophylline: Cats 10–20 mg/kg orally q12–24h, or 2–5 mg/kg slow i.v. in emergencies Dogs 10 mg/kg i.v. q6–8h, or 20 mg/kg orally q12–24h	
Glucocorticoids	To suppress tissue reaction associated with pulmonary contusion, smoke inhalation injury and volutrauma	Methylprednisolone: Feline asthma 1–2 mg/kg i.m. depot every 1–3 weeks Dogs (for CNS trauma) 30 mg/kg i.v. within 8 hours; then 15 mg/kg i.v., 2 and 6 hours later; then 2.5 mg/kg infused over 48 hours Prednisolone: Feline asthma 1mg/kg orally q12h for 10–14 days, tapering to 0.2 mg/kg q48h	Hypothalamic–pituitary axis depression
Antihistamines	Bronchoconstriction	Chlorphenamine: Small dogs 2–4 mg orally q8–12h Large dogs 4–8 mg/kg orally q8–12h Cats 2 mg/cat orally q12h	Sedation; potentiation of sedatives
Anti-tussives	Non-productive and exhausting coughing	Codeine: Dogs 0.5–2 mg/kg orally q12h Butorphanol: Dogs 0.05–0.1 mg/kg i.m., s.c. or 0.5–1 mg/kg orally q6–12h Cats 0.05–0.5 mg/kg i.m., s.c. q6–8h	Respiratory depression, sedation, potentiation of sedatives
Mucolytics	To facilitate clearance of viscid secretions	Bromhexine: Dogs 3–15 mg/dog i.m. q12h, 2–2.5 mg/kg orally q12h Cats 3 mg/cat i.m. q24h, 1 mg/kg orally q24h Acetylcysteine: Nebulize 50 mg as a 2% solution in saline over 30–60 minutes or instil 1–2 ml of a 20% solution into the trachea	

20.4 (continued) Drugs used for preoperative preparation of animals with pulmonary diseases.

Pre-anaesthetic medication with drugs with profound respiratory depressant effects should not be used. Acepromazine and low dose opioids are suitable in dogs and cats, while low dose ketamine (2.5–5 mg/kg) with or without midazolam may be used in cats. Animals must be preoxygenated. Ventilation should be controlled during anaesthesia: spontaneous ventilation tends to cause hypoventilation, which leads to further atelectasis and further shunting. Clearly, 100% oxygen should be given throughout to maximize diffusion gradients across abnormally large diffusion paths. Low inflation pressures must be used in any condition in which pulmonary damage is likely, e.g. trauma.

Pulmonary contusions

After blunt thoracic trauma, bleeding from ruptured pulmonary capillaries into the alveolar interstitium and spaces produces dyspnoea and areas of lung incapable of gas exchange. The ideal treatment is cage rest and oxygen enrichment of inspired gas. However, animals with pulmonary contusions may occasionally require anaesthesia for life-saving procedures, e.g. control of internal haemorrhage. A principal concern with pulmonary contusions is the limitation they place on blood volume restoration, which, if overzealous, leads to pulmonary oedema and a worsening of lung function. Contusions complicate the management of pulmonary oedema with furosemide, because, while the diuretic does not resolve the effects of extravasated erythrocytes, it *does* reduce the effective circulating blood volume and increase alveolar dead space. A disappointing response to oxygen therapy might prompt endotracheal intubation and IPPV; however, structural weaknesses in the lung make trauma from inflation more likely. If IPPV is attempted the inflation pressures must be the lowest consistent with lung expansion and the animal must not be allowed to 'fight' the ventilator.

Smoke inhalation

Animals with severe burn injuries may first require emergency surgery for vascular access, airway management and damage assessment. Later, repeated wound debridement and dressing, and skin grafting operations may be necessary. Smoke inhalation injury complicates anaesthesia in burn victims and, in conjunction with severe fluid loss, end-organ failure, hypercatabolism, pain and overwhelming sepsis, contributes greatly to morbidity and mortality.

Irrespective of burn severity, the initial approach to burns management is: airway protection, intravenous access, pain relief and fluid resuscitation. There may be significant problems with the acute pain of the injury (including an acute neuropathic element) so pain relief should be aggressive and prompt. Ketamine and morphine have much to commend their use, while cold, sterile water exerts an immediate effect. NSAIDs should be withheld until renal function is established. When severe burns are present, the infusion of drugs with pre-emptive analgesic effects, e.g. lidocaine, ketamine and morphine, should be instituted (see Chapters 9 and 13).

The airway may become critically compromised soon after burning. Oedema resulting from thermal injury of the respiratory epithelium and crystalloid resuscitation can rapidly result in complete airway obstruction. Emergency orotracheal intubation is required when severe dyspnoea is linked with facial burns, soot staining of the nostrils and singed vibrissae. Tracheotomy may seem a suitable option, but in human burn patients it is associated with a high incidence of infections and tracheal stenosis. Conditions for intubation are achieved after a period of preoxygenation using a combined mask/intravenous technique. The minimum effective dose of intravenous agents with analgesic properties (e.g. alfentanil or sufentanil and ketamine) should be favoured. The endotracheal tube should be sterile and have a high-volume, low-pressure cuff. Sterile lidocaine gel should be applied before intubation.

Direct thermal injury usually occurs above the glottis and is uncommon below the trachea, although a chemical tracheobronchitis resulting from inhalation of the incomplete products of combustion may develop in the distal airway. Inhalation injury can be complicated by aldehydes, carbon monoxide and cyanide toxicity. The last two combine irreversibly with haemoglobin and lower arterial oxygen content. Furthermore, their inhalation along with high carbon dioxide concentrations and low oxygen concentrations produces narcosis. Animals should be given 100% oxygen to breathe from the outset. Single high doses of methylprednisolone given soon after injury improves the outcome in human subjects (see Figure 20.4). Repeated doses are ill advised because burn victims are often critically immunosuppressed.

Airway damage after manifests 2–4 days as a necrotizing tracheobronchitis, characterized by copious exudation and coughing. Management now consists of oxygen inhalation, saline nebulization, coupage (judicious thumping of the chest wall in an attempt to loosen viscid airway secretion) and bronchodilators. Antibiotics are withheld until signs of bacterial infection are present and antibiotic sensitivity established. During this period, burn victims enter a profoundly hypermetabolic phase, in which oxygen and glucose consumption and carbon dioxide production are greatly elevated.

Profound sedation/anaesthesia are required for wound debridement and dressing changes at frequent intervals during this period. On these occasions, the implications of the animal's pulmonary dysfunction, hypermetabolism, immunosuppression and unstable volume state must be appreciated. However, achieving analgesia is a priority and this supports the aggressive use of opioids, ketamine and lidocaine in conjunction with volatile agents whenever an anaesthetic is required (see Chapters 9 and 13).

Chronic obstructive pulmonary disease

Chronic obstructive pulmonary disease refers to conditions in which chronic bronchitis and/or emphysema cause irreversible airflow limitations.

Chronic bronchitis

Chronic bronchitis describes conditions in which mucoid bronchial secretion production is increased. It is common in older dogs from urban environments. The presence of excessive mucus predisposes to infection, distal airway closure (atelectasis) and bronchopneumonia. Atelectasis causes chronic hypoxaemia, which results in polycythaemia and cor pulmonale. Hypoventilation results in chronic hypercapnia, which desensitizes the respiratory centres to the effects of carbon dioxide. Chronic bronchitis is characterized by:

- Hypersensitive respiratory reflexes (bucking, bronchospasm)
- Hypoxic respiratory drive. This is nearly abolished by anaesthetics and if animals breathe an oxygen mixture in recovery, hypercapnia and even carbon dioxide narcosis may occur
- Increased sensitivity to respiratory depressants.

Emphysema

In emphysema, abnormally large air spaces distal to the terminal bronchioles and destruction of alveolar walls cause loss of lung elastic recoil, resulting in overexpansion and early closure of airways during expiration, which causes gas trapping. Ventilation is usually well maintained, albeit by an exaggerated effort. Expiration is prolonged in emphysema.

Where appropriate, local anaesthetic techniques and sedation should be used in cases with advanced COPD because the risk from general anaesthesia is great. When general anaesthesia is unavoidable, extensive preparation is required. The objective of preoperative therapy is to make the pulmonary tree clean (sterile), dry and wide by using antibiotics, antispasmodics, mucolytics, steroids and bronchodilators. Drugs may be used to soften secretions, while coupage may prove beneficial. Other drugs used preoperatively to improve pulmonary function are described in Figure 20.4. Antibacterial treatments should also render the animal non-pyrexic. Anti-tussive drugs should not be given unless chronic coughing is unproductive and exhausting. Inspired gas enrichment with oxygen is desirable, although gases should be warmed and humidified using heated humidifiers or nebulizers. Cold, dry medical gases inspissate mucus and further impair its clearance by suppressing the activity of the mucociliary carpet.

Low dose acepromazine is suitable for pre-anaesthetic medication but may not always provide the degree of sedation required. Anti-sialagogues should be avoided as they inspissate secretions, while atropine inhibits the mucociliary carpet. Opioids should not be used for pre-anaesthetic medication because (with other CNS depressant drugs) they contribute to hypoventilation, and by suppressing the cough reflex they promote mucus accumulation. High doses should only be used if profound analgesia is desired and an effective means of tracheobronchial aspiration is available. Where possible, analgesia should be achieved with NSAIDs and local anaesthetic techniques. After pre-anaesthetic medication (and throughout the perioperative period), animals must be positioned so that purulent material from infected lung cannot drain into healthy tissue.

Induction should be smooth and a suitable level of anaesthesia achieved after induction, so that tracheal intubation does not stimulate hyperactive laryngeal and cough reflexes and bronchospasm. There is no ideal intravenous agent or technique for this purpose. Mask inductions (which involve the inspiration of high oxygen concentrations) may seem ill advised in the presence of impaired respiratory function; however, this should be weighed against the problems resulting from injectable agents, i.e. hypotension and apnoea.

During anaesthesia, ventilation should be controlled because:

- High inspired oxygen concentrations may depress ventilation
- Airway turbulence may critically increase the work of breathing and may impair lung expansion.

However, the ventilatory pattern should be modified:

- In chronic bronchitis high airway pressures are needed for lung inflation. However, the risks of volutrauma are real and high when emphysema is present
- A slow inspiratory cycle allows greater inspired gas dispersal through open and partially blocked airways
- A long expiratory pause is required to allow emphysematous lung units to empty
- The minute volume of ventilation should be increased to accommodate the increased alveolar deadspace volume.

If nitrous oxide is used, an inspired concentration of 50% should not be exceeded. Dry, cold medical gases make airway secretions more viscid, while many drugs and anaesthetics impair the function of the mucociliary carpet. Therefore, gases should be humidified and warmed and rebreathing systems should be used whenever possible. Heat and moisture exchangers inserted between the endotracheal tube connector and the breathing system inexpensively fulfil this function (see Chapter 5). Tracheobronchial suction should be performed as often as possible. An oesophageal stethoscope is a useful guide to the progression of accumulated secretion.

During recovery, the endotracheal tube should be left *in situ* for as long as possible in order to continue endobronchial suctioning. Postoperative pulse oximetry should be performed because inspired gas oxygen enrichment, while necessary, may suppress ventilation. Doxapram infusions may be useful in this context, although dose information does not exist for companion animals. Supplemental oxygen should be humidified, otherwise it will impair expectoration.

If there is any suspicion that respiratory disease is caused by infectious agents, breathing systems and endotracheal tubes must be sterilized or discarded.

Bronchoconstriction

In some conditions, including asthma in cats, bronchoconstriction occurs because of local chemical mediators initiating bronchospasm. Bronchoconstriction can also result from proliferative changes in the airway (chronic bronchitis). Preoperative bronchodilators may improve air flow in any condition in which the airway is narrowed by bronchoconstriction. Severe bronchospasm may critically limit bulk gas flow, while even minor disturbances will affect the distribution of gas to well perfused lung units.

Preoperative preparation aims to restore airway flow using antispasmodics, steroids, antihistamines and beta-2 agonists (see Figure 20.4). Handling must be conducted carefully as stress may precipitate bronchospasm. Animals that have been receiving glucocorticoids for prolonged periods may have suppressed adrenal function and require additional steroid treatment perioperatively.

Pre-anaesthetic medication with acepromazine and/or low dose ketamine is satisfactory; the former has antihistamine properties while the latter is a bronchodilator. Morphine or meperidine have a propensity to release histamine and should not be used. Atropine may be useful in some types of obstructive disorders because it causes bronchodilation, and it may reduce airway secretions.

Thiopental or alfaxalone (in the form of Saffan®) should probably not be used for induction as both can provoke bronchospasm. In sedated cats, a chamber induction with sevoflurane or halothane is probably ideal because there is little stress and both halothane and sevoflurane are potent bronchodilators. Alternatively, ketamine may be used: in human patients at least, it has potent bronchodilator effects.

If asthmatic problems arise during surgery, aminophylline or another phosphodiesterase inhibitor should be given intravenously. In emergencies, adrenaline at 0.22 mg/kg may be required. Beta-1 antagonists should not be used in animals prone to asthma.

References and further reading

Tobias K, Jackson AM & Harvey RC (2004) Effects of doxapram HCl on laryngeal function of normal dogs and dogs with naturally occurring laryngeal paralysis. *Veterinary Anaesthesia and Analgesia* **31**, 258–263

21

Thoracic surgery

Peter J. Pascoe

Introduction

Opening the thoracic cavity is still required for many procedures, but there is increasing use of less invasive techniques. Thoracoscopic approaches to pericardiectomy and lung lobectomy and using implantable coils to treat patent ductus arteriosus do not require a large intercostal incision. These advances may provide less surgical morbidity but the veterinary surgeon must still be cognizant of the underlying pathophysiology of the condition and the planned procedure in order to arrive at a suitable and safe anaesthetic technique.

Preoperative evaluation

Whenever the thoracic wall is breached, this has significant effects on the pulmonary system and so it is important to perform a careful evaluation of this before embarking on thoracic surgery. Preoperative evaluation is also covered in Chapter 2 but repetition here will help to reinforce the importance of thorough patient assessment before thoracic surgery.

History

Historical information about the patient is as important in the evaluation of respiratory disease as it is in any condition to aid in an accurate diagnosis. Chronic conditions may indicate a slowly changing condition, but often with pulmonary disease the physiological reserve is such that a chronically progressive disease may present acutely because the animal may show very few signs with small lesions in the lung or thoracic cavity. A question that is often not asked in small animal patients relates to exercise tolerance; this can give important information with regard to the likely risk of anaesthetizing the animal. The patient with poor exercise tolerance (due to some intrathoracic lesion) is at greater risk than the animal with normal tolerance. Another question that may provide some useful insight is whether the animal adopts any strange postures when it sleeps; an animal with a bilateral pleural effusion may have learned to sleep in a relatively upright position while an animal with unilateral changes may always sleep on one side.

Pulmonary function

When presented with a patient with a respiratory complaint, careful observation can help to establish the type of lesion. Patients with poor compliance of the lung (restrictive diseases such as pulmonary oedema, pneumonia, fibrosis or pleural effusion) tend to adopt a rapid shallow ventilatory pattern, whereas patients with obstructive diseases (laryngeal paralysis, collapsing trachea, small airway disease) tend to adopt a slower pattern with increased respiratory effort. In these cases trying to differentiate an inspiratory dyspnoea (usually extrathoracic causes) from an expiratory dyspnoea (intrathoracic lesions) may help to direct the clinician to the site of the lesion. Observing the movement of the chest and diaphragm may help to differentiate a problem with motor function from a pulmonary lesion. Arrhythmias of the diaphragm and intercostal muscles can lead to paradoxical breathing where the thoracic wall collapses on inspiration as the diaphragm moves caudally and the abdomen expands. This pattern could be associated with a severe respiratory obstruction, paralysis of the intercostal muscles or a lesion of the central nervous system (CNS) which has altered normal respiratory rhythm generation.

Examination of the mucous membranes for signs of cyanosis, flushing or slow capillary refill time may help to direct further examination. Mucous membrane colour has limitations for the diagnosis of hypoxaemia. Cyanosis, if present, is a strong predictor for hypoxaemia, although studies in humans have shown that clinicians are not very good at detecting cyanosis, even in patients with significant desaturation (Figure 21.1). The appearance of the membranes may be affected by ambient light (some fluorescent lights in particular) and it is also necessary for at least 15 g/l of desaturated haemoglobin to be present for cyanosis to be seen.

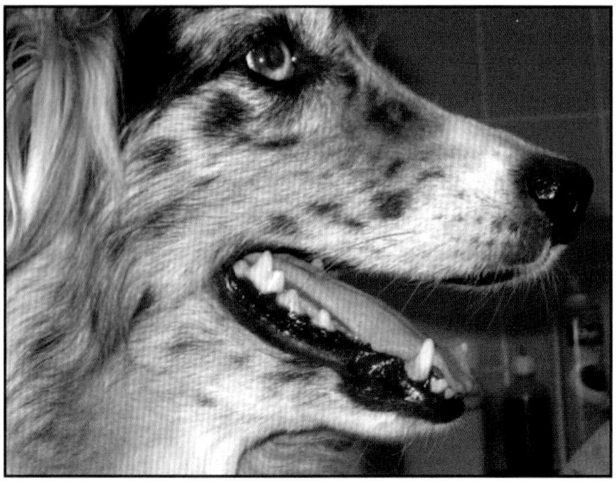

21.1 Cyanosis of the tongue in a dog with hypoxaemia.

Flushing of the mucous membranes may occur with hypercapnia, but there are other things that will cause this, and so it is not a pathognomonic sign. Capillary refill time, if definitely prolonged, is a reasonable indicator of poor circulation, but it too is a relatively insensitive test. Capillary refill time depends on ambient temperature, amount of pressure applied to the surface and the body temperature of the patient.

Auscultation of the lungs and trachea should be carried out to try to identify the location and nature of the lesion. Percussion of the lung field may also be helpful in detecting areas of hypo- or hyperresonance associated with fluid/solid masses or pneumothorax, respectively. If the examination of the patient at this point indicates the need for radiographic or ultrasonographic studies, these should be carried out. These studies may be better able to locate and define a lesion that has been difficult to elucidate on physical examination, and determine the surgical approach that is to be taken.

Preoperative measurement of respiratory volumes can be done relatively simply using a tight-fitting mask and a Wright's respirometer or an electronic spirometer. This may help to indicate whether the patient is hyper- or hypopnoeic (normal minute ventilation for dogs is 210 ± 56 ml/kg/minute and for cats is 175 ± 64 ml/kg/minute) but it does not define the extent of change that has occurred because the individual animal's normal minute ventilation is not known. There may also be alterations in the exchange of gas across the alveolar membrane due to the disease process, resulting in hypoventilation (increased P_aCO_2) despite an increase in minute volume.

Measurement of blood gases defines the degree of change in the respiratory system. Arterial samples can usually be obtained from a dorsal pedal or femoral artery. The validity of the results obtained from such a sample will depend, to some extent, on how the animal behaved during the collection of the sample. If the animal is greatly stressed by the procedure it tends to hyperventilate, which may mask the degree of hypoxaemia and decrease the arterial carbon dioxide tension (P_aCO_2). If a sample is to be taken from a dyspnoeic animal that objects to being restrained, the attempt should be abandoned. Venous samples can be used to obtain information with regard to acid–base status and P_vCO_2 if the sample can be obtained by free flow without occluding the vessel. A sample from the jugular vein is best used for this as it is the largest accessible vein and is least likely to collapse on to the needle during aspiration. These values may be significantly different from arterial values if there is a low cardiac output or a great increase in carbon dioxide production and should be interpreted with caution.

If a patient has any indication of fluid in the chest, a thoracocentesis should be performed to obtain a sample for further diagnostic investigations. A thoracocentesis is best carried out using a butterfly needle, teat cannula or intravenous catheter. A regular hypodermic needle is very sharp and is more likely to lacerate the lung. It is important to establish that the end of the needle/catheter has entered the thoracic cavity before a negative result is accepted, for example, where a short butterfly needle is used on an obese patient.

Cardiovascular function

Observation of the patient for venous distension and pulsations in the jugular vein should be carried out before handling the animal. Observation of vessels may not be feasible in many breeds because of long hair. Following this it is important to feel the pulse and get some sense of its character both centrally (femoral artery) and peripherally (dorsal pedal or radial arteries). A weak pulse is usually much more evident at a peripheral site than at the central vessel.

Auscultation of the heart must be carried out to characterize any abnormalities. If a murmur or arrhythmia is heard, the veterinary surgeon needs to decide whether further investigation is required. This must be predicated by the other lesions present in the animal and the resources of the client, but it is generally advisable to obtain as much information as possible about cardiac function prior to anaesthesia. This is particularly the case when a thoracic procedure is contemplated, as the surgery may have significant effects on cardiac function. Radiographs are helpful in delineating the size of the heart and whether left heart failure is present, but much more definitive information can be obtained from ultrasonography. M-mode or two-dimensional echocardiography can differentiate a pericardial effusion from an enlarged heart and can define the dimensions of cardiac structures and how they relate to normal. Doppler echocardiography can detect abnormal blood flow and be used to estimate the pressure gradient across stenotic vessels. Ultrasonography can also define the shortening fraction of the heart, which is a measure of contractility. The results from such tests should determine whether the animal is an appropriate candidate for surgical intervention or whether a period of medical therapy is warranted to ensure that myocardial activity is optimized. An electrocardiogram (ECG) helps to define both changes in the size of the heart (axis deviations) and any arrhythmias encountered during the examination.

An arterial blood gas sample should be taken if the investigation suggests any right-to-left shunting or low cardiac output. If an animal with a right-to-left shunt has a P_aO_2 of <60 mmHg (<8 kPa) on room air, great care is needed to ensure that a significant increase in right-sided pressures or decrease in left-sided pressures is not created, both of which could exacerbate the shunt.

Clinical pathology

Before undertaking such a major surgical intervention it is appropriate to obtain a complete blood count and biochemical profile to rule out further unrecognized intercurrent disease. An increased haematocrit may be evidence of a chronic hypoxaemia while a decreased value may represent chronic illness or blood loss. Anaemia may not be tolerated well in an animal with poor cardiac output, and it is imperative that this be taken into account when making a decision about preoperative or intraoperative transfusion. Dogs and cats tolerate a haematocrit of 0.15–0.2 l/l by increasing cardiac output so that oxygen delivery is maintained. However, an animal with a relatively fixed cardiac output (e.g. aortic stenosis) may barely survive at a haematocrit of 0.3 l/l.

Preparation

Pulmonary

Any conditions amenable to treatment before an animal is taken to surgery should be treated. If the animal has pneumonia that can be treated with antibiotics, without risk of developing a further infection, this should be done as long as the surgery can be delayed. If the pleural space, pericardium or abdomen is full of air or fluid, it should be drained as much as possible before carrying on with surgery. The animal with ascites has a decreased ability to ventilate and may show significant hypotension if put in dorsal recumbency. The fluid can usually be drained using a catheter (14–16 gauge) entering the abdomen 3–10 cm from the midline midway between the ribs and the pelvic limb on the right side. If the left side is used, care must be taken to avoid penetrating the spleen. Drainage of fluid in this way should be carried out slowly so that there is a slow change of pressure in the abdomen. An animal that has compensated for an increase in intra-abdominal pressure due to ascites may suffer from a massive hypotension and cardiovascular collapse if the intra-abdominal pressure is relieved too quickly. This is usually not an issue since it is hard to remove fluid rapidly with such a narrow access to the fluid (14 gauge catheter).

Pleural drainage can be achieved with minimal restraint in most animals, but cats with pleuritis are often extremely fractious and may need an analgesic prior to any attempt to carry out thoracic puncture. Opioids, such as hydromorphone (0.1 mg/kg i.m.) and butorphanol (0.2 mg/kg i.m.), provide analgesia while also giving some sedation, which is beneficial in these cases. After administering the opioid, the animal should be placed in an oxygen-rich environment and allowed to rest for 15–20 minutes before attempting to drain the chest. Ultrasonography can be used to guide placement of the drainage catheter, to minimize the risk of penetrating vital structures and assist in locating pockets of fluids if loculation has occurred. Animals with air or fluid in the pleural space should be evaluated for risk of a rapid return of the fluid after it has been drained. An animal with a pleural effusion could be tapped and drained several hours before thoracic surgery, with minimal chance of the fluid returning within that time frame. On the other hand, an animal which has a haemo- or pneumothorax may have such rapid recrudescence that the only option is to place a chest drain and apply continuous controlled suction. If it is not possible to maintain suction during transport to the operating room, the chest drain should be clamped off or connected to a water trap or Heimlich valve so that air cannot enter the pleural space. The chest drain should be a multifenestrated catheter which is directed toward the cranioventral quadrant of the thoracic cavity. It should be sutured in place using a technique which will ensure that the fenestrations cannot be pulled out and exposed to the atmosphere. A criss-cross (Roman bootlace, Chinese fingertrap) pattern is often used for this, but this may still allow for excessive movement in a dog with loose skin. A secure attachment can be achieved by passing the suture through the periosteum on one rib, thus ensuring that the chest tube will not retract very far from that site.

With any surgery involving entry into the thoracic cavity, it is essential to be able to ventilate the patient. This can be achieved simply by having someone squeeze the resevoir bag intermittently, but this is labour-intensive, so ventilation is usually achieved with the assistance of a mechanical device (see Chapter 6). Before anaesthetizing the patient, it is important to ensure that the ventilator is functioning and that it will work for that particular animal. This is likely to be a problem with some units when they are used on very small or very large patients; some machines are not able to provide small enough volumes for patients <5 kg, while others do not cope with giant breeds weighing 70–100 kg. Although not essential, the author has found it very helpful to be able to apply positive end expiratory pressure (PEEP) or continuous positive airway pressure (CPAP) to his patients once the thoracic cavity has been opened. Under normal circumstances the tendency of the lung to collapse is balanced by the tendency of the thoracic wall to spring outwards. Once the chest is opened the 'adhesion' between the chest wall and the lung is broken and the lung collapses to a smaller volume. Once this has happened it is necessary either to increase the tidal volume or to add PEEP/CPAP in order to maintain adequate gas exchange. In the author's experience, the addition of PEEP/CPAP has been helpful in reducing the atelectasis often associated with intrathoracic procedures. This effect can be achieved by adding a resistance to the expiratory limb of the circuit. The simplest method is to take the expiratory limb and pass it through a beaker of water, with the depth of the hose under the water determining the amount of PEEP; if the hose is 7 cm under water then the PEEP should be 7 cmH_2O. The same thing can be achieved by putting the scavenge hose from the ventilator under water, although this should be tested with the individual ventilator since some machines do not work properly when back pressure is exerted on this side of the circuit. This approach is often inconvenient because it can be hard to scavenge the gas after it has bubbled through the water. Commercial PEEP valves can be purchased which will apply a certain pressure. The valves usually come with preset values of 2.5, 5 and 10 cmH_2O and they can be used in sequence in order to provide 7.5 or 12.5 cmH_2O pressure. Some ventilators are equipped with a CPAP setting and the value required is dialled into the machine. With any of these techniques, a manometer placed in the circuit allows the measurement of the effect produced by the PEEP/CPAP manoeuvre. The author normally aims for a value of 3–7 cmH_2O on the basis of the effects on circulation, gas exchange and surgical access.

When preparing patients for a computed tomography (CT) scan, it is best to induce and maintain anaesthesia with the patient in sternal recumbency until the scans are complete. Small areas of atelectasis form rapidly in dogs and these denser areas of tissue may hide lesions that would be seen if the lung was fully expanded. With modern CT technology it is usually possible to scan a thorax in under 60 seconds, so it is feasible to breath-hold the animal for this procedure. The airway pressure is typically held at 15–20 cmH_2O for this period. This kind of intrathoracic pressure will significantly decrease venous return so it is important that the animal has a normal blood volume and that the veterinary surgeon monitors the effect on blood pressure during the scan.

When dealing with some tracheal surgeries, for example, surgeries involving tracheal resection, it may be necessary to place a tracheotomy tube during surgery and be able to continue the delivery of anaesthetic through this new tube. For these cases it is essential to have a range of sterile tracheostomy or endotracheal tubes and a sterile circuit available so that these can be placed in the surgical field without risk of contamination. Before proceeding with placement of a tracheostomy tube, check that all the connections between tubes are compatible to prevent any delays in switching from one circuit to the other.

If the patient has a pulmonary mass which may be an abscess or a tumour with a necrotic centre, it may be helpful to employ a bronchial blocker in order to prevent material from the lesion being expelled into the lower lung during the surgery. There are some endotracheal tubes designed for humans (e.g. TCB Univent), which can be used for this purpose in some small dogs (the maximum tube size has an internal diameter of 9.0 mm and the catheter used for occluding the bronchus is too short for larger dogs). By using the curves of the tube and catheter, it is possible to direct the catheter into the left or right mainstem bronchus blindly, although it is very difficult to know its exact location in the airway. The catheter also has an end-hole, so that it is possible to slowly deflate or reinflate the lung beyond the balloon occlusion. The main disadvantage with these tubes is that the main tube is a 'D' shape (in cross-section), which means that a very small endoscope is needed in order to visualize the placement of the catheter.

Another alternative is to use a Fogarty catheter; this can be placed in the airway before the endotracheal tube so that it goes down the side of the endotracheal tube. Once the animal is in position, an endoscope can be used to guide the Fogarty catheter into the appropriate bronchus, and then the balloon on the catheter can be inflated to occlude that airway. The two main disadvantages with this technique are that there is no end-hole in a Fogarty catheter, and that it is very easy for the catheter to become dislodged and slip back into the trachea. If this happens, an immediate total airway occlusion develops, which requires that the balloon be deflated and the catheter repositioned. A better version of this, the Arndt bronchial blocker, allows the catheter to be passed down the endotracheal tube with a loop over the endoscope (Figure 21.2). This system comes with an adapter that allows connection of the breathing system while the endoscope is passed through one port and the bronchial blocker through another. By passing the endoscope into the required bronchus, the blocker can be directed appropriately. One version of this catheter has a pear-shaped balloon that makes it less likely to dislodge from the airway. These catheters also have an end-hole to allow inflation/deflation of the blocked lung.

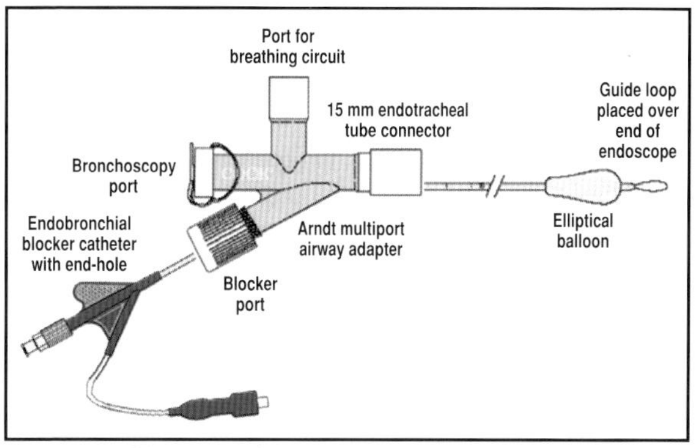

21.2 Diagram of the Arndt endobronchial blocker system. The adapter is connected to the endotracheal tube and the anaesthetic circuit is attached to the right-angled port. The endoscope can then be put down the central port while the endobronchial blocking catheter is fed down the angled side port. The loop is slipped over the end of the bronchoscope and the catheter and endoscope can be advanced together. The balloon is shown inflated to illustrate its shape but it would not normally be inflated until placed into the airway. Once it is in place the endoscope is removed and the central port closed. The screw cap on the side port is tightened to fix the catheter in place. The blocked lung can be deflated or PEEP can be applied through the catheter. Drawing adapted from Cook Medical diagrams.

The final approach for these cases is to use a double-lumen tube, which allows intubation of one mainstem bronchus and functional separation of the other. This has been described a number of times by various authors but has been difficult to apply clinically because of the anatomy of the canine respiratory tract (see section on thoracoscopy). If none of these approaches is possible, the surgeon should clamp the bronchus of the lobe nearest the lesion or, if that is not accessible, clamp the mainstem bronchus until the mass has been removed. Before the transected bronchus is closed, the airway should be suctioned to remove any material.

Cardiovascular

Before carrying out a thoracotomy on a patient with cardiovascular disease, it is important to optimize medical therapy that may improve the patient's condition, if the procedure can be delayed. If vasodilators, inotropes, diuretics or anti-arrhythmic drugs can improve the function of the cardiovascular system, this therapy should be instituted for long enough to make a difference. Cats with hyperthyroidism and associated cardiac changes should be given carbimazole or methimazole for at least 1 week before the surgery, as the mortality rate is much higher without such treatment.

For patients with bradycardia that is non-responsive to anticholinergic therapy, or that have sick sinus syndrome, it is advisable to place a temporary pacemaker until the permanent one can be implanted. This can usually be achieved by placing an introducer (a large thin-walled catheter) into a saphenous vein using local anaesthesia and then advancing the pacing lead up to the heart from this site. The author avoids using the jugular vein, if possible, when placing a temporary pacemaker prior to a permanent transvenous pacemaker, so that both vessels are available for this purpose if needed. If the patient is too small for a saphenous approach, the lead can be introduced via the jugular vein (Figure 21.3).

An animal with a pericardial effusion of sufficient magnitude to cause a restriction of myocardial function should have the fluid drained prior to surgery. This is typically carried out using a needle or catheter, and the intent is to drain enough fluid off to release any pressure in the pericardial sac. The animal is usually positioned in left lateral recumbency and access is gained through the right fourth to sixth intercostal space. An over-the-needle catheter with multiple fenestrations is ideal since the catheter can be left in place during the aspiration of fluid, minimizing the risk of trauma to the heart. This is best done using ultrasonographic guidance so that the myocardium is not traumatized.

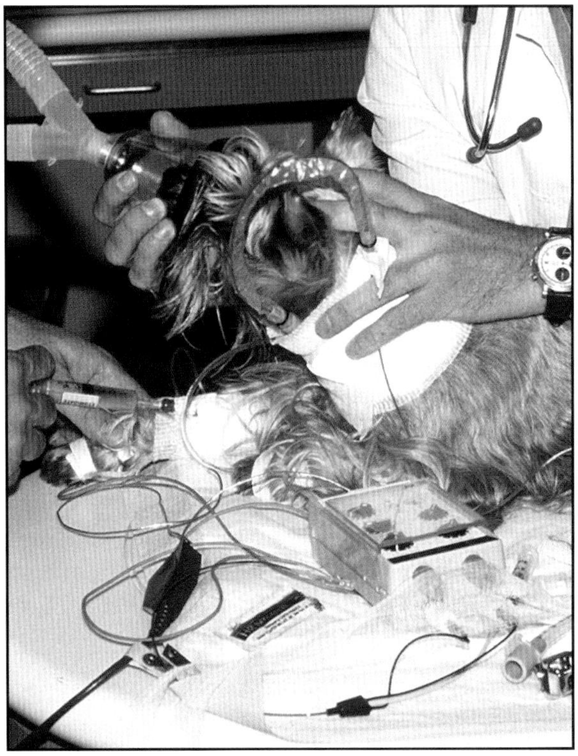

21.3 Temporary pacemaker inserted through an introducer in the jugular vein. The picture shows the pacing generator in the foreground. The animal has had the pacemaker inserted under sedation and will have a constant regulated heart rate during the induction and maintenance of anaesthesia.

The risk of surgical blood loss should be assessed prior to the procedure and, using the current haematocrit and cardiovascular status of the patient, a decision should be made as to whether blood is going to be needed. If blood is likely to be needed, the necessary arrangements should be made to obtain an adequate supply of cross-matched blood or packed red cells for that patient.

Surgical approach

Both a lateral and ventral approach to the chest involve some risk of damage to the underlying structures as the pleura is incised. The veterinary surgeon should establish controlled ventilation before the thorax is opened and should be able to stop ventilation for the brief period required to open the pleura. This reduces the risk of accidental injury to the lung during entry into the chest. A lateral thoracotomy may involve a single intercostal space or may entail the removal of one or more ribs. If surgery involves the heart, mediastinum or oesophagus, it is likely that the surgeon will need to pack off the lung in the surgical field. This should be done carefully so that minimal gas exchange surface area is lost, but it is also appropriate to compress the lung fairly completely since, by reducing the compliance of the upper lung, more gas will be directed to the lower lung field. However, it is expected that this manoeuvre will decrease the available exchange surface resulting in a decrease in the P_aO_2.

With a sternal approach, it is unlikely that the lung fields need to be compressed, but the alteration in the orientation of the heart can lead to some decrease in venous return, and it may be necessary to increase fluid therapy in order to increase central venous pressure (CVP; preload on the heart). As surgery proceeds, it is often noticed that certain manipulations cause a sudden dramatic decrease in arterial blood pressure. The surgeon and the anaesthetist should work together to define these deleterious events so that their effects can be minimized. It is more common to see cardiac arrhythmias with a ventral approach; this should be monitored carefully and therapy initiated if the arrhythmias appear to be detrimental to cardiovascular function.

Nitrous oxide (N_2O) is contraindicated during any thoracotomy because of the rapid accumulation of N_2O in gas pockets in the pleura. Since the pleural space is well vascularized and is in direct contact with the lung containing N_2O, the N_2O diffuses down the concentration gradient and can double the volume of a closed pneumothorax in 10–15 minutes.

Analgesia

Analgesia for thoracotomy can be provided in a number of ways. A lateral thoracotomy appears to cause less pain than a sternotomy, and many dogs will show few signs of pain after a single intercostal incision if other muscle groups have not been transected. An epidural injection of an opioid with or without a local anaesthetic certainly provides some analgesia for a thoracotomy, and it can be given before the surgery starts to provide some pre-emptive effect. This also provides bilateral analgesia so it is useful for both a lateral and sternal incision. An epidural catheter can be placed via the lumbosacral space and its tip advanced up to the mid-thoracic region. This can be used to deliver morphine and/or a local anaesthetic by intermittent boluses or by continuous infusion and can be left in place for several days after the surgery to provide ongoing analgesia. Intercostal nerve blocks have been used for a lateral approach and provide some analgesia, but when applied before surgery they are unlikely to give analgesia over more than half the thorax. This is because the dorsal branch of the intercostal nerve branches off close to the spinal cord, and it supplies the cutaneous structures to about halfway down the thoracic wall. The block can be done more effectively once the chest is opened, by injecting the nerves from inside the thorax aiming out towards the vertebrae where the nerves exit the canal. An interpleural block can be carried out after the chest has been closed. For a lateral thoracotomy, the animal is placed in dorsolateral recumbency and the local anaesthetic (usually 0.1–0.2% bupivacaine at 1–2 mg/kg) is injected through the chest drain. The anaesthetic tends to go to the part of the chest closest to the table and diffuse through the thoracic wall into the intercostal nerves. For a sternotomy, the local anaesthetic is injected through the chest drain with the animal in sternal recumbency. In both instances the animal should be left in that position for at least 10 minutes after the injection, so that the drug has time to get taken up into the relevant tissues.

Monitoring

Monitoring an animal undergoing a thoracotomy must allow the veterinary surgeon to establish the adequacy of ventilation, to diagnose arrhythmias and to provide information on changes in cardiac function, especially when the animal has cardiac disease. The monitoring of ventilation without being able to measure airway pressure, minute ventilation, end-tidal carbon dioxide ($PETCO_2$) or P_aCO_2 is difficult once the chest is open since the chest does not move in a manner that allows tidal volumes to be estimated. The list of monitoring techniques above is ordered in increasing desirability. Airway pressure indicates the force being applied to the pulmonary system but does not give any information about gas exchange. It is expected that peak pressures in the 10–15 and 10–20 cmH_2O range would be normal for the cat and dog, respectively. If higher pressures are required to achieve adequate inflation, it may be an indication of decreased airway compliance. Minute ventilation is a more accurate representation of how much gas is being moved in and out of the lungs but still does not tell us whether we have adequate exchange. End-tidal carbon dioxide should reflect the value for P_aCO_2, but there is often a discrepancy between the two values and this is not readily predictable. The two values are usually close enough in patients with normal lungs for clinicians not to be greatly under- or over-ventilating the patient, and a capnograph is a non-invasive monitor with continuous sampling that provides rapid feedback on changes in ventilation. Arterial or free-flow lingual venous blood gas samples will provide definitive assessment of ventilation. A pulse oximeter is very helpful in cases where desaturation may be expected (e.g. extensive pulmonary disease, right-to-left shunt) or where other techniques for measuring ventilation are not available. A pulse oximeter provides limited information on the early changes associated with ventilation/perfusion mismatching or alterations in shunt fraction, but if desaturation occurs it is likely to be sensed by the monitor and the veterinary surgeon warned before it is too late. A combination of capnography, arterial blood gas monitoring and pulse oximetry is ideal for these cases since the two non-invasive, continuous monitors can be checked intermittently by the measurement of blood gases, allowing more accurate interpretation of the values displayed. Electrocardiography is essential for these cases to allow diagnosis of arrhythmias. Early diagnosis and management may prevent progression to ventricular fibrillation.

Haemodynamic monitoring should include at least some measure of blood pressure, preferably with a transducer attached to an arterial catheter that also allows multiple sampling of blood for blood gas measurement. In some conditions it may also be beneficial to be able to monitor CVP and/or pulmonary arterial pressure.

Individual conditions

Trauma

Trauma to the chest wall requiring immediate surgical intervention includes a flail chest, puncture wounds to the thoracic cavity and intrathoracic bleeding. Delayed intervention may be made for fractured ribs although these are rarely repaired.

An animal with a flail chest may be unable to ventilate normally, and the flail segment is pulled inwards every time the animal inhales. This makes ventilation very inefficient and the animal may be hypoxaemic and hypercapnic. Some dogs and cats seem to cope quite well with a three- or four-rib flail segment and may not become hypoxaemic. While preparing to anaesthetize such a patient, the inspired gas should be supplemented with oxygen and the animal should be positioned with the flail segment down. This will minimize the ventilatory effects of the flail and improve ventilation. The anaesthetic technique should be aimed at gaining rapid control of the airway. This is best achieved using drugs with a rapid onset of action such as thiopental or etomidate. Propofol has a slower onset of action (1–2 minutes) and should be given slowly in order to minimize the respiratory depression and hypotension which can occur. Ketamine and tiletamine both take about 60 seconds to take effect, which is not ideal under these circumstances. Opioids, used for induction, also take at least 2 minutes to reach peak effect. Once the animal is intubated, it should be ventilated until the flail segment has been stabilized. Since a fractured rib could damage the lung, it is essential to monitor the patient carefully for signs of pneumothorax developing during this procedure.

Diaphragmatic hernia

Diaphragmatic hernias may be traumatic or congenital. Traumatic hernias are usually caused by an excessive force being applied to the abdomen, causing viscera to rupture through the diaphragm into the chest. Most of these patients present with dyspnoea, although some animals can be totally asymptomatic. The animal may be presented in extremis immediately post-trauma, or the hernia may be discovered as an incidental finding from abdominal radiographs or ultrasonograms. The liver is the most common organ to herniate and so some cases present with ascites and hepatic dysfunction. The severity of the dyspnoea usually relates to the loss of space in the chest for normal pulmonary function, and it may be helpful, when handling these animals, to lift them on to their hindlegs so that their back is perpendicular to the ground. Many of these animals have fractured limbs, pulmonary contusions and myocardial trauma, and these other lesions need to be assessed before proceeding with repair of the diaphragmatic hernia. The timing of surgical repair is controversial; one author suggests that one should 'never let the sun go down' on a diaphragmatic hernia, even in cases where the diagnosis has been made months after the traumatic incident. The justification for immediate repair is that it is quite possible for more abdominal content to shift into the thoracic cavity and for animals to become severely dyspnoeic, or even die, overnight, and this author has seen examples of such incidents. The disadvantages of carrying out the repair the same day may relate to scheduling conflicts and wanting to have the animal fully resuscitated and stable before proceeding with the repair. This author favours not delaying since there is usually time to provide adequate restoration of circulating volume (after trauma), while an animal that decompensates can die in a matter of minutes. Preoperative preparation of the patient is important: cases of acute trauma need to receive adequate fluid therapy and should be preoxygenated before induction.

Premedication with an opioid, at low doses, and with an anticholinergic is appropriate. In the recently traumatized patient (<5 days), acepromazine is avoided as it may exacerbate hypotension in such animals, and it can cause splenic enlargement. Preoxygenation should be carried out for 5 minutes, using a tight-fitting mask in order to increase the inspired oxygen concentration to >95%. The mask should be kept on during the induction until the animal is ready to be intubated. Induction with a dissociative agent, propofol or etomidate, is ideal; this allows rapid control of the airway so that the animal can be ventilated immediately. Thiopental commonly causes splenic enlargement, which could lead to severe respiratory distress if the spleen is wholly or partially in the chest.

Once the animal is intubated, positive-pressure ventilation should be initiated. It seems to be important not to re-expand atelectatic lung too rapidly, so the aim should be to use higher respiratory frequencies with lower peak airway pressures. Oxygenation of the arterial blood should be carefully monitored, as this author has found it difficult to avoid hypoxaemia if tidal volume is restricted excessively. The concern with rapid re-expansion of the lung is that this has been associated with pulmonary oedema. The pathophysiology of this condition is still not known but there is an increase in vascular permeability resulting from the production of reactive oxygen species. The contraction of endothelial cells responsible for the increased fluid leak can be blocked by an antagonist to the small guanosine triphosphatase (GTPase) signalling pathway (rho) and its target protein (rho-associated coiled-coil-forming protein kinase, ROCK). The aim with these cases is to provide adequate ventilation to prevent hypoxaemia and hypercapnia but *not* to re-expand the lung. Once the hernia has been repaired and the air evacuated from the chest, the lung will be expanded gradually by the animal, hopefully allowing enough time to prevent acute injury.

The usual approach to a diaphragmatic hernia is via a midline laparotomy, with extension of the incision into the sternum if necessary. Some advocate a lateral thoracotomy and repair of the hernia from the anterior surface of the diaphragm; this approach has been quite successful as long as the location of the hernia has been adequately defined (e.g. right lateral thoracotomy for a right-sided hernia). Before the hernia has been completely repaired, it is helpful to place a chest drain so that air can be drained from the thoracic cavity and the normal negative pleural pressure re-established.

Space-occupying lesions not associated with the cardiopulmonary system: thymoma

The most common tumours to be found in the thoracic cavity, which do not involve the heart or lungs, are thymomas. These can be of considerable size and interfere with pulmonary function by compression of the trachea, or affect venous return by compressing the cranial vena cava. Myasthenia gravis is also associated with thymoma and may be recognized by a history of regurgitation or by the presence of a megaoesophagus on thoracic radiographs. This condition may lead to aspiration pneumonia, and so extra care needs to be taken while handling these patients during induction and recovery (see sections in Chapters 22 and 26 for details on dealing with megaoesophagus). Patients with myasthenia are normally being treated with an anticholinesterase (physostigmine). This therapy should be given on the morning of surgery if the signs of myasthenia have been relatively severe. The presence of long-acting anticholinesterases may alter the duration of action of some opioids. The response to muscle relaxants is variable, but in general these patients tend to have an increased sensitivity to these drugs. If it is necessary to give a non-depolarizing relaxant (which is rarely necessary), the patient should receive small doses while the response is monitored (see Chapter 15).

The patient should be premedicated according to the severity of compromise caused by the thymoma. Routine premedication would be acceptable in a young active patient with few clinical signs, whereas a patient with prominent signs should be given minimal premedication. Before induction the patient should be preoxygenated and a suction apparatus should be immediately available if the animal has a megaoesophagus. The induction drug needs to have a rapid onset in cases of megaoesophagus, but if megaoesophagus is not present, the induction technique is not overly important. Maintenance with an inhalant would be typical. A second intravenous catheter should be placed in case more than one infusion is necessary. Some of these tumours wrap around the major blood vessels, so significant blood loss is possible, and there should be blood available for transfusion.

Oesophageal lesions including persistent right aortic arch

Access to the oesophagus in the thorax may require a thoracotomy. Congenital lesions, such as persistent right aortic arch (PRAA) or other aortic arch anomalies, may cause a restrictive lesion of the oesophagus. These animals are therefore prone to similar problems to those seen with megaoesophagus from other causes and should be handled as such.

While PRAA is usually an avascular remnant, some of the other anomalies causing oesophageal stricture may be associated with viable blood vessels, and significant blood loss can occur. The patient should have two venous catheters placed, and blood transfusions should be available. For oesophageal tears or foreign bodies, the greatest risks are from infection and pneumothorax. The latter can occur if the foreign object has damaged some lung as well as the oesophagus. If this is likely, due to the nature or position of the foreign body, the animal should have a chest drain placed before intermittent positive pressure ventilation (IPPV) is initiated.

Pulmonary lesions

Most of these cases will have some degree of respiratory compromise and will need preoxygenation prior to induction. Ideally, the mask should be left on for 5 minutes prior to induction, and during induction until the animal is ready to be intubated. If the mask is removed, the animal will begin to breathe room air and, since there are no oxygen 'stores' in the body, the benefit of preoxygenation will be lost within a few breaths. If the animal will not tolerate a mask, a bag over the head may be tolerated better: a plastic bag with an oxygen inlet can be placed over the head and closed on to the neck. If this technique is not feasible, it may be necessary to start the induction and place the mask as soon as the animal begins to lose consciousness. Although it may take up to 5 minutes to reach peak P_aO_2, the initial rise is steep and the animal will benefit from even a few breaths of 100% oxygen.

Pneumothorax is usually a result of damage to the lung or major airways. If there is any concern that air leakage may continue during the preparation period, a chest drain should be placed and the animal connected to a continuous suction device. If the amount of air in the thorax is minimal and there does not appear to be any ongoing leakage, it may be safe not to place a chest drain, as long as the time from induction to entrance into the thoracic cavity is short. If it is known that there will be significant ongoing air leakage from pulmonary tissue until the surgeon can oversew or remove the damage, a total intravenous anaesthetic technique should be considered. This is to avoid leakage of inhalant into the thoracic cavity so that surgeons and assistants do not have to breathe in waste anaesthetic gases. For this purpose, a propofol/opioid infusion technique is ideal; propofol is given at 0.1–0.3 mg/kg/minute while an opioid such as fentanyl can be given at 0.3–1.0 μg/kg/minute. In cats, the dose of fentanyl should not exceed 0.4 μg/kg/minute.

Animals with pulmonary contusions need to be ventilated very carefully, because there is some risk that the vessel rupture responsible for the contusion can be opened up again by stretching the lung excessively. Further haemorrhage into the lung may cause a significant loss of gas exchange area and lead to severe respiratory compromise. Ventilation of these animals should be with low tidal volumes and high frequencies (e.g. 20 breaths per minute, tidal volume 10 ml/kg).

Preoperatively, it is often difficult to differentiate between a pulmonary abscess and a tumour. If it is suspected that the lesion may be an abscess or a tumour with a necrotic centre, then the precautions described in the section on preparing patients with pulmonary disease should be taken. It is also wise to have a suction device available if the above measures fail to contain the pus. Any major drainage of pus into the lower lung carries a very poor prognosis for the patient.

Another concern with such lesions is that there may be adhesions between the lung and the parietal pleura, such that entry through the pleura results in entry into the lesion. The anaesthetist should be prepared to handle the blood loss or air leakage that can occur under these circumstances.

Lung lobe torsion is usually treated by excision of the lobe, and this is normally a relatively straightforward procedure, especially if it is done using advanced stapling techniques. Apart from the considerations above (preoxygenation, ventilation, etc.) there are no major new considerations for this surgery.

Chylothorax

Concerns with chylothorax and other pleural effusions relate to the amount of fluid in the chest and with adhesions that may have formed to the parietal pleura, increasing the chance of pulmonary injury when the thoracic cavity is opened. If possible, attempts should be made to drain the fluid off the chest before anaesthesia to improve intraoperative ventilation. Blood loss is minimal if the lymphatic duct is tied off or a drainage system is implanted into the diaphragm, but it can be substantial if a pleurodesis is performed.

Pericardiectomy

Pericardiectomy may be undertaken for a pericardial effusion or for a pericardial constriction. Animals with cardiac tamponade, where intrapericardial pressure approaches the right ventricular diastolic filling pressure, are at immediate risk of circulatory collapse. An intrapericardial pressure of 9 mmHg can cause a 60% reduction in cardiac output while pressures as high as 12–13 mmHg may be tolerated. Drainage of fluid from the pericardium should be carried out to relieve these symptoms before the animal is anaesthetized. The preferred approach for pericardiectomy is via sternotomy, since this gives the best access to the pericardium, but a lateral approach may be used in some cases. Pericardiectomy may also be amenable to endoscopic approaches (see below). If an animal with cardiac tamponade must be anaesthetized, it should be pretreated with fluids to ensure optimum venous return and a technique used which minimizes reductions in myocardial contractility and heart rate (heart rate is usually elevated in an attempt to maintain cardiac output in the presence of a reduced stroke volume). Etomidate would be the ideal induction drug for this purpose but an opioid induction could be used as long as care is taken not to allow the heart rate to decrease significantly. Once the animal is intubated, it is recommended that spontaneous ventilation be maintained to minimize any further reduction in venous return. However, it has also been shown that hypercapnia will further decrease cardiac output so it is better to use IPPV than to allow hypercapnia to develop. If IPPV is used, it is best to use higher breathing frequencies in order to limit peak airway pressures, and not to use PEEP. Dobutamine is probably the best drug to use to improve cardiac output, since it delays the onset of tissue hypoxia when compared with noradrenaline. However, dopamine also increases cardiac output and improves myocardial perfusion. Once the tamponade has been reduced, anaesthetic management of these patients during pericardiectomy is relatively straightforward. Ventricular arrhythmias are common during manipulation of the pericardium and so lidocaine should be on hand in case these begin to alter haemodynamic function. Haemorrhage may be marked if a decortication of the epicardium is undertaken and it is necessary to have adequate supplies of typed and cross-matched blood to cope with excessive blood loss.

Patent ductus arteriosus

Most animals anaesthetized for correction of a patent ductus arteriosus (PDA) (see also Chapter 19) are young and are usually in good health apart from the changes caused by the PDA. In the early stages, there are very few myocardial changes associated with a PDA. However, if the ductus is large and/or the lesion has not been recognized early, there can be significant enlargement of the left ventricle, with cardiac failure due to volume overload occurring terminally. If surgery is performed before significant changes have occurred, there are few concerns for the veterinary surgeon. Patients presented at an early age will have lower than adult blood pressures due to their stage of development and one should expect diastolic pressure to be very low before ligation of the ductus, because of the connection of the systemic circulation to the low-resistance pulmonary system. Because of this, phenothiazines and butyrophenones should be avoided for premedication because the alpha-blockade will tend to decrease systemic vascular resistance (SVR), decreasing diastolic pressure still further. The maintenance of diastolic pressure is important in the effectiveness of coronary perfusion. Systolic pressures are usually normal to high but, because of the low diastolic pressure, the mean pressure is also normal or reduced and is often in the 50–60 mmHg range during the approach to the ductus. Positive inotropes may increase systolic pressure and also increase mean pressure but should only be used if systolic pressures fall below 90 mmHg. Peripheral vasoconstrictors should not be used since an increased SVR will tend to increase the shunt through the ductus and may lead to pulmonary oedema.

If there are problems with the dissection of the ductus, it is possible to lose large quantities of blood very quickly. A second intravenous catheter should be placed so that fluids can be given rapidly if needed, although the outcome is rarely favourable if the ductus is ruptured. Before the ductus is ligated, it is wise to give an anticholinergic because the sudden change in blood pressure associated with ligation can elicit a strong baroreceptor reflex, which can even cause cardiac arrest. The anticholinergic blocks the vagal part of this reflex. The author typically uses the anticholinergic at the time of premedication, although it could be given closer to the time of ligation. Monitoring of direct arterial blood pressure in these cases enables assessment of moment-to-moment changes and is also of use in ensuring that the ductus has been ligated. Typically there is a sudden increase in diastolic pressure as soon as the ductus is tied off (Figure 21.4).

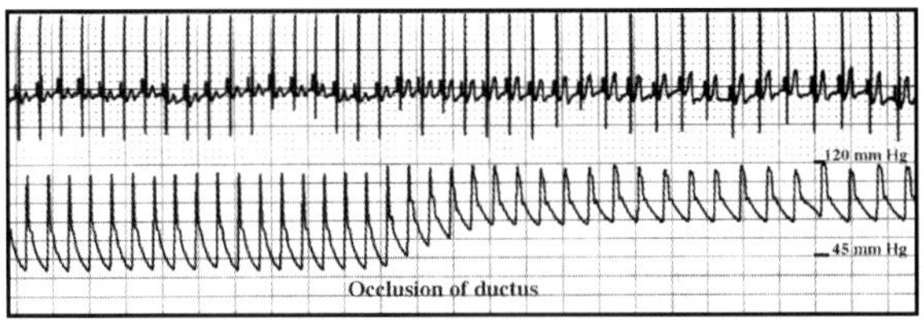

21.4 Arterial blood pressure and ECG tracing from a dog undergoing a patent ductus occlusion. Note the increase in diastolic pressure with minimal change in systolic pressure. The heart rate decreases from 128 to 108 beats per minute in response to the increased pressure (baroreceptor response). The trace is at 6.25 mm/second.

Patients with signs of cardiac failure or pulmonary oedema should be treated with diuretics and positive inotropes for 1–2 days prior to surgery. The anaesthetic technique should attempt to maintain myocardial function as much as possible and not cause further decreases in SVR. Premedication with an opioid–anticholinergic combination is useful, and induction with an opioid–benzodiazepine technique or etomidate with or without benzodiazepine is preferred. Maintenance of anaesthesia in these patients can be with a standard inhalant, unless signs of myocardial failure are present, in which case a balanced technique combining an opioid and/or a muscle relaxant with the inhalant would be in order. Patients with a right-to-left shunt are rarely amenable to surgical correction, since closure of the duct often results in right heart failure due to the pulmonary hypertension. If such an animal needs to be anaesthetized for part of the diagnostic work-up or for other reasons, the regimen described for the PDA with some degree of heart failure should be used. It is important to maintain or increase SVR while aiming to reduce (or at least not increase) pulmonary vascular resistance.

Non-surgical repair of the PDA is being used more often; for this procedure it is necessary to insert a catheter into the aorta from the femoral artery, or in very small dogs a carotid approach may be used. The tip of the catheter is positioned at the entrance to the PDA and a coil is released into the ductus. Anaesthetic techniques for these cases are similar to those described for the surgical approach except that a thoracotomy is not necessary, obviating the requirement for IPPV (although it may be needed for other reasons).

Pulmonic stenosis

Management of dogs with pulmonic stenosis is normally by balloon valvuloplasty, which does not require a thoracotomy. In small patients, or those with very narrow stenosis, surgery may be necessary. This can be done without cardiopulmonary bypass at normothermia: the usual technique is to place a patch over the pulmonary outflow and then cut through the stenosis, leaving the wall of the pulmonary artery open into the patch that has been applied.

Dogs with pulmonic stenosis usually present with right ventricular hypertrophy, although it is very rare for them to be in right heart failure. Animals with pressure gradients of <40 mmHg across the stenosis are at low risk for anaesthetic complications and may be handled in a relatively routine fashion. Animals with gradients >40 mmHg may have significant hypertrophy and should be regarded as having an increased anaesthetic risk, although it is uncommon to see problems with these cases until the gradient exceeds 80 mmHg. Right ventricular hypertrophy makes these animals more prone to reduced myocardial perfusion and ventricular arrhythmias. The anaesthetic technique chosen should aim to minimize the possibility of bradycardia; since the right ventricle is thick and non-compliant, cardiac output is more dependent on heart rate than in a normal animal. At the same time, a tachycardia tends to increase myocardial oxygen demand, while shortening diastole and reducing coronary perfusion. These two changes may lead to myocardial ischaemia and precipitate severe arrhythmias. Premedication should therefore aim to minimize anxiety and prevent tachycardia. Opioids combined with low doses of anticholinergics usually achieve this aim. Induction of anaesthesia can be carried out using etomidate with or without a benzodiazepine as the technique of choice, because there is minimal change in heart rate or contractility. An opioid–benzodiazepine technique can be used as long as an anticholinergic has been given previously, and the heart rate is monitored carefully during induction. Maintenance of anaesthesia can be with an inhalant such as isoflurane, or a balanced technique can be used with the addition of an opioid or N_2O. Lidocaine should be readily available as a first-line treatment for ventricular arrhythmias which may occur during therapy. Animals with a dynamic component to their stenosis should receive phenylephrine to treat hypotension as described below (aortic stenosis).

If a surgical approach is used for this condition, the anaesthetist should prepare as above but add a second venous access and have blood products available for rapid transfusion.

Aortic stenosis

Aortic stenosis (see also Chapter 19) is also associated with ventricular hypertrophy caused by a pressure overload. Balloon valvuloplasty for this condition has been very disappointing, and even results with surgical correction using cardiopulmonary bypass (beyond the scope of this text) appear to be no better than medical therapy. Closed aortic valvotomy has also been described. This requires a thoracotomy and carries a significant risk of haemorrhage and cardiac arrhythmias. If an animal with aortic stenosis must be anaesthetized for diagnostic procedures or non-cardiac surgery then most of the comments above (dealing with right ventricular hypertrophy) apply. However, there is more concern with reduction in SVR as coronary perfusion may be reduced if this occurs, and so the phenothiazines and butyrophenones are usually avoided. Management of intraoperative hypotension is also different. Many cases of aortic stenosis have a dynamic component, which is exacerbated if a positive inotrope is given. For these animals the author typically uses phenylephrine (2–5 μg/kg slow bolus i.v. followed by infusion of 0.1–1 μg/kg/minute) to treat hypotension, because the dose can be titrated to produce alpha-1 mediated vasoconstriction with minimal positive inotropic effect. For closed aortic valvotomy, the same techniques are used but the animal should be cross-matched before surgery and have at least two patent intravenous catheters. Lidocaine may be started prior to ventriculotomy.

Thoracoscopy

This may be used for diagnostic purposes (e.g. biopsy of a mass) or for surgical approaches (e.g. pericardiectomy, PDA, PRAA, thoracic duct ligation or lung lobectomy). The basic procedure involves the introduction of a rigid or flexible fibreoptic endoscope into the thoracic cavity, and the use of air or another gas to create a pneumothorax, allowing visualization of intrathoracic structures. One or more other ports are usually placed to allow the introduction of a gas or instruments required for the surgical manipulation. The approach may be made laterally with the animal in lateral recumbency, or ventrally (subxiphoid) with the animal in dorsal recumbency. For the lateral approach it is necessary to collapse the upper lung and so it is advantageous if selective one-lung ventilation (OLV) can be performed. In the dog, the right lung is about 1.5 times the size of the left lung and receives almost 60% of the blood supply. It is possible to achieve adequate ventilation of the animal using just the right lung although some desaturation can occur during the first few minutes. Some of the approaches to OLV are outlined above, but the preferred method is to use a double-lumen tube so that if a bilateral thoracoscopic procedure is undertaken, one can collapse each lung separately. The double-lumen tubes that have been used in dogs are the Robertshaw type (Figure 21.5), which have a long and short tube with two cuffs. The longer tube is placed in the bronchus while the shorter tube should remain in the trachea. Once the cuffs are inflated the right and left lungs should be functionally isolated from each other. The tubes are supplied as left and right versions: the right tube has an orifice in the side of the cuff that, in humans, is supposed to be placed at the entrance to the bronchus of the right upper lobe. This does not work well in dogs because of the position of the right apical lobe bronchus and it is difficult to place an endobronchial tube on the right side without losing ventilation to the right apical and cardiac (middle) lobes of the lung (Figure 21.5). Because of this difference in anatomy, it is usual to use a left-sided Robertshaw tube. The cuffs of these tubes are bright blue to improve visualization and an endoscope is necessary to ensure correct placement of the tube. Human studies have shown that blind positioning results in a high incidence of malpositioning (38–78%). The endoscope should be passed down both tubes to ensure that the ends of the tubes are in the correct place (not impacted against a bronchial wall and that the right tube has not slipped into the left main bronchus), and that the cuff is adequately

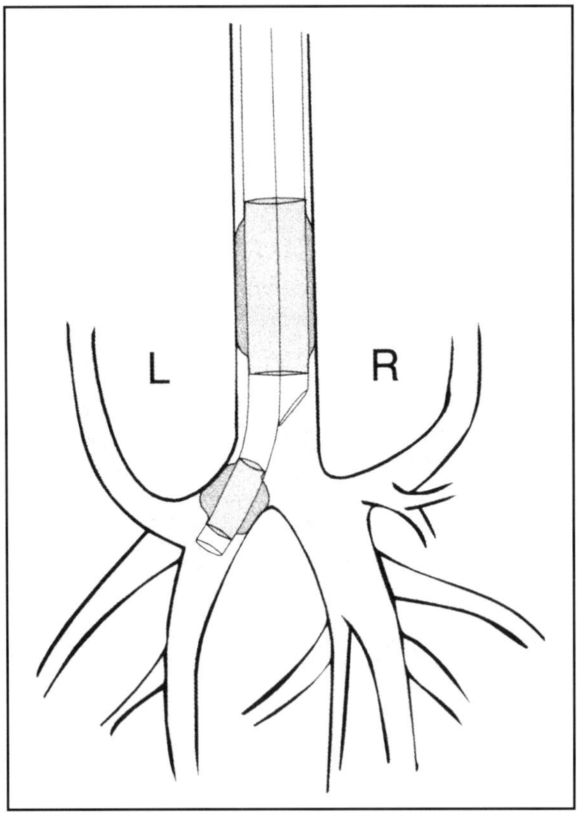

21.5 Diagram of the trachea and bronchi of the dog with the placement of a Robertshaw tube in the left mainstem bronchus. Note the proximity of the distal end of the tube to the bronchi in the left cranial lobe showing the likelihood of occluding one or more of these bronchi.

inflated in the correct position. For the larger sizes of tube (39 and 41 French) a 4.9 mm (outside diameter) bronchoscope will work, but something less than 4.2 mm will be needed for the smaller tubes (28–37 French). This technique remains impractical in many canine patients because Robertshaw tubes are designed for humans and are too short to be used in dogs over about 20 kg. This makes the Arndt endobronchial blockade technique the most practical and versatile approach for OLV (see Figure 21.2).

If a lateral approach is being used, then the dependent lung is ventilated while the upper non-dependent lung is collapsed. OLV appears to be adequate for the removal of carbon dioxide, but there is a significant risk of lower-than-normal P_aO_2 because of the loss of exchange area and shunting of blood through the non-ventilated lung. Studies examining OLV in normal animals have shown that despite the decrease in P_aO_2, delivery of oxygen to the periphery is unchanged because haemoglobin is still fully saturated and cardiac output does not change very much. However, it is common to perform thoracoscopy on animals with abnormal lungs and so hypoxaemia is always a concern. Strategies to improve oxygen exchange include:

- Application of PEEP to the dependent lung. The combination of gravity, weight of the heart and surgical manipulation all tend to induce collapse of the dependent lung. The application of PEEP is an attempt to minimize these changes and to hold the airways open. However, the ideal value of the PEEP is not easy to determine, since too low a value will not have any effect and too high a value will increase pulmonary intravascular pressure. Increased pulmonary intravascular pressure may decrease cardiac output and may also shunt blood into the upper unventilated lung. Nevertheless, in humans the application of 10 cmH_2O PEEP to the dependent lung has been shown to improve P_aO_2 in patients with a P_aO_2 <80 mmHg (<10.7 kPa). In normal dogs, 5 cmH_2O PEEP applied to the dependent lung does not significantly improve P_aO_2 or decrease cardiac output
- Application of CPAP to the non-dependent lung. This is applied to the upper lung before deflation is allowed to occur, or after a large tidal volume, so that the pressure is applied before the lung has collapsed. An adjustable, disposable CPAP valve can be bought for this application (Broncho-Cath® with CPAP system). The CPAP valve is applied to the upper lung endotracheal tube and oxygen is given at 5 l/minute. This approach allows some mass diffusion of oxygen into the upper lung and improves oxygenation more than the application of PEEP to the dependent lung alone
- Use of high-frequency ventilation to the non-dependent lung. In one human study, this gave comparable results to the application of CPAP in terms of P_aO_2 but interfered less with cardiac output, thus providing better oxygen delivery to the tissues. In this study, a high-frequency jet ventilator (HFJV) was used, set at a rate of 150 breaths per minute. The author has not had success with this technique in dogs.

If it is necessary to turn the dog over and examine the other hemithorax endoscopically, the use of a double-lumen tube enables the process to be reversed, so that the lung that was collapsed can be re-expanded while the other lung is deflated.

Using the subxiphoid approach (e.g. for pericardiectomy), it may be unnecessary to use a double-lumen tube since both sides may need to be kept at relatively low volumes in order to improve visualization. It is essential in these procedures for the surgeon and anaesthetist to coordinate their activities to achieve maximum visibility for the surgeon while maintaining adequate oxygenation. This often requires the use of hand ventilation to provide irregular ventilatory cycles between bouts of surgical activity. The use of a double-lumen tube may allow more flexibility in achieving the best ventilation with the least interference with surgery. Using PEEP/CPAP for this approach may also be beneficial in improving oxygenation.

Animals undergoing thoracoscopy should be monitored using pulse oximetry, so that any desaturation can be recognized and treated promptly. The addition of capnography, electrocardiography, direct arterial pressure and CVP measurement (CVP will be affected by the amount of air or carbon dioxide in the chest making it easier to recognize excessive pneumothorax) adds considerably to the ability to recognize problems early and treat them immediately. Once the thoracoscopic procedure has been finished, air should be removed from the chest and a chest drain placed, so that any remaining air can be removed or any subsequent haemorrhage or air leaks recognized.

Bronchoscopy

Most patients undergoing bronchoscopy are likely to have compromised pulmonary function, and therefore oxygen supplementation is important. As with cardiac conditions, it is helpful to reduce risks associated with bronchoscopy by providing supportive treatment before anaesthesia. In asthmatic cats, pretreatment with inhaled terbutaline can reduce the likelihood of acute bronchoconstriction. In larger animals, it is possible to use a standard endoscope and pass it through a diaphragm on an elbow attached to the endotracheal tube. A double-diaphragm arrangement is less likely to leak and will be less hazardous to the personnel managing the case (Figure 21.6). With this arrangement the animal can be kept anaesthetized with an inhalant delivered in oxygen, thus achieving the best oxygenation possible. It is also feasible to ventilate the animal should this be necessary. In smaller patients, where it is not possible to pass the endoscope through an appropriately sized endotracheal tube, or where the arrangement above is not available, it is necessary to maintain anaesthesia with an injectable technique. For short procedures this can probably be achieved with most of the injectable anaesthetics, but for longer procedures the author typically uses propofol. This drug will provide a rapidly adjustable depth of anaesthesia with a smooth recovery. For these cases oxygen can be supplied by three different methods:

- An oxygen source can be attached to one of the channels of the endoscope. This method will deliver oxygen deep into the lung, but supply may be limited to one lung (if the endoscope is in a bronchus) or may need to be discontinued if the endoscope's ports are needed for other equipment (e.g. suction or sampling)
- A catheter can be placed in the trachea and oxygen insufflated directly. This method provides high concentrations of oxygen but does nothing for removal of carbon dioxide. Care must be taken that the catheter is securely attached to the tubing supplying the oxygen so that it does not get dislodged into the trachea
- A catheter can be placed in the trachea and attached to an HFJV. This has the advantage of providing high concentrations of oxygen while also oscillating the gas in the airway, thus enhancing the removal of carbon dioxide. The author typically runs the HFJV at 180 breaths per minute and adjusts the pressure so that there is slight chest movement with each pulse; this often gives P_aCO_2 values in the normal range.

These patients should be monitored carefully and continuously. A pulse oximeter is ideal because desaturation often occurs, as the bronchoscope blocks off various portions of the lung. The bronchoscope should be moved or completely removed if desaturation occurs. When biopsies are being performed there may be significant haemorrhage into the airway, compromising gas exchange still further. Blood should be removed using the suction channel on the endoscope if possible. Occasionally a biopsy may rupture an airway or there may be sufficient pathology in the lower airway that spontaneous rupture occurs. This manifests as rapid desaturation, an increase in respiratory rate and a change in pulmonary compliance. Evacuation of air from the pleural space should be undertaken immediately and a chest drain placed to allow further removal of air over the next few hours.

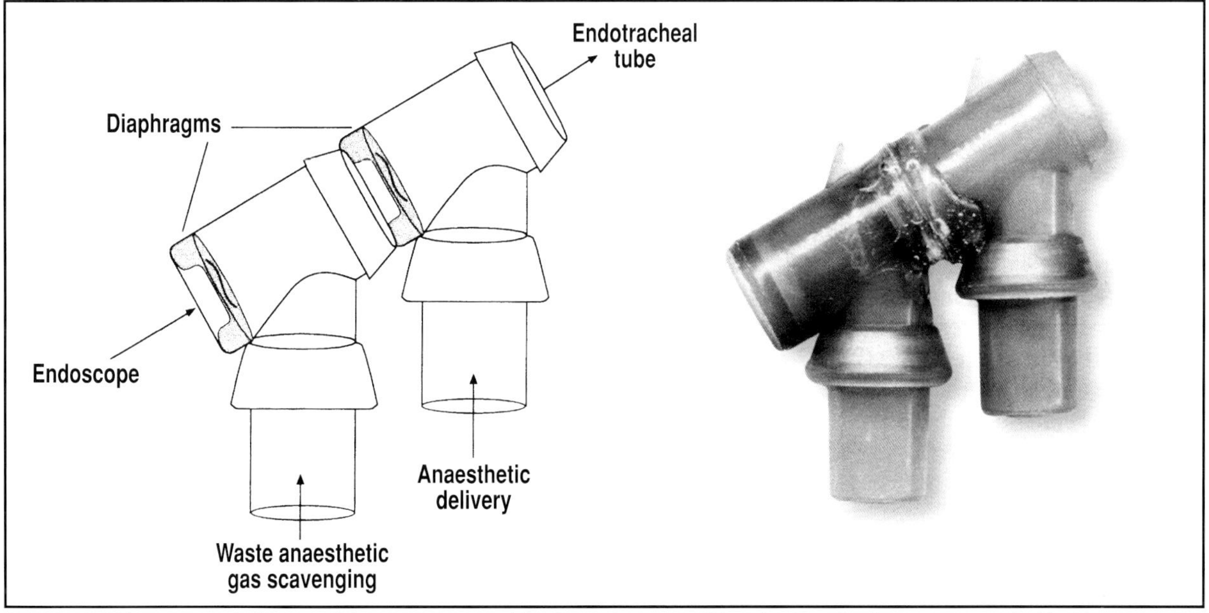

21.6 Diagram and picture of the adapter used for bronchoscopy. The double diaphragm created with this arrangement reduces the amount of anaesthetic spilling into the room while allowing the delivery of inhaled anaesthetics with positive pressure ventilation if needed.

Once the bronchoscopic examination is finished, the animal can be intubated and maintained on oxygen. An inhalant can be used to continue anaesthesia if necessary, or the animal can remain on oxygen until it is ready to be extubated. Continued monitoring with pulse oximetry and oxygen supplementation into the recovery period are essential for these patients to ensure that they do not become hypoxaemic.

Postoperative care

Many animals undergoing thoracic procedures are at risk for postoperative hypoxaemia. This can be minimized by taking the following precautions:

- Make every effort to ensure that the animal is normothermic by the time it is recovering. An animal that begins to shiver in order to warm itself up may increase its oxygen consumption by 300%. If the animal has poor pulmonary function, this extra demand may exacerbate any hypoxaemia
- Ensure that the animal has received analgesics (if necessary), and monitor the recovery carefully so that the animal emerges calmly from the anaesthetic. It may be necessary to give a tranquillizer if the animal becomes agitated during recovery. A rough recovery will be accompanied by huge increases in oxygen consumption, which may contribute to the hypoxaemia
- Place a chest drain and provide timely intermittent drainage or continuous suction if there is any risk of pneumo- or haemothorax. Remove the chest drain as soon as it is deemed safe to do so
- Provide an enriched supply of oxygen. A facemask can be used in the early postoperative period, as long as the animal tolerates it. A tight-fitting mask allows delivery of 100% oxygen but, unless the animal is deeply sedated, this requires someone to be with the animal all the time; most animals do not tolerate this technique for long. The delivery of 100% oxygen can also be achieved by placing a nasal insufflation catheter during the procedure and beginning oxygen insufflation as soon as the animal is extubated. This technique is less efficacious in larger animals, but does increase the inspired oxygen fraction (F_iO_2) to some extent and continues to deliver oxygen while the animal is being examined or treated. A more certain method of supplying high concentrations of oxygen is to place the animal in an oxygen cage. Inspired oxygen concentration can be adjusted according to the needs of the patient, but it is difficult to handle the animal without losing the benefit of the increased oxygen
- If surgery has been carried out on the heart or lungs, the animal must be monitored carefully for signs of respiratory distress, cardiac arrhythmias, congestive heart failure or shock.

References and further reading

Arndt GA, DeLessio ST, Kranner PW *et al.* (1999) One-lung ventilation when intubation is difficult – presentation of a new endobronchial blocker. *Acta Anaesthesiologica Scandinavica* **43**, 356–358

Bailey CS, Kitchell RL, Haghighi SS and Johnson RD (1984) Cutaneous innervation of the thorax and abdomen of the dog. *American Journal of Veterinary Research* **45**, 1689–1698

Baraff LJ (1993) Capillary refill: is it a useful clinical sign? *Pediatrics* **92**, 723–724

Barnett HB, Holland JG and Josenhans WT (1982) When does central cyanosis become detectable? *Clinical and Investigative Medicine* **5**, 39–43

Benumof J (1993) The position of a double-lumen tube should be routinely determined by fiberoptic bronchoscopy. *Journal of Cardiothoracic and Vascular Anesthesia* **7**, 513–514

Brasmer TH (1984) A is for Airway. In: *The Acutely Traumatized Small Animal Patient*, pp. 55–95. WB Saunders, Philadephia

Brownlie SE, Cobb MA, Chambers J, Jackson G and Thomas S (1991) Percutaneous balloon valvuloplasty in four dogs with pulmonic stenosis. *Journal of Small Animal Practice* **32**, 165–169

Cantwell SL, Duke T, Walsh JP *et al.* (2000) One-lung versus two-lung ventilation in the anesthetized dog: a comparison of cardiopulmonary parameters. *Veterinary Surgery* **29**, 365–373

Cohen E, Eisenkraft J, Thys D, Kirschner P and Kaplan J (1988) Oxygenation and hemodynamic changes during one-lung ventilation: effects of CPAP10, PEEP10, and CPAP10/PEEP10. *Journal of Cardiothoracic Anesthesia* **2**, 34–40

Cohen E, Thys DM, Eisenkraft JB and Kaplan JA (1985) PEEP during one lung anesthesia improves oxygenation in patients with low arterial PaO_2. *Anesthesia and Analgesia* **64**, 201

Comroe Jr JH and Botelho S (1947) The unreliability of cyanosis in the recognition of arterial anoxemia. *American Journal of Medical Science* **214**, 1–6

Dhokarikar P, Caywood DD, Ogburn PN, Stobie D and Burtnick NL (1995) Closed aortic valvotomy: a retrospective study in 15 dogs. *Journal of the American Animal Hospital Association* **31**, 402–410

Elliott AR, Steffey EP, Jarvis KA and Marshall BE (1991) Unilateral hypoxic pulmonary vasoconstriction in the dog, pony and miniature swine. *Respiration Physiology* **85**, 355–369

Fitzpatrick RK and Crowe DTJ (1986) Nasal oxygen administration in dogs and cats: experimental and clinical investigations. *Journal of the American Animal Hospital Association* **22**, 293–300

Fordyce WE and Tenney SM (1984) Role of the carotid bodies in ventilatory acclimation to chronic hypoxia by the awake cat. *Respiration Physiology* **58**, 207–221

Garcia F, Prandi D, Pena T *et al.* (1998) Examination of the thoracic cavity and lung lobectomy by means of thoracoscopy in dogs. *Canadian Veterinary Journal* **39**, 285–291

Gillespie DJ and Hyatt RE (1974) Respiratory mechanics in the unanesthetized dog. *Journal of Applied Physiology* **36**, 98–102

Gorelick MH, Shaw KN and Baker MD (1993) Effect of ambient temperature on capillary refill in healthy children. *Pediatrics* **92**, 699–702

Goss GA, Hayes JA and Burdon JG (1988) Deoxyhaemoglobin concentrations in the detection of central cyanosis. *Thorax* **43**, 212–213

Grifka RG, Miller MW, Frischmeyer KJ and Mullins CE (1996) Transcatheter occlusion of a patent ductus arteriosus in a Newfoundland puppy using the Gianturco-Grifka vascular occlusion device. *Journal of Veterinary Internal Medicine* **10**, 42–44

Kienle RD (1998a) Aortic stenosis. In: *Small Animal Cardiovascular Medicine, 1st edn*, ed. MD Kittleson and RD Kienle, pp. 260–272. Mosby, St. Louis

Kienle RD (1998b) Congenital pulmonic stenosis. In: *Small Animal Cardiovascular Medicine, 1st edn*, ed. MD Kittleson and RD Kienle, pp. 248–259. Mosby, St. Louis

Kitchell RL, Whalen LR, Bailey CS and Lohse CL (1980) Electrophysiologic studies of cutaneous nerves of the thoracic limb of the dog. *American Journal of Veterinary Research* **41**, 61–76

Koller ME, Smith B, Sjostrand U and Brevik H (1983) Effects of hypo-, normo-, and hypercarbia in dogs with acute cardiac tamponade. *Anesthesia and Analgesia* **62**, 181–185

LeFlore JL and Engle WD (2005) Capillary refill time is an unreliable indicator of cardiovascular status in term neonates. *Advances in Neonatal Care* **5**, 147–154

Linn K and Orton EC (1992) Closed transventricular dilation of discrete subvalvular aortic stenosis in dogs. *Veterinary Surgery* **21**, 441–445

Martin MWS, Godman M, Fuentes VL *et al.* (1992) Assessment of balloon pulmonary valvuloplasty in six dogs. *Journal of Small Animal Practice* **33**, 443–449

Martins JB, Manuel WJ, Marcus ML and Kerber RE (1980) Comparative effects of catecholamines in cardiac tamponade: experimental and clinical studies. *American Journal of Cardiology* **46**, 59–66

Mattila I, Takkunen O, Mattila P *et al.* (1984) Cardiac tamponade and different modes of artificial ventilation. *Acta Anaesthesiologica Scandinavica* **28**, 236–240

Meurs KM, Lehmkuhl LB and Bonagura JD (2005) Survival times in dogs with severe subvalvular aortic stenosis treated with balloon valvuloplasty or atenolol. *Journal of the American Veterinary Medical Association* **227**, 420–424

Morgan-Hughes JO (1968a) Fluorescent lighting and cyanosis. *Nursing Mirror and Midwives Journal* **126**, 51

Morgan-Hughes JO (1968b) Lighting and cyanosis. *British Journal of Anaesthesia* **40**, 503–507

Mure M, Domino KB, Robertson T, Hlastala MP and Glenny RW (1998) Pulmonary blood flow does not redistribute in dogs with reposition from supine to left lateral position. *Anesthesiology* **89**, 483–492

Nakatsuka M, Wetstein L and Keenan R (1988) Unilateral high-frequency jet ventilation during one-lung ventilation for thoracotomy. *Annals of Thoracic Surgery* **46**, 654–660

Orton EC, Herndon GD, Boon JA *et al.* (2000) Influence of open surgical correction on intermediate-term outcome in dogs with subvalvular aortic stenosis: 44 cases (1991–1998). *Journal of the American Veterinary Medical Association* **216**, 364–367

Pascoe PJ (1988) Oxygen and ventilatory support for the critical patient. *Seminars in Veterinary Medicine and Surgery (Small Animal)* **3**, 202–209

Pascoe PJ and Dyson DH (1993) Analgesia after lateral thoracotomy in dogs. Epidural morphine vs. intercostal bupivacaine. *Veterinary Surgery* **22**, 141–147

Popilskis S, Kohn D, Sanchez JA and Gorman P (1991) Epidural vs. intramuscular oxymorphone analgesia after thoracotomy in dogs. *Veterinary Surgery* **20**, 462–467

Popilskis S, Kohn DF, Laurent L and Danilo P (1993) Efficacy of epidural morphine versus intravenous morphine for post-thoracotomy pain in dogs. *Journal of Veterinary Anaesthesia* **20**, 21–25

Riegler FX, VadeBoncouer TR and Pelligrino DA (1989) Interpleural anesthetics in the dog: differential somatic neural blockade. *Anesthesiology* **71**, 744–750

Riquelme M, Monnet E, Kudnig ST, Gaynor JS, Wagner AE, Corliss D and Salman MD (2005a) Cardiopulmonary changes induced during one-lung ventilation in anesthetized dogs with a closed thoracic cavity. *American Journal of Veterinary Research* **66**, 973–977

Riquelme M, Monnet E, Kudnig ST *et al.* (2005b) Cardiopulmonary effects of positive end-expiratory pressure during one-lung ventilation in anesthetized dogs with a closed thoracic cavity. *American Journal of Veterinary Research* **66**, 978–983

Saunders AB, Miller MW, Gordon SG and Bahr A (2004) Pulmonary embolization of vascular occlusion coils in dogs with patent ductus arteriosus. *Journal of Veterinary Internal Medicine* **18**, 663–666

Sawafuji M, Ishizaka A, Kohno M *et al.* (2005) Role of Rho-kinase in reexpansion pulmonary edema in rabbits. *American Journal of Physiology. Lung Cellular and Molecular Physiology* **289**, L946–953

Schriger DL and Baraff LJ (1991) Capillary refill – is it a useful predictor of hypovolemic states? *Annals of Emergency Medicine* **20**, 601–605

Snaps FR, McEntee K, Saunders JH *et al.* (1998) Treatment of patent ductus arteriosus by placement of intravascular coils in a pup. *Journal of the American Veterinary Medical Association* **39**, 196–199

Staudte KL, Gibson NR, Read RA and Edwards GA (2004) Evaluation of closed pericardial patch grafting for management of severe pulmonic stenosis. *Australian Veterinary Journal* **82**, 33–37

Stokhof A (1986) Diagnosis and treatment of acquired diaphragmatic hernia by thoracotomy in 49 dogs and 72 cats. *Veterinary Quarterly* **8**, 177–183

Thompson SE and Johnson JM (1991) Analgesia in dogs after intercostal thoracotomy. A comparison of morphine, selective intercostal nerve block, and interpleural regional analgesia with bupivacaine. *Veterinary Surgery* **20**, 73–77

VadeBoncouer TR, Riegler FX and Pelligrino DA (1990) The effects of two different volumes of 0.5% bupivacaine in a canine model of interpleural analgesia. *Regional Anesthesia* **15**, 67–72

Wagner AE, Gaynor JS, Dunlop CI, Allen SL and Demme WC (1998) Monitoring adequacy of ventilation by capnometry during thoracotomy in dogs. *Journal of the American Veterinary Medical Association* **212**, 377–379

Wilson CW and Benumof J (2005) Anesthesia for Thoracic Surgery. In: *Miller's Anesthesia, 6th edn,* ed. RD Miller, pp. 1847–1940. Elsevier/Churchill Livingstone, Philadelphia

Wilson G and Hayes H (1986) Diaphragmatic hernia in the dog and cat: a 25-year overview. *Seminars in Veterinary Medicine and Surgery (Small Animal)* **1**, 318–326

Zhang H, Spapen H and Vincent JL (1994) Effects of dobutamine and norepinephrine on oxygen availability in tamponade-induced stagnant hypoxia: a prospective, randomized, controlled study. *Critical Care Medicine* **22**, 299–305

22

Gastrointestinal and hepatic disease

Rachel C. Bennett

Introduction

The principal function of the gastrointestinal tract is to supply the body with water, electrolytes and nutrients. Each division of the gastrointestinal tract is adapted for specific functions, e.g. passage of food in the oesophagus, the storage and initiation of digestion of food in the stomach and the digestion and absorption of nutrients in the small intestine and proximal colon.

Patients with diseases of the gastrointestinal tract often suffer from dehydration and malnutrition due to digestive impairment and increased metabolic demands due to the nature of their illness. Apart from the metabolic disturbances associated with gastrointestinal problems, these animals may be severely nauseous, and experiencing extreme discomfort or pain.

The presence of gastrointestinal disease has associated anaesthetic implications, e.g. hypoproteinaemia leads to reduced protein binding and an enhanced effect following drug administration. An emaciated patient with a reduced muscle mass and diminished fat stores may have an altered volume of distribution and a prolonged duration of drug action. Emaciated animals may develop hypothermia more rapidly than a normal healthy patient. Liver disease may impair the production of clotting factors, leading to coagulopathy and anaemia. Diseases of the endocrine pancreas lead to abnormalities in glucose homeostasis.

The assessment of patients with disease of the alimentary tract and associated organs should, therefore, anticipate the systemic effects of these diseases and how they may affect intraoperative management and postoperative care. It is the veterinary surgeon's responsibility to optimize the patient's condition before surgery. In human medicine it has been shown that nutritional support improves patient outcome, as well as reducing patient mortality. Information on perioperative nutritional support can be found in the *BSAVA Manual of Canine and Feline Emergency and Critical Care*.

There are very few prospective randomized clinical studies in veterinary medicine that have investigated the pros and cons of different anaesthetic techniques for use in patients with gastrointestinal, hepatic or pancreatic disease. Therefore much of the information discussed here is either anecdotal or extrapolated from the human field. Specific contraindications to drug use are discussed in the relevant sections of the chapter.

The oesophagus

Conditions of the oesophagus fall into three broad categories: obstruction, disorders of motility and inflammation.

Obstruction

Obstructive disorders can result from foreign bodies, strictures and vascular ring anomalies. Other possible differential diagnoses include extraluminal masses, gastro-oesophageal intussusception, oesophageal diverticulum and hiatal hernia.

Oesophageal foreign bodies are usually removed under general anaesthesia. These patients often appear to be very uncomfortable and depressed, particularly if the material has been present for some time. The provision of analgesia prior to anaesthesia will help to relieve the discomfort and subsequently reduce the dose of other anaesthetic drugs. Opioids are commonly used for this purpose: buprenorphine (0.01–0.02 mg/kg); methadone (0.2–0.5 mg/kg); or pethidine (meperidine) (2–5 mg/kg) would all be acceptable. Those drugs known to induce vomiting (e.g. morphine) should arguably be avoided. The use of non-steroidal anti-inflammatory drugs (NSAIDs) is inadvisable given the possibility of oesophageal mucosal damage.

Patients may present with some degree of dehydration. An intravenous catheter should be placed and fluid therapy given both prior to anaesthesia and during the procedure. The rate and type of fluid is dependent upon an assessment of hydration status at the time of initial presentation and the type of electrolyte disturbance, although replacement solutions such as 0.9% sodium chloride and lactated Ringer's (Hartmann's) solution are commonly used.

The presence of objects, e.g. bones, within the oesophagus prevents the passage of saliva and ingested material into the stomach. Fluid, saliva and food material can all accumulate cranial to the obstruction and may be regurgitated at the time of anaesthetic induction with the attendant risk of aspiration. Equipment for suction of the oropharynx should be available to remove food and fluid at this time.

Prior to the induction of anaesthesia, the animal should be positioned in sternal recumbency with its head elevated. The assistant should keep the head elevated until the patient's airway has been intubated and the cuff inflated. This reduces the risk of reflux of fluid and aspiration at a time when the patient has lost its protective laryngeal reflexes.

Anaesthesia is usually induced with propofol, although other rapidly acting drugs, such as thiopental, ketamine and etomidate (see Chapter 13), would also be suitable and can be titrated to effect. These induction drugs may be administered with diazepam or midazolam, thereby reducing the dose of the induction drug.

In humans the use of cricoid pressure is also implemented, i.e. pressure applied over the cricoid cartilage to occlude the oesophagus and prevent material passing into the oropharynx. This technique has not been documented in dogs or cats.

Once the endotracheal tube cuff has been inflated, suction can be used to remove any food or fluid from the oesophagus. Even with an endotracheal tube in place, material can still seep around the cuff. At the end of the procedure the endotracheal tube should ideally be removed with the cuff fully or partially inflated to withdraw any material that may have lodged proximal to it. If the patient attempts to vomit or reflux during induction, the head should be lowered below the level of the body allowing fluid to drain out. The pharynx should then be swabbed out and cleaned as much as possible before intubation is attempted.

Neuromuscular-blocking drugs can be used to aid removal of the foreign body. This is most effective in dogs, where the entire length of the oesophagus is made up of striated muscle. Neuromuscular-blocking drugs produce relaxation of the oesophageal muscle and aid removal of the object via the mouth or passage into the stomach. This technique can also be used in cats, although the caudal third of the oesophagus is composed of smooth muscle and therefore it is less likely to provide full relaxation if the foreign body is located in this region. A short-acting non-depolarizing muscle relaxant is most appropriate for this purpose (e.g. vecuronium 0.1 mg/kg). The duration of action is approximately 20 minutes, which should provide sufficient time for removal of the foreign material. An alternative option in cats would be mivacurium (see Chapter 15), but this drug is not suitable for use in dogs due to its prolonged duration of action in this species. The use of neuromuscular-blocking drugs necessitates artificial ventilation, either manually or mechanically.

Patients need to be assessed after the procedure to determine whether additional pain relief is required; this can be provided with further doses of an opioid, e.g. buprenorphine.

The longer the foreign body is present, the greater the likelihood of pressure necrosis leading to damage of the mucosa, submucosa and the external layers of the oesophageal wall. This can result in oesophagitis and ulceration and it may also affect oesophageal motility.

Oesophageal strictures may develop following foreign body obstruction, reflux of gastric contents (e.g. during general anaesthesia) or the ingestion of caustic substances. They are treated by gradual oesophageal dilation using either bougies or balloons inflated intraluminally. This procedure is always associated with the risk of oesophageal rupture and iatrogenic pneumomediastinum and pneumothorax (see below and Figure 22.1). The oesophageal mucosa can be immediately assessed endoscopically in an attempt to identify any perforations.

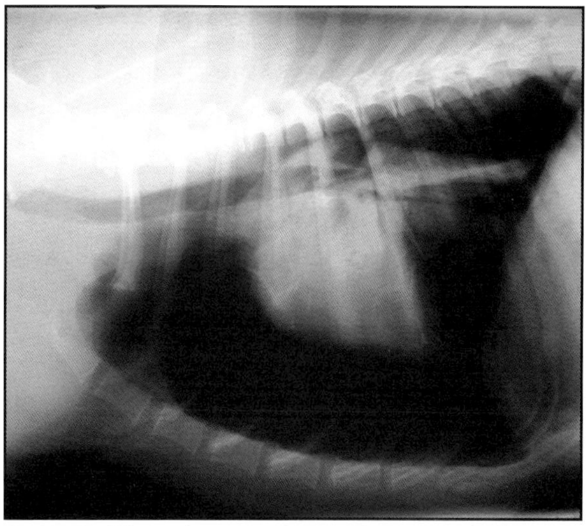

22.1 Bilateral pneumothorax after removal of an oesophageal foreign body in a dog. This was detected at the end of anaesthesia as a fall in oxygen saturation (S_pO_2) when the dog was breathing room air. Oxygen therapy via nasal catheter was required until thoracocentesis was performed.

It is important to assess the ventilatory pattern following removal of the foreign object. Signs of pneumothorax may include dyspnoea, decreased breath sounds on thoracic auscultation, resistance to manual inflation of the lungs, expansion of the thorax (i.e. movement of the chest wall outwards when the integrity of the pleural space has been breached) and hypoxaemia. A pulse oximeter is invaluable in assessment of oxygenation since it rapidly indicates changes. If any of these signs are present and appear to be progressive then rupture of the oesophagus must be considered. In this instance, the animal should be maintained under general anaesthesia using 100% oxygen. If time and facilities allow, thoracic radiography should be performed to confirm the diagnosis, although if it is impossible to take a radiograph then percutaneous drainage of the chest must be performed. This may simply mean drainage with a needle and syringe, or the use of chest drains, until oxygenation improves and ventilation reverts to a more normal pattern. Patients need to be monitored in recovery to ensure they are able to maintain their oxygenation and also to assess their ventilatory pattern. It is useful to place an intranasal catheter before the end of anaesthesia to allow administration of supplemental oxygen should the patient's condition subsequently deteriorate. It is also worthwhile leaving an intravenous catheter in place in case further anaesthesia or sedation is required.

Given the possible need for thoracic surgery in these patients, some veterinary surgeons recommend referral to institutions which have the means to deal with all of these possible sequelae.

Megaoesophagus

Motility problems of the oesophagus generally lead to megaoesophagus. Although surgical correction of this problem is rarely attempted, anaesthesia of animals with megaoesophagus may be required. Thoracic radiographs ideally should be taken prior to anaesthesia to assess whether aspiration pneumonia is present and to determine if further treatment is required prior to surgery (assuming the procedure is elective).

Opioids form the mainstay of premedication and anaesthesia is usually induced with propofol. The advantages of this drug are the rapid onset of action and the fact that it can be given to effect. The rapid and smooth recovery also means that animals are capable of protecting their airway as soon as possible after the procedure is completed. During the induction of anaesthesia, the patient should be managed in the manner described earlier, i.e. with the head elevated to reduce the risk of food material being regurgitated and aspirated (Figure 22.2). The airway should be intubated as soon as possible and the cuff of the endotracheal tube inflated to avoid material gaining access to the animal's airway. At the end of surgery it is worthwhile checking the oropharynx to identify any food material. This should be removed to reduce the risk of aspiration during recovery.

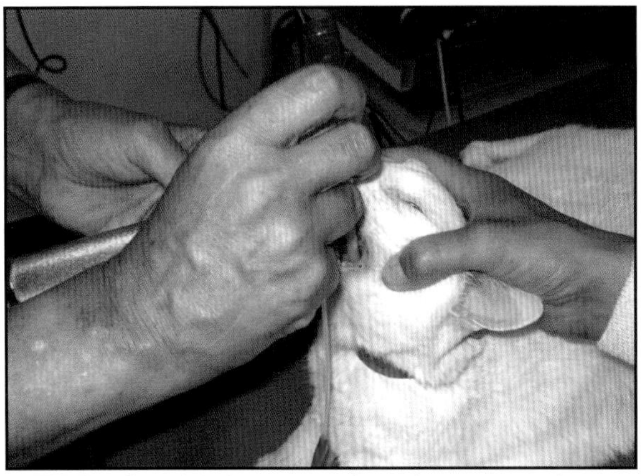

22.2 Cat with dysautonomia and megaoesophagus positioned for endotracheal intubation. Note that sternal recumbency and head elevation should be maintained until the trachea is intubated, and the endotracheal tube cuff inflated, to minimize the risk of regurgitation and aspiration.

Animals presenting for surgical correction of vascular ring anomalies may have some degree of megaoesophagus (Figure 22.3). The severity of this depends on the time taken to diagnose the condition. Anaesthetic management of patients for thoracic surgery is discussed in Chapter 21. Special consideration must also be given to the size and age of these patients.

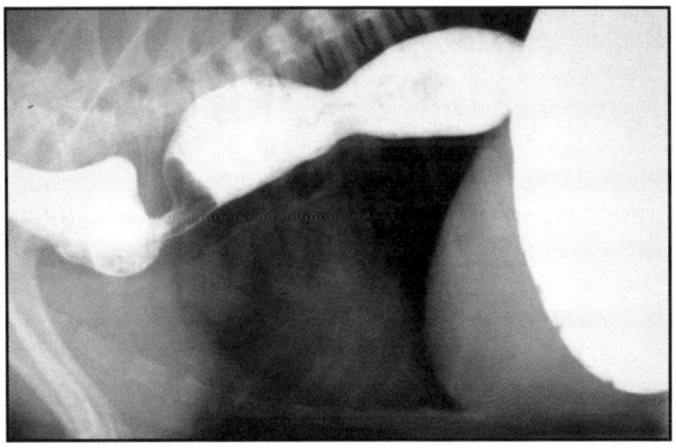

22.3 Chest radiograph of a dog with a vascular ring anomaly and megaoesophagus.

Oesophagitis

In veterinary patients, oesophagitis is associated with chronic vomiting, ingestion of caustic materials and gastro-oesophageal reflux (GOR) during anaesthesia. Oesophagitis following anaesthesia is a relatively rare occurrence, despite the fact that 16–17% of patients experience an episode of GOR during anaesthesia. However, if reflux does occur it can lead to oesophageal stricture formation. It is therefore important to lavage the oesophagus if gastric or intestinal fluid is regurgitated during anaesthesia. This can be done with a simple urinary catheter or alternatively with a double-lumen suction catheter, if available. The latter is better suited to this purpose but rather more expensive. Water or saline is infused until the aspirated material is clear and colourless. It is also advisable to give sucralfate and H_2-receptor antagonists (e.g. ranitidine) to try to protect the oesophagus from the effects of gastric or intestinal fluid.

Oesophagitis should be suspected when animals recovering from general anaesthesia salivate profusely, repeatedly attempt to swallow or show signs of pain during swallowing. These patients usually respond to treatment with sucralfate and ranitidine and these animals are generally fed by mouth. If oesophagitis is secondary to the presence of a foreign body, then it may be preferable to place a gastrostomy (PEG) tube and feed via this, thereby giving the oesophagus time to heal.

A recent study investigated the effect of administering metoclopramide to patients during general anaesthesia to determine whether this would prevent GOR from occurring (Wilson *et al.*, 2006). Administration of metoclopramide by bolus and constant rate infusion at doses much higher than commonly used reduces the incidence but does not totally prevent GOR in anaesthetized dogs undergoing orthopaedic surgery. In human anaesthesia, routine pretreatment of patients with an H_2-receptor antagonist and metoclopramide is not specifically recommended. At this time, it is unclear whether these drugs should be used in veterinary patients that have a previous history of oesophagitis or abnormal gastro-oesophageal motility.

Theoretically, anticholinergic drugs could increase the likelihood of reflux and the possibility of pulmonary aspiration, by decreasing lower oesophageal sphincter tone. There are no reports documenting this potential side effect and the human literature does not state that a history of reflux oesophagitis is a contraindication to the use of anticholinergic drugs.

The stomach and intestines

Surgery of the stomach and intestines can involve a wide range of conditions that may be acute in onset or more longstanding. The most common indications for anaesthesia and surgery in general practice are probably removal of gastrointestinal foreign bodies, treatment of gastric dilatation–volvulus (GDV) and performance of gastrointestinal biopsies.

Given the function of the gastrointestinal tract, alterations in extracellular volume are common and may be severe. Acute volume depletion can result from gastrointestinal bleeding, hypersecretion accompanied by inadequate fluid replacement, or third-space losses (e.g. as a result of GDV). In addition to hypovolaemia, gastrointestinal disease may lead to electrolyte and acid–base disturbances. The degree of dehydration should be assessed by clinical examination, and measurements of packed cell volume (PCV), total protein (TP), electrolytes and acid–base status before anaesthesia and surgery. The extent of the volume deficit guides the rate of volume administration prior to anaesthesia, whilst the nature of the loss enables more informed decisions to be made regarding fluid therapy (see Chapter 16). Ideally circulating blood volume should be restored before anaesthesia, thereby improving cardiovascular stability. 'High' gastrointestinal obstruction tends to lead to metabolic alkalosis due to the loss of acidic gastric contents, whereas loss of duodenal contents results in metabolic acidosis. Animals that are alkalotic benefit from an acidifying solution, such as 0.9% sodium chloride, whereas animals that are acidotic are usually treated with lactated Ringer's (Hartmann's) solution or acetated polyionic solutions.

Depending on the extent of volume depletion, multiple intravenous catheters may be required to allow the administration of crystalloids, colloids or blood products perioperatively. Central venous catheters may be indicated for the measurement of central venous pressure and an arterial catheter may be necessary for the measurement of arterial blood pressure.

The choice of drugs for premedication, and for induction and maintenance of anaesthesia, is dictated again by the severity of the condition and the degree of dehydration. Opioids usually form part of premedication and may also be used for the induction of anaesthesia. Propofol is arguably the most widely used induction drug nowadays and anaesthesia is usually maintained with either isoflurane or sevoflurane in oxygen. Nitrous oxide is not used routinely due to its tendency to cause further distension of the gastrointestinal tract.

Gastric dilatation–volvulus

GDV leads to hypovolaemic shock because of a reduction in venous return. The dilated stomach obstructs blood flow through the caudal vena cava, while the increase in gastric pressure decreases blood flow through the portal vein. The obstruction to blood flow in these two vessels leads to a decrease in venous return (and subsequently cardiac output) since venous return is the major determinant of cardiac output. Reduction of cardiac output results in a failure to maintain tissue perfusion, with the classical signs of shock: vasoconstriction leading to poor peripheral pulse quality, pallor of mucous membranes, cold extremities and tachycardia. Therefore it is essential to stabilize these patients before anaesthesia and surgery by deflating the stomach and administering intravenous fluids to restore circulating blood volume.

Blood samples taken prior to treatment provide an initial reference point and allow the efficacy of treatment to be assessed later. Typical blood tests include PCV, TP, urea, blood glucose and plasma electrolytes. Other laboratory tests that may be required include activated clotting time, colloid osmotic pressure and plasma lactate concentration. Volume resuscitation is usually performed with a balanced electrolyte solution given intravenously at a rate of 40–90 ml/kg per hour. Hypertonic saline may provide a more rapid means of volume resuscitation (4–6 ml/kg i.v.; see Chapter 16), but it must be followed by the administration of isotonic crystalloid solutions. Colloids may also be used and provide a more sustained restoration of circulating volume.

It is useful to have at least two intravenous catheters in place in order to allow both rapid volume resuscitation and easy access during surgery. They are also useful if several different drugs or fluids need to be administered during surgery, some of which may be incompatible, e.g. sodium bicarbonate cannot be given with dopamine or solutions containing calcium; blood products (where citrate has been used for anticoagulation) should not be given with solutions containing calcium such as lactated Ringer's (Hartmann's) solution.

Premedication may be achieved with an opioid. If the animal is very depressed, a reduced dose should be given. In cases where the animal is very debilitated, no premedication may be required, although analgesia will still be necessary postoperatively. Animals should be preoxygenated via a facemask. Wherever possible, monitoring equipment should be placed before the induction of anaesthesia. Electrocardiographic pads on the feet allow the heart rate and rhythm to be assessed continuously. A Doppler probe placed over a peripheral artery allows non-invasive measurement of blood pressure and also is an indicator of peripheral perfusion. If an arterial catheter has been placed, then direct blood pressure monitoring can be performed if facilities allow.

Anaesthesia may be induced with a combination of an opioid and benzodiazepine (e.g. fentanyl 0.01–0.02 mg/kg i.v. and diazepam 0.2–0.5 mg/kg i.v.; sufentanil 0.005 mg/kg and midazolam 0.1–0.6 mg/kg i.v.; hydromorphone 0.1–0.2 mg/kg i.v. and diazepam 0.2–0.5 mg/kg; or methadone 0.1–0.6 mg/kg i.v. and diazepam 0.2–0.5 mg/kg i.v.). Alternatively, etomidate may be used in combination with diazepam. These drugs have minimal impact on the cardiovascular system and for this reason they are commonly used in hypovolaemic animals undergoing surgery. Whichever technique is used, it is important to administer drugs slowly and to effect; in this way the risk of overdose is reduced. In theory ketamine and diazepam would be acceptable: ketamine causes a release of noradrenaline from postganglionic nerve terminals and thereby increases sympathetic tone. Blood pressure is maintained, there is little effect on myocardial contractility and ventilation is fairly well maintained. However, there is concern about the use of ketamine in patients who already have increased sympathetic tone. In these patients, a dramatic decrease in blood pressure can occur after the induction of anaesthesia. Ketamine should therefore be used judiciously in patients with GDV. Thiopental and propofol are known to cause hypoventilation and respiratory depression after intravenous administration. Thiopental is known to induce ventricular arrhythmias (ventricular bigeminy or trigeminy) and propofol may sensitize the myocardium to catecholamines. In these instances it is best to use drugs that are familiar and to give them slowly and to effect. In the recent CEPSAF (Confidential Enquiry into Perioperative Small Animal Fatalities) study performed in the UK, propofol did not appear to be better or safer than thiopental, although the need for emergency surgery was associated with an increased risk of mortality.

Maintenance of anaesthesia can be achieved with either isoflurane or sevoflurane in oxygen. Either of these drugs is preferable to halothane, which sensitizes the heart to the arrhythmogenic effects of catecholamines. Sevoflurane is less soluble than isoflurane, although it is still possible to achieve a rapid change in the depth of anaesthesia when either of these drugs is used. Both isoflurane and sevoflurane produce dose-dependent cardiovascular and respiratory depression, leading to hypotension and hypoventilation. Therefore, a balanced technique may be more appropriate in these patients using a potent short-acting opioid given by intravenous infusion (e.g. fentanyl, remifentanil) in addition to a neuromuscular-blocking drug. Opioids cause a significant reduction in the minimum alveolar concentration (MAC) of inhalants, but do not result in hypotension *per se*; in this way the unwanted side effects of the volatile anaesthetic may be minimized. Use of potent opioids causes profound respiratory depression, and patients generally require mechanical ventilation to prevent respiratory acidosis. Intermittent positive pressure ventilation (IPPV) causes a reduction in venous return and thereby leads to a drop in systemic arterial blood pressure; this effect is exacerbated in animals that are hypovolaemic, in which case further volume resuscitation will be required.

Anaesthetic monitoring should include electrocardiography, measurement of blood pressure (ideally measured directly), body temperature, arterial blood gases and acid–base status. If neuromuscular-blocking drugs are used, a peripheral nerve stimulator should ideally be available to monitor the blockade (see Chapter 15). This is particularly important in patients where there may be acid–base abnormalities.

Measurement of pH, arterial blood gases, bicarbonate and base excess allows the veterinary surgeon to determine the cause of an acidosis or alkalosis. Severe acidosis is commonly treated with sodium bicarbonate ($NaHCO_3$). The quantity of sodium bicarbonate to be administered can be calculated using the following formula:

$$NaHCO_3\,(\text{mmol}) = 0.3 \times \text{base excess (mmol/l)} \times \text{bodyweight (kg)}$$

It is common practice to calculate the deficit and then aim to replace one third of this over a 20–30-minute period. Rapid administration of sodium bicarbonate is associated with hypotension and acidosis of the central nervous system (CNS). Following treatment, the magnitude of the systemic acidosis can be reassessed and further sodium bicarbonate given if required. Administration of sodium bicarbonate leads to an increase in partial pressure of arterial carbon dioxide (P_aCO_2) and ventilation needs to be augmented if further respiratory acidosis is to be avoided.

Cardiac arrhythmias are associated with GDV in the dog. Monitoring of the electrocardiogram (ECG) allows the veterinary surgeon to detect arrhythmias and instigate treatment if required. Lidocaine is used to treat ventricular premature contractions. This can be given as a bolus (1–2 mg/kg), which can be followed by a constant rate infusion (50–100 μg/kg/minute). With infusions, the patient should be monitored for signs of lidocaine toxicity (e.g. muscle fasciculations, seizures) since the rate of elimination may be decreased in these animals. Procainamide may be used in those patients refractory to the effects of lidocaine (see Chapter 19).

It is useful to monitor PCV and TP during surgery as torsion of the stomach and spleen can sometimes cause rupture of major vessels. The extent of blood loss is not apparent until intravenous fluid administration restores blood volume and highlights an earlier period of blood loss. PCVs in the range of 10–12% have been measured in individuals that have bled preoperatively. Major haemorrhage requires administration of either packed red blood cells or fresh whole blood (see Chapter 16). Loss of large volumes of blood is also associated with the loss of clotting factors and platelets. Loss of clotting factors can be treated with fresh frozen plasma, fresh plasma or whole blood. Frozen plasma is deficient in the labile factors V and VIII. Low platelet numbers require treatment with platelet-rich plasma or fresh whole blood.

Gastroduodenoscopy

This is a diagnostic procedure commonly performed in dogs and cats. Patients often have a history of chronic vomiting or chronic diarrhoea and, although they can appear bright, there is usually some degree of dehydration. They may also be emaciated and often relatively old. Hydration status should be assessed at preoperative examination and intravenous fluid therapy administered overnight if the patient is clearly hypovolaemic and/or has electrolyte imbalance. A balanced electrolyte solution, such as lactated Ringer's (Hartmann's) solution, can be used for intravenous fluid therapy. If the patient is inappetent, fluids should be supplemented with potassium chloride (Figure 22.4). Care should be employed if these solutions are given during anaesthesia and it is advisable to use a separate intravenous catheter to avoid the administration of fluid boluses containing high concentrations of potassium.

Serum potassium (mmol/l)	Amount of KCl (mmol) to add to 250 ml fluid	Maximal fluid infusion rate (ml/kg/h)
<2.0	20	6
2.1–2.5	15	8
2.6–3.0	10	12
3.1–3.5	7	16

22.4 Intravenous fluid potassium supplementation to correct hypokalaemia. Data from Muir and Dibartola, 1983.

Patients are usually premedicated with an opioid for this procedure. A phenothiazine such as acepromazine (0.01–0.03 mg/kg) can be used, providing patients are not hypovolaemic and aged. Commonly used opioids include buprenorphine (0.01–0.02 mg/kg), butorphanol (0.1–0.4 mg/kg), pethidine (meperidine) (2–5 mg/kg) and methadone (0.2–0.5 mg/kg). The choice is dependent upon the temperament of the patient, age, severity of their condition and presence of concurrent illness. Some veterinary surgeons prefer to avoid the use of opioids, because of their tendency to increase gastroduodenal sphincter tone, and use acepromazine alone: in the author's experience this does not provide a sufficient degree of sedation/anxiolysis.

Propofol is commonly used for the induction of anaesthesia, combined with diazepam, although any of the other available induction agents could be used. Anaesthesia is maintained with isoflurane or sevoflurane in oxygen. Nitrous oxide is probably best avoided because of its ability to diffuse into gas-filled spaces, thus leading to further increases in gastric and duodenal volume during the procedure (there may also be health and safety implications if the nitrous oxide is removed and vented into the immediate vicinity at the end of the procedure).

Routine anaesthetic monitoring of these patients should include electrocardiography, indirect blood pressure measurement, capnography, pulse oximetry (for S_pO_2) and temperature. Measurement of S_pO_2 is particularly useful since inflation of the stomach can lead to cranial displacement of the diaphragm, leading to a reduction in functional residual capacity and hypoxaemia, identified as rapid desaturation. This can be rectified by deflation of the stomach until S_pO_2 improves. Irrespective of changes in S_pO_2, deflation should always be perfomed at the end of the procedure. Anaesthetic depth can change quite dramatically, especially when the endoscope is advanced into the duodenum. Supplemental doses of a short-acting opioid such as fentanyl may be used to obtund nociceptive reflexes. It is routine to place a gag in the animal's mouth to avoid any damage to the expensive and fragile endoscope. If regurgitation occurs during the procedure, the oesophagus should be lavaged with water and any material present in the oropharynx should be removed by suction.

Analgesics are not routinely administered following this procedure, although, if analgesia is required, opioids are the drugs of choice and NSAIDs should be avoided due to the risk of further gastric mucosal damage.

Inflammatory bowel disease

Management of anaesthesia requires preoperative evaluation of intravascular fluid volume and electrolyte status. Inflammatory bowel disease (IBD) in humans is associated with anaemia and liver disease and these should be identified prior to anaesthesia. If corticosteroids have been used in the previous medical management of the condition, further doses may be required during anaesthesia if there is any possibility that normal adrenal function has been suppressed (see Chapter 25). Underlying liver disease may dictate the anaesthetic drugs that can be used: alfaxalone may be preferable to propofol in cats with liver disease due to their inability to metabolize phenols, whilst isoflurane should be used for maintenance of anaesthesia.

Percutaneous placement of gastrostomy tubes

This is a relatively straightforward procedure to perform, although patients presenting for it can be extremely debilitated from inadequate food intake for days or even weeks. It is important to ensure that they are well prepared preoperatively. This may include restoration of circulating blood volume, increasing colloid osmotic pressure, and treating anaemia or coagulation defects. Opioids form the mainstay for premedication, e.g. buprenorphine (0.01–0.02 mg/kg) or methadone (0.2–0.5 mg/kg). Other sedatives or tranquillizers may not be required.

Gastric ulceration

The use of NSAIDs is the second most common cause of gastric ulcer formation in people; several studies have also investigated the occurrence of gastric ulceration in dogs given NSAIDS. In healthy dogs, meloxicam is not associated with gastric ulcers although concurrent administration with dexamethasone does lead to an increased incidence of ulceration, once again highlighting the importance of avoiding the administration of corticosteroids and NSAIDs simultaneously.

Dachshunds presenting with intervertebral disc prolapse have a high incidence of gastroduodenal ulceration, with a prevalence of 76% in one study. The administration of ulcerogenic medication prior to admission does not influence the prevalence (Dowdle *et al.*, 2003). Another study found no improvement when misoprostol (2 μg/kg orally q8h) or omeprazole (0.7 mg/kg orally q24h) were administered (Neiger *et al.*, 2000). However, the treatment was only used for a maximum of 6 days. This study confirmed the high incidence of gastrointestinal lesions in patients with intervertebral disc disease.

A comparison of ketoprofen, carprofen and meloxicam with control animals showed no statistically significant difference in the occurrence of gastrointestinal lesions between the three drugs and the control group. Animals receiving carprofen showed the fewest and least severe lesions. None of the dogs showed any clinical signs related to the gastrointestinal lesions (Forsyth *et al.*, 1998).

Certain breeds of dog (e.g. German Shepherd Dogs) seem to be particularly sensitive to the effects of ibuprofen on gastrointestinal ulcer formation, whilst Labrador Retrievers show a lower incidence of gastrointestinal ulceration (Poortinga and Hungerford, 1998). There are also many reports of gastrointestinal ulceration and perforation in dogs given NSAIDs for varying periods of time. The list of absolute contraindications for the use of NSAIDs include: gastric ulceration or gastrointestinal disorder of any kind; dehydration; hypotension associated with low effective circulating blood volume (congestive heart failure, ascites, diuretics); renal insufficiency; intervertebral disc disease; geriatric patients; trauma cases; patients in shock; thrombocytopenia; von Willebrand's disease; use of other NSAIDs or corticosteroids concurrently; and patients with severe or poorly controlled asthma (Mathews, 1996).

In humans, infection with *Helicobacter pylori* is a common cause of gastric and duodenal ulceration. Although *Helicobacter* spp. occur in both cats and dogs, there is no correlation between the existence of the bacteria and the occurrence of gastric ulcers in dogs and the link is tenuous in cats.

Dogs presenting with mast cell tumours are known to have elevated levels of plasma histamine, which leads to increased gastric acid secretion and an associated risk of gastric ulceration (Fox *et al.*, 1990). Therefore, it is routine in these animals to give H_1-receptor antagonists, such as chlorpheniramine or diphenhydramine, and H_2-receptor antagonists (e.g. ranitidine) before surgery. H_1-receptor antagonists also have sedative effects; giving them as part of the premedication allows any sedation to take effect prior to the induction of anaesthesia.

The large intestine, rectum and perineum

Constipation and obstipation are common clinical problems affecting both dogs and cats. Animals may have a history of vomiting, anorexia and weight loss. If the problem has been present for some time patients may be dehydrated, underweight and debilitated. Treatment depends on the severity of the condition, although general anaesthesia is often necessary to remove impacted material. If dehydration is present, then intravenous fluid therapy will be necessary prior to the anaesthetic. Blood samples should be taken to determine PCV, TP, electrolytes and acid–base status and the results should be used to guide fluid therapy. Some enema stimulants may precipitate vomiting, which will need to be managed during the anaesthetic. Severely constipated or obstipated animals may require multiple enemas or colectomy for the removal of impacted faeces. They can suffer from extreme discomfort and the use of epidural opioids may be warranted to ease their pain and aid defecation. Ketamine (0.5 mg/kg i.v.) has also been used to provide pain relief.

Megacolon is recognized in cats and sometimes in dogs. It may be the end result of chronic mechanical obstruction (e.g. healed, malaligned pelvic fractures) or functional colonic obstruction. Most cases of feline megacolon are idiopathic and represent end-stage colonic dysfunction. Colectomy is indicated in cases of megacolon, trauma, perforation, neoplasia and necrotic or irreducible intussusception. A pull-through resection of the colon is usually performed when an anastomosis must be made in the pelvic canal. Anaesthesia can be induced with any of the commonly available drugs such as propofol, alfaxalone/alfadolone, thiopental or ketamine. Analgesia can be provided by opioids and NSAIDs. An epidural injection can be given, although abnormal pelvic anatomy can make this more difficult.

Perineal hernias may be uni- or bilateral, and surgical correction can be prolonged. These patients are often geriatric, with an increased risk of concurrent disease. During the initial clinical examination, it is important to determine whether the urinary bladder has prolapsed into the hernia and blood biochemistry should be performed to rule out uraemia.

Premedication can be achieved with combinations of opioids and sedatives such as acepromazine. Anaesthesia can be induced with any of the commonly used induction drugs and maintained with isoflurane or sevoflurane in oxygen. Patients requiring surgery for perineal hernia repair are positioned in ventral recumbency with their rear end elevated and their head down. This results in diaphragmatic compression and impaired ventilation, which is exacerbated if the patient is overweight and aged. Intermittent positive pressure ventilation (IPPV) can be used from the start of surgery to avoid the inevitable hypoventilation. Alternatively, ventilation can be assessed using capnography and spirometry before making the decision to use IPPV. A sandbag is routinely placed under the pubis to prevent compression of the abdomen and thereby aid ventilation (Figure 22.5).

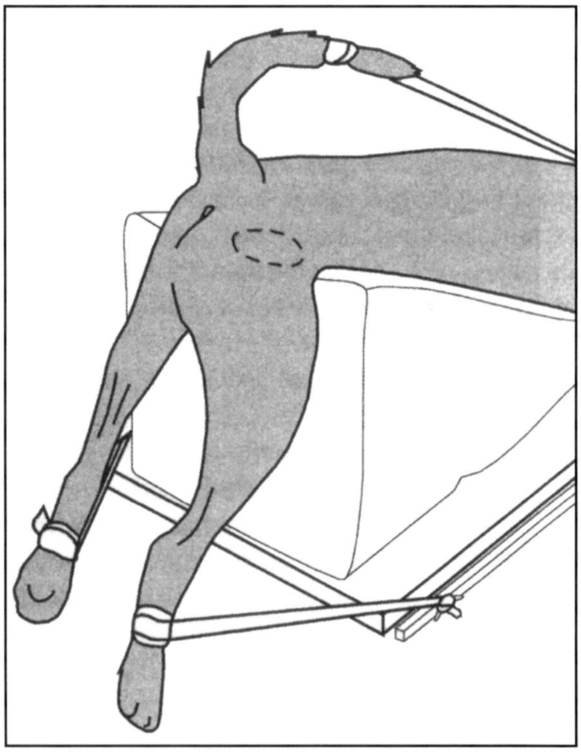

22.5 Positioning of a dog on a perineal stand for perineal surgery. Note the sandbag under the pubis (dashed circle). This raises the abdomen a little, decreases intra-abdominal pressure and permits the diaphragm to move more easily. Care must be taken to avoid too much tension on the leg ties to prevent nerve and muscle damage.

In contrast, animals presenting for correction of atresia ani are very young and often very small, with considerable potential for hypothermia and hypoglycaemia if the surgical time is prolonged.

Perianal fistulae are now treated with immunosuppressive therapy and rarely require surgery.

Anal gland (anal sac) resection is required when there is evidence of recurring infection or of anal gland adenocarcinoma. The latter may be associated with a paraneoplastic syndrome causing persistent hypercalcaemia and hypophosphataemia. This pseudohyperparathyroidism is attributed to the secretion of a parathyroid-like hormone by the tumour. Clinical signs of polyuria, polydipsia, muscle weakness, vomiting and constipation may be seen. The problem needs to be addressed prior to anaesthesia to prevent acute renal failure. Intravenous administration of 0.9% saline at maintenance rates (or higher) promotes diuresis and protects tubular epithelial cells from the toxic effects of hypercalcaemia.

Any of the conditions described above can result in pain, either as a direct result of the presenting complaint or secondary to a surgical procedure. Many of them are treated by the use of parenterally administered opioids and NSAIDs. The use of morphine given epidurally prior to the start of surgery is particularly beneficial, since many of these conditions are chronic and patients may have undergone repeated rectal examinations, adding to their discomfort and hypersensitivity. Epidural analgesia also makes it easier for them to defecate postoperatively.

The liver

The most common indications requiring anaesthesia of patients with hepatic conditions are performance of liver biopsy for diagnostic purposes, surgical correction of congenital portosystemic shunts and surgery for removal of hepatic tumours. Surgery of the biliary tract may be required following abdominal trauma or as a result of biliary tract obstruction.

Liver function

The liver is the site of production of albumin and also many of the coagulation factors. It is important in protein, lipid and carbohydrate metabolism and also the metabolism and excretion of many drugs. Therefore abnormal liver function due to congenital or acquired conditions can have an impact on any or all of these functions.

Albumin concentration is related to the synthetic capacity of the liver. Binding of a drug to plasma proteins restricts its distribution and may influence the elimination of the drug from the body. A reduction in the albumin concentration leads to an increase in the fraction of the unbound drug and an enhanced effect when highly protein-bound drugs are administered. This potential problem is avoided if drugs are given slowly, to effect. Plasma protein binding is classified as follows:

- High = >80%
- Moderate = 50–80%
- Low = <50%.

Propofol and diazepam are highly protein-bound, whereas thiopental is moderately protein-bound. In the dog ketamine has low plasma protein binding (45%), as does morphine (12%).

The liver is the production site for most of the clotting factors, apart from factor VIII (synthesized in endothelial cells and megakaryocytes), and for inhibitors of coagulation: antithrombin III, antiplasmin and fibrinolytic proteins, e.g. plasminogen. It is the site of vitamin K-dependent activation of factors II, VII, IX and X. Traditionally, measurement of clotting times, i.e. prothrombin time (PT) and activated partial thromboplastin time (APTT), has been used to determine whether clotting ability is impaired. Coagulation tests are relatively poor predictors of an animal's tendency to bleed and therefore it should be assumed that animals with hepatobiliary disease have a greater than normal risk of bleeding after procedures involving the liver. PIVKA (proteins induced by vitamin K absence or antagonists) has been shown to be a more sensitive indicator of clotting ability than the PT and APTT.

Hypoglycaemia can result due to impaired ability of the liver to synthesize glucose. It is worthwhile to measure this at the start of anaesthesia or preoperatively and supplement if it is low, e.g. 3.5 mmol/l or less.

One of the principal functions of the liver is the conversion of lipid-soluble compounds to water-soluble versions, which can be excreted in the urine or bile. Microsomal enzymes within the endoplasmic reticulum of the hepatocyte are responsible for drug metabolism. This is usually a two-stage process with initial oxidation or reduction, followed by conjugation with glucuronic or sulphuric acid. The microsomal enzymes referred to as the *mixed function oxidase system* utilize oxygen and cytochromes. Diseases of the liver can impair the activity of these enzymes leading to a prolonged duration of drug action. For this reason, it is important in cases of liver disease to use drugs that are either short acting or readily reversible. Severely jaundiced patients are more likely to develop acute renal failure and sepsis postoperatively. In human patients, it is advocated that diuresis be established with mannitol preoperatively and antibiotic therapy started.

Hepatic dysfunction does not alter the elimination of atracurium, presumably because of the role of Hofmann degradation in the cessation of its effects (see Chapter 15). The elimination of vecuronium in the presence of hepatic dysfunction or biliary tract obstruction is not increased until the dose exceeds 0.1 mg/kg in humans.

In humans, it is still unclear what the ideal drug choices and techniques are for patients with liver disease. However, patients with chronic liver disease have decreased hepatic blood flow caused by increased vascular resistance in the portal vein. Therefore, hepatic blood flow and hepatocyte oxygenation are more dependent on hepatic arterial blood flow than is the case in normal patients. The portal venous system is essentially a passive vascular system, such that intraoperative decreases in systemic arterial pressure and cardiac output can result in reductions in portal vein blood flow. In animal models, hepatic blood flow appears to be adequately maintained during the administration of isoflurane, desflurane and sevoflurane but not of halothane. The ability of the hepatic artery to vasodilate in response to decreases in portal vein blood flow is blunted by high volatile and intravenous anaesthetic concentrations. It is therefore advisable to use balanced anaesthetic techniques, combining volatile anaesthetics with nitrous oxide and short-acting opioids.

Hepatic injury and volatile anaesthetics

Halothane hepatitis is a rare but life-threatening form of hepatic dysfunction, which is believed to be an immune-mediated condition in genetically susceptible human patients. The major evidence for this is the presence of IgG antibodies in the majority of patients diagnosed with the condition. The antibodies are directed against liver microsomal proteins on the surfaces of hepatocytes, which have been covalently modified by the reactive oxidative trifluoroacetyl halide metabolite of halothane. The acetylation of liver protein changes these proteins from 'self' to 'non-self', which results in the formation of antibodies against this new protein and a form of autoimmune hepatitis. It is thought that the subsequent antigen–antibody interactions are responsible for the liver injury described as halothane hepatitis. There is one report of halothane hepatitis in the dog. Like halothane, the fluorinated volatile anaesthetics isoflurane, enflurane and desflurane may form trifluoroacetyl metabolites, resulting in cross-sensitivity with halothane. The incidence of hepatitis after these anaesthetics is lower than after halothane because the degree of metabolism is so much less. There are no reports of hepatitis following the use of isoflurane. The chemical structure of sevoflurane is such that it does not undergo metabolism to trifluoroacetylated metabolites in dogs or cats. Instead it is metabolized to hexafluoroisopropanol, inorganic fluoride and formaldehyde. Theoretically, patients sensitized to either halothane, isoflurane or desflurane could be anaesthetized safely with sevoflurane.

Volatile anaesthetics may produce mild postoperative liver enzyme abnormalities, which probably reflect alterations in hepatic oxygen delivery relative to demand leading to inadequate hepatocyte oxygenation. In humans the cytosolic liver enzyme α-glutathione S-transferase is a more sensitive marker of hepatocellular damage than other liver enzyme markers. This enzyme has been shown to increase following anaesthesia using isoflurane, desflurane and sevoflurane.

Liver biopsy

Before this procedure is undertaken all dogs and cats should have PT and APTT measured, and ideally also a platelet count. Impaired prothrombin production (due to biliary obstruction and the absence of bile salts to facilitate gastrointestinal absorption of vitamin K) is usually reversed by parenteral vitamin K therapy. Because of the high frequency of vitamin K deficiency in hepatic disease, many clinicians routinely pretreat all patients with parenteral vitamin K for 24 hours prior to liver biopsy. Biopsy is contraindicated in the presence of severe coagulopathy, with associated abnormalities in the PT and APTT; in this instance the administration of fresh frozen plasma is required to provide coagulation factors. Ultrasound-guided liver biopsy carries less risk of haemorrhage and also less risk of infection than other techniques.

After biopsy, animals should be checked for any signs of bleeding using ultrasonography. They are hospitalized overnight and pulse rate and quality and mucous membrane colour are monitored to ensure that haemorrhage is not pronounced and ongoing.

Patients can be premedicated with an opioid such as pethidine (meperidine), which has a reasonably short duration of action. This allows assessment of whether the hepatic disease will result in a prolonged duration of action. It is also considered to be a good sedative and analgesic drug. It has been advocated in the past because it reduces the tendency of patients to pant and allows better visualization of the liver by the ultrasonographer. Anaesthesia can be induced with propofol and maintained with isoflurane in oxygen. Benzodiazepines are not used because their effects can be prolonged in animals with hepatic dysfunction. Intravenous fluids are routinely used in these patients.

Ligation of portosystemic shunts

Animals with portosystemic shunts (PSS) tend to have increases in bile acids, total bilirubin, fasting ammonia concentrations, white blood cell count and hepatic enzymes (alkaline phosphatase (ALP), aspartate transaminase (AST) and alanine aminotransferase (ALT)). In some cases these patients have prolonged bleeding times, although this is uncommon. Blood urea, blood glucose and total protein concentrations and PCV tend to decrease, often with low albumin values. Dogs and cats with PSS are also prone to hepatic encephalopathy, which can manifest as anything from mild depression to coma. Medical management should be instigated prior to surgery, and usually includes antibiotics, lactulose and a low-protein diet (with an increased ratio of branched chain to aromatic amino acids), in an attempt to optimize the patient's condition and reduce the likelihood of postoperative complications.

Patients with hepatic disease often have an exaggerated response to centrally acting drugs. Increased cerebral sensitivity results from an increase in the number of central gamma-aminobutyric acid (GABA) receptors during chronic liver failure. Hepatic dysfunction results in a decrease in the ability of the liver to metabolize and inactivate drugs. A low plasma protein concentration means that the volume of distribution of drugs that bind to albumin is reduced, leading to a relative drug overdose. The clearance of drugs with a high hepatic extraction ratio is affected by reduction in hepatic blood flow, which occurs in PSS and cirrhosis.

Preoperatively, haematology and serum biochemistry should indicate whether intraoperative colloids and/or blood products will be required. Animals with intrahepatic shunts are more likely to lose blood during surgery, and a cross-match should be performed for whole blood or packed red cells with a suitable donor. It is important that blood should be relatively fresh (i.e. less than 1 week old) since ammonia concentrations increase with storage time, and administration of more ammonia may compromise neurological outcome. Similarly, plasma products should be fresh or fresh frozen to reduce the ammonia burden given. Brain ammonia concentrations may be increased with an alkalosis, so it is important not to hyperventilate these patients.

Animals with PSS have a poorly developed liver with abnormal circulation. This may result in altered uptake, metabolism and elimination of drugs, with variable consequences. Opioids are commonly used since they generally provide good cardiovascular stability. The liver is the major site of biotransformation for most opioids, with the major metabolic pathway being oxidation. The exceptions are morphine and buprenorphine (which primarily undergo glucuronidation) and remifentanil (which is cleared by ester hydrolysis). Although glucuronidation is considered to be less affected than oxidative metabolism in human patients with cirrhosis, the clearance of morphine is decreased and oral bioavailibility increased in these patients. The consequence of reduced drug metabolism is drug accumulation in the body, especially with repeated administration. One study performed in dogs with clinical hepatic disease showed an increased duration of action and altered elimination of pethidine (meperidine). Use of pethidine can result in the accumulation of the metabolite norpethidine, which can cause seizures. On the other hand, the analgesic activity of morphine relies on transformation into the active metabolite. If metabolism is decreased in patients with chronic liver disease, the analgesic action of these drugs may be compromised. Finally, the disposition of a few opioids, such as fentanyl, sufentanil and remifentanil, appears to be unaffected in liver disease. Therefore it is recommended that low doses and/or short-acting drugs be used. Patients should be assessed carefully before administering further doses of drug in order to avoid accumulation. Ideally, one should select agents that may be reversed.

Premedication is usually with an opioid (e.g. methadone 0.2–0.3 mg/kg) with or without an anticholinergic. Young animals are readily sedated with low doses of opioids. The use of phenothiazines is not recommended, due in part to their relatively long duration of action and their effects on systemic blood pressure. The use of alpha-2 agonists is not recommended due to their profound effects on the cardiovascular system.

Anaesthesia can be induced either with propofol, or with isoflurane or sevoflurane in oxygen, delivered by facemask. The animal is intubated and anaesthesia maintained with a volatile anaesthetic. Studies performed in people suggest that either isoflurane or sevoflurane should be suitable for maintenance of anaesthesia. Thiopental may result in prolonged recoveries; while ketamine could be used, it is not ideal because of the CNS side effects produced and because it is usually given with a benzodiazepine. Isoflurane is considered to be the drug of choice in patients with liver disease due to the minimal hepatic metabolism and little effect upon hepatic blood flow. Sevoflurane would also be an appropriate choice since it too undergoes little hepatic metabolism and studies in human liver transplant patients have demonstrated alternative sites of metabolism. The use of mask induction obviates the need for the injectable anaesthetic drugs and their hepatic metabolism. Since sevoflurane is less irritant to the airways, induction of anaesthesia with this drug can be smoother than that seen with isoflurane. Both of these agents are relatively insoluble and therefore induction time is short.

Patients with PSS are often hypotensive even at light levels of anaesthesia and therefore a balanced anaesthetic technique is helpful. Neuromuscular-blocking drugs can be used to provide muscle relaxation without the need for high vaporizer settings. Atracurium is the drug of choice because it undergoes Hofmann elimination.

A peripheral intravenous catheter allows the administration of intravenous fluids. If total protein is low (<50 g/l) a synthetic colloid or fresh frozen plasma can be administered throughout anaesthesia and surgery at 5 ml/kg/h. This provides intravascular volume support, helps to maintain colloid osmotic pressure and also allows the administration of clotting factors if fresh frozen plasma is used. It may be useful to place a second intravenous catheter either peripherally or centrally. A central venous catheter allows measurement of CVP during shunt ligation. Nowadays most single extrahepatic shunts are treated by application of an ameroid ring and there are fewer dramatic changes in venous return and arterial blood pressure. Another technique used for treatment of these aberrant blood vessels is transvenous coil embolization. There is little information on the anaesthetic management used for this procedure, although the same considerations exist.

Arterial catheters allow rapid measurement of arterial blood pressure although the Doppler technique can also be used if an arterial catheter cannot be placed. The dorsal pedal artery is most commonly used but auricular, radial and lingual arteries can all be catheterized percutanously. An intra-arterial catheter allows not only measurement of blood pressure but also sample collection for blood gas analysis and measurement of TP, PCV and blood glucose. Blood glucose should also be measured after the induction of anaesthesia and hypoglycaemia is treated by the administration of 5% glucose solution in the intravenous fluid. A peripheral nerve stimulator should be placed before the administration of neuromuscular-blocking drugs. This can be located over the facial nerve or the radial or ulnar nerve, whichever is easiest to access.

Monitoring body temperature is also important in small patients since they have a large surface area to volume ratio and readily lose core body heat due to the open abdominal cavity and the solutions used for surgical preparation. Body temperature can be maintained using warm water blankets or hot air blankets placed around the patient; those designed for use with babies are especially useful.

Postoperative analgesia is provided by use of parenterally administered opioids and also via the administration of epidural morphine. Lumbosacral epidural injection is usually performed after the induction of anaesthesia. Preservative-free morphine is given at 0.1 mg/kg, diluted to a volume of 0.3 ml/kg to a maximum volume of 6 ml. This seems to provide satisfactory analgesia despite the fact that surgery is via a cranial abdominal approach.

Postoperative monitoring is required to ensure portal hypertension does not occur. This is unlikely if an ameroid ring has been used. Seizures may occur postoperatively and there are reports of treatment with low dose propofol infusions (1–3.5 mg/kg boluses followed by infusion at 0.05–0.25 mg/kg/minute).

Removal of hepatic tumours

Surgery for removal of hepatic tumours can be challenging: the major anaesthetic and surgical problem is haemorrhage. Reductions in venous return may also occur due to occlusion of the caudal vena cava during surgical manipulation of the liver. Coagulation times should be assessed prior to surgery and ideally fresh frozen plasma and blood should be available. The surgical approach may require a large incision and this should be borne in mind when postoperative analgesia is selected. If there is no indication of coagulopathy, the use of epidural analgesics, such as preservative-free morphine, can provide long-lasting and profound analgesia.

It is routine to place two intravenous catheters to enable the administration of multiple forms of intravenous fluid therapy, e.g. crystalloids and blood. Ideally, an arterial catheter and central venous catheter should also be placed to allow rapid assessment of arterial blood pressure and central venous pressure, thus guiding volume replacement.

Opioids form the mainstay of postoperative pain control. NSAIDs arguably should be avoided if there is any concern about adequate liver function, which makes multimodal pain control more difficult. Alternative modalities would include lidocaine infusion, which seems to be effective in the control of visceral pain (see below). However, one should bear in mind that lidocaine is metabolized in the liver.

Feline hepatic lipidosis

Many cats with hepatic lipidosis may require anaesthesia for placement of oesophagotomy or gastrostomy tubes (Figure 22.6). It is recommended that injectable agents requiring hepatic metabolism are avoided. Prolonged anaesthetic recovery is reported to occur in such patients following administration of oxymorphone (and probably hydromorphone), propofol, diazepam, etomidate and ketamine. Life-threatening haemolytic anaemia has been found to occur following injection of etomidate and diazepam preparations (which contain propylene glycol), as well as injection of propofol. Therefore, premedication is provided with a relatively short-acting opioid such as pethidine (meperidine) at a low dose. Doses in the range of 0.1–0.2 mg/kg have been advocated by other authors. It is recommended that anaesthesia is induced and maintained with isoflurane (or sevoflurane) given

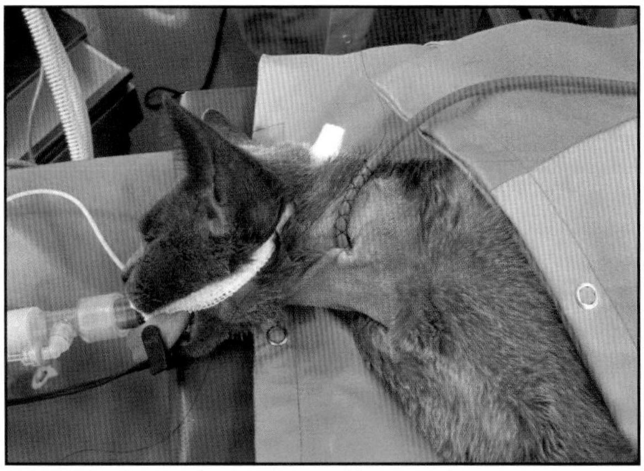

22.6 Anaesthetized cat with oesophagotomy tube. This patient had suffered a road traffic accident a week before and had been inappetent since then. Hepatic lipidosis developed and the cat was anaesthetized for oesophagotomy tube placement to allow enteral feeding.

by mask initially until the patient can be intubated. Anticholinergics should also be avoided because they reduce gastrointestinal motility and this can impair the effectiveness of any nutritional support.

Anticonvulsant therapy and anaesthesia

The incidence of epilepsy in the canine population is estimated to be 2% and a proportion of these animals will receive anticonvulsant therapy. It is not uncommon to anaesthetize patients who are receiving anticonvulsant drugs such as phenobarbital and potassium bromide. Liver enzymes should be monitored during therapy as a routine precaution to assess liver damage/function along with plasma drug concentrations. These drugs can cause microsomal enzyme induction leading to an increased anaesthetic drug requirement and a shorter duration of action. In the author's experience this does not appear to have a clinically perceptible effect.

Diseases of the biliary tract

Emergency surgery for acute cholecystitis or common bile duct obstruction is often associated with vomiting and may require volume and electrolyte replacement. Chronic cholestasis can impair the absorption of fat-soluble vitamins, such as vitamin K. Coagulation times, ideally PT, APTT and PIVKA, should be measured prior to surgery. If PT and/or PIVKA are prolonged then parenteral supplementation with vitamin K is required. Treatment may take 24–48 hours of repeated intramuscular injections to be effective. If surgery needs to be performed sooner, the use of fresh frozen plasma should be considered in order to replace factors II, VII, IX and X. These patients can have ileus and should be considered to be at an increased risk for pulmonary aspiration of gastric contents.

Morphine causes constriction of the sphincter of Oddi with an increase in pressure within the common bile duct. The pressure may increase 10-fold with a duration of effect of 2 or more hours. For this reason morphine is contraindicated in patients with conditions of the gallbladder and biliary tract. Pethidine and fentanyl may also increase constriction at the sphincter of Oddi, although pressures in the bile duct do not increase to the same extent as those seen with morphine. Pentazocine increases sphincter constriction, but nalbuphine and buprenorphine seem to have minimal effect. Butorphanol increases the pressure more than nalbuphine but less than fentanyl.

Pancreatic disease

Anaesthetic management of patients with diabetes mellitus and insulinoma is covered in Chapter 25.

Pancreatitis

Uncommonly, patients presenting with acute pancreatitis require anaesthesia and surgery. This is generally based on ultrasonographic signs of pancreatic abscessation. The incidence of pancreatitis in the canine and feline population is currently unknown and is the subject of ongoing research. The aetiology is also believed to differ between human and canine patients. Pancreatitis is considered to be one of the most painful conditions encountered in small animal medicine and pain management is problematic. In humans alcohol abuse and gallstones are aetiological factors in 60–80% of patients with acute pancreatitis; 10% of cases are idiopathic; and the other 10% are due to miscellaneous causes (e.g. trauma, inherited conditions and vascular abnormalities). In dogs, genetic factors appear to have the greatest influence on the aetiology of the condition.

In humans, there are case reports of pancreatitis developing after short-term and prolonged propofol administration. This is thought to be associated with hypertriglyceridaemia, which may occur as a result of propofol administration or be pre-existing. In animals with pancreatitis, it may be wise to avoid the use of drugs that contain lipid emulsion (e.g. propofol and diazepam). However, studies in healthy rats have failed to demonstrate any direct relationship between propofol and pancreatitis. There are also reports in human medicine of pancreatitis developing in patients with Cushing's disease and arguably drugs solubilized in a lipid emulsion should also be avoided in these individuals. A study performed at the Queen's Veterinary School Hospital, University of Cambridge, failed to show any link between the use of propofol for the induction of anaesthesia and elevation in pancreatic enzyme levels, although triglyceride levels were increased.

Pancreatic pain can be extremely difficult to treat successfully. It may be unresponsive to opioids or NSAIDs and other alternatives are under investigation, e.g. lidocaine infusions, ketamine infusions and epidural analgesia. In humans, the coeliac ganglion can be anaesthetized although this has never been attempted in veterinary species.

Peritonitis

Patients with peritonitis are generally extremely ill and they should arguably be referred to a practice with the means to provide intensive care pre- and postoperatively. Diagnosis is based on the history, clinical signs, ultrasonography and abdominocentesis. Intravenous fluid therapy is indicated prior to surgery in an attempt to stabilize the cardiovascular system. Hypoproteinaemia is often present and this should be treated with colloids, such as hetastarch at 1–3 ml/kg/h. Multiple intravenous catheters are required to allow rapid fluid administration and to overcome the problems of giving fluids which are incompatible with one another. A multilumen jugular catheter is useful, not only for fluid administration but also for measurement of central venous pressure. Arterial catheters allow accurate measurement of arterial blood pressure and aid anaesthetic management, although they are difficult to place in severely hypovolaemic, endotoxaemic patients. In this instance arterial blood pressure can be measured using a Doppler technique.

Anaesthesia can be induced with a combination of a short-acting opioid (e.g. fentanyl, 10 µg/kg) and diazepam at 0.5 mg/kg. Maintenance may be achieved with isoflurane or sevoflurane in oxygen, combined with a fentanyl infusion at 0.3–0.7 µg/kg/minute and/or lidocaine at 25–50 µg/kg/minute.

It is common to place a PEG tube to ensure an adequate food intake postoperatively, since these animals are frequently inappetent following surgery. A urinary catheter is required to allow measurement of urine output and to guide fluid therapy postoperatively. This should always be placed using an aseptic technique.

Visceral pain control

Documentation of pain in animals with medical conditions of the abdomen or neoplasia of the abdominal organs is sparse, despite the fact that pain is often the major presenting sign in human patients. Combinations of opioids and NSAIDs are frequently used for the treatment of visceral pain, most commonly following ovariohysterectomy or castration. Buprenorphine (0.01–0.02 mg/kg) and carprofen (4 mg/kg i.v. or s.c.) or meloxicam (0.2 mg/kg i.v. or s.c. in dogs and 0.3 mg/kg s.c. in cats) are often used.

Newer drug treatments are now being used for the alleviation of visceral pain originating from the abdominal cavity. These include:

- Lidocaine at 1 mg/kg i.v., followed by a constant rate intravenous infusion at 25–50 µg/kg/minute
- Ketamine at 0.5 mg/kg i.v. followed by 10 µg/kg/minute during anaesthesia (reduced to 2 µg/kg/minute following surgery) (Wagner *et al.*, 2002)
- Medetomidine at 1 µg/kg/h
- Morphine at 0.1 mg/kg/h.

Other drugs are also currently under investigation. Constant rate infusions generally require the use of syringe drivers to ensure accurate delivery, although all of the drugs listed above can be added to a 500 ml bag of 0.9% saline and given with the maintenance fluid therapy (Figure 22.7).

Drug (concentration)	Dose for intravenous infusion (μg/kg/minute)	Amount of drug (mg) to add to 0.5 l of 0.9% saline	Amount of drug (mg) to add to 1.0 l of 0.9% saline	Infusion rate (ml/kg/h)
Morphine (10 mg/ml)	3	30	60	3
Lidocaine (20 mg/ml)	50 (give loading dose of 1 mg/kg slowly intravenously before starting infusion)	500	1000	3
Ketamine (100 mg/ml)	3 (give loading dose of 0.5 mg/kg i.v. before starting infusion)	30	60	3
Medetomidine (1 mg/ml)	0.01–0.02 (give loading dose of 0.3–1 μg/kg i.v. before starting infusion)	0.2	0.4	2–3

22.7 Intravenous infusions for relief of visceral pain in dogs. Morphine, lidocaine and ketamine may be administered individually or in combination (they may be mixed in the same bag of 0.9% saline). Medetomidine should be administered alone. The bag should be mixed well after drug addition and labelled clearly. With lidocaine infusions, the patient should be assessed for signs of toxicity such as muscle fasciculations or seizures. The infusion should be stopped after 24 hours to reassess the patient. This is also important because some drugs are cumulative (e.g. alpha-2 agonists, ketamine) whilst others have active metabolites (morphine, ketamine). Solutions should be discarded after 24 hours and new solutions made.

References and further reading

American Society of Anesthesiologists Task Force on Preoperative Fasting (1999) Practice guidelines for preoperative fasting and the use of pharmacologic agents to reduce the risk of pulmonary aspiration: application to healthy patients undergoing elective procedures: a report by the American Society of Anesthesiologists Task Force on Preoperative Fasting. *Anesthesiology* **90**, 896–905

Boston SE, Moens NM, Kruth SA and Southorn EP (2003) Endoscopic evaluation of the gastroduodenal mucosa to determine the safety of short-term concurrent administration of meloxicam and dexamethasone in healthy dogs. *American Journal of Veterinary Research* **64(11)**, 1369–1375

Dowdle SM, Joubert KE, Lambrechts NE, Lobetti RG and Pardini AD (2003) The prevalence of subclinical gastroduodenal ulceration in Dachshunds with intervertebral disc prolapse. *Journal of the South African Veterinary Association* **74**, 77–81

Elwood C (2006) Diagnosis and management of canine oesophageal disease and regurgitation. *In Practice* **28**, 14–21

Forsyth SF, Guilford WG, Haslett SJ and Godfrey J (1998) Endoscopy of the gastroduodenal mucosa after carprofen, meloxicam and ketoprofen administration in dogs. *Journal of Small Animal Practice* **39**, 421–424

Fox LE, Rosenthal RC, Twedt DC *et al.* (1990) Plasma histamine and gastrin concentrations in 17 dogs with mast cell tumors. *Journal of Veterinary Internal Medicine* **4**, 242–246

Heldmann E, Holt DE, Brockman DJ, Brown DC and Perkowski SZ (1999) Use of propofol to manage seizure activity after surgical treatment of portosystemic shunts. *Journal of Small Animal Practice* **40(12)**, 590–594

Hiebert C (1977) The recognition and management of gastric-oesophageal reflux without hiatal hernia. *World Journal of Surgery* **1**, 445

Hugonnard M, Leblond A, Keroack S, Cadore JL and Troncy E (2004) Attitudes and concerns of French veterinarians towards pain and analgesia in dogs and cats. *Veterinary Anaesthesia and Analgesia* **31**, 154–163

Mathews K (1996) Nonsteroidal anti-inflammatory analgesics in pain management in dogs and cats. *Canadian Veterinary Journal* **37**, 539–545

Muir WW and Dibartola SP (1983) Fluid therapy. In: *Current Veterinary Therapy VIII*, ed. RW Kirk, pp. 28–40. WB Saunders, Philadelphia

Neiger R, Gaschen F and Jaggy A (2000) Gastric mucosal lesions in dogs with acute intervertebral disc disease: characterization and effects of omeprazole or misoprostol. *Journal of Veterinary Internal Medicine* **14**, 33–36

Poortinga EW and Hungerford LL (1998) A case-controlled study of acute ibuprofen toxicity in dogs. *Preventive Veterinary Medicine* **35**, 115–124

Rombeau JL, Barot LR, Williamson CE and Mullen JR (1982) Preoperative total parenteral nutrition and surgical outcome in patients with inflammatory bowel disease. *American Journal of Surgery* **143(1)**, 139–143

Wagner AE, Walton JA, Hellyer PW, Gaynor JS and Mama KR (2002) Use of low doses of ketamine administered by constant rate infusion as an adjunct for postoperative analgesia in dogs. *Journal of the American Veterinary Medical Association* **221**, 72–75

Wilson DV, Evans AT and Mauer WA (2006) Influence of metoclopramide on gastroesophageal reflux in anesthetized dogs. *American Journal of Veterinary Research* **67(1)**, 26–31

23

Urogenital disease

Petro Dobromylskyj

Introduction

Patients with urogenital disease present a range of challenges to the veterinary surgeon. Problems range from the stable chronic renal failure patient through to the ruptured pyometra case. For non-urgent cases, preoperative stabilization may be planned well in advance, whereas for the acute emergency patient minimal time will be available. In these cases there must be clear-cut priorities before induction of anaesthesia. In addition, some patients may present with severe problems, such as acute renal failure, which require medical management. Anaesthesia for correction of any concurrent surgical problem will be delayed.

Renal failure

Pathophysiology

In addition to the excretion of waste products, the kidneys have a major role in controlling the volume and composition of blood and tissue fluids. Abnormalities of renal function can produce life-threatening changes in these variables over both the long and short term. In addition, a number of pathological conditions of the urogenital system can have major effects on cardiovascular function, many of which are mediated through the kidneys.

Healthy kidneys convert approximately 5% of cardiac output into primitive urine, the vast majority of which is reabsorbed. Selective reabsorption and secretion of plasma components and metabolic waste products determine the changes in composition of the blood produced by the kidneys. As this system fails, the ability of the veterinary surgeon to manipulate these plasma variables becomes necessary for patient survival. Manipulation of electrolyte values into normal reference ranges is achieved through appropriate fluid selection. As measurement of blood volume is technically difficult, the aim is to produce a circulation that delivers adequate oxygenated haemoglobin to the tissues.

Fluid therapy, therefore, becomes an essential tool for controlling blood volume, pH and electrolyte status. This applies across the range of problems, from a patient with stable chronic renal failure undergoing an elective procedure to one with acute postrenal obstruction. While estimations of fluid disturbances can often be made from clinical examination and patient history, the accuracy of these estimates can be markedly improved by the ability to measure electrolytes and acid–base status. Even so, simple acceptance of the results needs tempering with the knowledge that they may not reflect whole body status, and that they may change rapidly with therapy.

In *chronic renal failure* (CRF), the patient is often polyuric, polydipsic and uraemic, with weight loss, depression, halitosis, anorexia, anaemia and occasional vomiting and diarrhoea. The remaining functional nephrons can only cope with limited sodium and water loads. Approximately 30% of patients with chronic renal failure may be hypertensive (defined as a systolic blood pressure >180 mmHg) and receiving medication for this, normally a calcium channel-blocking agent. Hypertension makes the patient intolerant to the anaesthetic state, with swings between hypertension and, more likely, severe hypotension. The lowest acceptable figure for mean arterial pressure should also be set higher for uncontrolled hypertensive patients (i.e. 80–90 mmHg rather than 60 mmHg). A patient with compensated CRF can decompensate with use of anaesthetic drugs and in the presence of hypovolaemia and hypotension. It is important to be sure the kidneys are producing urine before anaesthesia is induced and therapy should be planned for correction of deficits and replacement of ongoing losses.

In addition to controlling blood volume and composition, the kidney is the source of erythropoietin and chronic renal failure is frequently associated with a non-regenerative anaemia. There is also a tendency for an animal in renal failure to develop gastric ulceration and bleeding, and thus a reduced haematocrit is very likely. If mild, this may simply emphasize the need to avoid hypoxaemia at all stages of anaesthesia and recovery. If severe, then intervention to improve oxygen-carrying capacity is needed. Oxyglobin®, packed red blood cells or whole blood administration are the options available (see Chapter 16). Oxygen delivery to the tissues can also be maximized by maintaining cardiac output (heart rate and stroke volume).

There are several physiological changes that have effects on drug action in renal failure. It is common for albumin levels to be low ('nephrotic syndrome'), so highly protein-bound agents such as thiopental and propofol may need marked dose reductions. The ability to titrate administration of an induction agent closely to effect, even if that involves administration over several minutes, can minimize the problem of relative overdose under these circumstances. Slow titration also facilitates the dose reductions needed due to the presence of uraemia and metabolic acidosis. Relatively few drugs are primarily excreted in the urine. The two most problematical in the past were the neuromuscular-blocking drugs gallamine and pancuronium, but these have minimal use in current veterinary anaesthesia. Of more concern are drugs such as morphine, ketamine and diazepam, all of which have active metabolites that are primarily excreted via the kidneys. Hydromorphone is normally rapidly excreted through the kidneys as parent drug and metabolites (6-hydroxy epimers).

Non-steroidal anti-inflammatory drugs (NSAIDs) all act by blocking the production of prostaglandins and leukotrienes, which control renal blood flow autoregulation and glomerular filtration pressure. Inhibition of this control system can result in marked deterioration of renal function. Opioid analgesics and regional analgesia using local anaesthetics are devoid of this effect and are the preferred analgesic techniques.

Preoperative assessment and stabilization

Patients with compensated CRF should, in addition to their routine clinical examination, have renal function, electrolytes (including sodium, potassium, chloride, bicarbonate and inorganic phosphate) and packed cell volume (PCV) measured. Arterial blood pressure can be estimated preoperatively using a Doppler or oscillometric technique. Hypertension should be controlled, most commonly by using amlodipine, although calcium channel blockers may promote further hypotension under anaesthesia. Medication should, however, be continued up to and including the day of anaesthesia, providing it can be administered without food.

Urinalysis, including specific gravity, protein concentration and bacteriology, is useful for assessing patient status.

For an elective procedure, hypokalaemia should be corrected with oral potassium supplementation. Metabolic acidosis can be corrected with oral sodium bicarbonate, although bicarbonate precursors, such as potassium citrate, can be used to combine treatment for hypokalaemia with treatment for acidosis. Hyperphosphataemia should be controlled with oral phosphate-binding agents. Uraemia can be partly managed by dietary changes appropriate for a renal failure patient. As dietary management is rarely effective in advanced renal failure, a period of peritoneal dialysis may be needed prior to general anaesthesia. In urgent circumstances, correction using potassium-enriched intravenous fluids should be performed with caution, typically not extending the infusion rate beyond 0.5 mmol/kg/h and monitoring the electrocardiogram (ECG) for markers of potassium overdose. Repeated plasma potassium measurement will increase the safety of potassium administration. Glucose-containing solutions should be used with care, as the insulin response produced will lower plasma potassium concentration further.

Metabolic acidosis can be controlled preoperatively with intravenous sodium bicarbonate as needed. Accurate dosage requires plasma bicarbonate measurements and care must be taken to avoid hypernatraemia.

Uraemia may be reduced by ensuring an adequate preload is maintained with intravenous fluids, but in severe renal failure the only effective method for reducing uraemia preoperatively may be dialysis. Peritoneal dialysis is effective and practicable using a glucose-rich sodium chloride-based dialysate. In addition to removing metabolic waste products, dialysis will also remove fluid from the circulation and provide glucose. Fluid balance must be maintained with intravenous replacement and potassium concentration monitored closely, particularly as the hyperglycaemia will be associated with an insulin response, which will result in a net movement of potassium into the intracellular compartment. Haemodialysis is a referral procedure in those countries where it is available.

Hyperkalaemia is a rare finding in CRF (more common in acute renal failure) but must be corrected preoperatively as discussed below.

A patient in *acute renal failure* (ARF) with hyperkalaemia and in uraemic crisis is severely compromised and should not be anaesthetized. Fluid deficits, electrolyte imbalances, increased level of uraemia and decreased urine production should be corrected over the 24 hours before anaesthesia is induced.

For emergency procedures, the essentials are restoration of an adequate blood volume and a potassium concentration within the normal physiological range, correction of metabolic acidosis and reduction of uraemia.

Anaesthetic management

Intravenous access is mandatory for patients in renal failure to allow closely controlled fluid and drug administration. For patients undergoing major or prolonged surgery, measurement of central venous pressure (CVP) is useful to assess circulating volume status. Placement of a central venous catheter is normally performed after induction of anaesthesia, unless the patient is moribund. While the absolute value of CVP may be of limited clinical significance (see Chapter 7), trend analysis will allow avoidance of volume overload from over-aggressive fluid therapy. Inadequate correction of volume loss manifests as a progressive fall in CVP. A progressive rise in central venous pressure with fluid therapy combined with a low urine output is highly suggestive of acute renal failure.

Arterial blood pressure may be monitored invasively for major procedures or non-invasively for minor procedures. Doppler techniques have the advantage of providing qualitative information about trends in peripheral blood flow and are not reliant on a stable cardiac rhythm, unlike oscillometric methods. Underestimation of systolic pressure by Doppler techniques is quite marked in cats and the value obtained is closer to mean arterial pressure than systolic pressure. While underestimation acts as a 'safety net' against hypotension, it could potentially result in volume overload and this must be considered before aggressive fluid therapy is used to treat a perceived hypotension problem.

Pulse oximetry is particularly useful in recovery, where drug-induced hypoxaemia can easily be eliminated using supplementary oxygen. This is essential when dealing with a severely anaemic patient where oxygen delivery is compromised despite full haemoglobin saturation and arterial desaturation would lead to rapid worsening of tissue hypoxia.

Capnography allows detection of hypoventilation and facilitates accurate setting of the ventilator (if one is used). Anaesthetic gas monitoring is useful if low-flow circle circuits are used with larger patients, although ultimately the cardiovascular variables are more likely to dictate inhalation agent concentration.

Because many chronic renal failure patients are very thin, protection against hypothermia is also essential. Active warming, reflective coatings, insulation and heat and moisture exchangers all have a role in maintaining normothermia. It is also essential to keep the anaesthetic time to a minimum.

Premedication

Preoperative preparation of these patients will have frequently involved placement of an intravenous catheter some time before general anaesthesia. Under these circumstances, premedication for chemical restraint is often not needed and the benefits of sedation should be weighed against the disadvantages of possible prolonged duration of action, or failure to clear metabolites of the sedative.

Analgesia with a mu agonist opioid may be beneficial; morphine (0.1–0.3 mg/kg i.m., s.c.), hydromorphone (0.05–0.1 mg/kg i.m., s.c.) or methadone (0.1–0.2 mg/kg i.m., s.c.) are the preferred agents. NSAIDs are in general best avoided. Carprofen might be used if an NSAID is considered essential, but may be better administered postoperatively when the blood volume and pressure changes associated with anaesthesia and surgery are stable.

In view of the frequent cardiovascular problems present in these patients, alpha-2 agonists are probably best avoided. For uncooperative cats, a chamber induction may be necessary. This can also be used to allow blood sampling and catheter placement in very fractious cats. Acepromazine at low dose rates (0.01–0.03 mg/kg) may allow less stressful management of these patients with minimal effect on blood pressure.

Induction

Selection of an induction agent may be influenced by the need to avoid both hypotension and sympathetic nervous system activation, in order to prevent diversion of blood from the renal circulation:

- A low dose of midazolam (0.1 mg/kg i.v.) immediately followed by a slow infusion of propofol (1–3 mg/kg i.v.) over several minutes has much to recommend it, provided that oxygen is administered throughout the process
- Thiopental is probably best avoided in patients with low muscle mass and little fat reserve as there is minimal scope for recovery by redistribution
- Etomidate (0.25–1.0mg/kg i.v.) following diazepam (0.25–0.5 mg/kg i.v.) has minimal cardiovascular side effects
- Alfaxalone (Saffan®; Alfaxan®) has an excellent safety record but may, in common with rapidly administered propofol, be associated with unacceptably low mean arterial blood pressure.

Whichever induction agent is chosen, attention to oxygenation is obligatory. A mask or chamber induction will normally provide excellent oxygenation at the cost of poor airway control.

Inhalant anaesthetics

Sevoflurane metabolism results in production of some fluoride ions, although no renal or hepatic changes are found in healthy dogs. Prolonged use of this agent is probably best avoided in patients with severe renal compromise. Isoflurane would appear to be the preferred choice in view of cardiac rhythm stability (when a catecholamine infusion may be required for both inotropic and vasopressor effects) and good recovery profile. Nitrous oxide can be used to minimize the concentration of volatile agent and the attendant cardiorespiratory depression. While volatile agents depress renal nerve sympathetic activity (vasodilation), nitrous oxide can increase sympathetic activity (vasoconstriction). The improvement in cardiac output from decreased volatile agent administration may offset the vasoconstriction caused by nitrous oxide.

Normocapnia (35–45mmHg (4.6–6 kPa)) is desirable to avoid hypercapnia-induced sympathetic nervous system activation and intermittent positive pressure ventilation (IPPV) may be needed to achieve this. Long-term IPPV reduces renal blood flow and causes fluid retention. The benefits of short-term IPPV during anaesthesia are the elimination of drug-induced respiratory acidosis and effective control of volatile agent uptake and elimination. The risk:benefit ratio is determined by the needs of the individual patient. Short-acting opioids, such as fentanyl and its derivatives, are appropriate for intraoperative reflex suppression, but IPPV will be mandatory with these agents.

Muscle relaxants

With the commonly used neuromuscular-blocking drugs, there are only minor concerns in patients with renal failure. Vecuronium is longer acting in patients with CRF than in normal patients, but the effect is small. Atracurium duration is unaffected, although, in humans, renal failure may predispose to the build-up of the toxic metabolite, laudanosine, if prolonged use is undertaken. This is unlikely to be a problem with the duration of administration likely to be needed in veterinary patients.

Postoperative care

Analgesia

Analgesia needs will be determined by the surgery performed. Local anaesthetic blocks may be particularly appropriate, and epidural administration of morphine is also useful. Epidural opioids will generally have no effect on either arterial blood pressure or renal prostaglandin metabolism. Inclusion of a local anaesthetic may result in unacceptable hypotension due to blockade of the spinal sympathetic outflow, but can reduce sympathetic discharge to renal arteries. If hypotension is managed, then local anaesthetics could be used. Arterial blood pressure should be monitored and hypotension treated with intravenous fluids, vasopressors and/or inotropes (see below).

Supplementary pure agonist opioids can be given parenterally should epidural morphine produce inadequate pain control. In the immediate recovery period, the intravenous route of administration is preferred in order to obtain rapid control of emergence pain. Histamine release with clinical doses of intravenous morphine appears to be rare and has not been recorded with methadone or hydromorphone. Later increments may be given subcutaneously, provided fluid balance is controlled.

Morphine is extensively metabolized to both morphine 6-glucuronide and morphine 3-glucuronide and both of these may accumulate in renal failure patients. As morphine 6-glucuronide is analgesic and morphine 3-glucuronide can produce hyperalgesia and neuroexcitation, careful observation of the effects of supplementary doses is needed. For systemic dosing, methadone may have some advantage in that it has no active metabolites, in the dog at least. Hydromorphone can also be used in cats and dogs (0.05–0.1 mg/kg i.m.). The situation in cats is less clear as they do not normally use glucuronide conjugation for drug elimination; buprenorphine (0.01 mg/kg) has been shown to be more effective in experimental models than morphine (0.2 mg/kg). In the late postoperative period, when pain is less severe, buprenorphine is probably the drug of choice for both dogs and cats due to its longer duration of action compared to pure agonist opioids.

Fluid therapy

Intravenous fluid therapy should continue in recovery. While lactated Ringer's (Hartmann's) solution is normally appropriate for intraoperative cardiovascular support, it will provide an excessive sodium load for a patient in renal failure. Use of a half-strength sodium chloride solution (0.45%) or a 0.18% sodium chloride solution with 4% dextrose is more logical. All fluids should contain at least 5 mmol/l of potassium, and more may be added based on measured plasma potassium levels (see also Chapters 22 and 25).

Decreased urine output intra- or postoperatively is a serious problem in CRF patients, and may indicate the development of ARF. Correction of reduced renal perfusion pressure using a bolus of lactated Ringer's solution with monitoring of central venous and arterial pressures may correct the situation. The use of adrenaline or noradrenaline infusions (initially 0.1–1.0 μg/kg/minute, then titrated to effect) to support the cardiovascular system does not appear to cause the anticipated problem of renal vasoconstriction in human studies.

Cardiovascular support with an inotrope appears to be better for minimizing renal damage than leaving hypotension untreated. If the cardiovascular system is stable and anuria persists, urine output may be re-established with osmotic diuretics (glucose and mannitol are readily available). Of the loop diuretics, furosemide is the most commonly used. Low dose dopamine is an effective method of stimulating urine output in humans that has been used extensively in the past. Unfortunately, although diuresis may be useful in managing volume overload incurred during cardiovascular management, there is little evidence that this diuresis is protective of renal function. In particular, low dose dopamine is rarely used in human anuric patients; furosemide is preferred if volume overload needs correction.

Postrenal failure: urethral obstruction and bladder rupture

Pathophysiology

Complete urethral obstruction and rupture of the urinary tract are the two commonest causes of postrenal failure in cats and dogs. Both of these are primarily surgical problems requiring anaesthesia for their correction. Postrenal failure results in a wide range of metabolic derangements which are life-threatening yet potentially reversible, particularly hyperkalaemia and metabolic acidosis. In addition, many patients will have been vomiting and, in some, this may be severe enough that the loss of gastric acid may counterbalance the underlying renal metabolic acidosis. Respiratory acid–base disturbances may include either alkalosis (secondary to pain-induced tachypnoea) or acidosis from restriction of diaphragmatic movement (due to uroperitoneum or grossly distended bladder).

Preoperative assessment and stabilization

Assessment and treatment of hyperkalaemia is the initial priority. In addition, sodium, chloride, haematocrit, urea and creatinine measurements are useful. Assessment of acid–base disturbance needs a minimum of pH and bicarbonate measurements, if these are available.

In the absence of potassium measurements, some indication of potassium status may be available from the ECG (Figures 23.1 and 23.2). ECG changes do not in general become obvious until plasma potassium concentration is >7 mmol/l, and therefore visible ECG abnormalities indicate that potassium management is urgently needed before anaesthesia.

Small or absent P waves
Peaked T wave
Prolonged P–R interval
Increased duration of QRS complex
Shortened Q–T interval

23.1 ECG markers of hyperkalaemia. These are detectable with a plasma potassium >7 mmol/l and become progressively more obvious, particularly with potassium concentrations >9 mmol/l.

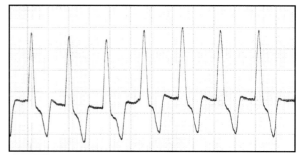

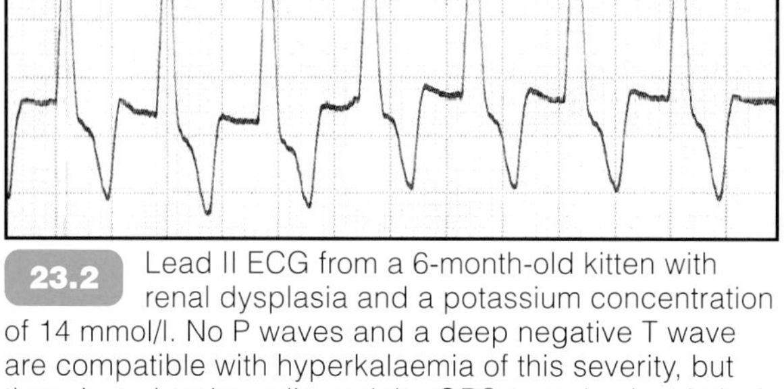

23.2 Lead II ECG from a 6-month-old kitten with renal dysplasia and a potassium concentration of 14 mmol/l. No P waves and a deep negative T wave are compatible with hyperkalaemia of this severity, but there is no bradycardia and the QRS complex is relatively normal in duration.

Of the management options available (Figure 23.3), the use of a calcium salt as a physiological antagonist to the effect of hyperkalaemia on cardiac myocytes is probably the most straightforward approach, although it does not lower potassium concentration. The effect is rapid and can be followed on ECG. While the duration of effect is short, it does allow time to instigate measures that do lower plasma potassium concentration. Clearly, dilution with potassium-free fluids will achieve this more rapidly than use of lactated Ringer's (Hartmann's) solution, but the administration of fluid containing 5 mmol/l potassium will still reduce a plasma potassium concentration of 9 mmol/l. However, because many patients are mildly hyponatraemic, dextrose-supplemented normal saline will correct this while promoting endogenous insulin secretion to drive potassium back into the intracellular domain. A commercial 0.9% saline solution with 5% glucose is available, or alternatively a 10% glucose solution can be prepared by adding 200 ml of a 50% glucose solution to a litre of 0.9% saline.

Calcium gluconate 10% (0.5 ml/kg slowly i.v. (over 10–20 minutes) with ECG monitoring)
50% Dextrose (1–2 ml/kg i.v.); allows endogenous insulin production to lower blood potassium
Sodium bicarbonate (1–2 mmol/kg i.v.); corrects or reduces metabolic acidosis
Insulin (neutral) (0.25 IU/kg i.v. plus 2 g/IU dextrose i.v., followed by intravenous fluids containing glucose). Monitor for hypoglycaemia
Drain peritoneal urine if appropriate; peritoneal dialysis
Dilute potassium with potassium-free intravenous fluids

23.3 Methods for management of hyperkalaemia.

Correction of metabolic acidosis with bicarbonate will produce similar intracellular movement of potassium (see Chapter 16).

Several therapeutic approaches may be combined. In cases of ruptured urinary tract, the drainage of potassium-rich urine from the abdomen is beneficial; once a peritoneal catheter is placed, it can be used to irrigate the peritoneum with a warmed potassium-free solution. Direct loss of fluid into the inflamed peritoneum will contribute to hypovolaemia, and fluid loss in excess of the estimated urine volume will need to be replaced as part of management. In cases of urethral obstruction, cystocentesis will provide immediate temporary management. Placement of a prepubic balloon-tipped cystostomy tube will allow repeated drainage of urine if surgery must be delayed for any significant period. Some urgency is still required for relief of urinary obstruction, as progressive damage to the urethral lining will occur with prolonged calculus retention. It is also occasionally practical to pass a fine gauge urinary catheter past relatively small or porous stones and so establish short-term urinary flow before anaesthesia, at the cost of some increased urethral trauma.

Anaesthetic management

Premedication

Chemical restraint is not always required as part of premedication, as patients will already have intravenous access from preoperative stabilization. Alpha-2 agonists are contraindicated, due to their effects on the cardiovascular system and their suppression of endogenous insulin production, thus permitting hyperglycaemia. This insulin suppression will interfere with the use of glucose in the management of hyperkalaemia as insulin is required for the treatment to work. Phenothiazines may be safe at low dose rates but there is little indication for their inclusion. Opioids will be essential perioperatively and benzodiazepines may be used both for their anaesthetic-sparing and muscle relaxant effects, with minimal effect on the cardiorespiratory system.

Induction

Uraemic patients are likely to be extremely sensitive to anaesthetic induction agents. Drugs that can be administered very slowly, to effect, are preferred and hence propofol is particularly useful. Etomidate may also be used in view of its good cardiovascular profile. Alternatively ketamine (2.5–5.0 mg/kg i.v.) combined with diazepam (0.1–0.2 mg/kg i.v.) may be used for induction as the initial recovery from ketamine is due to redistribution rather than either metabolism or excretion, so a single dose of 5 mg/kg or less is unlikely to produce a protracted recovery. Co-administration of an opioid or benzodiazepine will further reduce the dose of induction agent required. Rapid-onset, short-acting opioids such as fentanyl (3 μg/kg i.v.) or alfentanil (10 μg/kg i.v.) are the most useful in dogs but are of limited use in cats. Occasional intense bradycardia associated with these agents can lead to profound hypotension; an anticholinergic included in premedication will avoid this problem, or it can be used as treatment.

Preoxygenation should protect against hypoxaemia during the period of respiratory depression invariably associated with slow parenteral inductions, particularly those involving opioids.

Maintenance

During maintenance of anaesthesia, there is no benefit from a respiratory acidosis superimposed on a metabolic acidosis, so IPPV is the preferred method of ventilation. The use of capnography to monitor the effectiveness of ventilation is extremely useful. Isoflurane is probably superior to halothane because of its reduced tendency to provoke arrhythmias if inotrope infusions are needed. It is unclear whether sevoflurane would have any significant advantage over isoflurane in these patients.

Good oxygenation is paramount and at least 50% inspired oxygen is preferred until a reliable pulse oximeter reading is available, at which point increased inspired nitrous oxide may be used to minimize the need for volatile agent. Alternatively pure oxygen may be used as the carrier gas and an opioid, administered by incremental bolus or infusion, substituted for nitrous oxide.

Neuromuscular blockade is not needed for either feline patients with urethral obstruction, or for simple retropulsion of uroliths in dogs where the plan is for delayed cystotomy. For cystotomy, or for repair following rupture of the bladder or urethra, neuromuscular blockade may be of marked benefit for surgical access.

Atracurium or vecuronium may be used. A modest increase in duration of action of vecuronium may occur but this is unlikely to be significant at normal dose rates or durations of administration. Prolonged administration would make monitoring with a peripheral nerve stimulator obligatory (see Chapter 15).

Arterial blood pressure, preferably estimated by Doppler for short procedures, or by direct measurement for major procedures, gives an overall picture of the effect of the anaesthetic on the cardiovascular system. Oscillometers may be useful when the pulse is regular. Electrocardiography is essential for analysis of arrhythmias in those patients with abnormal potassium concentrations. Repeated measurements of plasma potassium and acid–base status allow logical management of fluid therapy. It is particularly important to avoid over-treatment of hyperkalaemia, as the resulting hypokalaemia has its own associated problems.

Cardiovascular collapse

Cardiovascular collapse can occur quite suddenly in these patients and is particularly probable in poorly stabilized patients. Drainage of large volumes of peritoneal fluid/urine under anaesthesia can remove hydrostatic pressure from the peritoneal cavity and allow marked loss of protein-rich fluid through the inflamed peritoneal lining. During anaesthesia for cystocentesis or urethral catheterization, the sudden loss of severe visceral nociceptive input from the distended bladder may precipitate a marked fall in plasma catecholamine levels, with associated cardiovascular collapse. Immediate resuscitation with fluids (90 ml/kg/h initially) and inotropes (adrenaline or noradrenaline at 0.1–1.0 μg/kg/minute, titrated to effect) will be needed, combined with appropriate reassessment of anaesthetic delivery.

Postoperative care

Analgesia provided by opioids will be needed for all patients. Any opioid-induced tendency to urinary retention will be immaterial, as an indwelling urinary catheter should be placed to allow monitoring of urine output. In general, a urine output of >1 ml/kg/h is acceptable.

Some patients will show a marked postoperative diuresis, which may need fluid therapy well in excess of maintenance requirements. Monitoring of electrolytes and acid–base status should be continued for at least 24 hours after anaesthesia, and until normal oral intake is restored.

Pyometra

Pathophysiology

The majority of reproductive tract surgery in female animals requires access to the abdominal cavity. The commonest indication for emergency ovariohysterectomy is undoubtedly pyometra. Animals may be presented with a range of metabolic disturbances, from minimally affected physiology through to extreme abnormalities of fluid, electrolyte and acid–base balance. Concurrent prerenal failure is common and will normally require volume replacement. Endotoxaemia is also possible in severe cases and will require aggressive antibiotic treatment and cardiovascular support.

Acid–base disturbances may range from alkalosis (secondary to chloride loss from persistent vomiting) to acidosis (secondary to profound hypovolaemia). Under these conditions there is no logical method of determining acid–base status without in-house measurement. Electrolyte disturbances are equally important, with particular attention paid to plasma potassium concentration. While uncorrected acid–base disturbances may be tolerable for short periods, extremes of hypo- or hyperkalaemia, either primary or secondary to pH changes, are never acceptable.

The dehydration produced by continuous dilute urine output with concurrent severe vomiting is capable of producing extreme plasma volume deficits. Clinical assessment can be aided by haematocrit measurement (see Chapter 16). Many dogs with chronic pyometra will have pre-existing anaemia secondary to chronic infection before crisis, coupled with acute blood loss into the uterine contents. Relatively normal haematocrit values in dehydrated patients may drop rapidly following fluid resuscitation.

The reproductive cycle of the bitch, with elevated blood progesterone levels in the postoestrous period, predisposes to insulin resistance and the increased likelihood of new-onset diabetes in the postoestrous period. As this is the commonest time for the development of pyometra, the possibility of concurrent diabetes should be considered in all cases. Emergency ovariohysterectomy in a critically ill patient without detecting and managing any concurrent diabetes is likely to result in severe ketoacidosis and poor outcome. Endotoxaemia is associated with marked insulin resistance and will further complicate management.

Preoperative assessment and stabilization

On the basis of the above considerations it would appear that clinical assessment of dehydration, haematology, electrolytes, renal function, blood and urine glucose and, if available, acid–base measurements are the preferred tools for assessing the morbidity of a pyometra patient. Preoperative assessment may reveal a clinically healthy patient that requires little more than an elective ovariohysterectomy with the normal careful attention to fluid balance appropriate to a patient undergoing a laparotomy. Intravenous access, fluid therapy and appropriate monitoring are essential.

For critically ill patients major resuscitation is appropriate preoperatively. There is little justification for immediate surgery without at least partial correction of fluid deficits and potassium abnormalities. Hyperkalaemia does not appear to be as common as in postrenal failure patients, but conversion of a normal potassium concentration to a hypokalaemic value can be inadvertently achieved. This can even occur while using lactated Ringer's (Hartmann's) solution, despite its potassium content of 5 mmol/l, especially if therapy corrects an unmeasured metabolic acidosis.

For patients with a large estimated volume deficit, central venous access is desirable. Central venous catheters have the advantages of a potentially larger bore relative to peripheral venous lines, and are less likely to be contaminated with either vomit or vaginal discharge.

While a single central venous pressure measurement is of relatively little use because of the large variation in values found in dogs, response to a fluid challenge can be a useful guide to the efficacy of therapy. A prompt rise, followed by return to baseline, can be taken as an indication that fluid administration can be continued. A sustained rise following a bolus suggests caution and close monitoring for signs of pulmonary oedema (see Chapter 7).

Although polydipsia and polyuria are common signs of pyometra, severe hypovolaemia (which can occur rapidly once vomiting limits water intake) can result in anuria due to prerenal failure. Restoration of urine output is essential in these patients prior to anaesthesia. The advantages of an indwelling urinary catheter must be weighed against its presence in a highly contaminated vagina. In general the problems of iatrogenic cystitis are probably less than those caused by undetected anuria, so a urinary catheter can be justified.

Patients with a ruptured pyometra require aggressive treatment prior to anaesthesia as they will have septicaemia and frequently have severe hypotension that is refractory to fluid therapy. In addition to fluid and antibiotic therapy, support with inotropes may be needed. When open drainage of the abdomen is required, attention to fluid and electrolyte balance and enteral nutrition are essential, as massive loss of protein-rich fluid will be ongoing for several days.

Anaesthetic management

Premedication

Premedication may be varied to suit the severity of the illness. Moribund patients require little if any premedication. Apparently healthy patients may be premedicated as routine, for example with very low dose acepromazine (0.01–0.03 mg/kg) and an opioid.

Induction and maintenance

Induction of anaesthesia should be performed slowly, titrating the induction agent carefully to effect. Propofol may have some advantage under these circumstances as administration over several minutes is usually excitement free and allows continued oxygen administration by mask throughout the process. Boluses of propofol should be avoided as they are frequently associated with a marked fall in blood pressure. Induction of anaesthesia with propofol is associated with an increased risk of postoperative wound infections and might be better avoided in septicaemic patients.

Seriously ill dogs are best managed with a high-dose opioid, or diazepam–etomidate induction, or an opioid followed by ketamine/benzodiazepine (see Chapter 13). High dose opioid inductions are generally associated with cardiovascular stability but marked respiratory depression. All mu agonist opioids produce profound bradycardia at those dose rates used to minimize the requirement for other induction agents. Therefore, a small dose of atropine or glycopyrronium may be needed immediately prior to induction. Choosing a rapid-onset opioid with minimal tendency to cause histamine release allows bolus administration. Methadone, fentanyl, sufentanil or alfentanil are useful agents. Even hydromorphone (0.15 mg/kg i.v.) can be used. Preoxygenation by close-fitting facemask is started before opioid administration. Time is allowed for the opioid to take effect and small increments of propofol or midazolam are then given until intubation is possible. Midazolam has poor ability to suppress swallowing reflexes, even if the patient is surgically unresponsive. This is much less noticeable when propofol or ketamine/diazepam is used for induction.

Following intubation, the patient is then ventilated mechanically (or manually) with enough volatile agent to produce good surgical conditions and a stable cardiovascular system. In general, short-acting opioids need to be administered by either constant rate infusion or frequently repeated boluses to maintain stable operating conditions. Longer-acting drugs such as methadone or hydromorphone will often provide intense analgesia for the duration of surgery.

Monitoring

Monitoring during anaesthesia should follow normal protocols for major surgery. Arterial blood pressure is the main guide for avoiding relative overdose of anaesthetic agents in these critically ill patients. Capnography will demonstrate when spontaneous ventilation is adequate, although in the absence of a ventilator one is limited to manual support of breathing if hypercapnia is detected. Although pulse oximetry provides limited information about a healthy patient breathing high concentrations of oxygen, if there is serious lung pathology hypoxaemia may occur. However, in all patients, pulse oximetry is particularly useful to detect hypoxaemia during recovery. Measurement of anaesthetic gas and inspired oxygen concentrations is helpful if low-flow circle systems are used.

Septicaemic patients can develop severe hypotension during anaesthesia due to a combination of hypovolaemia, depressed cardiac output and peripheral vasodilation. These patients will be critically ill and require both central venous and arterial pressure monitoring to guide management of the circulation. Initial management of hypotension with crystalloid may be supplemented with colloid preparations (see Chapter 16). In those patients where anaemia is present, whole blood or Oxyglobin® provide combined colloid and oxygen-carrying capacity.

When adequate fluid therapy and appropriate anaesthetic management cannot produce an acceptable blood pressure, inotropes and vasopressors are needed to provide an adequate perfusion pressure for vital organs. Adrenaline is the most readily available agent suitable for cardiovascular support. As a combined alpha- and beta-adrenoceptor agonist, it increases both cardiac output and peripheral vascular resistance. An initial infusion rate of 0.1 μg/kg/minute can be titrated upwards to 1.0 μg/kg/minute depending on response. Noradrenaline can be used at the same dose rate as adrenaline and has greater selectivity for alpha adrenoceptors; it will also effectively raise blood pressure. There is some concern that using vasoconstrictive agents compromises blood flow to the splanchnic and renal beds, as it undoubtedly does in healthy animals. Under conditions of endotoxaemia with marked peripheral vasodilation, this is less relevant and improvement in perfusion pressure appears to override vasoconstriction-induced compromise. Dobutamine may be used at 5–10 μg/kg/minute provided preload is adequate, but results with this agent in dogs appear variable.

Postoperative care

The main requirements in recovery are analgesia and a stable cardiorespiratory system. If a high dose of long-acting opioid or an ongoing opioid infusion is used, there is the possibility of drug-induced respiratory depression in recovery. Drug-induced hypoxaemia is easily corrected with supplementary oxygen, but it must be borne in mind that this does not correct the associated hypercapnia. Modest hypercapnia is of less significance than hypoxaemia in the immediate postoperative period.

Ongoing fluid therapy with continual electrolyte and acid–base assessment are also essential postoperatively, depending on the condition of the patient. In the postoperative period, critically ill patients may be given parenteral feeding via the central venous line used for fluid administration and CVP measurement. Alternatively, feeding though an oesophagostomy or gastrostomy tube placed during surgery is a more physiological route of nutrition, provided vomiting has stopped. Oral intake of food and water are the most reliable markers for discontinuation of intravenous support.

Other genital conditions

There are several other reproductive problems that require a similar approach to the classic pyometra case. In particular, prostatic abscesses in male dogs may be large and associated with septicaemia. Although these are primarily managed medically in the initial stages, they may eventually require anaesthesia for drainage or marsupialization. As for the pyometra patient, this requires good abdominal access in a seriously ill animal and management as for pyometra would be appropriate.

Paraprostatic cysts may require anaesthesia for marsupialization but do not usually involve septicaemia. A routine protocol for major abdominal surgery would be appropriate. However, if paracentesis has been involved in their investigation, there is always the possibility of iatrogenic infection in the cyst with major septic consequences.

Testicular torsion is a rare occurrence in normal entire male dogs, but somewhat more common if there is a testicular tumour. Although these patients have lost minimal blood volume, they are likely to present in extreme pain, which will need aggressive management preoperatively and prompt surgery. Postoperative management should be routine.

References and further reading

Caulkett NA, Cantwell SL and Houston DM (1998) A comparison of indirect blood pressure monitoring techniques in the anesthetized cat. *Veterinary Surgery* **27**, 370–377

Cone EJ, Phelps BA and Gorodetzky CW (1977) Urinary excretion of hydromorphone and metabolites in humans, rats, dogs, guinea pigs, and rabbits. *Journal of Pharmacology* **66**, 1709–1713

Davies G, Kingswood C and Street M (1996) Pharmacokinetics of opioids in renal dysfunction. *Clinical Pharmacokinetics* **31(6)**, 410–422

Dyson D (1992) Anesthesia for patients with stable end-stage renal disease. *Veterinary Clinics of North America Small Animal Practice* **22(2)**, 469–471

Ishida Y, Tomori K, Nakamoto H, Imai H and Suzuki H (2003) Effects of antihypertensive drugs on peritoneal vessels in hypertensive dogs with mild renal insufficiency. *Advances in Peritoneal Dialysis* **19**, 10–14

Kalthum W and Waterman AE (1990) The renal excretion of pethidine administered postoperatively to male dogs. *British Veterinary Journal* **146(3)**, 243–248

Ma H and Zhuang X (2002) Selection of neuromuscular blocking agents in patients undergoing renal transplantation under general anesthesia. *Chinese Medical Journal (Engl)* **115(11)**, 1692–1696

Martis L, Lynch S, Napoli MD and Woods FF (1981) Biotransformation of sevoflurane in dogs and rats. *Anesthesia and Analgesia* **60(4)**, 186–191

Milne RW, McLean CF, Mather LE *et al.* (1997) Influence of renal failure on the disposition of morphine, morphine-3-glucuronide and morphine-6-glucuronide in sheep during intravenous infusion with morphine. *Journal of Pharmacology and Experimental Therapeutics* **282(2)**, 779–786

Par-Soo CK, Wang C, Chakrabarti MK and Whitwam JG (2001) Comparison of the effects of inhalational anaesthetic agents on sympathetic activity in rabbits. *European Journal of Anaesthesiology* **17(5)**, 311–318

Robertson SA, Hauptman JG, Nachreimer RE and Richter MA (2001) Effects of acetylpromazine or morphine on urine production in halothane-anesthetized dogs. *American Journal of Veterinary Research* **62(12)**, 1922–1927

Schenk HD, Radke J, Ensink FB *et al.* (1995) Interactions between renal and general hemodynamics in fentanyl, droperidol, ketamine, thiopental and in peridural anesthesia – animal studies. *Anaesthesiology and Reanimation* **20(3)**, 60–70

Sun L, Suzuki Y, Takata M and Miyasaka K (1997) Repeated low flow sevoflurane anesthetic effects on hepatic and renal function in beagles. *Matsui* **46(3)**, 351–357

Wright M (1982) Pharmacologic effects of ketamine and its use in veterinary medicine. *Journal of the American Veterinary Medical Association* **180**, 1462–1471

Yeh SY, Krebs HA and Changchit A (1981) Urinary excretion of meperidine and its metabolites. *Journal of Pharmaceutical Science* **70(8)**, 867–870

24

Caesarean section

Robert E. Meyer

Introduction

Although much has been published on the subject of Caesarean section anaesthesia for dogs and cats, there are limited case-based data available to support or recommend best veterinary practice. The purpose of this chapter is to review the recent veterinary literature on small animal Caesarean section, to review the relevant pharmacological and physiological changes that occur in the parturient small animal patient, and make best-practice recommendations for maternal and neonatal patient care.

Review of outcome studies in small animals

Dogs

Puppy mortality rates are slightly higher for Caesarean section accompanying dystocia than for normal birth. In problem-free vaginal deliveries, the normal proportion of dead-born puppies is reported to be between 2.2 and 4.6% and the proportion of puppies that die in the immediate neonatal period is similar. When dystocia is not followed by Caesarean section, 15.6% of puppies are stillborn and 7.9% of live puppies may die soon after birth.

Moon *et al.* (1998), in a multicentre prospective case series study, reported perioperative management and mortality rates for 808 bitches undergoing Caesarean section in North America between December 1994 and February 1997. For 3410 puppies delivered by Caesarean section, survival rates were 92% immediately following delivery, 87% at 2 hours and 80% at 7 days. In 76% of the litters (614/807), all puppies delivered by Caesarean section were born alive. By comparison, the survival rates for 498 puppies born naturally during the study were 86% immediately following delivery, 83% at 2 hours and 75% at 7 days. Maternal mortality rate was reported to be 1% (9/808); however, 5 of these deaths (56%) were attributed to pneumonia. Given the study design, it is not known at what stage the pneumonia occurred, but aspiration seems the likely cause. Surgery was performed on an emergency basis in 58% of the cases (453/776), most commonly on the Bulldog, Labrador Retriever, Boxer, Corgi and Chihuahua breeds. Breeds associated with elective surgery were Bulldog, Labrador Retriever, Mastiff, Golden Retriever and Yorkshire Terrier. The most common methods of anaesthesia were administration of isoflurane for induction and maintenance (34%), and administration of propofol for induction followed by administration of isoflurane for maintenance (30%).

A later analysis of the same data showed that the following factors increased the likelihood of all puppies surviving following delivery:

- Surgery was not an emergency
- Dam was not brachycephalic
- Four puppies or fewer in the litter
- No naturally delivered or deformed puppies
- All puppies breathed spontaneously at birth
- At least one puppy vocalized spontaneously at birth
- Neither methoxyflurane nor xylazine was part of the anaesthetic protocol.

Methoxyflurane (used by four practices on 19 litters) and the alpha-2 agonist xylazine (used by seven practices on 23 litters) were associated with dead-born puppies. However, 13/23 litters exposed to xylazine were also exposed to ketamine. The authors acknowledge that xylazine may have adversely influenced the ketamine data in their study. No other anaesthetic drugs were either positively or negatively associated with puppy survival at time of birth. It must be noted that methoxyflurane and halothane are no longer available in the USA.

Similarly, no anaesthetic agents were positively or negatively associated with neonatal survival at 2 hours, suggesting there were no differences in residual anaesthetic effects at this time. This finding runs counter to the clinical impression that anaesthetic drugs with a longer duration of action (e.g. long-acting opioids, cyclohexamines, benzodiazepines) might influence puppy survival, when residual depressant effects have been reported in human babies and in primates after Caesarean section. The authors speculate that differences between drugs were not apparent at 2 hours because all dams and puppies were still experiencing generalized depression following anaesthesia and surgery. Both propofol and isoflurane were associated with improved neonatal viability at 7 days, although the authors acknowledge that these agents may have been positively influenced by the presence of spontaneous vocalization and by litter size in their analysis.

Using the same data set, Moon-Massat and Erb (2002) reported factors affecting puppy 'vigour', defined as spontaneous breathing and vocalizing within

2 minutes of delivery. The use of inhaled anaesthetics decreased the odds that all puppies would be breathing or any puppies would be moving at delivery, emphasizing the need for light levels of inhalation anaesthesia. The use of ketamine decreased the odds that all puppies would be breathing spontaneously at delivery. Thiobarbiturates were associated with no puppies spontaneously moving at birth. This finding is consistent with other prospective and retrospective veterinary reports, but runs counter to recommendations for human obstetrical practice (see below). Moon-Massat and Erb were not able to determine the reason for this difference between puppies and human infants within the confines of their retrospective study. Although the use of inhaled anaesthetics, ketamine and thiobarbiturates adversely influenced puppy vigour at delivery, these drugs did not influence neonatal mortality.

Neonatal survival rates following propofol induction and isoflurane maintenance were reported by Funkquist *et al.* (1997) in a prospective clinical study where 141 bitches underwent emergency Caesarean section. Anaesthesia was induced with propofol (6.5 mg/kg i.v.) followed by isoflurane in 65% nitrous oxide and 35% oxygen for maintenance. An intentional 20-minute delay was permitted following induction and before delivery of puppies to allow time for propofol clearance. Of 412 puppies delivered by Caesarean section, 71% (293) survived, 3% (13) were born alive but died within 20 minutes of delivery, and 26% (106) were stillborn. Puppy viability was described as 'often...alert on delivery; most typically, however, they were initially lethargic but suddenly became lively and remained so after massaging and respiratory stimulation'. Funkquist *et al.* retrospectively compared their propofol–isoflurane results with their own prior work, where Caesarean section was performed using epidural lidocaine anaesthesia or intravenous thiopental administered to effect followed by immediate delivery of puppies (Figure 24.1). The data were further subdivided into groups depending on whether puppies had been born prior to Caesarean section. The puppy mortality rate during the first 24 hours was highest with thiopental (20%) and lowest with propofol–isoflurane (6%) and epidural anaesthesia with lidocaine (4%). These rates include puppies that died within the first 20 minutes after delivery (e.g. no spontaneous ventilation). Consideration was not specifically given in the analysis to duration of time that the dam had been in labour prior to Caesarean section, but this was mitigated somewhat by group classification based on the number of live and dead puppies born prior to Caesarean section. When no puppies had been born prior to Caesarean section (Figure 24.1), subsequent postoperative puppy survival rates reported by Funkquist *et al.* for propofol–isoflurane anaesthesia (89%) are similar to the overall survival rates (92%) reported by Moon *et al.* (1998).

In a prospective clinical study, Luna *et al.* (2004) examined the effect of four different anaesthetic combinations on neurological and cardiorespiratory activity in puppies at birth. Chlorpromazine (0.5 mg/kg i.v.) was administered to 24 at-term bitches. Six bitches were in each group and received either thiopental (8 mg/kg i.v.), midazolam (0.5 mg/kg i.v.) with ketamine (2.0 mg/kg i.v.) or propofol (5 mg/kg i.v.) prior to enflurane maintenance, or epidural anaesthesia with lidocaine (2.5 mg/kg; 2% solution) and bupivacaine (0.625 mg/kg; 0.5% solution) with adrenaline prior to Caesarean section. Puppy neurological reflexes were reported to be least depressed by epidural anaesthesia, followed by propofol–enflurane, thiopental–enflurane and midazolam–ketamine–enflurane. There was no difference in puppy heart rate at delivery between groups, although respiratory rate was highest in puppies delivered after epidural anaesthesia and lowest in the propofol group and the midazolam–ketamine group. Two of 21 puppies from dams receiving midazolam–ketamine died within the first 24 hours after surgery and one of the 24 puppies from dams receiving propofol–enflurane died 1 hour after anaesthesia. The authors concede that differences in mortality between groups cannot be attributed solely to the anaesthetic induction agents because other factors, such as duration of labour and puppy condition, may contribute to mortality.

Conventional wisdom holds that prolonged anaesthesia time or a long delivery time are both associated with increased neonatal mortality due to fetal exposure to anaesthesia as well as reduction in uterine perfusion associated with surgical incision and

Group	Percentage of puppies alive at delivery		
	Epidural lidocaine n = 372 pups	**Thiopental** Immediate surgical removal after induction n = 121 pups	**Propofol–isoflurane/N_2O** 20 minute delay after induction n = 380 pups
Group 1 (no puppies born prior to Caesarean section)	83% (229/277)	56% (32/57)	89% (197/221)
Group 2 (only live puppies born prior to Caesarean section)	72% (46/64)	34% (12/35)	70% (55/79)
Groups 3 (both live and dead puppies born prior to Caesarean section) and 4 (only dead puppies born prior to Caesarean section)	71% (22/31)	7% (2/29)	68% (54/80)

24.1 Results of the study by Funkquist *et al.* (1997) comparing puppy survival rates from three different anaesthetic protocols.

manipulation. Indeed, when propofol was used for induction, Funkquist *et al.* (1997) allowed 20 minutes to elapse prior to puppy delivery in order to permit fetal clearance; in contrast, in their earlier study delivery was immediately initiated following thiopental induction in an attempt to limit fetal exposure. Luna *et al.* (2004) initiated surgical delivery 20 minutes following injectable induction and the start of inhalant maintenance, and 30 minutes following epidural anaesthesia. Surprisingly, Moon-Massat and Erb (2002) found no evidence that a very short time between induction of anaesthesia and delivery was advantageous, and puppy survival was not affected by either long anaesthesia time (defined as >45 minutes) or a long delivery time (>10 minutes).

Cats

In contrast to dogs, very few outcome data are available for feline Caesarean section. In one study of feline dystocia, 123 Caesarean sections were performed but no outcome data were given for either maternal or fetal survival. In another study, 26 cats underwent Caesarean section accompanied by *en bloc* resection of the ovaries and uterus. A 58% incidence of dead-born kittens was reported in this group of cats; of live-born kittens, 10% died during the first week *ex utero*. One queen died 9 days after surgery as a result of an ongoing coagulopathy. Without scientific data to support a best-practice approach, anaesthetic choice for feline Caesarean section will continue to depend largely on the drugs and facilities available, as well as the veterinarian's understanding of the physiological and pharmacological changes accompanying pregnancy.

Applied physiology of pregnancy

A number of physiological changes are present in the parturient patient that significantly impact upon anaesthetic management. These changes are detailed below and summarized in Figure 24.2.

Physiological change	Potential effect	Potential complication	Preventive action
Respiratory			
Decrease in FRC, TLV	Closer to alveolar closing capacity	Atelectasis	Intermittent sighs during surgery
Higher oxygen requirements and an increase in V_A	If apnoea occurs	Hypoxaemia occurs quickly	5–7 minutes of preoxygenation with mask at a rate of 5–6 l/minute; oxygen supplementation during surgery
Decreased FRC and increased V_A	Uptake of inhalant anaesthetics is more rapidly achieved	Inhalational overdose possible	Vigilant attention to anaesthetic depth
Cardiovascular			
Increases in cardiac output and blood volume	If not maintained, hypotension	Decreased blood flow to the fetus	Blood pressure monitoring, intravenous fluids intraoperatively ± pre- and postoperatively
Delay in compensatory cardiovascular reflexes to blood loss and hypovolaemia	Less responsive to therapeutic measures	Continued hypoperfusion in face of standard treatment; anaemia as a result of volume loading	Prophylactic therapy; immediate aggressive treatment
Neurological			
Sedative effects of progesterone; oestrogen and progesterone-activated pain transmission prevention	Anaesthetic requirements and drug clearance decreased	Apparent sensitivity to anaesthetics, overdose with injectables or inhalants possible	Vigilant attention to anaesthetic depth
Gastrointestinal			
Delayed gastric emptying	Increased likelihood of stomach ingesta		Rapid induction technique and protection of the airway
Decreased oesophageal sphincter tone	Increased incidence of regurgitation	Regurgitation and aspiration on induction or recovery causing aspiration pneumonia with increased pulmonary damage	Extubate when laryngeal reflexes present
Increased gastrin levels	Low pH of gastric fluid		
Mechanical			
Enlarged abdomen	Diaphragm pushed forward	Hypoventilation, hypotension	Assist ventilation; give oxygen and intravenous fluids

24.2 Physiological changes that occur during pregnancy and affect the anaesthetic management of the patient. FRC = Functional residual capacity; TLV = Total lung volume; V_A = Alveolar ventilation. Adapted from Pascoe and Moon (2001).

Oxygen consumption is increased by 20% in the parturient patient. To meet this increased oxygen demand, tidal volume is increased by 40% and respiratory frequency by 10%, to provide a 50% increase in alveolar ventilation. In addition, cranial displacement of the diaphragm reduces total lung volume and functional residual capacity by 20% due to reductions in both the expiratory reserve and residual volumes. The sum of these respiratory changes means:

- Without supplemental oxygen, the parturient will desaturate quickly should apnoea occur
- Induction with inhaled anaesthetics, and subsequent changes in anaesthetic depth, will occur much faster than in the non-parturient patient.

Maternal plasma volume increases more than red blood cell volume, leading to the 'relative anaemia' of pregnancy. Anaemia is greater as the number of fetuses increases. Cardiac output increases 40%, with increased stroke volume accounting for two thirds of the increase and heart rate for the rest. Autoregulation of fetal blood flow does not occur, as uteroplacental perfusion is pressure-dependent. Compensatory cardiovascular reflexes to blood loss and hypovolaemia may be delayed, and the parturient patient may be less responsive to vasopressor or chronotrope therapy. Colloids may be more effective in treating hypotension than crystalloids for intravenous fluid loading. Ephedrine treatment of hypotension in the parturient patient is controversial. In women undergoing Caesarean section, the use of ephedrine to treat hypotension associated with spinal anaesthesia resulted in fetal acidaemia and lower umbilical artery pH. Although dorsal recumbency leads to aortocaval depression and reduced uterine perfusion in women, anatomical differences and greater collateral circulation tend to preserve uterine perfusion in small animals. Because of these circulatory changes:

- Maternal blood pressure should be routinely monitored during Caesarean section
- If maternal hypotension occurs, fetal perfusion will be reduced
- Intravenous fluid loading is the first choice for treating maternal hypotension.

Anaesthetic requirement is reduced 25–40% during pregnancy. This is due to a combination of increased progesterone and progesterone metabolite levels, which are potent positive allosteric modulators of gamma-aminobutyric acid type A ($GABA_A$) receptors, and increased hormonal prevention of pain transmission, activated by oestrogen and progesterone during pregnancy. Epidural veins are engorged due to increased collateral blood flow, which decreases the epidural and cerebrospinal fluid spaces by 30–50%. As a result:

- Anaesthetic overdose is more likely unless inhaled or injectable anaesthetic doses are appropriately reduced
- A smaller volume of local anaesthetic is required for lumbosacral epidural or spinal anaesthesia to ascend to a specific dermatome.

Increased progesterone levels during pregnancy lead to delayed gastric emptying, increased gastric volume and reduced gastro-oesophageal sphincter tone. The increasing physical size of the uterus causes displacement of the pylorus, and increased gastrin levels result in lowered gastric pH. These gastrointestinal changes can result in:

- Reduced lung volumes
- Increased risk of regurgitation and aspiration during induction or recovery
- Increased pulmonary damage following accidental aspiration.

Pharmacological considerations

Placental transfer occurs with every anaesthetic in common use, regardless of whether the drug is injected or inhaled. The endotheliocortical placenta of dogs and cats allows rapid transfer of drugs from the mother to the fetus. Puppies and kittens delivered by Caesarean section will therefore be exposed to whatever anaesthetics have been administered to their mother.

The amount of drug delivered to the placenta depends on placental blood flow and maternal protein binding, while the amount of drug available to the fetus depends on placental uptake and fetal metabolism and clearance. Drugs cross biological membranes by simple diffusion as governed by the Fick principle, which states:

$$Q/t = \mathrm{K}A\,(C_{\mathrm{m}} - C_{\mathrm{f}})/D$$

where Q/t = rate of diffusion, K = diffusion constant, A = available surface area for exchange, C_{m} = concentration of free drug in maternal blood, C_{f} = concentration of free drug in fetal blood, and D = diffusion barrier thickness. The diffusion constant (K) is determined by factors such as molecular size, lipid solubility and ionization. Drugs with molecular weights <500 Daltons readily cross the placenta, while drugs of 500–1000 Daltons will be more restricted. Most anaesthetic drugs have molecular weights that permit unimpeded transfer.

Highly lipid-soluble drugs cross biological membranes more easily. Non-ionized forms of drugs are more lipophilic than their ionized forms, and thus cross membranes more readily. Opioids and local anaesthetics are weak bases, with relatively low ionization and considerable lipid solubility. This means that maternal-to-fetal concentration gradients are important with these agents, as only 'free', non-protein-bound, drug is available for transfer. At equilibrium, the concentrations of non-ionized drug in the fetal and maternal circulations will be similar. In an acidotic fetus, however, there is a tendency for a weak base to exist in the ionized form, which cannot diffuse back across the placenta into the maternal plasma. This is known as 'ion trapping' and can cause drug accumulation of opioids or local anaesthetics within fetal tissues and plasma, especially with high or repeated dosing.

Anaesthetic recommendations

Specific anaesthetic recommendations for Caesarean section in dogs and cats are provided in Figure 24.3. In general, when faced with an elective or emergency Caesarean section in a small animal, one should:

- Choose drugs with short duration of action or drugs with specific antagonists available (Figure 24.4)
- Use the lowest possible dose of injectable or inhaled anaesthetic agents, realizing that the parturient patient has substantially lower anaesthetic requirements. A general rule of thumb is to reduce anaesthetic dose by 30–60%
- Use local anaesthetic techniques when possible and appropriate
- Monitor blood pressure and provide intravenous fluid support
- Provide supplemental oxygen to all patients
- Provide endotracheal intubation if general anaesthesia is used.

When faced with an emergency Caesarean section, it may be better to use a familiar technique rather than one not used before, even if the familiar technique is less than ideal for this purpose. For general anaesthesia, one can either mask with an inhalant or induce with an injectable agent and maintain with an inhalant. When general anaesthesia is selected, the airway should be secured as quickly as possible to prevent maternal aspiration. The advantage of mask induction is that it is a simple technique that most practitioners are familiar with and fetal depression is rapidly reversed after delivery with the onset of spontaneous breathing. The disadvantages are that maternal aspiration is a possibility prior to endotracheal intubation, and personnel are exposed to waste anaesthetic gases. Although the health effects of long-term exposure to trace concentrations of anaesthetics in the operating room environment appear minimal, it remains prudent to continue to recommend control measures that reduce occupational exposure without compromising patient safety. The author's personal choice is mask induction for cats and very small dogs, and injectable induction followed by inhalant maintenance for larger dogs.

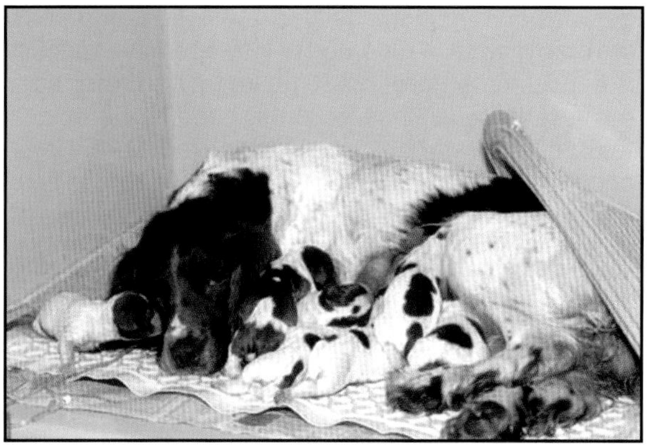

24.4 Anaesthetic agents promoting rapid recovery of the mother allow her to care for her puppies as soon as possible, but puppies should not be placed with mothers still under anaesthetic effects.

The use of premedication will depend on the situation. By relieving maternal anxiety and distress, premedicants can help maintain uterine perfusion. They also reduce the maternal dose of induction and maintenance agents, thus helping to reduce fetal drug exposure. A healthy animal presenting for elective Caesarean section will probably need premedication, while a depressed, toxic animal presenting as an emergency will need much less, if any.

Mu agonist opioids

The mu agonist opioids (e.g. morphine, pethidine (meperidine), methadone, hydromorphone, fentanyl) can provide preoperative sedation and supplemental intraoperative analgesia with minimal cardiovascular effects. Disadvantages include maternal respiratory

Elective	Emergency patient in good health	Emergency patient in poor health	Precautions/concerns
Local anaesthetic techniques			
Opioid premedication plus epidural lidocaine	Opioid premedication plus epidural lidocaine	± Opioid premedication plus epidural lidocaine	May induce hypotension – measure blood pressure and be prepared to treat
	Opioid premedication plus local infiltration of the abdominal wall	Local infiltration of the abdominal wall	May not provide adequate analgesia – be prepared to induce general anaesthesia
General anaesthetic techniques			
Mask induction and maintenance	Mask induction and maintenance	Mask induction and maintenance	Be aware of regurgitation/aspiration risk and only use if risk is low
Opioid premedication plus propofol/inhalant	Opioid premedication plus propofol/inhalant	Propofol/inhalant	Propofol may cause significant hypotension in patient in poor health
Opioid premedication plus etomidate/inhalant	Opioid premedication plus etomidate/inhalant	± Opioid premedication plus etomidate/inhalant	May see myoclonus with etomidate – add low dose diazepam (0.01–0.02 mg/kg) or fentanyl (2–5 μg/kg) intravenously

24.3 Recommended techniques of anaesthesia for Caesarean section in dogs and cats. Adapted from Pascoe and Moon (2001).

depression requiring assisted ventilation, and possible bradycardia. If repeated or intraoperative redosing is expected, fentanyl (3–10 μg/kg i.v.) is preferred as it is less likely to become ion-trapped in the acidotic fetus than longer-acting opioids. Bradycardia often occurs following opioid administration; atropine is the antimuscarinic of choice as glycopyrronium does not cross the placenta and the neonates will probably be bradycardic as well. The antagonist naloxone can be used to reverse neonatal opioid depression (0.01–0.02 mg/kg); if needed, naloxone should be specifically administered to the neonate following delivery to avoid reversing maternal analgesia. Concurrent benzodiazepine administration and mu agonist opioid for anaesthetic premedication or induction is not recommended for bitches undergoing Caesarean section (see later).

Phenothiazines

Phenothiazines (e.g. acepromazine, chlorpromazine) are not ideal premedication agents. The neonate has reduced ability to metabolize drugs hepatically, and phenothiazines have properties of prolonged sedation and alpha-1 mediated vasodilation leading to the possibility of hypotension in the mother. Nonetheless, these agents do not seem to be associated with increased maternal or neonatal mortality and, if judged necessary, can be used effectively at low doses.

Propofol

Propofol induction is associated with better neonatal outcome. Propofol crosses the placenta and reaches the fetus within 2 minutes of administration. Maternal levels are three times higher than fetal levels following a single bolus intravenous dose and six to nine times higher following 1 hour of continuous infusion, demonstrating a placental barrier effect. Mean residence times (mean time that a drug resides in the body) are similar for the mother and fetus following a single intravenous bolus but increased in the fetus with continuous infusion. Fetal elimination is prolonged following a single bolus or continuous infusion, with half-lives more than twice those observed for the mother. Plasma protein binding for propofol is higher in the mother than in the fetus, and this tends to limit placental transfer as only unbound drug can pass. However, as propofol may bind less to fetal plasma proteins than to maternal plasma proteins, it is speculated that the free fraction of fetal drug may be higher and likely to be pharmacologically active. Based on the above, the use of continuous infusion or multiple bolus injections of propofol for Caesarean section anaesthesia cannot be recommended.

Propofol can have significant adverse cardiovascular effects and should be used cautiously in depressed or critically ill patients to avoid reduction of cardiac output and uterine perfusion.

Thiobarbiturate

Recent outcome studies have shown reduced puppy vigour and increased puppy mortality following thiobarbiturate administration. The ultra short-acting barbiturate thiopental is quite lipid soluble and readily crosses the placenta following intravenous administration. In human infants, however, ultra short-acting barbiturates are associated with higher Apgar scores (see later) and less neonatal depression at birth than either midazolam or propofol, due to rapid decline in fetal levels. Induction to umbilical cord clamp times of approximately 10 minutes coincide with declining fetal levels of these agents, and therefore little human neonatal depression occurs when delivery is delayed for at least 10 minutes. It cannot be determined from Moon *et al*'s retrospective analyses when thiobarbiturates were administered relative to time of delivery. In light of the human medical experience, however, one can speculate that puppy outcome may have improved in the thiopental group in the Funkquist *et al.* (1997) report if more time had been allowed to pass prior to delivery.

Like propofol, the ultra short-acting barbiturates can have significant adverse cardiovascular effects and should be used cautiously in depressed or critically ill patients.

Etomidate

In critically depressed canine patients, a small intravenous dose of fentanyl can be given prior to induction with etomidate. If etomidate is not available, a reasonable alternative would be to substitute a low intravenous dose of propofol (1–2 mg/kg) or thiopental (2–5 mg/kg) together with lidocaine (0.25–1 mg/kg i.v.) to facilitate endotracheal intubation, to start an inhaled anaesthetic such as isoflurane or sevoflurane, and wait at least 10 minutes prior to surgical delivery for fetal levels to decline.

Alfaxalone/alfadolone

Alfaxalone/alfadolone (Saffan®; 4–6 mg/kg) has been recommended for use in cats undergoing Caesarean section because it undergoes rapid clearance from the circulation and produces minimal respiratory depression. Anecdotally, kittens delivered by Caesarean section using alfaxalone/alfadolone are reported to appear sleepy. There are currently no outcome studies evaluating the use of alfaxolone/alfadolone for feline Caesarean section.

Benzodiazepines

Benzodiazepines should be used cautiously, if at all, in dogs and cats presenting for Caesarean section. Benzodiazepines are lipophilic, undissociated agents that readily penetrate membranes. Rapid placental transfer with significant fetal uptake occurs with these agents and elimination from the newborn is quite slow. In veterinary medicine, these agents are used mainly for their centrally mediated muscle relaxant effects and are frequently combined with other injectable anaesthetics, such as the dissociative ketamine. In human obstetrical practice, maternal benzodiazepine administration during labour is associated with lower Apgar and neurobehavioural scores and 'floppy infant syndrome', with symptoms ranging from mild sedation, hypotonia and reluctance to suck, to apnoeic spells, cyanosis and impaired metabolic responses to cold stress. Similar depression of neurological reflexes following midazolam–ketamine–enflurane anaesthesia has been observed in puppies. It is not known whether neonatal kittens are neurologically depressed by benzodiazepines, but this seems likely. A specific antagonist, flumazenil (0.01–0.03 mg/kg; 0.1 mg/ml), is available. Although flumazenil does not seem to be effective in cats, it can be tried.

Ketamine

Ketamine provides better maternal cardiovascular stability, especially in sick or depressed animals, but provides more fetal depression, necessitating intensive resuscitation. Although ketamine does not affect puppy survival, ketamine depresses puppies delivered by Caesarean section, reduces spontaneous breathing at birth and reduces puppy neurological reflexes. Because ketamine and other dissociative anaesthetics, such as Telazol® (tiletamine/zolazepam), require concurrent benzodiazepine administration, these agents should also be used only if absolutely necessary and then only at the lowest practical dose.

Alpha-2 agonists

The alpha-2 agonists increase puppy mortality, probably by reducing uterine perfusion. Moon *et al.* (2000) found that puppies were more likely to be dead at delivery when xylazine was administered. Bradycardia, hypertension and hypoxia lasting 20 minutes occurred in fetal lambs when xylazine was administered to awake pregnant ewes. Goats receiving 40 μg/kg of medetomidine i.m. (equivalent to a canine dose of 33 μg/kg) demonstrated a 50% reduction in uterine blood flow, resulting in fetal hypoxaemia and acidosis. The alpha-2 agonists should be avoided in small animal Caesarean section.

Local anaesthetics

Local anaesthetic techniques are generally considered the 'gold standard' in terms of optimal fetal and maternal viability, although neonatal puppy survival rates are equivalent with epidural lidocaine and propofol–isoflurane general anaesthesia. When deciding to use local anaesthetic techniques, it is necessary to take into account the time and skill required as well as the amount of adjunctive sedative or tranquillizer drugs that may be necessary to gain maternal cooperation. On the other hand, local blocks can effectively augment analgesia and reduce the amount of more depressing systemic agents required when given concurrently with general anaesthesia.

Caesarean section can be performed using a simple local infiltrative line block (up to 2 mg/kg lidocaine diluted to the volume required to infiltrate the incision site); once the puppies or kittens have been delivered, an inhaled anaesthetic with or without an opioid can be administered if needed for closure.

Jones (2001) recently reviewed epidural anaesthesia in small animals. Lidocaine (2–3 mg/kg, up to 6 ml maximum volume) is the preferred agent for Caesarean section due to its quick onset and relatively short duration of action; adrenaline (5 μg/ml) may be added to prolong maternal analgesia and further reduce systemic uptake. Should the dura mater be penetrated by the needle and cerebrospinal fluid obtained, as is likely in cats and small dogs, an attempt can be made to replace the needle into the epidural space; alternatively, 50% of the calculated epidural dose can be administered into the subarachnoid space. Care must be taken not to push the needle to the floor of the spinal canal and penetrate the distended epidural veins.

Hypotension secondary to temporary midthoracic sympathetic blockade may occur with spinal anaesthesia, and respiratory compromise or arrest can occur should the block ascend to the cervical region. Hypotension associated with spinal anaesthesia can reduce uterine blood flow and umbilical cord pH more than epidural or general anaesthesia. Local anaesthetics can cause fetal depression when ion-trapped within an acidotic fetus, but this is usually a problem only when very high or repeat doses are administered.

Postoperative analgesia

Both the non-steroidal anti-inflammatory agents (NSAIDs) and the opioids are useful drugs for controlling maternal post-Caesarean pain. The NSAIDs are particularly attractive as they are unlikely to produce maternal depression, identified by Moon *et al.* (2000) as a cause of reduced litter survival. NSAIDs (carprofen, meloxicam) should be administered prior to surgery for optimal postoperative pain control. Although platelet aggregation is reduced by NSAIDs, bleeding times are not increased following ketoprofen, meloxicam or carprofen. Both NSAIDs and opioids will partition into breast milk, however the amounts are very low such that postoperative use of these drugs for maternal pain control is considered safe for breast-feeding human infants.

Fluids

A balanced isotonic crystalloid solution (e.g. lactated Ringer's solution) should be administered intravenously at 5–10 ml/kg/h during surgical procedures to maintain uterine perfusion. As previously stated, colloids (e.g. 6% hetastarch) may be more effective in treating hypotension (see Chapter 16).

Neonatal resuscitation

A warm, dry box should be prepared ahead of time to receive the neonates. Immediately following delivery, the neonate should be placed on a clean dry warm towel and any membranes and fluid cleared from its nose and mouth. Suction equipment is useful, but cotton-tipped swabs and a bulb syringe can be used effectively. Vigorous body rubbing is used to dry the neonate and to stimulate spontaneous breathing. Swinging the neonate to clear fluids probably does not help much and may even be harmful. Mouth-to-mouth resuscitation can be used if there is difficulty taking the first breath, or the trachea can be intubated to permit positive pressure ventilation.

A slow heart rate, as determined by auscultation, palpation, or Doppler ultrasonography, may indicate neonatal hypoxia. Neonatal oxygen therapy has the potential to raise newborn arterial oxygen tension significantly. Growing evidence from both animal and human studies, however, suggests that 100% oxygen may have adverse effects on neonatal breathing physiology and cerebral circulation due to free radical formation. Room air is seemingly as effective as 100% oxygen for neonatal resuscitation, with reduced neonatal mortality reported in human infants resuscitated with room air, and no evidence of harm. Oxygen should still be available during resuscitation, however, especially for compromised neonates (Figure 24.5).

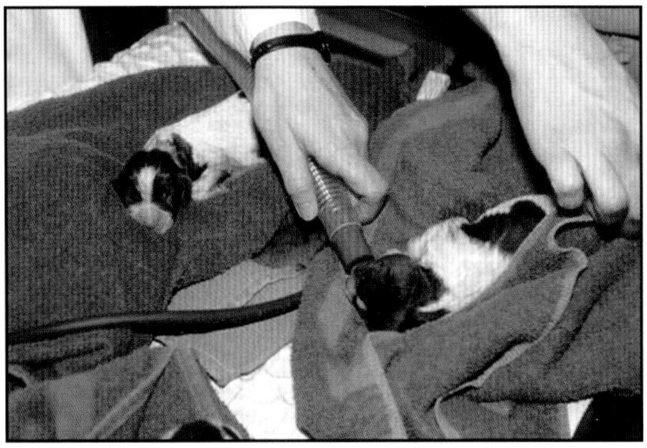

24.5 Puppies hypoventilating from the effects of anaesthetic agents may require supplemental oxygen using the 'flow-by' technique which rarely raises the inspired oxygen to 100%.

Although opioids were not identified during Caesarean section as risk factors, naloxone (1–10 µg/kg) can be administered intramuscularly, into the neonatal umbilical vein, or dripped sublingually to reverse opioid depression, if deemed necessary. It is difficult to recommend the routine use of doxapram, an analeptic used as a respiratory stimulant, for neonatal resuscitation. Doxapram is rarely used in resuscitation of human infants, is not effective during hypoxaemia, and is unlikely to result in a positive response when administered to a neonate that is hypoxaemic due to hypoventilation.

Acupuncture stimulation of the governor vessel 26 point (GV 26) has been successfully used to resuscitate neonatal kittens following Caesarean section. A hypodermic 25 gauge 1.6 cm needle can be used instead of a traditional acupuncture needle. The needle is inserted in the midline of the most dorsal aspect of the area between the upper lip and the nose (philtrum). The needle hub is held between the thumb and index finger and the needle pressed 2–4 mm into the skin and subcutaneous tissue. Vigorous needle stimulation is continued until signs of arousal are observed. Acupuncture treatment of GV 26 may stimulate the sympathetic nervous system, as well as the respiratory and cardiovascular systems.

Seymour (1999) suggested applying Apgar scoring to examine neonatal survival following Caesarean section in small animals. Apgar scores, named after the medical anaesthetist Virginia Apgar, are used to assess the condition of human infants at birth. Each of five physical signs traditionally used by anaesthetists to monitor patient condition: heart rate, respiratory effort, muscle tone, reflex irritability and colour, are scored at 1, 5 and 10 minutes following birth. The scores provide a snapshot of the newborn's status and the effectiveness of resuscitation over time. The Apgar score is sufficiently sensitive to detect differences between newborns whose mothers received spinal *versus* general anaesthesia for Caesarean section, but is not specific for the effects of anaesthesia on neonates. Although a complete Apgar score for each puppy in a litter would be impractical, Luna *et al.* (2004) applied an Apgar-like evaluation system (heart and respiratory rate; the withdrawal, suction and anogenital reflexes; and the magnum and flexion reflexes) to evaluate neonatal depression effectively following elective Caesarean section. Similar studies in cats undergoing Caesarean section using such a scoring system would be very useful in improving patient care.

Anaesthesia for pregnant patients not undergoing Caesarean section

The objectives for managing anaesthesia in parturient patients undergoing non-obstetrical operative procedures are preservation of maternal safety and avoidance of intrauterine fetal hypoxaemia and acidosis due to reduced uterine perfusion. In this situation, the fetus is a passive recipient of maternal anaesthesia and is generally only affected indirectly by maternal haemodynamic or ventilatory changes. No anaesthetic, opioid, sedative–hypnotic or anxiolytic drug appears to be teratogenic nor safer than another drug for this purpose.

When the fetuses are to be killed at the time of ovariohysterectomy, the goal is to anaesthetize the fetuses *in utero* so that they can be euthanased without distress. The anaesthetic plan for the dam should take into consideration all the physiological and pharmacological changes associated with pregnancy. As stated previously, the fetuses will be passively anaesthetized by maternal exposure to the induction and maintenance agents. An overdose of pentobarbital is administered intraperitoneally or intravenously via the umbilical vein to each fetus immediately after the uterus has been removed from the dam to ensure death.

References

Andaluz A, Tusell J, Trasserres O *et al.* (2003) Transplacental transfer of propofol in pregnant ewes. *Veterinary Journal* **166**, 198–204

Andersen AC (1957) Puppy production in the weaning age. *Journal of the American Veterinary Medical Association* **130**, 151–158

Baka NE, Bayoumeu F, Boutroy MJ and Laxenaire MC (2002) Colostrum morphine concentrations during postcesarean intravenous patient-controlled analgesia. *Anesthesia and Analgesia* **94**, 184–187

Brock N (1996) Anesthesia for canine cesarean section. *Canadian Veterinary Journal* **37**, 117–118

Celleno D, Capogna G, Emanuelli M *et al.* (1993) Which induction drug for cesarean section? A comparison of thiopental sodium, propofol, and midazolam. *Journal of Clinical Anesthesia* **5**, 284–288

D'Alessio JG and Ramanathan J (1998) Effects of maternal anesthesia in the neonate. *Seminars in Perinatology* **22**, 350–362

Deneuche AJ, Dufayet C, Goby L, Fayolle P and Desbois C (2004) Analgesic comparison of meloxicam or ketoprofen for orthopedic surgery in dogs. *Veterinary Surgery* **33**, 650–660

Edwards JE, Rudy AC, Wermeling DP, Desai N and McNamara PJ (2003) Hydromorphone transfer into breast milk after intranasal administration. *Pharmacotherapy* **23**, 153–158

Ekstrand C and Linde-Forsberg C (1994) Dystocia in the cat: a retrospective study of 155 cases. *Journal of Small Animal Practice* **35**, 459–464

Erden V, Yangin Z, Erkalp K *et al.* (2005) Increased progesterone production during the luteal phase of menstruation may decrease anesthetic requirement. *Anesthesia and Analgesia* **101**, 1007–1011

Fresno L, Moll J, Penalba B *et al.* (2005) Effects of preoperative administration of meloxicam on whole blood platelet aggregation,

buccal mucosal bleeding time, and haematological indices in dogs undergoing elective ovariohysterectomy. *Veterinary Journal* **170**, 138–140
Funkquist PME, Nyman GC, Lofgren A-MJ and Fahlbrink EM (1997) Use of propofol-isoflurane as an anesthetic regimen for cesarean section in dogs. *Journal of the American Veterinary Medical Association* **211**, 313–317
Gin T, Yau G, Jong W *et al.* (1991) Disposition of propofol at caesarean section and in the postpartum period. *British Journal of Anaesthesia* **67**, 49–53
Gintzler AR and Liu NJ (2001) The maternal spinal cord: biochemical and physiological correlates of steroid-activated antinociceptive processes. *Progress in Brain Research* **133**, 83–97
Hale TW, McDonald R and Boger J (2004) Transfer of celecoxib into human milk. *Journal of Human Lactation* **20**, 397–403
Herman NL, Li AT, Van Decar TK *et al.* (2000) Transfer of methohexital across the perfused human placenta. *Journal of Clinical Anesthesia* **12**, 25–30
Hickford FH, Barr SC and Erb HN (2001) Effect of carprofen on hemostatic variables in dogs. *American Journal of Veterinary Research* **62**, 1642–1646
Ilkiw JE, Farver TB, Suter C, McNeal D and Steffey EP (2002) The effect of intravenous administration of variable-dose flumazenil after fixed-dose ketamine and midazolam in healthy cats. *Journal of Veterinary Pharmacology and Therapeutics* **25**, 181–188
Johnston SD and Raksil S (1987) Fetal loss in the dog and cat. *Veterinary Clinics of North America: Small Animal Practice* **17**, 535–554
Jones RS (2001) Epidural analgesia in the dog and cat. *Veterinary Journal* **161**, 123–131
Lascelles BD, Cripps PJ, Jones A and Waterman-Pearson AE (1998) Efficacy and kinetics of carprofen, administered preoperatively or postoperatively, for the prevention of pain in dogs undergoing ovariohysterectomy. *Veterinary Surgery* **27**, 568–582
Lemke KA, Runyon CL and Horney BS (2002) Effects of preoperative administration of ketoprofen on whole blood platelet aggregation, buccal mucosal bleeding time, and hematologic indices in dogs undergoing elective ovariohysterectomy. *Journal of the American Veterinary Medical Association* **220**, 1818–1822
Littleford J (2004) Effects on the fetus and newborn of maternal analgesia and anesthesia: a review. *Canadian Journal of Anesthesia* **51**, 586–609
Luna SPL, Cassu RN, Castro GB *et al.* (2004) Effects of four anaesthetic protocols on the neurological and cardiorespiratory variables of puppies born by caesarean section. *Veterinary Record* **154**, 387–389
McElhatton PR (1994) The effects of benzodiazepine use during pregnancy and lactation. *Reproductive Toxicology* **8**, 461–475
Meyer RE (1999) Anesthesia hazards to animal workers. *Occupational Medicine* **14**, 225–234
Moon PF, Erb HN, Ludders JW, Gleed RD and Pascoe PJ (1998) Perioperative management and mortality rates of dogs undergoing cesarean section in the United States and Canada. *Journal of the American Veterinary Medical Association* **213**, 365–369
Moon PF, Erb HN, Ludders JW, Gleed RD and Pascoe PJ (2000) Perioperative risk factors for puppies delivered by cesarean section in the United States and Canada. *Journal of the American Animal Hospital Association* **36**, 359–368
Moon-Massat PF and Erb HN (2002) Perioperative factors associated with puppy vigor after delivery by cesarean section. *Journal of the American Animal Hospital Association* **38**, 90–96
Pascoe PJ and Moon PF (2001) Periparturient and neonatal anesthesia. *Veterinary Clinics of North America: Small Animal Practice* **31**, 315–341
Perez R, Sepulveda L and SantaMaria A (1991) Xylazine administration to pregnant sheep: Effects on maternal and fetal cardiovascular function, pH, and blood gases. *Acta Veterinaria Scandinavica Supplement* **87**, 181–183
Reynolds F and Seed P (2005) Anaesthesia for Caesarean section and neonatal acid-base status: a meta-analysis. *Anaesthesia* **60**, 636–653
Robbins MA and Mullen HS (1994) En bloc ovariohysterectomy as a treatment for dystocia in dogs and cats. *Veterinary Surgery* **23**, 48–52
Sakamoto H, Kirihara H, Fujiki M, Miura N and Misumi K (1997) The effects of medetomidine on maternal and fetal cardiovascular and pulmonary function, intrauterine pressure and uterine blood flow in pregnant goats. *Experimental Animals* **46**, 67–73
Seymour C (1999) Caesarean Section. In: *Manual of Small Animal Anaesthesia and Analgesia*, ed. C Seymour and R Gleed, pp.217–222. British Small Animal Veterinary Association, Cheltenham
Skarda RT (1999) Anesthesia case of the month: Dystocia, cesarean section and acupuncture resuscitation of newborn kittens. *Journal of the American Veterinary Medical Association* **214**, 37–39
Spigset O and Hagg S (2000) Analgesics and breast-feeding: safety considerations. *Paediatric Drugs* **2**, 223–238
Stoelting RK and Dierdorf SF (2002) Diseases associated with pregnancy. In: *Anesthesia and Co-existing disease, 4th edn*, p. 672. Churchill Livingston, New York
Tan A, Schulze A, O'Donnell CP and Davis PG (2005) Air versus oxygen for resuscitation of infants at birth. *Cochrane Database of Systematic Reviews* **18**, CD002273

25

Endocrine disease

Craig Johnson and Elizabeth J. Norman

Introduction

The endocrine system plays a major role in the maintenance of the body's internal environment and the regulation of growth and development. Many important physiological systems, such as glucose and calcium homeostasis, are controlled by the endocrine system, which utilizes complex negative feedback loops based on the release of hormones into the blood. The target organs of different hormones can vary from small groups of cells in specific tissues (e.g. the prostaglandins of the female reproductive cycle) to all the cells of the body (e.g. insulin). This means that the effects of various hormones can be widespread and dramatic and also that disorders of the endocrine system can have far-reaching effects upon the body.

The endocrine system is important in anaesthesia in two ways:

- Its function is affected by physiological insults such as surgical procedures. An endocrine response to surgery, which is usually called the stress response, is seen to a greater or lesser extent in healthy patients
- The alterations in function caused by disorders of the endocrine system can alter the response of the patient to anaesthesia and cause additional perioperative management problems for the veterinary surgeon.

The stress response

The 'stress response' is the term used to cover the response of a normal endocrine system to a noxious stimulus. In general terms, the stress responses elicited by different noxious stimuli are qualitatively similar and only vary in their magnitude and duration. Stress responses can be caused by a variety of noxious stimuli in various combinations. The stimuli (or stressors) are detected by the body in various ways and the response is orchestrated by the hypothalamo-pituitary axis, which acts as a common pathway in the generation of the response. The sensory and effector arms of the stress response are illustrated in Figures 25.1 and 25.2.

The stress response initiates a number of alterations in metabolic activity that can persist for several days after the stress of surgery. The changes are

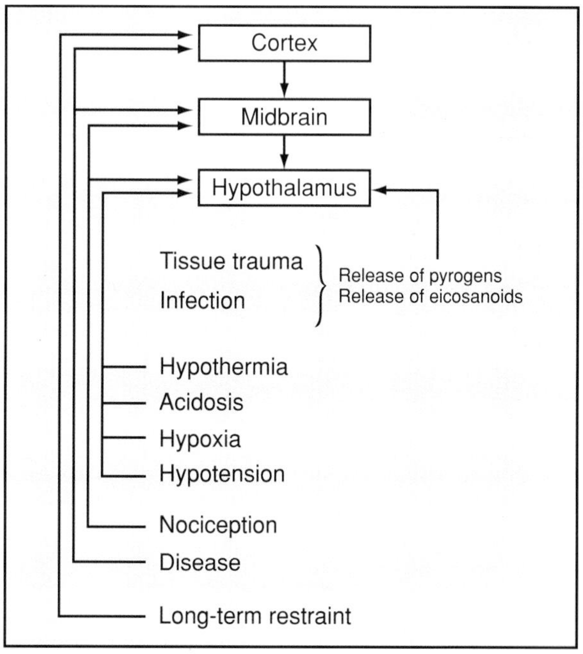

25.1 The sensory arm of the stress reponse.

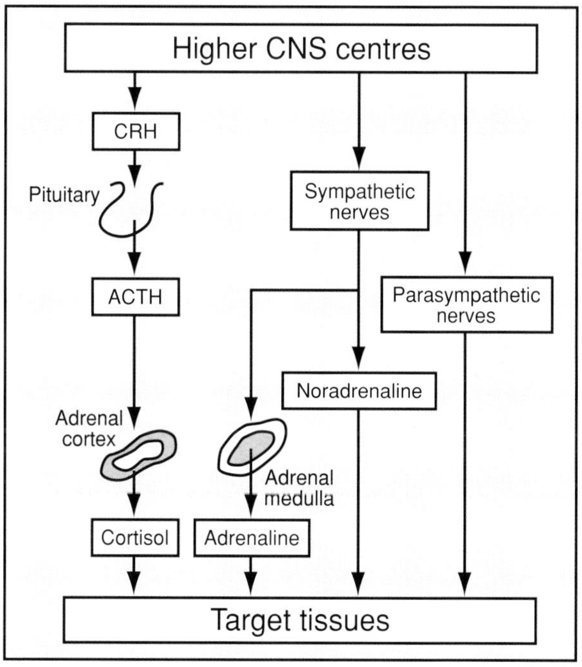

25.2 The effector arm of the stress response. ACTH = Adrenocorticotrophic hormone; CRH = Corticotropin-releasing hormone.

aimed at preserving homeostasis in the face of stimuli that are a serious threat to life. In the initial phase of the stress response, the body conserves sodium and water and enters a catabolic state with negative nitrogen balance. Later in the course of the response, an anabolic phase is entered.

The first phase aims to preserve blood volume (and thus tissue perfusion) and ensures that there are adequate metabolic substrates in the blood for the continuation of function of the vital organs. Increased plasma catecholamine concentrations form an integral part of this phase of the stress response by diverting blood flow to the essential organs of the body. There are also increases in other catabolic hormone concentrations, such as glucagon and cortisol, and concomitant decreases in anabolic hormone concentrations, such as insulin and testosterone.

The second phase of the stress response begins the process of healing damaged tissues. Metabolism becomes largely anabolic, with the increased cellular uptake of substrates and the manufacture of proteins. The changes in plasma hormone concentrations and metabolic nitrogen balance that occur in both phases of the stress response are summarized in Figure 25.3. The two phases are sometimes referred to as the ebb and flow of the stress response.

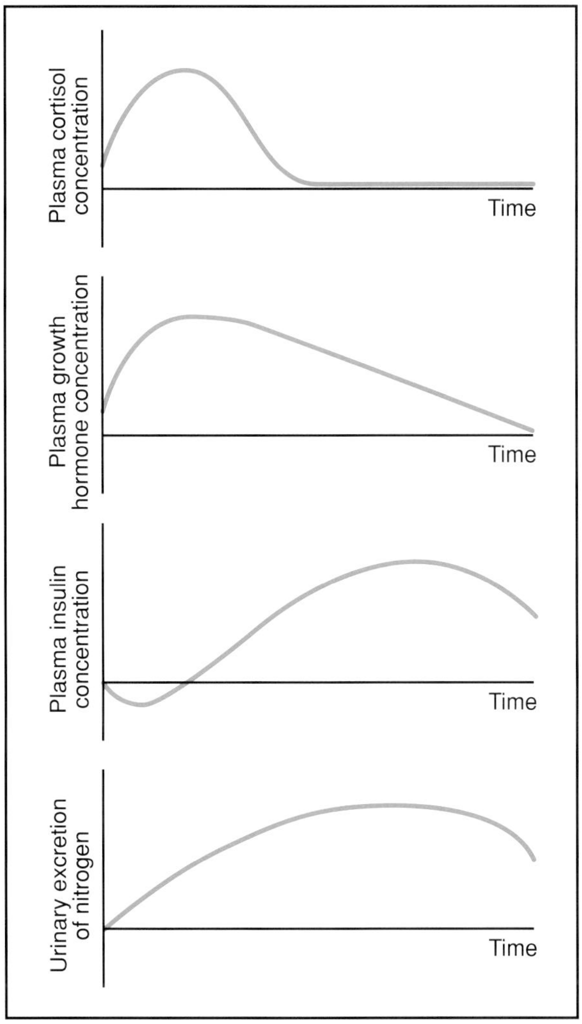

25.3 Metabolic and hormonal changes associated with the stress response.

The alterations in endocrine function that comprise the stress response are appropriate to the preservation of life after 'natural' insults such as severe trauma. Unfortunately, many of the stimuli that initiate a stress response (see Figure 25.1) occur in the surgical patient. In this situation the stress response may be less appropriate. For example, where careful attention is paid to perioperative fluid balance, the sodium conservation seen in the stress response is not required. It may actually be detrimental to the patient and can exacerbate such conditions as congestive heart failure and acute renal failure.

The stress response can be decreased by reducing the number and magnitude of noxious stimuli to which a patient is subjected during anaesthesia. Good anaesthetic practice should ensure that stressors such as hypoxaemia, hypothermia, hypotension, acidosis, etc. are minimized throughout the course of the anaesthetic. In addition, the perception of nociceptive stimuli can be minimized by the use of carefully planned multimodal analgesia.

Some anaesthetic agents, such as the alpha-2 agonists and etomidate, seem to block the stress response in the effector arm rather than reduce sensory input. This direct blocking of the response itself, rather than reduction by the removal of stressors, can be detrimental to the patient. It seems that the inability to mount a stress response in situations where the body perceives that one is required can be very dangerous and even result in the death of the patient. It may be advisable to stimulate a stress response artificially by the administration of glucocorticoids in patients where the endogenous stress response may be inhibited by, for example, hypoadrenocorticism, hyperadrenocorticism or chronic steroid therapy. In these cases, production of endogenous corticosteroid is not regulated by the normal mechanisms and so the endocrine changes that characterize the stress response may only be triggered in response to an increase in steroid hormone concentrations greater than that which the body is able to produce. Exogenous steroids can be used to initiate the stress response, allowing the patient to respond to the stressful situation in a relatively normal way.

Anaesthesia for some specific endocrinopathies

The adrenal gland

The adrenal glands are composed of two parts: the inner medulla and the outer cortex. The medulla secretes the catecholamines adrenaline and noradrenaline, while the cortex secretes cortisol, aldosterone and over 30 other steroid hormones. The cortical hormones are involved in many regulatory processes such as sodium homeostasis and the stress response. Diseases of the adrenal glands usually involve release of too much or too little of one or more of the above hormones. The wide range of target organs of the adrenal hormones means that these diseases can have dramatic effects upon the patient.

Cushing's syndrome (hyperadrenocorticism)

Cushing's syndrome results from the secretion of excessive amounts of glucocorticoids by the adrenal cortex. This may be due to adrenal neoplasia or to the overstimulation of a normal adrenal gland by excessive amounts of adrenocorticotrophic hormone (ACTH) produced by a pituitary tumour. Although treatment of Cushing's syndrome is usually achieved by medical therapy, animals with this condition often require anaesthesia and present particular problems for the veterinary surgeon.

The main physiological changes are listed in Figure 25.4. Dogs with hyperadrenocorticism have alveolar–arterial oxygen gradients above normal, and significant resting hypoxaemia is common. Factors likely to contribute to this ventilatory dysfunction include respiratory muscle weakness, abdominal enlargement, pulmonary mineralization and interstitial disease, and pulmonary thromboembolism.

Cushing's disease (hyperadrenocorticism)	
Slow tissue healing Polydipsia/polyuria Hypercoagulability Muscle wasting Skin changes	Lethargy Hypoxaemia Polyphagia Abdominal enlargement
Addison's disease (hypoadrenocorticism)	
Bradycardia Dehydration Syncope Polydipsia/polyuria	Weight loss Weakness Lethargy
Diabetes mellitus	
Loss of glucose homeostasis Ketoacidosis	Polydipsia/polyuria Weight loss
Diabetic ketoacidosis	
Dehydration Hypovolaemia Metabolic acidosis Sodium deficiency Total body potassium deficit	Severe hyperglycaemia Vomiting Anorexia CNS depression Underlying serious illnesses
Hyperthyroidism	
Hypertrophic cardiomyopathy Hypertension Tachyarrhythmias Tachypnoea and dyspnoea Nervous or aggressive behaviour	Compromised renal function Weight loss Polyuria and polydipsia Vomiting Polyphagia
Hypothyroidism	
Obesity Lethargy Hypothermia	Reduced drug metabolism Bradycardia Intraoperative hypotension
Phaeochromocytoma	
Intermittent weakness Intermittent hypertension Intermittent tachycardia Intermittent tachypnoea or panting Intermittent anxiety	Arrhythmias Reduced blood volume Polyuria/polydipsia Acute collapse Acute haemorrhage
Oestrogen-secreting neoplasia	
Non-regenerative anaemia Thrombocytopenia	Pyrexia Immunosuppression

25.4 Major physiological changes of the common endocrinopathies relevant to the veterinary surgeon.

Most untreated and inadequately treated dogs with hyperadrenocorticism are hypertensive and some 12% are severely so, with systolic pressures above 190 mmHg. The cause of hypertension is not well understood and multiple mechanisms may be involved, such as activation of mineralocorticoid receptors by high levels of glucocorticoids, increased myocardial sensitivity to catecholamines, activation of the renin–angiotensin system and increased vasopressor responsiveness. In spite of the potential for water and sodium retention in these cases, polyuria and polydipsia are extremely common in dogs with hyperadrenocorticism. When deprived of water, most can concentrate their urine, but this response may be inadequate. Replacement fluid therapy is therefore important to avoid hypovolaemia and dehydration, but must be carefully balanced to ensure that any hypertension is not worsened.

In these patients the veterinary surgeon should concentrate on the maintenance of adequate perfusion and the avoidance of perioperative hypertension and hypoxaemia. Preoxygenation and the provision of increased inspired oxygen tensions postoperatively are very important. When good fluid balance has been assured, premedication with a low dose of acepromazine combined with an opioid will reduce afterload and provide a useful reduction in the dose requirements of other anaesthetic agents, although doses that provide noticeable sedation should be avoided because of the concomitant respiratory depression.

Abdominal enlargement is common, reflecting a combination of hepatomegaly, increased abdominal fat, a large bladder and abdominal muscle weakness. During anaesthesia, care should be taken to position the animal so that the weight of the abdominal contents does not compromise respiratory function or blood flow in the vena cava.

Alterations in the structure of connective tissue can have implications for the ability of the tissues to heal after surgery. Skin thinning and reduced elasticity can make placement of intravenous cannulae difficult. Care should be taken with cannulae or other intravenous injections, as alterations in collagen formation can make patients prone to bruising.

Animals with hyperadrenocorticism are at increased risk of pulmonary thromboembolism. Circulating concentrations of procoagulant factors are increased and the anticoagulant antithrombin III is decreased, producing a hypercoagulable state. The predisposition to thromboembolism is further exacerbated by hypertension and sepsis as well as factors that promote vascular stasis such as increased haematocrit, obesity and prolonged periods of recumbency. Preoperative assessment of antithrombin III concentrations may aid in determining the degree of risk of thromboembolism. Prophylaxis with plasma to increase antithrombin III levels combined with heparin and hetastarch to reduce clotting may be indicated, especially when a major surgical procedure, such as adrenalectomy, is planned. A regimen recommended by Feldman and Nelson (2004a) is to administer a transfusion of plasma with 35 IU/kg of heparin added.

Heparin is continued subcutaneously after surgery, with an initial dose of 35 IU/kg tapering over 4 days, and on the fifth postoperative day a single hetastarch transfusion is administered. The anaesthetic and analgesic plan should aim to encourage early ambulation in the patient so that prolonged recumbency is avoided. Postoperative analgesia should be based around continued opioid therapy; non-steroidal anti-inflammatory drugs (NSAIDs) should only be considered with extreme caution as they may precipitate renal failure or gastrointestinal ulceration in animals with high endogenous steroid concentrations.

Dogs that develop pulmonary thromboembolism usually have acute onset of dyspnoea, tachypnoea and cyanosis. Radiographic changes include pleural effusion, pulmonary infiltrates, increased diameter and blunting of pulmonary arteries, decreased vascularity of affected lung lobes and increased vascularity of unaffected lung lobes. At times, however, no radiographic abnormalities are seen. Blood gas analysis usually reveals hypoxaemia (P_aO_2 <70 mmHg; <9.3 kPa) and hypocapnia (P_aCO_2 12–30 mmHg; 1.5–4 kPa). Treatment is symptomatic and should be aimed at increasing inspired oxygen fraction and supporting the cardiac output. Heparinization will prevent the formation of new clots, but will not dissolve those that have already formed. There are many suggested protocols for heparin therapy, with different doses and routes of administration being suggested. One protocol is to give an initial dose of 50 IU/kg heparin i.v. and continue with an infusion of 5–50 IU/kg/h. The aim is to prolong the activated partial thromboplastin time (APTT) by 1.5 or 2 times the reference value. Regular monitoring of APTT is very important to ensure that anticoagulation is adequate but not excessive.

In dogs and cats undergoing adrenalectomy, steroid replacement therapy will be needed during anaesthesia. If bilateral adrenalectomy is performed, both glucocorticoid and mineralocorticoid supplementation will be required. When unilateral adrenalectomy is performed to remove a functioning adrenocortical tumour, glucocorticoid replacement is always required acutely, but mineralocorticoid replacement is not usually required. Chronic suppression of pituitary ACTH secretion will have resulted in atrophy of the adrenal zona fasciculata and zona reticularis in the contralateral gland, but the zona glomerulosa (and hence aldosterone secretion) is usually spared. Preferences for the type of glucocorticoid and the route used vary. Suggested protocols include dexamethasone 0.05–0.1 mg/kg as an intravenous infusion over 6 hours and hydrocortisone continuous infusion at 625 µg/kg/h. However, a higher hydrocortisone dose may be more appropriate since the plasma cortisol concentrations obtained by continuous hydrocortisone infusion in dogs with chronic hypercortisolaemia are significantly less than those seen in normal dogs. A reducing dose of glucocorticoids is then administered in the days after surgery, depending on the degree of adrenal suppression. Mineralocorticoid support can be provided during surgery by the use of sodium-replete intravenous fluids and/or hydrocortisone (which has both glucocorticoid and mineralocorticoid activity). For longer term mineralocorticoid support postoperatively, parenteral desoxycorticosterone pivalate (DOCP) (2.2 mg/kg every 25 days) or oral fludrocortisone (0.01–0.02 mg/kg/day) can be used.

The need for glucocorticoid support during stressful procedures or surgeries also needs to be remembered in dogs on long-term medical therapy for hyperadrenocorticism. Dogs well controlled on mitotane are functionally hypoadrenocorticoid and are unable to respond appropriately with increased glucocortiocoid secretion during stress. Even though trilostane is a relatively short-acting enzyme blocker, it can produce prolonged adrenal suppression in some dogs and steroid supplementation may also be needed during anaesthesia.

Addison's disease (hypoadrenocorticism)

The main clinical signs relevant to the veterinary surgeon are listed in Figure 25.4. Most patients with Addison's disease will have been previously stabilized with medical therapy at the time of surgery. The main problem is their inability to mount an appropriate stress response to surgery similar to that seen in healthy animals. Healthy patients undergoing major surgery develop a 5–10-fold increase in cortisol production. If the patient is unable to produce this increase in endogenous glucocorticoid, it is important that exogenous therapy is provided to prevent adrenal crisis and circulatory collapse in the perioperative period. It should be noted that resuscitation with fluids and positive inotropes may be ineffective in the absence of sufficient plasma steroids and this in itself may increase the suspicion that Addison's disease is responsible for the cardiovascular failure.

It is estimated that the adrenal glands of normal unstressed dogs secrete approximately 1.0 mg/kg of cortisol each day. Bearing in mind the relative glucocorticoid potencies of various synthetic steroids, this corresponds to a dose of 1.0 mg/kg/day of hydrocortisone, 0.25 mg/kg/day prednisolone or 0.03 mg/kg/day of dexamethasone. During the stress of surgery, doses 5–10 times higher should be provided. For minor surgery, a quick return to maintenance requirements is likely, whereas for major procedures at least 3 days of high glucocorticoid requirements should be anticipated. If complications such as fever or ongoing blood or protein loss continue, then 'stress doses' should be continued until these have resolved. After resolution, a weaning dose regimen can be used to return to maintenance requirements. A suggested protocol for glucocorticoid replacement during surgery in dogs with adrenal insufficiency is given in Figure 25.5. Despite the importance of perioperative glucocorticoid administration, the drug should be withdrawn as soon as possible after surgery as side effects may include delayed healing and immunosuppression, leading to an increased risk of postoperative infection.

Animals receiving chronic doses of corticosteroids (including progestogens) for treatment of non-adrenal conditions will also have a less than normal adrenal response to stress and may be at risk of circulatory collapse if not adequately supplemented. The degree of adrenal suppression will vary depending on the type, dose and duration of steroid therapy and also upon individual factors. An ACTH stimulation test prior to

Minor surgery	Major surgery
Preoperatively *either* • Hydrocortisone 4–5 mg/kg *or* • Dexamethasone 0.1–0.2 mg/kg *or* • Prednisolone sodium succinate 1.0–2.0 mg/kg	Preoperatively *either* • Hydrocortisone 4–5 mg/kg *or* • Dexamethasone 0.1–0.2 mg/kg *or* • Prednisolone sodium succinate 1.0–2.0 mg/kg
Immediately postoperatively *either* • Hydrocortisone 4–5 mg/kg *or* • Dexamethasone 0.1–0.2 mg/kg *or* • Prednisolone sodium succinate 1.0–2.0 mg/kg	Immediately postoperatively *either* • Hydrocortisone 4–5 mg/kg *or* • Dexamethasone 0.1–0.2 mg/kg *or* • Prednisolone sodium succinate 1.0–2.0 mg/kg
Post recovery Back to normal maintenance regimen	Post recovery for 3 days *either* • Prednisolone/prednisone 0.5 mg/kg twice daily *or* • Cortisone/hydrocortisone 2.5 mg/kg twice daily *or* • Dexamethasone 0.1 mg/kg once daily for 3 days Day 4 Back to normal maintenance regimen

25.5 Suggested protocol for glucocorticoid supplementation during surgery in dogs with adrenal insufficiency (adapted from the recommendations of Peterson *et al.*, 1984). Similar doses may be administered by any route.

elective procedures may be useful to help judge the degree of suppression and guide the need for supplementation. When severe suppression is present, a protocol similar to that used for primary hypoadrenocorticism as described above would be suitable during the stress of surgery.

Phaeochromocytoma

This is a rare tumour of the cells of the adrenal medulla, which secretes catecholamines. Many of the clinical features of phaeochromocytoma are a result of activation of alpha and beta adrenergic receptors by secreted catecholamines, but signs may also result from tumour metastasis, obstruction of vessels such as the posterior vena cava, or haemorrhage from the tumour. Secretion of catecholamines may be episodic or continuous. The factors causing catecholamine release in a particular patient are variable and unpredictable. These tumours are not innervated and release of catecholamines from them may occur independent of increased sympathetic activity. Applying pressure to or handling the tumour can lead to catecholamine release. Various drugs, including tricyclic antidepressants, droperidol, glucagon, metoclopramide, phenothiazines, naloxone and tyramine-containing foods, such as some cheeses, are reported to precipitate hypertensive episodes in humans with phaeochromocytoma. Times of particular risk in dogs are during anaesthetic induction and surgical manipulation of the tumour.

The veterinary surgeon should be ready to deal with sudden, unpredictable and severe changes in heart rate and blood pressure, tachy- and bradyarrhythmias and haemorrhage. Blood pressure may reach values of 300 mmHg and heart rate over 250 beats per minute. Various arrhythmias may occur, including ventricular premature contractions, atrial tachycardia and third-degree heart block. Hypotension following tumour excision is a common problem and may require unusually high volume fluid replacement. Hypotension is multifactorial, arising from a combination of the sudden withdrawal of catecholamines, hypovolaemia and impaired sympathetic reflexes.

Preoperative stabilization for 1–2 weeks with alpha adrenergic-blocking agents is currently recommended to reduce hypertension, restore circulating fluid volume and promote a smoother anaesthetic induction in dogs. Phenoxybenzamine can be administered at doses of 0.25 mg/kg twice daily and the dose gradually increased until either a maximum dose of 2.5 mg/kg twice daily is reached, or signs of hypotension or adverse drug reactions occur. Severe tachycardia can be treated with beta adrenergic blockers, such as propranolol 0.2–1 mg/kg three times daily or atenolol 0.2–1 mg/kg once or twice daily. It is very important that beta adrenergic blockade only be performed after initiation of alpha adrenergic blockade, as a reduction in beta receptor-mediated vasodilation could severely exacerbate hypertension.

Such preoperative therapy significantly improves surgical outcomes in humans but does not completely prevent complications. Electrocardiography and arterial blood pressure monitoring during anaesthesia are essential and it is useful to have appropriate drugs and fluids ready before the induction of anaesthesia. Preanaesthetic and anaesthetic drugs with the potential to increase complications in animals with phaeochromocytoma include morphine, atropine, acepromazine, chlorpromazine, droperidol, halothane, suxamethonium (succinylcholine) and atracurium. However, the choice of agents used is less important than good preoperative management, careful induction and monitoring.

Intraoperatively, alpha adrenergic blockade can be continued with phentolamine to counter hypertension.

A loading dose of 0.1 mg/kg i.v. is followed by a continuous infusion at 1–2 µg/kg/minute. If hypertension, tachycardia or arrhythmias persist with this therapy, beta blockade with the short-acting drug esmolol can be given. A loading dose of 0.1 mg/kg i.v. is followed by a continuous infusion at 50–70 µg/kg/minute. Magnesium sulphate can also be used to reduce hypertension at a dose of 30 mg/kg over 10 minutes. Treatment of hypotension involves reduction or discontinuation of phentolamine and volume expansion with crystalloids or colloids. These measures are usually effective in countering hypotension and alpha adrenergic agonist therapy is not usually required. In addition to these drugs, a selection of anti-arrhythmics, such as lidocaine, propranolol and verapamil, should be readily available. Complications can continue into the postoperative period, and careful monitoring, including blood pressure, should be continued for 24–48 hours.

Disorders of glucose homeostasis

The two most common conditions in this group are diabetes mellitus and insulinoma. These conditions result in either a functional lack of (diabetes mellitus), or abundance of (insulinoma) circulating insulin. In both cases the normal homeostatic mechanisms are breached, and the animal loses its ability to regulate blood glucose concentration adequately. Long-term effects upon the body's metabolic processes can be dramatic, resulting in various conditions such as chronic intermittent hypoglycaemia, ketoacidosis and dehydration. During the perioperative period, there can be sudden alterations in plasma glucose concentration, which are masked by anaesthesia and so can go unnoticed. In the worst instance, severe brain damage can occur which does not become apparent until the end of anaesthesia.

The metabolic and endocrine changes caused by anaesthesia and surgery alter the balance of glucose homeostasis, and so the maintenance of perfect balance is not a realistic goal even in patients that are well controlled by medical therapy. The aims of the veterinary surgeon should be first to prevent hypoglycaemia at any time during management of the case, to prevent prolonged or severe hyperglycaemia (and the development of ketoacidosis) and to maintain normal fluid and electrolyte balance.

Diabetes mellitus

Diabetic patients present for anaesthesia for a variety of procedures: some procedures are an essential part of the management of the condition (e.g. a bitch in season requiring ovariohysterectomy), some are indirectly related to the condition (e.g. cataract removal) and some are unrelated to the diabetes. Where possible, anaesthesia should only be undertaken once the diabetes is adequately controlled by medical management. Animals that are not properly controlled may be ketoacidotic and/or have unpredictable changes in blood glucose concentrations during anaesthesia. Ketoacidotic patients often have severe metabolic dysfunction, including altered protein binding and hepatic function. This can make them unusually sensitive to anaesthetic agents and can greatly increase the duration of action of these drugs. Poor perioperative glycaemic control may also increase the risk of postoperative infection. The main physiological changes relevant to the veterinary surgeon are listed in Figure 25.4. There are no particular limitations on the type of anaesthetic agents that can be used in diabetic animals, and a regimen should be chosen which suits the experience of the veterinary surgeon and the concurrent disorders being investigated or treated. Short-acting agents have the advantage of allowing the animal to resume eating as soon as possible after the procedure. The use of regional anaesthetic techniques for surgery involving limbs, pelvis and eyes may reduce the hormonal and hyperglycaemic response to stress. The management of blood glucose in the perioperative period is the main additional task of the veterinary surgeon.

Although continued insulin administration during fasting may cause concern about the risk of hypoglycaemia developing, insulin activity is still important during fasting to enable tissue uptake of nutrients. In addition, release of stress hormones such as corticosteroids and catecholamines promotes gluconeogenesis and glycogenolysis and will increase insulin requirement. Thus, insulin should not be withheld unless there is evidence of residual insulin activity from the previous dose. Close monitoring of blood glucose and balancing of insulin activity with dextrose infusion are used to maintain blood glucose in the target range of 8.3–14 mmol/l in the perioperative period. Surgery should be scheduled for the morning. This reduces the need for a long period of fasting and allows better management of the early postoperative period.

Various recommendations are made regarding the proportion of the animal's normal insulin dose to administer on the morning of anaesthesia. Feldman and Nelson recommend doses varying from one quarter to half the animal's usual dose, according to the morning pre-insulin blood glucose concentration (Figure 25.6).

Morning presurgery insulin dose
Pre-insulin blood glucose <5.5 mmol/l: no insulin administered, begin 2.5–5% dextrose infusion Pre-insulin blood glucose 5.5–11 mmol/l: one quarter usual insulin dose, begin 2.5–5% dextrose infusion Pre-insulin blood glucose >11 mmol/l: half usual insulin dose, withhold dextrose infusion until blood glucose <8.3 mmol/l
Blood glucose monitoring
Every 30–60 minutes Goal 8.3–14 mmol/l
Dextrose infusion
Blood glucose <8.3 mmol/l, increase/begin dextrose infusion Blood glucose 8.3–14 mmol/l, maintain dextrose infusion rate Blood glucose >14 mmol/l, reduce dextrose infusion rate Blood glucose >16 mmol/l, discontinue dextrose infusion
Regular/crystalline insulin intramuscularly
Administered if blood glucose remains >16 mmol/l for more than 1 hour after cessation of dextrose infusion Give 20% of usual insulin dose in the form of soluble insulin intramuscularly Repeat no more frequently than every 4 hours

25.6 Protocol for blood glucose management during anaesthesia of diabetic cats and dogs recommended by Feldman and Nelson (2004d).

No insulin is given to animals in which the pre-insulin blood glucose is low, indicating persistent activity of previously administered insulin. In cats, it has been recommended that the full usual insulin dose be given as long as glucose can be measured before and during surgery. Of more importance than the initial dose given is the careful monitoring of blood glucose. This should be checked every 15 minutes during anaesthesia, reducing to every 30 minutes for the rest of the perioperative period. A 2.5–5% dextrose infusion can be administered at rates varying around 2–4 ml/kg/h to lower or raise blood glucose. If severe hyperglycaemia (>16 mmol/l) occurs, indicating the need for additional insulin, short-acting soluble (neutral) insulin can be administered either intramuscularly or by continuous infusion. Continuous infusion of insulin may have advantages in enabling closer control of blood glucose than intermittent administration, but requires the use of an infusion or syringe pump.

Animals on twice-daily insulin can often be returned to their usual insulin and feeding regimen on the evening of surgery. Animals which remain inappetent can be maintained on a dextrose infusion and regular insulin given every 6 hours (depending on blood glucose concentrations) until their condition improves. If a long procedure and recovery are anticipated, potassium supplementation in fluids should also be provided according to the guidelines in Figure 25.7.

Serum potassium concentration (mmol/l)	Final potassium concentration of intravenous fluids (mmol/l)
3.0–3.5	40
2.5–3.0	50
2.0–2.5	60
<2.0	80

25.7 Guidelines for potassium supplementation of intravenous fluids for anorexic animals on insulin therapy. Note that potassium administration rates should never exceed 0.5 mmol/kg/h.

Cats stabilized on glipizide should not receive this on the morning of surgery; blood glucose should be monitored and treated with short-acting soluble insulin and dextrose as outlined for diabetics on insulin. Sulphonylureas interfere with the mechanisms which protect the heart against ischaemic events and, for this reason, it has been recommended that human patients be restabilized on insulin prior to major procedures in which cardiac perfusion may be compromised. It is not known whether such effects are clinically important in diabetic cats.

Diabetic ketoacidosis

Ketoacidotic diabetic patients have severe metabolic abnormalities, which make them very poor candidates for anaesthesia (see Figure 25.4). They are usually dehydrated, hypovolaemic, acidotic and sodium-deficient. There is a total body potassium deficit, but the blood potassium concentration will vary according to the state of renal perfusion and may not reflect this. They are severely hyperglycaemic but fortunately the concurrent presence of hyponatraemia usually prevents severe hyperosmolarity. Magnesium and phosphorus deficiencies may be present or may develop with therapy for ketoacidosis. An underlying serious illness frequently coexists. Common underlying conditions in dogs and cats include pancreatitis, bacterial infection including sepsis, cholangiohepatitis, renal failure, cardiac disease, hyperadrenocorticism and dioestrus.

Elective procedures requiring anaesthesia should not be undertaken if ketonuria is present, although it is reasonably safe to proceed with emergency anaesthesia once improvements in tissue perfusion and acid–base status have been achieved and blood glucose concentration has declined to <16 mmol/l.

In emergency patients, stabilization of cardiovascular status is a priority and will, in itself, begin to address the most life-threatening changes associated with diabetic ketoacidosis. Electrolyte and acid–base status should be determined frequently and fluid therapy should be tailored to correct imbalances. Use of hypotonic solutions (such as 0.45% NaCl) should be avoided. The metabolic acidosis does not usually require specific treatment, as it often resolves with fluid and insulin therapy. Potassium supplementation will be needed in all patients, but may need to be delayed in some if blood potassium levels are initially high. Specific therapy with insulin and glucose can follow this initial fluid and resuscitative therapy. Protocols for insulin therapy in diabetic ketoacidosis involve administration of soluble (neutral) insulin intermittently, given either by intramuscular injection or by continuous intravenous infusion. Dextrose infusions are used to maintain blood glucose between 11 and 14 mmol/l during insulin therapy. It is important to recognize that, even if initial therapy has reduced blood glucose to this target level without the use of insulin, insulin must still be administered in order to reverse ketosis. Close monitoring of central nervous system (CNS) status, blood glucose, electrolytes, urine output and other cardiovascular parameters is needed, as well as blood gas analysis if this is available. Dextrose and insulin therapy can be continued during surgery and into the postoperative period as necessary. These patients often have greatly impaired hepatic function, and any drugs that rely upon hepatic metabolism should be used cautiously.

Insulinoma

Insulinomas are adenocarcinomas of the beta cells of the islets of Langerhans. They secrete insulin, resulting in intermittent bouts of hypoglycaemia that may be accompanied by seizures, weakness, collapse, ataxia, muscle fasciculations and behavioural changes. Episodes may be precipitated by fasting, eating, excitement or exercise. Insulinomas tend to be small, and exploratory surgery is often required to confirm a diagnosis, as well as for treatment. Insulinomas often metastasize to the liver, but removal of the pancreatic tumour can result in remission for 12 months or more.

Surgical resection of an insulinoma presents several challenges for the veterinary surgeon. Affected dogs are usually old and may have concurrent disorders that need consideration, although the main concern specific to insulinoma is the prevention of severe hypoglycaemia. Although animals with chronic hypoglycaemia may become adapted and display few clinical signs, further decreases in blood glucose, even small ones, can result in CNS damage and possibly death.

Preoperative management of blood glucose can usually be achieved with small frequent meals and corticosteroid therapy. During pre-anaesthetic fasting, intravenous fluid therapy with 2.5–5% dextrose should be provided and blood glucose monitored frequently. The aim is to maintain blood glucose concentration above 2.2 mmol/l, but euglycaemia does not have to be attained. It is important not to cause hyperglycaemia, which may provoke release of excessive quantities of insulin from the tumour. For this reason, fluids containing >5% dextrose should not be used. If 2.5–5% dextrose infusion is insufficient to prevent hypoglycaemia, addition of 0.5–1.0 mg/kg of dexamethasone over 6 hours in intravenous fluids may be helpful and if hypoglycaemia persists glucagon can be administered by constant rate infusion at 5–10 ng/kg/minute. Frequent monitoring of blood glucose should continue throughout the operative period and following surgery. Animals may be hypoglycaemic, normoglycaemic or hyperglycaemic after surgery. Hyperglycaemia that occurs following removal of insulinoma tissue is a reflection of insufficient insulin release by the atrophied non-neoplastic beta cells that remain. This hyperglycaemia is usually transient, but insulin therapy may be required if it persists for more than a few days.

Postoperative pancreatitis is a common complication of pancreatic handling during surgery. The veterinary surgeon can help to minimize the risk of pancreatitis by ensuring that fluid therapy prior to and during surgery is sufficient to encourage good pancreatic circulation, and that intraoperative hypotension is avoided. Following surgery, it should be assumed that animals do have pancreatitis and food withheld for the first 1–2 postoperative days.

The anaesthetic management for pancreatic surgery and for patients with pancreatitis is described in Chapter 22.

The thyroid glands

Feline hyperthyroidism

Hyperthyroidism (see also Chapter 19) is commonly seen in old cats with thyroid adenomas or adenomatous hyperplasia. The physiological changes resulting from chronic thyroid hormone excess involve all body systems and can create a fragile metabolic and cardiorespiratory state. Preoperative medical therapy is desirable to stabilize patients before either elective procedures or definitive treatment with surgery or radioiodine. On occasion, however, sedation of uncontrolled hyperthyroid cats must be undertaken before diagnosis in order to facilitate sample collection or other diagnostic procedures. Cats with hyperthyroidism are frequently hyperactive, nervous and aggressive, and they may become severely dyspnoeic and develop tachyarrhythmias with restraint.

The physiological changes of most importance to the veterinary surgeon are listed in Figure 25.4. Cardiac abnormalities are common and may range from systolic murmur, tachyarrhythmia, cardiac gallop, or hypertension to congestive heart failure. Cardiac effects arise as a consequence of increased cardiac output required to meet the demands of the increased metabolic rate and gradually lead to hypertrophic cardiomyopathy. Mild hypertension is common in hyperthyroid cats but severe hypertension may be limited to cats with concurrent renal disease. Respiratory muscle weakness and decreased pulmonary compliance contribute to tachypnoea and dyspnoea at rest. The development of congestive cardiac failure may lead to pleural effusion and worsen dyspnoea.

Hyperthyroid cats have increased renal blood flow and glomerular filtration rate with polyuria with compensatory polydipsia. The presence of concurrent renal failure may be masked by the effect of increased glomerular filtration rate and by loss of muscle mass, which reduces serum creatinine concentration. Urea tends to increase due to increased protein catabolism. Despite the frequent elevation of hepatic enzymes in hyperthyroid cats, histological examination of liver tissue reveals only mild to moderate changes and decreased hepatic function is unlikely in the absence of concurrent liver disease. Rather, the veterinary surgeon should anticipate enhanced hepatic metabolism of drugs because of the increased metabolic rate. Ionized hypocalcaemia is found in 27–50% of untreated hyperthyroid cats (although total calcium concentrations remain normal) and hyperphosphataemia in the absence of azotaemia occurs in 20–43%.

Treatment with thiourylenes (carbimazole or methimazole) for 6–12 weeks to reduce total thyroxine concentrations to within the reference range before thyroidectomy significantly reduces perioperative mortality. In cats where tachycardia and arrhythmias are not controlled by thiourylene therapy alone, propranolol or atenolol should be given for at least 3–5 days prior to surgery. A dose of propranolol of 2.5–5 mg every 8 hours has been recommended, but hyperthyroid cats have increased absorption and decreased clearance of propranolol: a low dose should therefore be used initially and gradually increased if needed. Heart rate is a good indicator of the adequacy of beta adrenergic blockade. For atenolol, a dose of 2 mg/kg or 6.25 mg/cat once daily is recommended. Propranolol may cause bronchospasm in cats with a history of asthma or reactive airway disease (as a result of beta-2 adrenergic blockade).

The details of the final anaesthetic plan will vary from case to case, depending upon the relative severity of the clinical signs. In cats with a relatively healthy cardiovascular system, opioid-based premedication can be followed by induction of anaesthesia with propofol or alfaxalone. Atropine should never be given to these cases (except as an emergency drug) as the increase in myocardial oxygen consumption and arrhythmogenicity caused by parasympathetic blockade can be catastrophic. Ketamine should also be avoided because it causes central stimulation of the sympathetic system, which may facilitate cardiac arrhythmias. When the cat's temperament or degree of cardiomyopathy would make restraint for intravenous cannulation dangerously stressful, an induction chamber can be used with sevoflurane or isoflurane to produce a slow and relatively stress-free induction. When induction of anaesthesia proceeds before intravenous access is secured, a cannula should be placed as soon as possible because sudden changes in cardiovascular function may require the urgent administration of intravenous drugs. Throughout anaesthesia, careful attention should be paid to general homeostatic mechanisms such as fluid balance and thermoregulation. The clinical condition of these cases can change with alarming rapidity and attention to detail can pay dividends in minimizing later complications.

Anaesthesia should be monitored very closely to ensure that an adequate plane is achieved without a dangerous degree of cardiovascular depression. Optimal anaesthesia will reduce the incidence of cardiac arrhythmias; a reduction in inhalation agent and increase in inspired oxygen tension should be considered if arrhythmias do occur. Even so, sudden changes can occur and it is advisable to have a number of drugs drawn into syringes readily to hand. Atropine (an anticholinergic), a beta adrenergic antagonist (e.g. esmolol) and an intravenous anaesthetic agent (e.g. propofol) will cope with bradycardia, tachycardia and inadequate anaesthesia, respectively. It is advisable to have an emergency resuscitation box to hand in case of more severe complications.

Hypocalcaemia following thyroidectomy occurs in 15–82% of cats undergoing bilateral thyroidectomy, depending on the surgical technique used, and is likely to be due to manipulation and stretching of parathyroid vessels, with subsequent thrombosis. However, while calcium concentrations should be monitored postoperatively, treatment is not needed unless the cat develops clinical signs of hypocalcaemia. Therapy with calcium and vitamin D should be aimed at resolving clinical signs of hypocalcaemia while keeping serum calcium levels as low as possible. Hypocalcaemia commonly occurs within 1–3 days of surgery and blood calcium concentrations should be monitored once or twice daily for 5 days postoperatively. If serum calcium is still within the reference range 48 hours after surgery, development of hypocalcaemia is unlikely.

In some circumstances, hyperthyroid cats may require sedation for routine procedures such as blood sampling or radioiodine administration. Pethidine (meperidine) at a dose of 2–4 mg/kg i.m. has proved to be safe and effective in these cases.

Canine hypothyroidism

Hypothyroidism is a common endocrinopathy of dogs. Thyroid hormone deficiency affects most body tissues, although changes are insidious and tend not to compromise homeostasis severely. There is a decrease in basal metabolic rate with a reduction in the rate of synthesis, mobilization and degradation of protein, carbohydrate and lipids. Heat production and energy expenditure are reduced. In most affected dogs, dermatological signs are accompanied by signs of decreased metabolism, including lethargy, exercise intolerance, weight gain and weakness. A mild anaemia is present in about one third of cases. Several other signs are infrequently reported including polyneuropathy, vestibular disease, facial paralysis, bradycardia, vomiting and diarrhoea. Cardiac effects are usually subtle. Loss of the inotropic and chronotropic effects of thyroid hormone leads to reductions in stroke volume, heart rate, arterial blood pressure and contractility. Peripheral vascular resistance is increased and blood volume is reduced. These changes reduce blood flow to tissues but this is balanced by decreased peripheral oxygen requirement. Hypothyroidism may worsen pre-existing cardiac disease, but on its own is unlikely to cause clinically significant cardiac dysfunction. Assumptions about the causal nature of associations between many signs such as megaoesophagus, laryngeal paralysis, bleeding disorders, cardiomyopathy and reproductive and behavioural abnormalities are unfounded and probably reflect a common breed disposition. The veterinary surgeon need not be concerned that these conditions are any more likely in a hypothyroid dog than in another of the same age and breed.

For elective procedures, stabilization of the hypothyroid state with thyroxine therapy is recommended. Improvement in some signs, such as lethargy, occurs within a week, but other signs can take weeks to months to resolve. Cardiovascular signs, such as reduced heart rate and contractility, may only be partially improved over an 8-week period and therefore it may be unrealistic to delay surgery until full resolution of all signs has occurred. In practice, anaesthesia even in uncontrolled hypothyroid dogs carries little additional risk when care is taken. Of main concern is the delay in metabolism and excretion of drugs; this may prolong recovery and may require adjustments in dosage. It is particularly noticeable with drugs that are metabolized by the hepatic cytochrome P450 enzymes. Because so many drugs share this metabolic pathway, it is difficult to design an anaesthetic protocol that avoids such metabolism entirely. The most important principle is to choose short-acting agents and to use minimal doses. Close attention to patient monitoring will assist in optimizing this aspect of anaesthesia.

Negative inotropic drugs should be avoided. This is particularly true of halothane, which can cause a pronounced reduction in contractility since sarcoplasmic calcium uptake can already be reduced. The reduced heat production in the hypothyroid state will predispose to hypothermia and this needs to be anticipated. In humans, other complications occurring in severely hypothyroid patients include perioperative hypotension and gastrointestinal hypomotility. Hypoventilation may also occur as a result of the abdominal contents causing pressure on the diaphragm, and remedial steps should be taken if the end-tidal carbon dioxide is too high.

Male feminizing syndrome (Sertoli cell tumours)

Male feminizing syndrome is produced by testicular tumours that produce excessive quantities of oestrogens or their precursors. Sertoli cell tumours are most commonly associated with this syndrome, and it is more likely to affect dogs with abdominally located testes. Clinical signs include dermatological and feminizing signs, although of principal concern to the veterinary surgeon is the possibility of bone marrow suppression, which occurs in some affected dogs.

Haematological changes are characterized by an initial neutrophilia, followed by a severe pancytopenia. Clinical signs of anaemia, haemorrhage and infection may be present and stabilization with blood products (see Chapter 16) is likely to be required before surgery. Despite castration and supportive care, most cases in which pancytopenia develops are fatal.

Summary

The above discussion has dealt with anaesthesia for patients with common endocrine disorders. There are many more unusual disorders of this system. When planning management strategies for these cases, the best starting point is a thorough understanding of the underlying pathophysiology of the condition. In most cases, the major concern is how best to monitor and compensate for a specific failure of the patient's homeostatic mechanisms. It should, however, be remembered that these animals may be unable to compensate for major stressors, and so the anaesthetic protocol should be chosen to minimize the metabolic insult of the surgical procedure.

References and further reading

Archer FJ and Taylor SM (1996) Alkaline phosphatase bone isoenzyme and osteocalcin in the serum of hyperthyroid cats. *Canadian Veterinary Journal* **37(12)**, 735–739

Atkins CE (1997) Thyrotoxic heart disease. In: *Consultations in Feline Internal Medicine, 3rd edn,* ed. JR August, pp. 279–285. WB Saunders Company, Philadelphia

Barber PJ and Elliott J (1996) Study of calcium homeostasis in feline hyperthyroidism. *Journal of Small Animal Practice* **37(12)**, 575–582

Behrend EN (1999) Medical therapy of feline hyperthyroidism. *Compendium on Continuing Education for the Practicing Veterinarian* **21(3)**, 235–244

Berry CR, Hawkins EC, Hurley KJ and Monce K (2000) Frequency of pulmonary mineralization and hypoxemia in 21 dogs with pituitary-dependent hyperadrenocorticism. *Journal of Veterinary Internal Medicine* **14(2)**, 151–156

Birchard SJ, Peterson ME and Jacobson A (1984) Surgical treatment of feline hyperthyroidism: results of 85 cases. *Journal of the American Animal Hospital Association* **20(5)**, 705–709

Church DB, Emslie DR and Watson ADJ (1999) Plasma cortisol concentrations following cortisone infusion in dogs before and after treatment with cortisone acetate. *Australian Veterinary Journal* **77(10)**, 671–673

DiBartola SP and Brown SA (2000) The kidney and hyperthyroidism. In: *Kirk's Current Veterinary Therapy XIII: Small Animal Practice*, ed. JD Bonagura, pp. 337–339. WB Saunders, Philadelphia

Dluhy RG, Lawrence JE and Williams GH (2003) Endocrine hypertension. In: *Williams Textbook of Endocrinology, 10th edn,* ed. P Reed Larsen *et al.*, pp. 552–585. WB Saunders Company, Philadelphia

Elliott J, Barber PJ, Syme HM, Rawlings JM and Markwell PJ (2001) Feline hypertension: clinical findings and response to antihypertensive treatment in 30 cases. *Journal of Small Animal Practice* **42(3)**, 122–129

Feldman EC and Nelson RW (2004a) Canine hyperadrenocorticism (Cushing's syndrome). In: *Canine and Feline Endocrinology and Reproduction, 3rd edn,* ed. EC Feldman and RW Nelson, pp. 252–357. WB Saunders, Philadelphia

Feldman EC and Nelson RW (2004b) Disorders of the testes and epididymides. In: *Canine and Feline Endocrinology and Reproduction, 3rd edn,* ed. EC Feldman and RW Nelson, pp. 961–976. WB Saunders, Philadelphia

Feldman EC and Nelson RW (2004c) Feline hyperthyroidism (thyrotoxicosis). In: *Canine and Feline Endocrinology and Reproduction, 3rd edn,* ed. EC Feldman and RW Nelson, pp. 152–218. WB Saunders, Philadelphia

Feldman EC and Nelson RW (2004d) Pheochromocytoma and multiple endocrine neoplasia. In: *Canine and Feline Endocrinology and Reproduction, 3rd edn,* ed. EC Feldman and RW Nelson, pp. 440–463. WB Saunders, Philadelphia

Fischer JR, Smith SA and Harkin KR (2000) Glucagon constant-rate infusion: a novel strategy for the management of hyperinsulinemic-hypoglycemic crisis in the dog. *Journal of the American Animal Hospital Association* **36(1)**, 27–32

Flanders JA (1994) Surgical therapy of the thyroid. *Veterinary Clinics of North America: Small Animal Practice* **24(3)**, 607–621

Flanders JA, Harvey HJ and Erb HN (1987) Feline thyroidectomy. A comparison of postoperative hypocalcemia associated with three different surgical techniques. *Veterinary Surgery* **16(5)**, 362–366

Gilson SD, Withrow SJ and Orton EC (1994) Surgical treatment of pheochromocytoma: technique, complications, and results in six dogs. *Veterinary Surgery* **23(3)**, 195–200

Jacobs G, Whittem T, Sams R, Calvert C and Ferguson D (1997) Pharmacokinetics of propranolol in healthy cats during euthyroid and hyperthyroid states. *American Journal of Veterinary Research* **58(4)**, 398–403

Jacoby RC, Owings JT, Ortega T, Gosselin R and Feldman EC (2001) Biochemical basis for the hypercoagulable state seen in Cushing's syndrome. *Archives of Surgery* **136(9)**, 1003–1007

James MP (1989) Use of magnesium sulphate in the anaesthetic management of phaeochromocytoma: a review of 17 anaesthetics. *British Journal of Anaesthesia* **62(6)**, 616–623

Kemppainen RJ (1986) Principles of glucocorticoid therapy in nonendocrine disease. In: *Current Veterinary Therapy IX. Small Animal Practice,* ed. RW Kirk, pp. 954–962. WB Saunders, Philadelphia

Kobayashi DL, Peterson ME, Graves TK, Lesser M and Nichols CE (1990) Hypertension in cats with chronic renal failure or hyperthyroidism. *Journal of Veterinary Internal Medicine* **4(2)**, 58–62

Maher ER and McNeil EA (1997) Pheochromocytoma in dogs and cats. *Veterinary Clinics of North America: Small Animal Practice* **27(2)**, 359–380

Mooney CT (2001) Feline hyperthyroidism. *Irish Veterinary Journal* **54(8)**, 397–406

Nichols R (1997) Complications and concurrent disease associated with canine hyperadrenocorticism. *Veterinary Clinics of North America: Small Animal Practice* **27(2)**, 309–320

Ortega TM, Feldman EC, Nelson RW, Willits N and Cowgill LD (1996) Systemic arterial blood pressure and urine protein/creatinine ratio in dogs with hyperadrenocorticism. *Journal of the American Veterinary Medical Association* **209(10)**, 1724–1729

Panciera DL (1997) Treatment of hypothyroidism: consequences and complications. *Canine Practice* **22(1)**, 57–58

Panciera DL (2001) Conditions associated with canine hypothyroidism. *Veterinary Clinics of North America: Small Animal Practice* **31(5)**, 935–950

Peterson ME, Birchard SJ and Mehlhaff CJ (1984) Anesthetic and surgical management of endocrine disorders. *Veterinary Clinics of North America: Small Animal Practice* **14(4)**, 911–925

Peterson ME, Kintzer PP, Cavanagh PG *et al.* (1983) Feline hyperthyroidism: pretreatment clinical and laboratory evaluation of 131 cases. *Journal of the American Veterinary Medical Association* **183(1)**, 103–110

Rand JS and Martin GJ (2001) Management of feline diabetes mellitus. *Veterinary Clinics of North America: Small Animal Practice* **31(5)**, 881–913

Reed Larsen P and Davies TF (2002) Hypothyroidism and thyroiditis. In: *Williams Textbook of Endocrinology, 10th edn,* ed. PR Larsen *et al.*, pp. 423–455. WB Saunders, Philadelphia

Robertshaw HJ, McAnulty GR and Hall GM (2004) Strategies for managing the diabetic patient. *Best Practice and Research Clinical Anaesthesiology* **18(4)**, 631–643

Shapiro LE and Surks MI (2001) Hypothyroidism. In: *Principles and Practice of Endocrinology and Metabolism, 3rd edn,* ed. KL Becker, pp. 445–454. Lippincott Williams and Wilkins, Philadelphia

Thoday KL and Mooney CT (1992) Historical, clinical and laboratory features of 126 hyperthyroid cats. *Veterinary Record* **131(12)**, 257–264

Welches CD, Scavelli TD, Matthiesen DT and Peterson ME (1989) Occurrence of problems after three techniques of bilateral thyroidectomy in cats. *Veterinary Surgery* **18(5)**, 392–396

26

Neurological disease

Elizabeth Leece

Introduction

Neurological disease may be caused by intracranial disease, spinal disease or neuromuscular disease. Anaesthesia may be performed for diagnostic investigation, surgical intervention or supportive management of neurological disease, whilst other patients with neurological non-related problems may require anaesthesia for other conditions. As ever, a thorough understanding of pathophysiology and the effects of anaesthesia in each situation is important in designing an appropriate anaesthetic protocol.

Intracranial disease

The most common intracranial disease in veterinary patients is epilepsy, although other conditions, such as head trauma and neoplasia, may be presented for diagnosis and treatment. Good understanding of neuroanatomy and physiology allows appropriate anaesthetic handling.

Pathophysiology

The function of the brain is dependent on maintenance of cerebral circulation within the restricted space of the cranium. Intracranial disease or injury interferes with the control of cerebral circulation, predisposing to further ischaemic damage. Anaesthesia should maintain normal neurophysiology whilst limiting the extent of secondary damage. There are four intracranial constituents:

- Brain
- Cerebrospinal fluid (CSF)
- Arterial blood
- Venous blood.

These structures are essentially non-compressible, although CSF and venous blood are connected to low-pressure systems outside the cranium and can be displaced if intracranial pressure (ICP) rises (Figure 26.1). Increased ICP may occur because of trauma, haematoma, oedema or space-occupying lesions (SOLs). Initially, displacement allows good compensation and a relatively stable ICP with increasing volume. However, once compensation is exhausted, ICP will rise rapidly (Figure 26.2). Since space is limited in the posterior fossa, ICP increases relatively early in the case of SOLs in this area and secondary hydrocephalus may occur due to CSF outflow obstruction. Tentorial and tonsillar herniation of the brain matter may occur at the upper limit of ICP or if sudden increases in ICP occur.

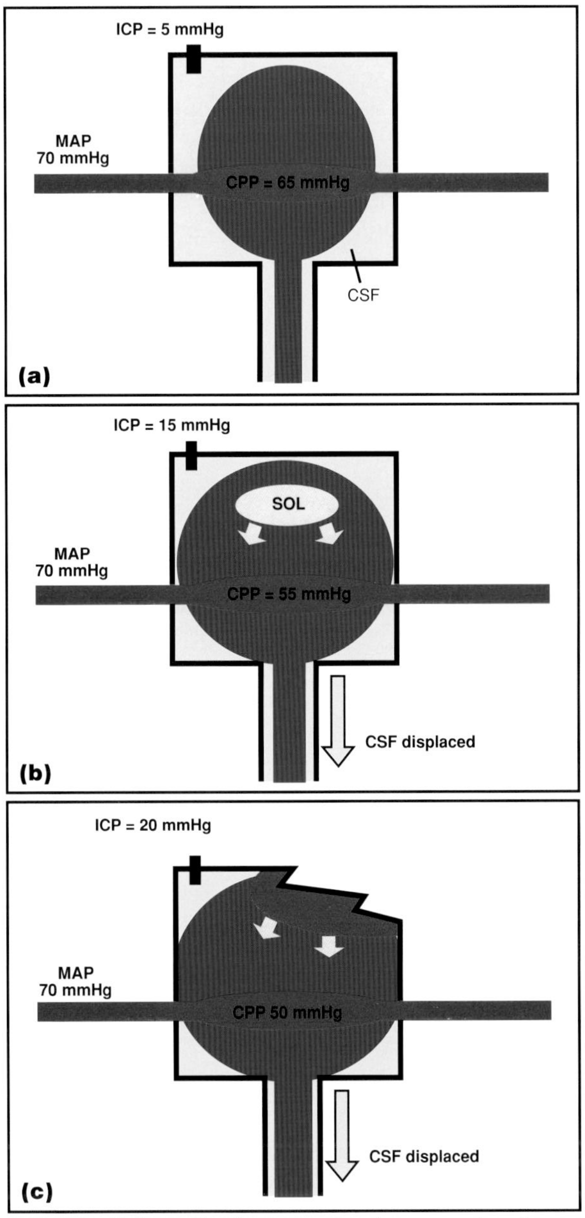

26.1 Schematic diagrams showing normal and raised ICP. **(a)** The normal intracranial compartments made up of the brain (80%), CSF (10%) and blood (10%) and their communication with the low-pressure systems. As the brain is displaced by either **(b)** a space-occupying lesion (SOL) or **(c)** by trauma and haematoma, CSF volume is reduced. As ICP increases, it opposes the driving pressure of the mean arterial blood pressure (MAP) and cerebral perfusion pressure (CPP) falls.

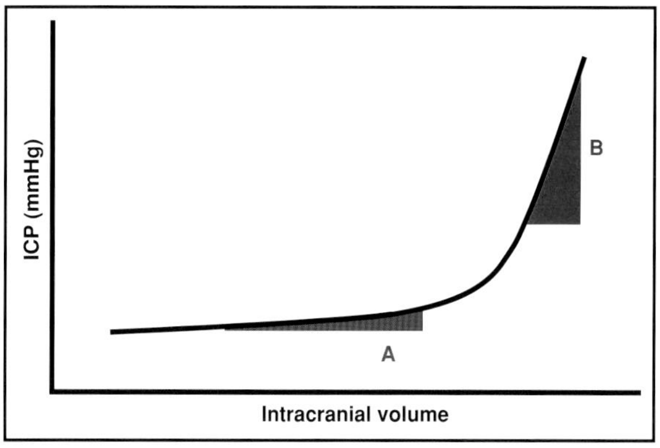

26.2 Initially, compensatory mechanisms accommodate increases in intracranial volume and ICP remains relatively stable (A). Once these mechanisms are exhausted, ICP rises dramatically with only small volume increases (B).

The aim of neuroanaesthesia is to optimize physiology with specific aims, including:

- Maintenance of cerebral perfusion pressure (CPP)
- Maintenance of autoregulation
- Maintenance of flow–metabolism coupling
- Maintenance of carbon dioxide reactivity
- Reduction in ICP
- Avoidance of sudden increases in ICP
- Cerebral protection minimizing primary and secondary damage.

Cerebral blood flow

The primary goal of anaesthesia is to maintain cerebral blood flow (CBF), which is related to CPP and cerebral vascular resistance (CVR):

$$\text{CBF} = \frac{\text{CPP}}{\text{CVR}}$$

Many factors affecting these variables can be manipulated by the veterinary surgeon.

Cerebral perfusion pressure

CPP is determined by the mean arterial blood pressure (MAP), opposed by the intracranial pressure:

$$\text{CPP} = \text{MAP} - \text{ICP}$$

Perfusion is directly dependent on MAP and the anaesthetist should pay particular attention to blood pressure monitoring, and maintenance of cardiac output and systemic vascular resistance. Cardiovascular depression should be minimized, whilst fluid therapy is important in maintaining venous return and blood volume. It is advisable to maintain CPP above 70 mmHg in patients with intracranial pathology, which correlates to a MAP of 70–80 mmHg. The head should not be elevated more than 30 degrees, otherwise a higher MAP would be required.

Cerebral vascular resistance

Autoregulation: In the normal brain, blood flow is maintained at a constant level over a wide range of perfusion pressures (50–150 mmHg). Outside this range, blood flow is dependent on mean arterial blood pressure (Figure 26.3). Autoregulation may be impaired in the injured brain and sudden changes in blood pressure, such as increases in response to surgery, should be avoided. Drugs that maintain autoregulation should be administered.

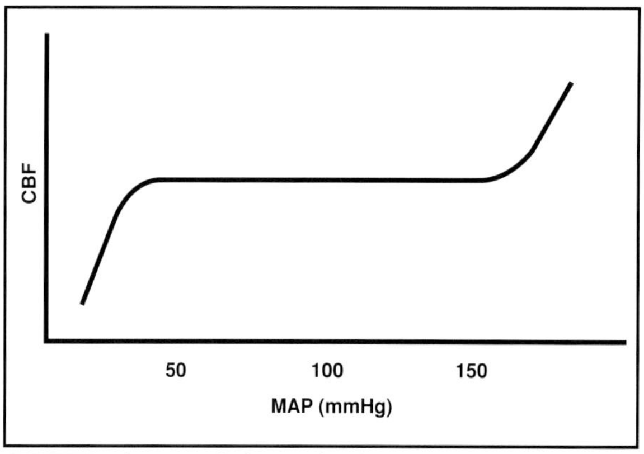

26.3 Autoregulation maintains a constant cerebral blood flow (CBF) over a wide range of perfusion pressures (CPP or MAP) in the healthy brain. Outside this range, or in an injured brain where autoregulatory mechanisms are lost, CBF is directly related to the perfusion pressure.

Flow–metabolism coupling: Cerebral blood flow is normally well matched to metabolic requirements although certain agents may interfere with this coupling.

Chemical: As arterial carbon dioxide levels (P_aCO_2) increase, cerebral vasodilation occurs in a linear fashion (Figure 26.4). At the other extreme, maximal vasoconstriction occurs at low levels. Prolonged, severe hyperventilation (P_aCO_2 <26 mmHg (<3.5 kPa)) has been shown to be detrimental in human head trauma patients, although short periods of hyperventilation (P_aCO_2 26–30 mmHg (3.5–4.0 kPa)) may be beneficial in deteriorating patients whilst other therapy is instigated. In general, P_aCO_2 should be maintained between 30 and 33 mmHg (4.0 and 4.5 kPa) with intermittent positive pressure ventilation (IPPV).

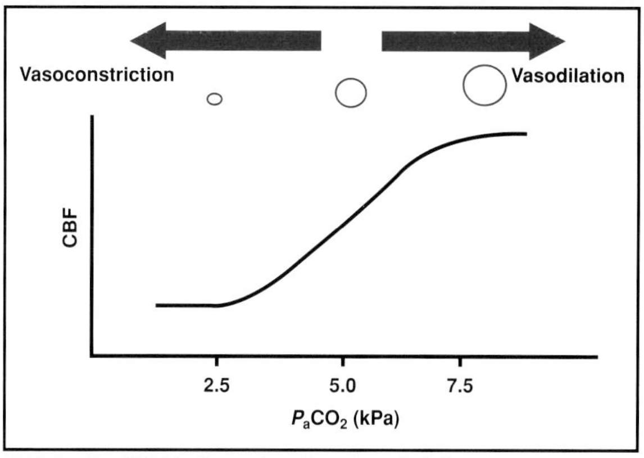

26.4 CBF is linearly related to P_aCO_2, apart from extreme hypo- or hypercapnia when maximum vasoconstriction or vasodilation occurs. Maintenance of P_aCO_2 at the low end of the normal range is useful in reducing blood volume without the risk of excessive vasoconstriction and ischaemia.

Hypoxaemia results in vasodilation of cerebral vasculature and should be avoided perioperatively.

Some anaesthetic agents alter vascular tone. Inhalational agents cause a dose-dependent vasodilation although carbon dioxide reactivity is maintained with sevoflurane and isoflurane to a similar degree, with maintenance of normocapnia counteracting vasodilation. Propofol causes vasoconstriction, so it is recommended in neuroanaesthesia.

Intracranial pressure

Normal ICP is 0–10 mmHg.

Clinical signs of raised ICP include depression, pupillary changes, alterations in respiratory pattern and cardiovascular abnormalities. Currently ICP is rarely monitored clinically in veterinary patients. Magnetic resonance imaging (MRI) findings may be suggestive of raised ICP (Figure 26.5).

With severely raised ICP, vital medullary centres may be compressed, resulting in the *Cushing's triad* (hypertension, bradycardia and respiratory disturbances). The patient aims to maintain perfusion by increasing blood pressure. Hypertension, with a concomitant bradycardia, is seen and ventricular arrhythmias commonly occur in veterinary patients. It is imperative that therapy is instituted to decrease ICP and maintain CPP in these cases, as opposed to treating the secondary cardiovascular effects.

Adequate CPP is more important than ICP *per se*, but the anaesthetist can decrease ICP in a number of ways:

- Positioning: head slightly elevated (no more than 30 degrees)
- Avoiding increases in central venous pressure (CVP) (avoid jugular occlusion, give pelvic support, minimize peak inspiratory pressure during IPPV and use a smooth intubation technique with no coughing)
- Mannitol (0.2–1 g/kg i.v. over 10–20 minutes)
- Furosemide (0.5–1 mg/kg i.v., constant rate infusion (CRI) 1 mg/kg/h)
- IPPV to maintain normocapnia
- Intravenous lidocaine has been shown to decrease ICP in veterinary patients.

Diuretics are classically used to reduce raised ICP although it is important to maintain hydration with appropriate fluid therapy:

- Mannitol decreases blood viscosity by increasing blood volume. Improved rheology increases oxygen delivery to the brain resulting in vasoconstriction and a rapid reduction in ICP. After 15–30 minutes, fluid will move down the increased osmotic gradient from the extravascular to the intravascular fluid compartment resulting in reduced brain volume. Low doses of mannitol are used (0.2–1 g/kg i.v. over 10–20 minutes) and may be repeated as required. CRIs of mannitol do not produce the same osmotic effect and bolus administration is preferred
- Loop diuretics reduce CSF production as well as reducing brain fluid. Furosemide (0.5–1 mg/kg i.v.) has been used in conjunction with mannitol in patients with life-threatening increased ICP.

Pre-anaesthetic considerations for patients with raised ICP

If raised ICP is suspected, mannitol administration may be beneficial. A full range of haematology and biochemical tests should be performed. Many cats with intracranial disease may be dehydrated. Electrolyte abnormalities are common and alterations in sodium should be corrected; the time period over which this should be performed depends on the rapidity of onset. A baseline urine specific gravity measurement is useful to guide fluid therapy.

Premedication will depend on the mental status of the patient. Opioids are useful and do not cause respiratory depression in these patients at low clinical doses. Morphine should not be used since this may result in vomiting and lead to a massive increase in ICP. Occasionally more profound sedation may be required, particularly in cats, and low doses (1–5 μg/kg) of medetomidine have been used although their effects on cerebral vasculature are not well documented (Figure 26.6).

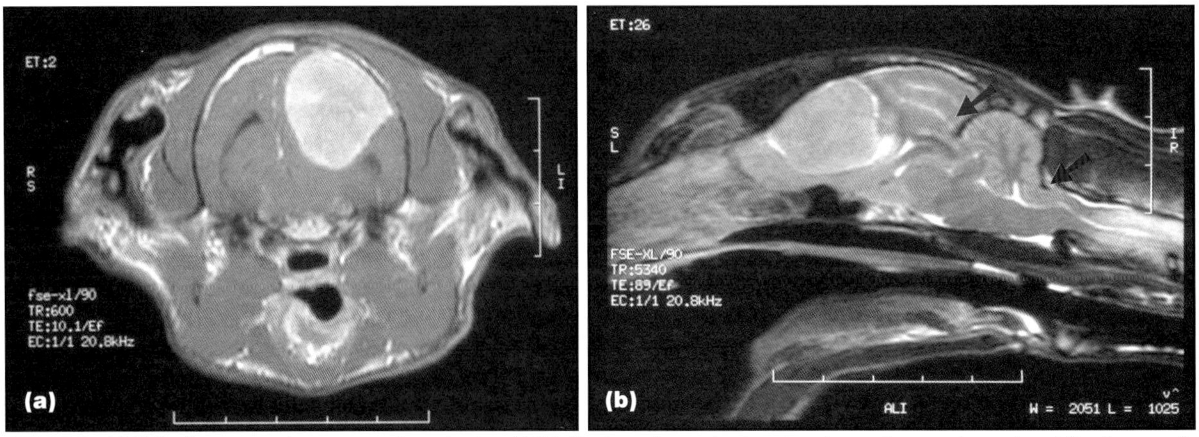

26.5 MRI findings may be suggestive of raised ICP. Reduced ventricular size, loss of normal gyral architecture and midline shift are good indicators of raised ICP on **(a)** the transverse scan, whilst **(b)** a sagittal scan is important to rule out subtentorial (red arrow) or tonsillar (blue arrow) herniation. The degree of oedema may also be assessed as a guide for treatment.

Agent	ICP	Seizure threshold	Neurological effects	Suggested doses in raised ICP
Acepromazine	–	↓	Clinically relevant doses do not appear to affect incidence of seizures	10–30 µg/kg i.m.
Medetomidine	↓	↓–	Cerebral vascular effects not fully understood Dose-dependent systemic cardiovascular effects (i.v. > i.m.) so use with caution with raised ICP. May cause vomiting Decreases flow–metabolism coupling	1–5 µg/kg i.m.
Opioids	–	–	No direct effect on ICP (high doses may cause hypoventilation, ↑ P_aCO_2) Avoid morphine which may cause vomiting Bradycardia with bolus administration therefore CRI more suitable during maintenance (Figure 26.7)	Methadone 0.1–0.2 mg/kg i.m. Butorphanol 0.2–0.5 mg/kg i.m. Buprenorphine 10–20 µg/kg s.c./i.m. Fentanyl 2–5 µg/kg i.m./i.v. q20minutes Fentanyl patch 3–5 µg/kg/h
Benzodiazepines	↓	↑	Potentiate respiratory depression seen with induction agents	0.1–0.2 mg/kg i.v.

26.6 Summary of the neurological effects of commonly used agents for premedication.

Anaesthetic considerations for patients with raised ICP

Patients should be preoxygenated to minimize hypoxaemia during induction. It is important that an adequate plane of anaesthesia is achieved prior to attempts to intubate the trachea. Coughing will cause a profound increase in ICP, whilst the cardiovascular changes associated with poor intubation need to be avoided. Lidocaine, 1 mg/kg i.v. given 1 minute prior to induction, may be used to minimize these responses. Lidocaine has also been shown to decrease ICP. Care should be taken when intubating patients with caudal fossa disease since abnormal head position may be detrimental. Both propofol and thiopental are suitable induction agents and may be combined with opioids such as fentanyl to decrease the response to intubation (Figure 26.7). IPPV and capnography should be implemented immediately following intubation and end-tidal carbon dioxide maintained between 30 and 33 mmHg (4 and 4.5 kPa) throughout. The minimal peak inspiratory pressures required to maintain optimal carbon dioxide levels should be used during IPPV to minimize increased intrathoracic pressure and, therefore, central venous pressures.

Total intravenous anaesthesia (TIVA) has been suggested as the preferred anaesthetic technique in humans and dogs although there is now emerging evidence suggesting sevoflurane may be the ideal agent. A variable rate infusion (VRI) of propofol 0.1–0.4 mg/kg/minute with alfentanil 0.5–2 µg/kg/minute provides good cardiovascular stability during craniectomy in dogs. Remifentanil is well suited to neuroanaesthesia due to its rapid elimination and recovery of respiratory function. In humans, sevoflurane is emerging as the most suitable anaesthetic for neuroanaesthesia and has been used in cats and dogs in association with opioid infusions. Opioid infusions are useful to minimize the amount of anaesthetic required whilst obtunding abrupt changes in MAP in response to surgery. Nitrous oxide should be avoided. A summary of maintenance agents in neuroanaesthesia is given in Figure 26.8.

Extensive monitoring, including direct blood pressure, is vital, particularly during surgery when abrupt changes in cardiovascular parameters may indicate associated brainstem compromise. Increased CVP is avoided as it opposes jugular drainage. CVP is a guide for fluid replacement following haemorrhage. Jugular catheters may be used for this purpose although occlusion during placement can be detrimental. Peripherally inserted central catheters may be introduced into the thoracic caudal vena cava via the medial saphenous vein (Figure 26.9). The use of neuromuscular-blocking agents, such as vecuronium or atracurium, will help decrease peak inspiratory pressure whilst minimizing movement. Low heart rates are commonly seen in neuroanaesthesia, particularly with TIVA, and should not be treated with the administration of anticholinergic agents unless MAP is affected. These drugs will mask changes in cardiovascular status associated with surgery or brainstem compression.

Agent	ICP	Seizure threshold	Comments	Dose
Propofol	↓↓	↑	Should be administered slowly to effect to avoid profound respiratory depression	1–8 mg/kg i.v.
Thiopental	↓↓	↑	Not suitable for CRI	5–10 mg/kg i.v.
Ketamine	↑	↓	Larger doses may increase ICP due to muscle rigidity and increase sympathetic tone Avoid in patients with seizures Has been used in aggressive cats for premedication with midazolam at low doses	2–5 mg/kg i.m. combined with benzodiazepine

26.7 Summary of the neurological effects of induction agents.

Agent	ICP	Seizure threshold	Comments	Doses
Fentanyl	–	–	Good cardiovascular stability May accumulate with prolonged CRI	Bolus 1–2 µg/kg i.v. CRI 2–5 µg/kg/h i.v.
Alfentanil	–	–	Can be used for prolonged CRIs Provide analgesia before discontinuing CRI	0.5–2 µg/kg/minute i.v.
Remifentanil	–	–	Does not rely on liver metabolism and so is rapidly eliminated Provide analgesia before discontinuing CRI	0.2–0.5 µg/kg/minute i.v.
Propofol	↓	↑	Cerebral vasoconstriction results in good operating conditions Prolonged CRIs should be avoided in cats	0.1–0.4 mg/kg/minute i.v.
Sevoflurane	↓	↑	Maintains autoregulation and flow–metabolism coupling Improved cardiovascular characteristics and easily titratable to effect Indicated for neuroanaesthesia	<2x MAC
Isoflurane	↓	↑	Similar to sevoflurane but less favourable neuroanaesthesia characteristics	<1.5x MAC
Halothane	↑	↑	Interferes with flow–metabolism coupling Vasodilation cannot be regulated by IPPV and so should not be used	Not recommended
Enflurane	↑	↓	Do not use in neuroanaesthesia	Not recommended
Nitrous oxide	↑	–	Increases cerebral metabolic demand and CBF	Not recommended

26.8 Summary of the neurological effects of agents used for the maintenance of anaesthesia.

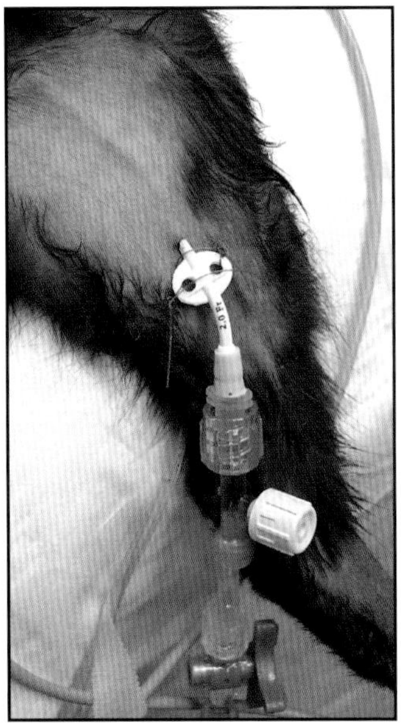

26.9 A peripherally inserted central catheter in a cat. The catheter is measured to the correct length from the point of the insertion in the medial saphenous vein to just caudal to the heart base prior to placement via a 'peel away' technique. Central jugular catheters may also be used but occlusion of the vessel during placement may decrease venous drainage from the brain.

Intraoperatively, normal (0.9%) saline is usually chosen over lactated Ringer's (Hartmann's) solution, Normosol or Plasmalyte as these are slightly hypotonic (see Chapter 16). Lactated Ringer's also contains calcium, which is implicated in secondary brain injury. Hyperchloraemic acidosis may occur with prolonged infusions of normal saline. Routine surgical fluid rates (10 ml/kg/h) are usually used unless higher rates are required, for example during haemorrhage. Hypotension and haemorrhage may be treated with colloids or hypertonic saline. Haemoglobin oxygen carriers (Oxyglobin®) may be used in severe haemorrhage to maintain oxygen delivery although its effects on cerebral vasculature are poorly understood. Cats should be blood typed prior to surgery in case a blood transfusion is required. Placement of an indwelling urinary catheter for urine output measurement is useful.

Postoperative care

Following surgery, the patient should remain anaesthetized until it is normothermic and any haemorrhage has been corrected. Prolonged anaesthesia and ventilation may be beneficial in patients where there has been marked surgical retraction or haemorrhage (Figure 26.10). Patients with severely raised ICP and those undergoing craniotomy under TIVA may have prolonged recoveries. If ventilation is to be continued, a mixture of air and oxygen should be used. Ideally a smooth, rapid recovery is desirable to allow early neurological assessment and sevoflurane provides these favourable characteristics. Good analgesia is required during this time.

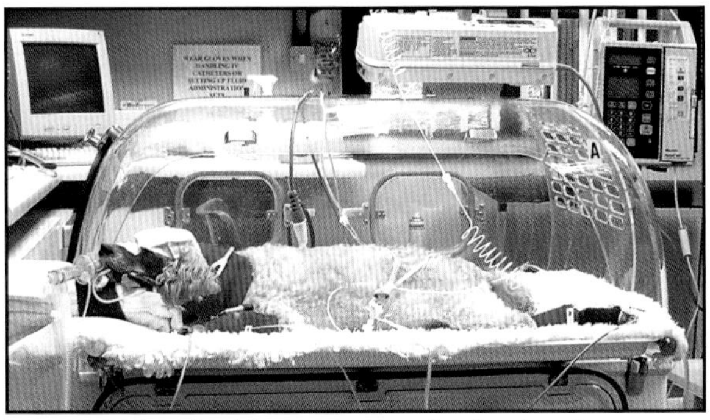

26.10 A patient in recovery maintained under anaesthesia using TIVA. Patients may be recovered in either sternal or lateral recumbency. Sternal recumbency may allow better spontaneous ventilatory function, although care must be taken in arthritic patients, and jugular occlusion should be avoided.

The risk of megaoesophagus and dysphagia due to cranial nerve damage, particularly with caudal fossa surgery, makes it advisable to withhold food for 24 hours. Percutaneous endoscopic gastrostomy (PEG) tubes should be placed for nutritional support in cases of head trauma and caudal fossa surgery.

Dementia, seen as inappropriate behaviour or circling, may be encountered following surgical trauma or haemorrhage and must be differentiated from pain. Sedation is often required in these patients, with acepromazine (5–10 μg/kg) or propofol (0.1–0.4 mg/kg/minute) proving useful. Many of these patients also display hypertension, which may exacerbate haemorrhage. If MAP approaches 140 mmHg, beta-blockers such as esmolol (50–100 μg/kg i.v. bolus or 50–200 μg/kg/minute CRI) or labetalol (0.1 mg/kg slow i.v. bolus repeated to effect or 0.1 mg/kg/h CRI titrated to effect) may be used, whilst acepromazine can also help decrease blood pressure.

Seizure activity should be controlled. Transfrontal approaches carry the risk of sneezing and aspiration, and pharyngeal packs should be placed preoperatively. Subcutaneous emphysema may develop, whilst pneumocephalus presents with neurological deterioration. Constipation may be seen postoperatively, particularly in cats, and straining to defecate massively increases ICP. Patients that may be dehydrated and receive opioids should be rehydrated and warm saline enemas are occasionally administered under anaesthesia.

Analgesia

Humans report headaches following craniotomy and it is not unreasonable to assume that similar pain is experienced by veterinary patients. Caudal fossa surgery is more painful than the supratentorial approach. Patients with increased ICP appear depressed, whilst cats are often aggressive, perhaps suggesting pain. A multimodal approach to analgesia should be adopted in these cases. Opioids may be used at clinical doses, although morphine should be avoided due to vomiting. Care must be taken in severely obtunded patients and drugs titrated to effect. Pupil size and responsiveness may be affected, particularly in cats, interfering with neurological assessment. Non-steroidal anti-inflammatory drugs (NSAIDs) may be used if the patient is not receiving steroids; paracetamol (acetaminophen) may be a useful additional agent for neurological pain in dogs. Following craniotomy, local anaesthetic infiltration around the surgical wound provides immediate postoperative analgesia. Intravenous lidocaine infusions may also be useful for analgesia due to a reduction in ICP.

Anaesthetic considerations for specific conditions

Anaesthesia for head trauma

The first 48 hours following head trauma are critical, with delayed deterioration occurring due to secondary injury and ongoing haemorrhage and inflammation or oedema. Anaesthesia may be required for management of the case, imaging or treatment of other injuries. Thorough systematic evaluation must establish the presence of other injuries. Rapid resuscitation is vital to maintain adequate perfusion to meet metabolic requirements. Analgesia is also required and may aid in patient assessment. Hypotension and hypoxaemia are associated with a poor outcome in humans and aggressive monitoring and therapy are required. Morbidity and mortality is significantly reduced if a CPP >70 mmHg is targeted. Fluid therapy should be administered to improve MAP and CVP and to normalize heart rate. Small volumes of hypertonic saline (1–4 ml/kg) or colloids are initially preferred for resuscitation, thus avoiding large volumes of relatively hypotonic crystalloids. Mild haemodilution (PCV 30–35%) is desirable because it improves cerebral oxygen delivery. Oxygen supplementation is beneficial during initial assessment and prior to anaesthesia.

Hyperventilation can be detrimental in the compromised brain due to vasoconstriction, although mild hyperventilation may be beneficial in the short term during stabilization.

The use of steroids is *contraindicated* in head trauma and they may in fact be detrimental. In particular they will cause hyperglycaemia. Severity of head trauma in veterinary patients correlates with the degree of hyperglycaemia and, since glucose is linked to increased brain injury, steroids and glucose-containing fluids should be avoided. Occasionally, diabetes insipidus may result from head trauma, and careful monitoring of urine output and specific gravity is helpful.

Postoperatively, seizure activity may develop and should be controlled to limit further injury. Nutritional support should be provided for comatose patients and those with facial fractures.

Anaesthesia for patients with space-occupying lesions

Steroids are often used preoperatively to reduce peritumour oedema and, in this situation, can dramatically improve clinical signs. Their use should be continued perioperatively. Positioning for caudal fossa surgery involves flexion of the neck (Figure 26.11) and armoured tubes (see Chapter 5) are useful. Jugular obstruction should be avoided.

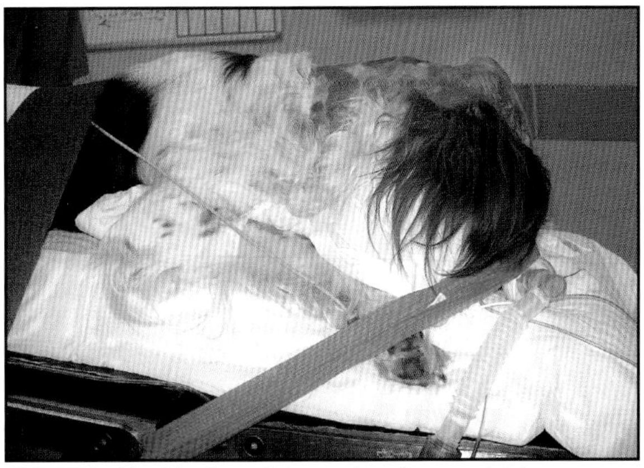

26.11 Positioning of the patient for caudal fossa surgery or suboccipital craniectomy involves flexion of the neck. An armoured endotracheal tube avoids kinking and airway occlusion. Jugular occlusion must be prevented, whilst endotracheal tube connectors must be secure. Capnography is useful for detection of disconnection from the circuit.

Brain relaxation is important to allow surgical access without excessive traction on the tissue. Mannitol can be administered prior to dural opening, to aid relaxation. Meningioma removal can be associated with marked haemorrhage, particularly in cats, which can be minimized by reducing CVP.

Hydrocephalus

Patients may be presented for shunt placement to direct CSF from the ventricular system to the peritoneal cavity. Preoperative stabilization of patients includes reducing CSF production. Intraoperative use of opioids is advisable to avoid stimulation from the tunnelling of the catheter subcutaneously.

Anaesthesia for epileptic patients

Seizure activity should be differentiated from syncopal attacks and extracranial causes, such as hypoglycaemia or hepatic disease. Anti-epileptic drugs alter biochemistry results: phenobarbital increases alkaline phosphatase and decreasing calcium levels, whilst potassium bromide will falsely elevate chloride values. These drugs cause polydipsia, and water should be available until premedication. Intravenous access should be secured and patients observed, allowing prompt seizure treatment. Anti-epileptic medications should *not* be discontinued perioperatively.

Premedication should minimize stress whilst providing analgesia. Manufacturers of acepromazine advise that the drug should not be used in epileptic patients, since high doses of a similar drug reportedly caused a reduction in seizure threshold. However, acepromazine has been used at clinically relevant doses (5–70 μg/kg i.v., i.m.) in epileptic patients and does not alter the incidence of seizures (Tobias *et al.*, 2006). Opioids provide good sedation and analgesia without altering seizure activity, whilst low dose alpha-2 agonists improve sedation in excitable patients. Benzodiazepines can cause dysphoria in non-seizuring patients and should not be used alone. Propofol and thiopental are suitable induction agents, whilst ketamine should be avoided. Sevoflurane and isoflurane have less detrimental effects on neurophysiology than does halothane and they are the inhalational agents of choice. TIVA with propofol is suitable for maintenance and is used for long-term control of status epilepticus. Mask induction may result in excitement and is best avoided. Patients should be monitored carefully in a quiet recovery environment.

Anaesthesia for seizure management

Control of prolonged seizure activity (status epilepticus or cluster seizures) prevents further neurological damage and minimizes hypoxaemia, hypoglycaemia and hyperthermia. Initially diazepam (0.2–2 mg/kg i.v. or rectally) or midazolam (0.05–0.5 mg/kg i.v. or i.m.) may be used whilst loading with other anti-epileptic agents is achieved. Refractory seizure activity may require further sedation or anaesthesia. Propofol (4–8 mg/kg i.v. followed by sedation with CRI 0.1–0.4 mg/kg/minute) is useful, although respiratory monitoring is required. Pentobarbital may also be used initially at 2–15 mg/kg i.v., followed by CRI 0.1–0.2 mg/kg/minute. Occasionally muscle tremors may be seen during recovery from intravenous sedation. These are often localized to the head and neck. Patients should be monitored closely during this time for worsening of such activity, which may indicate actual seizure activity. Temperature and glucose levels should be checked prior to weaning these patients off the infusions. Sevoflurane or isoflurane may also be administered for prolonged seizure control, although endotracheal intubation and careful monitoring are required. Heavily sedated patients require a high level of supportive care including:

- Airway management
- Respiratory monitoring
- Adequate bedding
- Turning every 4 hours
- Bladder care, preferably by placing an indwelling urinary catheter
- Eyes should be lubricated at least every 6 hours
- If intubated, oral hygiene should be addressed including cuff deflation and repositioning, changing endotracheal tube (tubes with low-pressure, high-volume cuffs are preferred) and moistening of the mouth.

Anaesthesia for patients with vestibular disease

Anaesthesia for vestibular disease will often result in a degree of decompensation for 24–48 hours postoperatively and owners should be warned of this. The use of short-acting agents is advisable, with low dose medetomidine and propofol resulting in rapid and complete recoveries. Nausea may be seen following anaesthesia.

Spinal disease

Spinal cord injury may occur because of intervertebral disc disease, fibrocartilagenous embolism, neoplasia, trauma or congenital instability. Anaesthesia may also be required for the diagnosis of discospondylitis or meningitis. Destabilization of the spinal column or surgical trauma may result in further deterioration of neurological signs. Patients will encounter varying degrees of pain and can develop severe neuropathic pain, which can be extremely difficult to manage.

Anaesthesia for spinal disease

Patients may exhibit pain due to compression of neuronal tissue. Analgesia should be provided in the premedication to allow placement of intravenous catheters without the need for excessive restraint. A multimodal analgesic protocol should be adopted, including opioids and NSAIDs with additional drugs as required. This is particularly important for patients with severe neck pain, especially during intubation. An accessible, wide-bore intravenous catheter should be available for rapid fluid replacement where haemorrhage is anticipated.

Careful positioning for the different procedures is important to minimize excessive venous pressure, which may exacerbate venous haemorrhage (see below). Judicious use of IPPV may be beneficial for control of P_aCO_2 because ventilation is often impaired by excessive surgical pressure. Hypercapnia causes vasodilation and may contribute to blood loss. IPPV also maintains a rhythmical respiratory pattern, thus helping the surgeon.

Intraoperative analgesia may be supplemented with intravenous infusions of short-acting opioids, such as fentanyl and alfentanil. Ketamine infusions are proving to be extremely useful during and after spinal surgery and also provide neuroprotection (Figure 26.12). Occasionally, marked autonomic responses are encountered during drilling, when distortion of the vertebral column can cause dynamic compression at the site of intervertebral disc extrusion, and also during manipulation of disc material. This is more common in chronic conditions with nerve root entrapment. The use of opioid boluses or intravenous lidocaine (loading dose 1 mg/kg followed by CRI 25–50 μg/kg/minute) may be helpful.

Many drugs have neuroprotective properties, although this has not translated into clinical benefits in humans. The only agent shown to be of benefit in spinal trauma is high dose methylprednisolone (MPSS) if given within 8 hours after injury, due to free radical scavenging properties during this specific time period, rather than anti-inflammatory actions. MPSS should not be used in the presence of voluntary motor function, since prognosis is good without steroid use. If given after 8 hours, steroids may in fact be detrimental to the patient, with many side effects reported. There is absolutely no indication for their use at this time. Despite documented side effects in veterinary species, many spinal injury patients receive steroids due to the anti-inflammatory action; however, NSAIDs should be the primary choice. Suggested protocols for MPSS are shown in Figure 26.13.

Haemorrhage is commonly encountered during spinal surgery and blood loss, and MAP should be monitored. Hypothermia develops during prolonged procedures in smaller patients and should be minimized.

Analgesia for patients with spinal disease

Neuropathic pain is now well recognized in human patients but may be difficult to identify in animals. Neuropathic pain may be difficult to treat with standard analgesic techniques such as opioids and NSAIDs and a multimodal approach needs to be adopted. Neuropathic pain may result from a variety of reasons, including traumatic injury to nerves, nerve root entrapment, neoplasia (such as brachial plexus neoplasia), discospondylitis and meningitis. Animals manifest pain in several ways, such as depression and withdrawal from human interaction, anorexia, aggression or hyperaesthesia. Many protocols have been used for these patients, including *N*-methyl-D-aspartate (NMDA) antagonists, systemic local anaesthetics, alpha-2 adrenoceptor agonists, gabapentin and tricyclic antidepressants (Figure 26.14). If management is not satisfactory with high dose opioids and NSAIDs, a combination of intravenous lidocaine and ketamine can prove extremely useful whilst the underlying cause is investigated and treated. Lidocaine infusions can be continued for several days in normovolaemic patients without liver disease, although tolerance may develop. Once treatment for the underlying condition has been initiated, a gradual tapering of the dose allows assessment of pain.

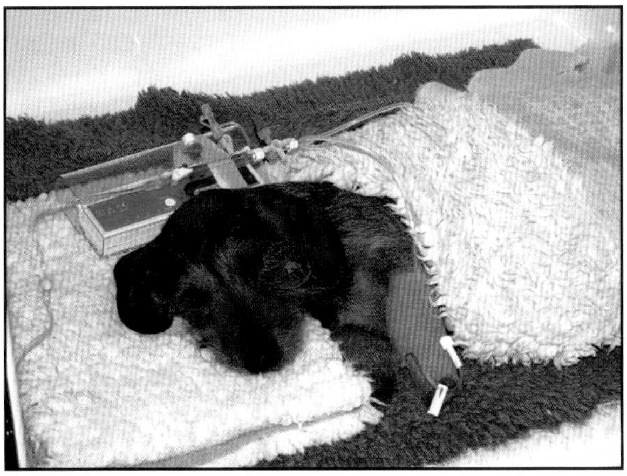

26.12 Ketamine infusions may be continued postoperatively for 12–24 hours and appear substantially to reduce opioid requirements.

Time after injury	MPSS protocol
Up to 3 hours	30 mg/kg i.v. followed by 15 mg/kg i.v. at 2 and 6 hours after initial injection 30 mg/kg i.v. followed by 5.4 mg/kg/h for 24 hours
3–8 hours	30 mg/kg i.v. followed by 15 mg/kg i.v. at 2 and 6 hours after initial injection then 2.5 mg/kg/h for 42 hours 30 mg/kg i.v. followed by 5.4 mg/kg/h for 48 hours
Over 8 hours	Contraindicated

26.13 Suggested protocols for the use of MPSS in patients with acute spinal trauma within the first 8 hours following injury (adapted from Bracken, 2002). Gastric protectants should be used concomitantly with steroid treatment.

Drug	Dose	Comments
Opioids	Methadone 0.2–0.5 mg/kg s.c./i.m. Morphine 0.2–0.5 mg/kg s.c./i.m./i.v. 0.1–0.4 mg/kg/h CRI following loading dose Fentanyl CRI 0.02–0.2 μg/kg/minute Buprenorphine 20 μg/kg s.c./i.m./i.v. Fentanyl patch 3–5 μg/kg/h	Good for inflammatory pain but not very effective for neuropathic pain. High doses may be required Methadone may have some NMDA antagonist effects and so may be indicated for use in neuropathic pain. May accumulate with repeated administration Fentanyl patches have a long onset time and may not achieve significant plasma levels

26.14 Analgesic agents and doses used in acute and/or chronic neuropathic pain. (continues) ▶

Drug	Dose	Comments
NSAIDs	Carprofen 4 mg/kg orally/s.c./i.v. Meloxicam: Dogs 0.2 mg/kg s.c./orally then 0.1 mg/kg q24h Cats 0.3 mg/kg s.c./orally then 0.1 mg/kg q24h for 4 days	Should be used in conjunction with other analgesic modalities
Paracetamol (acetaminophen)	10 mg/kg orally/i.v. q12h	May be useful for meningitis or pain caused by intracranial disease. May be used in conjunction with opioids. **Do not use in cats**
Lidocaine	Loading dose 1 mg/kg i.v. followed by CRI 25–50 µg/kg/minute i.v.	Tolerance may develop during prolonged infusions. Dose should be decreased in hypovolaemic patients or those with liver disease
Ketamine	50–100 µg/kg i.m./i.v. bolus 5–10 µg/kg/minute i.v. infusion	NMDA antagonist
Alpha-2 agonists	Medetomidine: 2–5 µg/kg i.m. Loading dose 1 µg/kg i.v. followed by CRI 1–2 µg/kg/h i.v.	Tolerance may develop during prolonged infusions and so dose may need to be adjusted. Infusions >48 hours may have decreased efficacy
Gabapentin	5 mg/kg orally q12h	Side effect of mild sedation. Drug should not be discontinued abruptly
Amitriptyline	Cats 0.25–1 mg/kg orally q24h Dogs 1–2 mg/kg orally q12h	Side effects include nausea and depression

26.14 (continued) Analgesic agents and doses used in acute and/or chronic neuropathic pain.

Preservative-free morphine (0.1 mg/kg) or hydromorphone (0.05 mg/kg) can be applied topically to the spinal cord prior to closure in dorsal procedures, although efficacy has not been assessed in animals. Spinal and epidural morphine are undergoing investigation for analgesia following spinal surgery.

Postoperative care

Movement should be restricted, minimizing the risk of further haemorrhage, haematoma formation and resultant neurological deterioration. Some patients require sedation, which can be achieved with opioid analgesic agents, alpha-2 agonists or acepromazine. Recumbent patients should be turned every 4 hours to minimize positional atelectasis, and padded bedding should be provided to minimize bruising and the development of pressure sores. If prolonged recumbency or bladder dysfunction is expected an indwelling urinary catheter should be placed.

A small percentage of patients with cervical spinal disorders require postoperative ventilatory support. Patients undergoing surgery or suffering injury at this level should be assessed at the end of the anaesthetic for adequate ventilatory function. Cyanosis may be seen if the patient is not receiving oxygen supplementation, although hypercapnia is a more reliable indicator of such dysfunction.

Anaesthetic considerations for specific spinal surgeries

Cervical spondylopathy

'Wobbler' surgery is often performed on Dobermanns and a buccal mucosal bleeding time test should be performed prior to surgery, along with von Willebrand's assessment if possible. Patients with von Willebrand's disease should be managed with desmopressin and plasma transfusions where appropriate (see Chapter 16) whilst drugs affecting platelet function should be avoided, such as acepromazine and certain NSAIDs.

Dorsal approach to the spinal cord

Haemorrhage is the most common complication of laminectomy. The anaesthetist can help minimize blood loss by reducing venous pressures. Minimal peak inspiratory pressure should be used in ventilated patients and excessive abdominal pressure avoided by positioning and emptying the bladder (Figure 26.15).

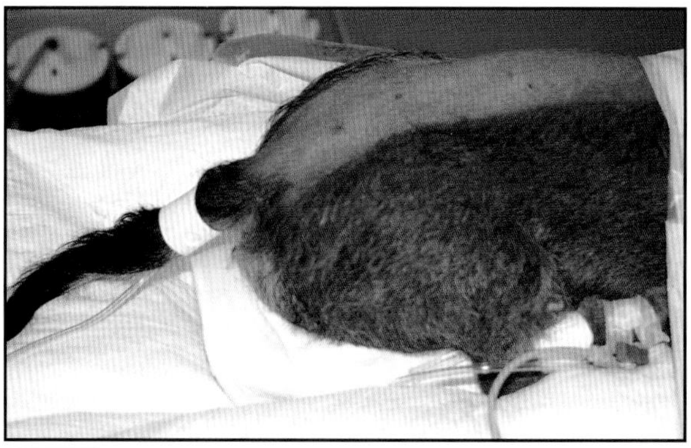

26.15 Abdominal pressure should be minimized in sternal recumbency by placing a support (sandbag or padding) underneath the pelvis to elevate it. The bladder should also be emptied prior to surgery. Decreased intra-abdominal pressure will improve venous drainage from the vertebral canal, minimizing bleeding at surgery.

Ventral slot surgery

During ventral slot surgery, the trachea and vagal trunk are retracted to allow surgical access. Neuromuscular-blocking agents may allow improved surgical access. Excessive traction on the trachea may affect airway patency and alter ventilator setting requirements if pressure-cycled ventilators are used. Iatrogenic damage to the recurrent laryngeal nerves will affect laryngeal function postoperatively. Vagal stimulation may cause bradycardia and retractors should be repositioned. Anticholinergic drugs are rarely required. The patient is positioned with the neck fully extended (Figure 26.16) and care must be taken not to allow the head to be lower than the body since this may exacerbate haemorrhage. The head should not be higher than the body, as air embolism may occur during venous haemorrhage. Direct or indirect blood pressure monitoring is advisable since haemorrhage is commonly encountered on the ventral approach, due to the anatomy of the venous sinuses. Surgery at the level of the cervical vertebrae may result in respiratory compromise and should be monitored with capnography and pulse oximetry. Arterial blood gas analysis may also be helpful.

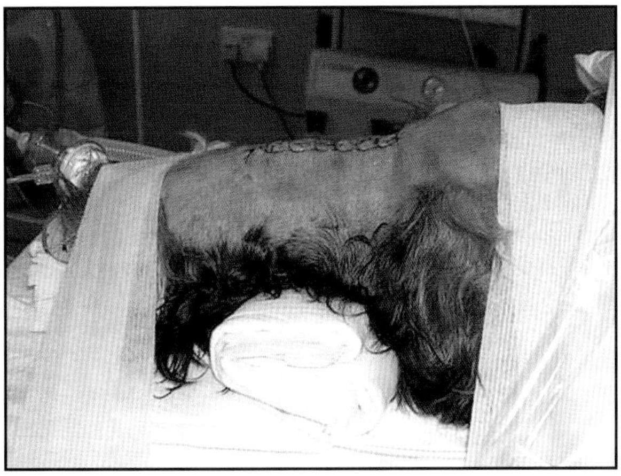

26.16 Patient positioning for ventral slot surgery usually involves severe neck extension.

Atlantoaxial subluxation

Atlantoaxial subluxation is perhaps one of the most challenging spinal conditions for anaesthetists. Typically a congenital or developmental condition affecting immature toy breed dogs, it causes instability of the atlantoaxial joint with acute or chronic cord compression. Damage at this level can cause respiratory compromise or failure and patients must be handled with great care, particularly at induction. Adequate sedation will allow intravenous catheter placement with minimal restraint. Struggling at this time could result in rapid deterioration. A rapid, intravenous induction technique causing minimal respiratory depression is desirable and either propofol or thiopental are suitable. It is advisable to avoid benzodiazepines, since profound muscle relaxation may result in further destabilization of the joint. Preoxygenation should be carried out by the 'flow by' technique prior to induction if tolerated. The head and neck should be supported in a neutral position during induction and the patient positioned in lateral recumbency for intubation. The head and neck should be kept in the horizontal plane and the upper jaw supported with the head remaining in a neutral position for intubation (Figure 26.17). The use of a laryngoscope is extremely useful during intubation.

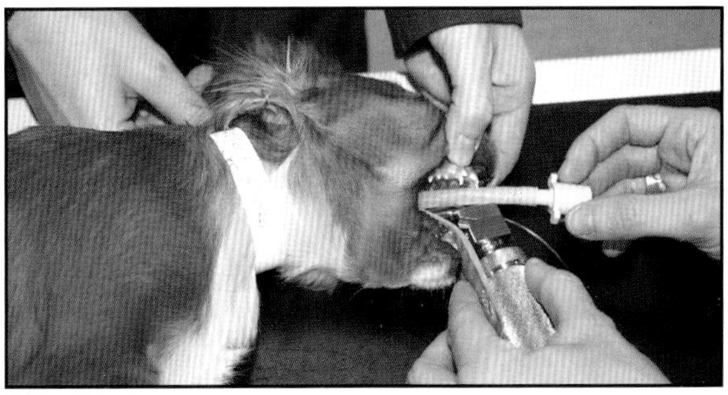

26.17 Positioning for intubation of suspected atlantoaxial subluxation is vital. The head and neck are kept in a horizontal plane and in a neutral position. Preoxygenation is worthwhile in these patients whilst a laryngoscope can aid intubation.

Care must also be taken when positioning for imaging. A supportive neck brace is applied (Figure 26.18) to stabilize the patient whilst allowing growth prior to surgical intervention. This presents further problems for the anaesthetist during recovery and should not be too tight, avoiding compression of the pharyngeal area. If the brace is too tight or poorly positioned, the patient may also experience difficulty in swallowing, potentially resulting in upper airway obstruction or aspiration pneumonia. When anaesthetizing these patients prior to surgery, the bandage supporting the brace should be cut prior to induction to allow rapid removal of the entire brace if difficulty intubating is encountered. Suction should be available.

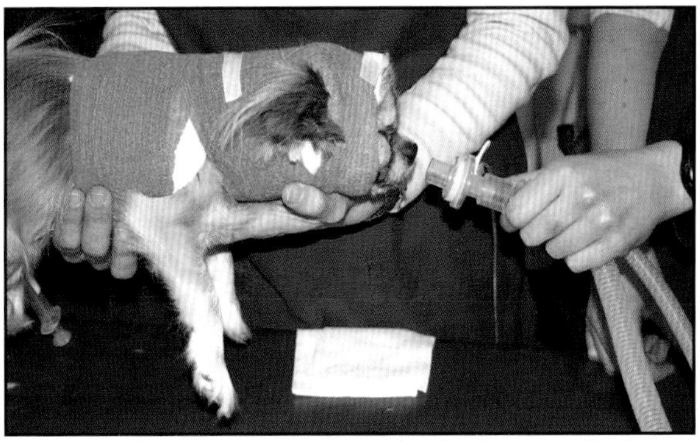

26.18 Oxygen supplementation is often required during recovery or prior to induction of patients with neck braces. If cyanosis develops the neck brace should be loosened or reapplied. During induction the supporting bandage should be cut to allow rapid removal if difficulties arise at intubation.

Spinal trauma

Cases with spinal trauma should be stabilized on a board prior to transport. Life-threatening conditions, such as ruptured bladder, haemorrhage, lung or myocardial contusions and pneumothorax, should be ruled out. Intravenous access should be secured, fluid therapy instigated and analgesia administered, ideally using intravenous opioids in the first instance. Cardiopulmonary parameters should be stabilized prior to anaesthesia.

Meningitis

Patients with meningitis may be extremely difficult to restrain due to severe pain and hyperaesthesia. The judicious use of low dose medetomidine (1–5 μg/kg i.m.)

in combination with an opioid should allow handling for catheter placement. Intravenous analgesic agents such as lidocaine or ketamine may be used, whilst low dose medetomidine may be required in animals suffering extreme pain.

Neuropathies and neuromuscular disease

Animals may present with focal or generalized muscular weakness due to neuropathies or neuromuscular disease. Neuromuscular disease may present as muscular rigidity in tetanus, necessitating anaesthesia to provide supportive care such as ventilation and nutrition.

It is important to rule out treatable metabolic causes prior to anaesthesia, such as electrolyte abnormalities. Myopathies may be associated with steroid use, as well as certain endocrinopathies such as hypothyroidism and hyperadrenocorticsm (see Chapter 25).

Immune-mediated myasthenia gravis (MG) is one of the common neuromuscular diseases affecting dogs and cats. The disease may be focal or generalized, with some animals presenting in acute fulminating MG requiring anaesthesia. A reduction in functional postsynaptic acetylcholine receptors causes muscular weakness with sustained activity. Megaoesophagus and dysphagia are common findings in MG and have important implications for anaesthesia. MG is associated with mediastinal thymoma and this should be ruled out before surgical excision (see Chapter 21). Surgical stress may exacerbate MG causing deterioration.

General anaesthesia is preferred to heavy sedation to allow airway control and ventilatory support. Benzodiazepines and alpha-2 agonists exacerbate muscular weakness and should be avoided. Opioids will provide sedation with or without acepromazine, although morphine should be avoided in patients with suspected megaoesophagus. Radiographs to rule out megaoesophagus should be taken prior to induction of anaesthesia. Following preoxygenation, a rapid intravenous induction technique using propofol or thiopental allows rapid airway control. The patient should be maintained in sternal recumbency prior to intubation, with the head kept in an elevated position to prevent regurgitation and aspiration (Figure 26.19). The trachea should be intubated rapidly and the cuff inflated before the head is lowered. Cricoid pressure may be performed during intubation by applying pressure either side of the trachea just below the larynx to minimize regurgitation. Suction should be available to clear any pharyngeal fluid or material. In dysphagic patients, excessive volumes of saliva may be present in the oropharynx and dry swabs are extremely helpful for tongue retraction, whilst suction or the use of sponge swabs may also be required.

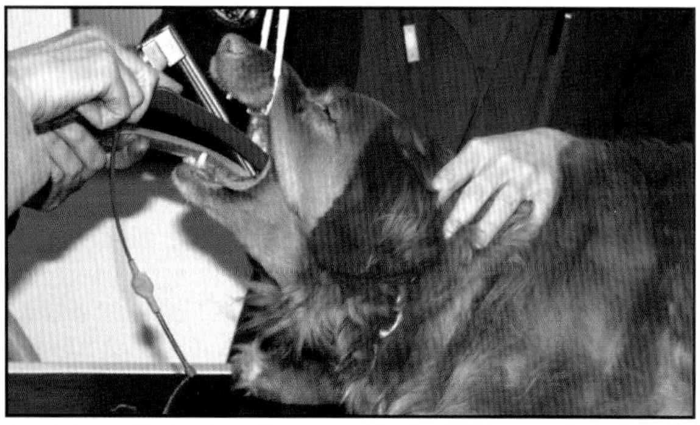

26.19 Patients with suspected megaoesophagus should be maintained in sternal recumbency with the head elevated for intubation to prevent aspiration. The cuff should be fully inflated before the head is lowered and suction should be available.

Intraoperative monitoring of ventilation is important and IPPV is required if hypoventilation occurs. Breathing systems should have minimal resistance. The use of inhalant agents results in rapid elimination and recovery, minimizing respiratory depression and improving airway protection. In MG patients, the palpebral reflex may diminish with repeated stimulation and may not be a reliable indicator of depth of anaesthesia.

Neuromuscular-blocking agents may be used at low doses in patients with neuromuscular disease (see Chapter 15). Monitoring using a nerve stimulator is mandatory.

In severely affected patients undergoing diagnostic procedures, postoperative supportive care should be planned. In animals with megaoesophagus or dysphagia, a PEG tube should be placed for nutrition, whilst those with severe ventilatory compromise may require tracheotomy to allow prolonged ventilatory support. Nasogastric and oesophagostomy tubes are avoided in patients with oesophageal dysfunction. Baseline thoracic radiographs should be taken in case aspiration pneumonia develops.

Anaesthesia for patients with tetanus requires the same general considerations as above. It is important to provide a quiet, darkened recovery area to minimize stimulation. In severely affected patients, tracheotomy is advisable for both airway management and IPPV. Sedatives such as acepromazine have been used to decrease response to stimulation.

Partial inflation of the endotracheal tube cuff during extubation allows secretions to be drawn into the oropharynx from the airway. The pharynx should be supported higher than the nose allowing secretions or regurgitant fluid to drain through the mouth, minimizing the risk of aspiration (Figure 26.20). Adequate

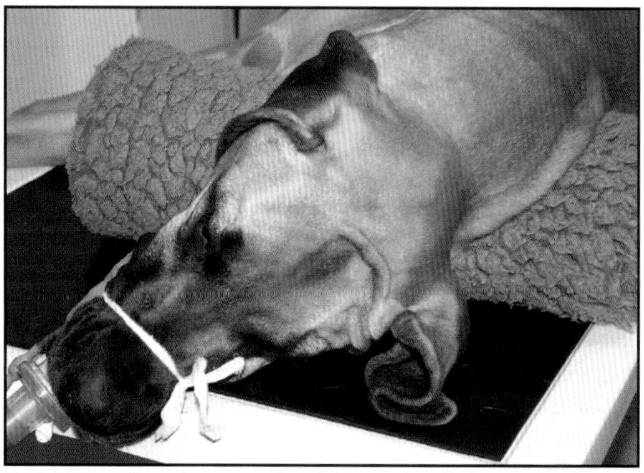

26.20 The pharynx should be raised above the level of the nose to allow fluid to drain from the oropharynx following extubation of patients with megaoesophagus or dysphagia.

analgesia should always be provided because severely affected patients may not be able to exhibit normal signs of pain. In certain conditions steroids may be required for treatment, so NSAIDs should be avoided. Patients may be unable to generate heat by shivering and postoperative hypothermia may result.

Patients should be turned regularly to minimize atelectasis. Pulse oximetry is a useful monitor of ventilation in patients not receiving oxygen supplementation and may be used as a guide for oxygen therapy. Arterial blood gas analysis is an invaluable monitoring tool for impending respiratory failure as P_aCO_2 increases and can be used as a guide for the implementation of IPPV.

Anaesthesia for neurological diagnostic procedures

Anaesthesia for cerebrospinal fluid sampling

CSF may be sampled from the atlanto-occipital space or lumbar intervertebral spaces. Cervical sampling carries increased risk due to spinal cord trauma and the proximity to the brainstem. If raised ICP is suspected, CSF sampling should be avoided, although the risk of tonsillar herniation can be minimized by the judicious use of hyperventilation, sometimes in combination with osmotic diuretics. The patient should be adequately anaesthetized to prevent movement during collection and ideally an armoured tube should be used (see Chapter 5) and 100% oxygen supplied during the procedure. Ventilatory effort and the capnograph should be observed for signs of respiratory tract obstruction, as older endotracheal tubes may 'kink' during flexion of the neck.

Anaesthesia for electromyography

This technique generally involves patients with neuromuscular disease and there should be particular emphasis on ventilatory monitoring and support. Environmental electrical interference may be a problem. An adequate plane of anaesthesia minimizes patient interference and reaction to nerve conduction velocity studies.

Anaesthesia for myelography

Myelography is a relatively safe diagnostic tool for spinal cord disease. Intrathecal injection of contrast medium causes mild meningitis whilst more serious side effects include seizures, apnoea, hyper- and hypotension, tachypnoea, tachycardia, bradycardia, arrhythmias and cardiac arrest. The resultant meningeal irritation should be managed with anti-inflammatory agents.

Seizures may be the result of chemotoxicity and hyperosmolality, with newer contrast media theoretically being less epileptogenic. Generalized seizures most commonly occur in the first hour of recovery, although may be seen some hours later. Dogs over 20 kg have a higher incidence of seizures following myelography, possibly due to the relatively larger volume of injectate compared to CSF volume. Cervical injection of contrast carries a higher risk than lumbar injection and the latter technique should be performed where possible. Rostral flow of contrast to the basal subarachnoid space and ventricular system is minimized by slow injection over 1–2 minutes and maintaining the head in an elevated position afterwards. It may also be advisable to avoid the use of agents that may lower the seizure threshold (see Figures 26.6 and 26.7). Seizures are normally successfully controlled with intravenous or rectal diazepam.

Anaesthesia for computed tomography

Accessibility is the major problem encountered during computed tomography (CT) scanning. Often patients are heavily sedated for this short procedure with drug combinations such as medetomidine and an opioid. Patients with suspected raised ICP should be anaesthetized and IPPV provided. It is important to ensure intravenous access, whilst monitoring should be as standard. Some endotracheal tubes have radio-opaque markers that can interfere with scan quality.

Anaesthesia for magnetic resonance imaging

Anaesthesia for MRI has the problem of accessibility, plus limitations regarding MRI compatible equipment. All staff should be fully trained to avoid accidental use of ferromagnetic material, which can become projectile, causing injury to patients, personnel and equipment.

Most patients should be anaesthetized, since scan times are long and patient movement causes motion artefacts, which may be more significant during certain sequences and in different planes. Occasionally comatose patients undergo brain MRI without any anaesthesia. These patients are positioned in sternal or lateral recumbency, avoiding compression of the jugular veins, and are monitored as normal since rapid decompensation may necessitate ventilation. Induction of anaesthesia should be performed outside the scanner room if possible.

Hypothermia occurs in smaller patients and is significant in those undergoing surgery. Good insulation should be provided and MRI fans turned off.

The intravenous contrast agents may occasionally result in an anaphylactoid reaction and monitoring is vital, with a progressive fall in the end-tidal carbon dioxide giving the first indication. Cardiopulmonary resuscitation is impossible within the magnet and the patient should be removed.

MRI anaesthetic and monitoring equipment

These topics are covered in Chapters 4 and 5.

References and further reading

Bracken MB (2002) Steroids for acute spinal cord injury. *Cochrane Database of Systematic Reviews* **3**, CD001046

Tobias KM, Marioni-Henry K and Wagner R (2006) A retrospective study on the use of acepromazine maleate in dogs with seizures. *Journal of the American Animal Hospital Association* **42**, 283–289

27

Paediatric patients

Daniel Holden

Introduction

Newborn dogs and cats are termed neonates until 4 weeks of age and paediatric until 12 weeks old. Although patients of this age range are not common candidates for anaesthesia, situations do arise where an anaesthetic may be necessary (investigation and surgical correction of congenital abnormalities, restraint for diagnostic procedures, blood sampling, cannulation). The differences in anatomy, physiology and pharmacology between neonatal/paediatric patients and adults should be appreciated. Equipment selection is also important.

Comparative anatomy, physiology and pharmacology

Some values for selected physiological measurements in paediatric dogs and cats are shown in Figure 27.1.

Parameter	Normal value
Rectal temperature	35.4–36°C (96–97°F) Increases to 37.7°C (100°F) after 4 weeks of age
Heart rate	210–300 beats/minute
Arterial blood pressure	Systolic 70–82 mmHg Mean 56–66 mmHg Diastolic 40–52 mmHg
Haematocrit	35–45% at birth 25–35% at 28 days
Haemoglobin	110–140 g/l at birth 80–90 g/l at 28 days
Respiratory rate	20–36 breaths/minute

27.1 Normal values for selected physiological parameters in puppies and kittens.

Cardiovascular system

Systemic vascular resistance rises and pulmonary vascular resistance falls abruptly immediately after birth. As the alveoli inflate, a more rigid scaffold for pulmonary vessels is created and vascular tone falls as oxygen tension increases. Rapid cessation of placental blood flow causes the rise in systemic vascular resistance. These changes in vascular tone combine to reverse blood flow through the (still patent) ductus arteriosus, and exposure of the ductal intima to oxygenated blood causes contraction of its muscular layer, resulting in attenuation and closure. The resulting increase in left atrial pressure causes closure of the foramen ovale. These changes are shown in diagrammatic form in Figure 27.2. The changes are initially functional and do not normally become anatomical for several weeks, and major changes in arterial oxygen tension or acid–base status may increase pulmonary vascular resistance and re-open fetal circulatory pathways.

Cardiac output in the paediatric patient is primarily rate dependent. This is due to the relatively large percentage of non-contractile cardiac mass and low ventricular compliance. As a result, stroke volume is effectively fixed and increases in preload and afterload

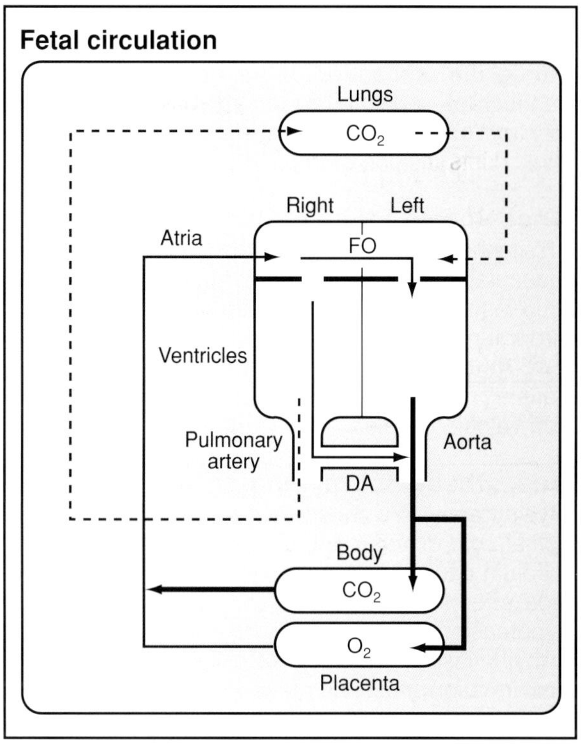

27.2 Schematic representation of the fetal circulation as compared with the adult circulation. In the fetus, relatively little blood goes to the lungs (dashed line) compared with that passing through the placenta, where oxygenation occurs. A considerable amount of blood passes from the right to the left atrium through the foramen ovale (FO) and from the pulmonary artery to the aorta through the ductus arteriosus (DA). Reproduced from Brown and Kozlowski (1997) with permission from the publisher. (continues) ▶

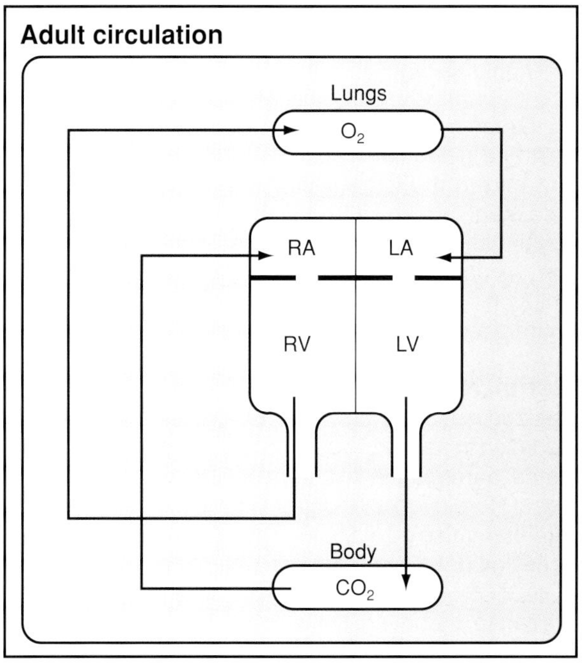

27.2 (continued) Schematic representation of the fetal circulation as compared with the adult circulation. In the fetus, relatively little blood goes to the lungs (dashed line) compared with that passing through the placenta, where oxygenation occurs. A considerable amount of blood passes from the right to the left atrium through the foramen ovale (FO) and from the pulmonary artery to the aorta through the ductus arteriosus (DA). LA = Left atrium; LV = Left ventricle; RA = Right atrium; RV = Right ventricle. Reproduced from Brown and Kozlowski (1997) with permission from the publisher.

are poorly tolerated. The parasympathetic dominance that exists in the immature heart also means that the bradycardic effects of drugs such as opioids and alpha-2 agonists may induce severe hypotension. As a result of these factors, paediatric patients are less well able to tolerate blood loss than adults and losses of as little as 5 ml/kg may cause significant hypotension.

Haemopoiesis does not effectively commence until 2–3 months of age; before this haemoglobin concentrations are lower than those of adults, further reducing the tolerance to surgical haemorrhage.

Respiratory system

Differences in anatomy, compared with adults, are marked. The tongue is relatively large and the upper airway narrow, meaning that airway obstruction is likely without intubation. Airway resistance and work of breathing are also increased. Functional residual capacity (FRC) is low and may be lower than the closing volume (volume at which small airways close). Lung and chest wall compliance is high. These factors mean that airway closure and hypoventilation are major risks, especially in the presence of potent respiratory depressants such as anaesthetic agents.

Tissue oxygen demand is two to three times greater in paediatric patients; resting respiratory rate is higher and the respiratory pattern is sinusoidal with little or no end-expiratory pause. Hypoxaemia and rebreathing are therefore potential risks unless adequate fresh gas flows through anaesthetic breathing systems are employed. Intermittent positive pressure ventilation (IPPV) is also strongly recommended in patients under 6–8 weeks, although great care should be taken to avoid barotrauma. Most ventilators suitable for patients of this size are pressure cycled to avoid such problems (see Chapter 6).

Hepatic function

Of main relevance to the anaesthetist is the immaturity of the hepatic microsomal enzyme systems responsible for the metabolism and transformation of many anaesthetic and analgesic drugs. These systems are not considered fully functional until at least 8 weeks of age and therefore drugs undergoing extensive hepatic metabolism should be avoided; if this is not possible, doses should be reduced and significantly longer elimination half-lives should be expected.

Glycogen storage in the neonatal and paediatric liver is minimal and any excessive fasting or delay in feeding after anaesthesia results in rapid exhaustion of stores, leading to hypoglycaemia. Glucose-containing fluids may be required during prolonged surgical procedures.

Renal function and fluid balance

Adult plasma albumin levels are not fully attained until approximately 8 weeks of age and therefore highly protein-bound drugs (e.g. propofol) will exert a greater immediate effect due to the greater proportion of free drug in circulation.

Total body water content and extracellular fluid volume are higher than in adult animals, resulting in an increased volume of distribution of many water-soluble drugs. A greater tendency to dehydrate with smaller fluid losses also exists

Renal function is also reduced in the first 6–8 weeks of life; paediatric patients cannot tolerate large volumes of fluid administered rapidly and are less well able to concentrate urine than adults. Rapidly administered solute loads are tolerated poorly and all intravascular fluids should be given carefully via syringe pump or burette infusion set. Flow regulators placed in the administration line (Figure 27.3) are also useful to avoid overtransfusion.

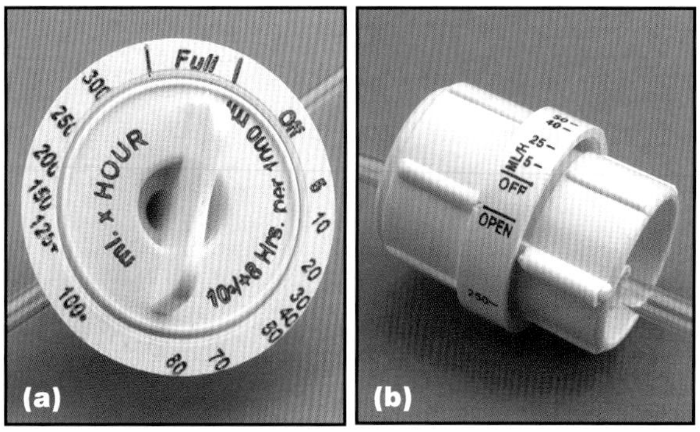

27.3 Flow regulators. Note that the flow rates indicated on the regulator should be used for reference only, as considerable variation can occur between indicated and actual flow rate. **(a)** Dial-faced flow regulator. **(b)** Twist-action flow regulator. (Courtesy of Mark Lever, Infusion Concepts Ltd.)

Temperature regulation

Low subcutaneous fat reserves, a high surface area:body mass ratio, poor thermoregulatory ability, less ability to shiver and a higher critical temperature (the point at which metabolic activity is required to maintain a normal core temperature) all mean that paediatric and neonatal patients are at major risk of developing hypothermia during and after anaesthesia and surgery. Every attempt should be made to minimize anaesthetic and surgical time. The importance of insulating materials, warming devices, minimal use of surgical preparation solutions and the maintenance of a high ambient temperature cannot be overemphasized. Warm water mattresses and warm air blower devices such as the Bair Hugger® (see Chapter 3, Figure 3.5) are extremely useful.

Preoperative preparation and premedication

It is both unnecessary and unwise to withhold food from unweaned puppies and kittens prior to anaesthesia. Excessive fasting may promote hypoglycaemia and predispose to hypothermia. Patients over 6 weeks old may require starvation for a maximum of 2–3 hours; withholding of water is not required.

The decision to give a premedicant drug depends upon many factors (such as underlying disease, duration of surgery and familiarity with the drugs used), but in general the potential reduction in dose of induction and maintenance agents, as well as the benefit of providing intra- and postoperative analgesia, make some form of premedication seem a sensible option. The main classes of drug which may be considered for use as premedicants are:

- Sedatives
- Opioid analgesics
- Anticholinergics.

Drugs used for sedation, analgesia and chemical restraint in paediatric patients (and appropriate doses) are shown in Figure 27.4. The importance of accurate weighing (and therefore accurate dosage) of such small patients cannot be overemphasized. If necessary, drugs may need to be diluted in an appropriate solution (usually 5% dextrose or 0.9% saline) to allow more accurate dosing.

Sedatives

Benzodiazepines can provide consistently effective sedation in paediatric patients (unlike adults), although some paradoxical excitement may occasionally be seen. Cardiovascular depression is minimal with good skeletal muscle relaxation, but some respiratory depression does occur and apnoea may be a problem if other depressant drugs (especially opioids) are given. Because these agents undergo extensive hepatic metabolism, care should be taken to avoid overdosage in patients less than 8 weeks of age. Of the available agents (none of which are licensed for use in veterinary species in the UK), diazepam and midazolam are the most common (see Chapter 12). Flumazenil is a specific benzodiazepine antagonist available for human use which may prove useful should perioperative respiratory insufficiency occur; its short duration of action (approximately 1 hour) may mean that repeat doses (10–30 μg/kg i.v.) are required to reverse the effects of the initial drug.

Acepromazine is probably the most common routine premedicant in use in veterinary practice and can be used effectively to sedate healthy paediatric

Drug	Dose (mg/kg)	Route	Comments
Acepromazine	0.01–0.03	s.c./i.m./i.v.	Avoid in patients under 8 weeks or in debilitation/dehydration
Diazepam	0.1–0.4	s.c./i.m. (emulsion i.v.)	Non-intravenous uptake may be variable
Midazolam	0.1–0.25	i.m./i.v.	Shorter duration than diazepam
Flumazenil	0.1	i.v.	Benzodiazepine antagonist; short duration (50–60 minutes)
Xylazine	1–2	s.c./i.m./i.v.	Marked cardiorespiratory side effects; avoid under 12 weeks
Medetomidine	0.005–0.04	s.c./i.m./i.v.	More potent and longer-acting than xylazine
Atipamezole	0.2–0.4	i.m.	Alpha-2 antagonist
Pethidine (meperidine)	1–4	s.c./i.m. (NOT i.v.)	Rapid onset; 2–3 hour duration
Morphine	0.05–0.3 (epidural: 0.1 in 0.25ml/kg NaCl)	s.c./i.m./slow i.v.	4–5 hour duration. May cause bradycardia; use with an anticholinergic
Buprenorphine	0.01–0.03	s.c./i.m./i.v.	Slow onset of action (35–40 minutes)
Butorphanol	0.05–0.3	s.c./i.m./i.v.	Useful sedative; analgesic efficacy uncertain
Naloxone	0.01–0.1	i.m./i.v.	Opioid reversal agent; will reverse analgesia. Short duration (30–60 minutes)
Ketamine	0.5–3 (i.v.), 5–10 (i.m.)	i.m./i.v.	Analgesic; very useful with benzodiazepines
Atropine	0.02–0.04	s.c./i.m./i.v.	Rapid onset; used for therapy of bradycardia
Glycopyrronium	0.01–0.02	s.c./i.m./i.v.	Slower onset; does not cross blood–brain barrier?

27.4 Drugs used for sedation, chemical restraint and analgesia in paediatrics.

patients at doses no greater than 0.03 mg/kg. In very young (less than 8 weeks) or debilitated patients, acepromazine can cause profound and long-lasting sedation, together with cardiovascular collapse and hypothermia due to peripheral vasodilation; its use is contraindicated in these circumstances.

The alpha-2 agonist agents are very effective sedatives with some analgesic properties, but can produce dramatic bradycardia (of particular importance in these patients due to their highly rate-dependent cardiac output) and respiratory depression. These drugs are also extensively metabolized in the liver, and their use should probably be avoided in anything other than fit healthy adult patients.

Opioid analgesic agents

Opioid analgesic agents are capable of providing profound analgesia both intra- and postoperatively, and will also reduce the dose of other agents required to induce and maintain anaesthesia. The onset and duration of drug effects will vary considerably according to which agent is used. The two most potentially serious side effects of opioids in paediatric patients are bradycardia (which can result in marked falls in cardiac output and blood pressure due to the rate dependency of these parameters) and respiratory depression (which may be compounded by administration of other agents). Shorter-acting agents, such as pethidine (meperidine) which has a duration of action of 2–3 hours, may be more versatile. It may be prudent to have pure antagonist agents such as naloxone available if excessive respiratory depression occurs.

Opioids are most commonly administered by intramuscular injection, but the use of subcutaneous, epidural or even intra-articular routes should be considered to provide analgesia while minimizing side effects.

Anticholinergic agents

The parasympathetic dominance and high rate dependency of cardiac output make the pre-anaesthetic administration of an anticholinergic agent a sensible option, although there is some evidence to suggest that these agents may not be effective in puppies and kittens less than 2 weeks of age due to autonomic immaturity. Glycopyrronium and atropine are the most common anticholinergic agents in use. In addition to reducing the incidence and severity of bradycardia, they also reduce respiratory tract secretions, thereby reducing the potential for airway obstruction. In spite of its slower onset of action, glycopyrronium may be preferable to atropine because of its longer duration and decreased tendency to produce sinus tachycardia, although both drugs may be used intravenously to treat acute bradyarrhythmias.

Induction of anaesthesia

Volatile anaesthetic agents

In the vast majority of neonatal patients, the accepted induction method of choice is by mask using a volatile agent such as isoflurane or sevoflurane, as intravenous catheter placement in these individuals is often technically challenging and is most easily accomplished after induction and endotracheal intubation. Induction of anaesthesia with volatile agents is rapid due to the low FRC and relative increase in alveolar ventilation. The ideal facemask should conform reasonably well to the patient's face because ill-fitting masks effectively increase deadspace and may prolong induction of anaesthesia.

The most common volatile agents currently employed in veterinary practice are isoflurane and sevoflurane. A more detailed discussion of both agents can be found in Chapter 14, but there are some aspects of its pharmacology that make sevoflurane very suitable for paediatric anaesthetic cases. Its blood/gas partition coefficient (0.68) is significantly lower than that of isoflurane (1.43), meaning that uptake and elimination (and therefore induction and recovery) are likely to be much more rapid. The decrease in blood solubility is matched by a decrease in potency, with a minimum alveolar concentration (MAC) of 2–2.6%, meaning that higher vaporizer settings are required. Sevoflurane produces dose-dependent respiratory and cardiovascular depression in a manner similar to isoflurane, although heart rate may be better maintained. In contrast to isoflurane, sevoflurane has a relatively mild, inoffensive odour that makes it more suitable for mask induction, although some early studies in adult animals suggests that this might not be significantly superior to other agents. Due to its considerable expense, many clinicians choose to induce anaesthesia in paediatric patients by mask with sevoflurane, and then switch to isoflurane for maintenance once intubation is achieved. It should be remembered that mask or chamber inductions with any agent significantly increase atmospheric pollution with anaesthetic gases.

For those patients with significant dyspnoea or other evidence of hypoxaemia, or those at increased risk of regurgitation and subsequent aspiration upon induction, administration of a rapidly acting intravenous induction agent with rapid endotracheal intubation is preferable.

Regardless of the induction technique employed, a wide range of endotracheal tube sizes and an effective laryngoscope (Miller or Robertshaw blade size 0 or 00 are very useful) or other light source should be readily available in order to establish a patent airway. Commercially available endotracheal tubes are made down to 1.0 mm; anything smaller is best constructed in advance from an intravenous catheter or similar. All intubations should be performed with the utmost care, as damage to delicate structures and subsequent laryngeal oedema and spasm are easily produced.

Intravenous anaesthetic agents

Of the available agents, propofol and ketamine are probably the most commonly used. Because of their low muscle and fat mass, relatively low plasma protein levels and immature hepatic enzyme pathways, neonatal and paediatric animals may show increased sensitivity to, and prolonged recovery from, barbiturate anaesthesia. This group of drugs is therefore best avoided in animals under 8–10 weeks of age.

Propofol is an ultra short-acting hypnotic that may be used for induction and maintenance of anaesthesia by incremental dosage or infusion (see Chapter 13). Prolongation of recovery may be a problem in neonates, as the drug is highly lipid soluble and requires hepatic metabolism (although extrahepatic metabolism has been described in the dog). Slower hepatic clearance of propofol in cats compared with dogs may mean slower recovery times in this species.

Ketamine should be used in combination with some form of sedative agent, with benzodiazepines being the most suitable in paediatric patients. Ketamine is an attractive agent for use in these individuals due to its analgesic properties and relative lack of cardiopulmonary depressant effects, but the drug does undergo extensive hepatic metabolism (with active metabolites) and renal elimination and should therefore be used with care in neonates and paediatric patients. Although laryngeal reflexes are maintained under ketamine anaesthesia, marked salivation can occur, which may compromise an unprotected airway. Its use should probably be restricted to induction of anaesthesia, or use in lower doses together with benzodiazepines to provide immobilization for minor procedures.

Maintenance of anaesthesia

Constant and meticulous attention should be paid to maintenance of a patent airway and adequate ventilation, because drug-induced respiratory inadequacy and airway obstruction are common complications. Oxygen should always be provided even if anaesthesia is maintained with intravenous agents. Nitrous oxide can be used to hasten induction via the 'second gas' effect (see Chapter 14), but the high oxygen consumption of the neonatal animal may mean that its use throughout the surgical procedure may not be desirable because it reduces the inspired oxygen concentration. If nitrous oxide is used, it should not constitute greater than half of the inspired gas mixture.

The anaesthetic breathing system used should have minimal apparatus deadspace, a low circuit volume and minimal internal resistance to gas flow. The Jackson-Rees modification of Ayre's T-piece is usually suitable; some 20–30 variations of the T-piece have been described, but the valveless models are most suitable. Scavenging from an open-ended bag can be difficult and torsion of the bag about its long axis can lead to occlusion and barotrauma; the bag should therefore be in constant view of the veterinary surgeon and taped in a safe position if necessary. More recently, a valved T-piece (Mapleson D; see Chapter 5) has become popular; this has a closed bag with an exhaust valve between the bag and expiratory limb. Use of the T-piece requires high fresh gas flows (2.5–3 times minute volume to completely avoid rebreathing during spontaneous ventilation) which will precipitate hypothermia. Patients over 5 kg in weight can be maintained using other non-rebreathing systems such as the Bain, Lack or Magill, or human paediatric circle absorber systems. The Bain system can still be used in patients <5 kg in countries where the T-piece is not available. Positive pressure ventilation should not be performed with the Lack or Magill systems for long periods as marked rebreathing can occur. If automatic ventilators are being used, pressure-cycled systems are more suitable for paediatric patients to avoid the risk of barotrauma (see Chapter 6). Preset airway pressures should not exceed 15–20 cmH_2O.

Every effort to conserve body temperature should be made. Insulating blankets, bubble wrap and warmed cotton wool can all be wrapped around the patient and a surgical window prepared. Surgical preparation solutions should be applied with sterile swabs to minimize evaporative heat loss. The ambient temperature of the operating area should be kept as high as possible and all intravenous fluids should be warmed. Heat and moisture exchangers (see Chapter 5) can be used but may increase the work of breathing in small subjects, as well as adding to apparatus deadspace.

Intraoperative fluid administration is desirable in order to replace insensible losses, as well as to provide haemodynamic support. Puppies and kittens are relatively intolerant of an acute fluid load and therefore rates of administration should not exceed 10 ml/kg/h. The use of syringe drivers or infusion pumps greatly facilitates accurate fluid therapy in these patients, although burette-type giving sets are equally effective. Dextrose-containing low-salt solutions (e.g. 0.18% sodium chloride in 4% glucose or 5% dextrose in water) are the most suitable, although in the event of significant blood loss (more than 10% of blood volume) an equal volume of colloid or fresh whole blood is indicated for restoration of circulating volume. Surgical swabs can be weighed to assess blood loss: 1 ml of blood weighs approximately 1.3 g. Although isotonic crystalloid fluids can be administered subcutaneously, the intravenous or intraosseous routes are infinitely preferable for longer-term or more rapid administration.

Monitoring during anaesthesia

Monitoring of the paediatric patient should be attentive and adverse trends should be identified and acted upon early. Although an increasing array of sophisticated electronic monitoring equipment is available for veterinary anaesthesia, there is no substitute for the constant physical presence of an attentive, knowledgeable individual actively monitoring the patient's vital signs.

It should also be remembered that total anaesthetic time can be significantly increased by the setting up of various monitoring systems and introduction of invasive monitoring lines, particularly if the veterinary surgeon is unfamiliar with them.

Monitoring of respiratory and cardiac sounds is best achieved with a precordial or oesophageal stethoscope, and an electrocardiograph will allow assessment of cardiac rhythm. Several devices are available for the non-invasive oscillometric measurement of arterial blood pressure; vagaries in patient limb dimensions relative to cuff size may produce very variable results in some patients, especially at low pressures. The cuff width should be approximately 40% of limb circumference. Use of a Doppler flow probe with a sphygmomanometer cuff (see Chapter 7) gives reliable readings of systolic pressure but not of diastolic pressure.

Invasive monitoring of arterial blood pressure is not only technically demanding (requiring cannulation of an undoubtedly small peripheral artery) but potentially expensive due to the equipment required. Assessment of the adequacy of the circulation in practice is therefore often somewhat qualitative and relies on subjective assessment of pulse pressure, capillary refill time, urine output and mucous membrane colour. This can be difficult in a small patient draped up for surgery, so preparation should ensure that adequate visibility under the drapes is maintained.

Basic monitoring of respiratory function consists of assessing respiratory rate and depth by visualization of chest wall excursions (the surgeon should be actively discouraged from leaning on the patient or leaving surgical instruments resting on the patient's chest or abdomen) and movement of the reservoir bag, together with sounds heard via the stethoscope. Simple respiratory monitors that detect temperature changes or movement of gases in the airway are available; however, false values may be registered due to passive movement of air caused by manipulation of the patient's thorax, and some patients may be too small to generate sufficient air movement to register a breath.

Pulse oximeters provide a useful method of non-invasive respiratory monitoring in veterinary anaesthesia. These devices require a peripheral pulse to be present in order to function, and therefore any peripheral vasoconstriction or reduction in pulse pressure can result in a loss of signal. Many of the probes are sprung in order to maintain tissue contact; in delicate tissues such as the tongue of a puppy or kitten, the pressure produced by the spring within the probe may effectively eliminate blood flow at the probe site, again resulting in loss of signal. The majority of available probes will not read through excessively hairy or pigmented skin, making effective probe placement difficult, although oesophageal and rectal reflectance probes are also available.

Adequacy of ventilation can be monitored by capnography. Constant capnographic monitoring is expensive but allows rapid and accurate monitoring of ventilation and early detection of apnoea, disconnection, severe cardiovascular complications, venous air embolism, airway obstruction and low cardiac output. Capnography in small patients may be hampered by the small tidal volumes in neonates and paediatric animals, as sampled gas is subject to great potential dilution by fresh gas flows from breathing systems. This may result in 'peaking' of the waveform and an artificially low end-tidal carbon dioxide value. This problem can be ameliorated by the use of capnographs with a lower gas sampling rate; newer models may sample as little as 5–10 ml/minute. In addition, use of a smaller deadspace volume side-stream adaptor, or inserting a needle through the wall of the endotracheal tube, will create a more normal capnogram, but the needle may become blocked or aspirate moisture. Mainstream capnography avoids gas sampling artefacts but many of the adapters produce excessive apparatus deadspace between the breathing system and endotracheal tube; this can be avoided by using neonatal adaptors which have a much smaller deadspace volume (as little as 0.5 ml).

As previously mentioned, maintenance of adequate body temperature is essential. Core temperature should be monitored frequently via a deep rectal or oesophageal probe. Soil temperature probes or thermistor probes designed for catering can often be purchased cheaply and adapted for use at minimal cost. Comparisons can be made with peripheral (e.g. interdigital) temperature readings in order to assess the adequacy of peripheral perfusion; a core–periphery gradient of greater than 4°C is indicative of inadequate peripheral perfusion.

Postoperative care

As with any patient, constant attention should be paid to the airway, breathing and circulation. Human neonatal incubators are ideal for recovery because they allow constant visualization of the patient and enable a warm, humid and oxygenated environment to be maintained without the need for physical restraint. If necessary the airway should be cleared of secretions and extubation performed as late as possible. Oxygen supplementation should be provided until recovery from anaesthesia is complete and normal body temperature is achieved. If respiration appears inadequate, or there is evidence of hypoventilation or desaturation, positive pressure ventilation with 100% oxygen should be instituted until the patient is capable of maintaining normal ventilation.

The danger of postoperative hypothermia and its attendant complications in paediatric and neonatal patients has already been emphasized. However, rewarming of the hypothermic neonate should be done slowly, as aggressive external heating may not only cause thermal injury but may also precipitate a hypotensive crisis due to rapid peripheral vasodilation. Installation (and removal after 5 minutes) of 10 ml/kg warmed isotonic fluids into the rectum may be useful to elevate core temperature; lavage of the urinary bladder with warm fluids has also been described and appears clinically effective. Thermal support should be maintained after normal body temperature has been reached, as relapse into hypothermia can occur in young patients.

Postoperative analgesia is a major concern in neonates and paediatric patients, not only because significant pain is morally and ethically unacceptable, but also because it may inhibit normal feeding behaviour. Treatment of pain in very young animals is also complicated by differences in neonatal pain behaviour patterns compared with those of adult animals, which may not be as obvious. This may make recognition of the characteristic signs of pain difficult, but does not mean that pain is experienced to a lesser degree. The preoperative use of opioids, such as pethidine (meperidine), morphine or buprenorphine, provides excellent analgesia postoperatively but excessive or supplemental doses may produce respiratory depression. This is not a contraindication to their use, but does mean that doses should be carefully calculated and administered. Consideration should also be given to other techniques such as local anaesthetic blocks (see Chapter 10). Local anaesthetic solutions should be diluted by 50% to reduce the potential for overdosage. Bupivacaine is a relatively long-acting local anaesthetic agent with a duration of up to 8 hours that can be used for effective regional anaesthesia. Care should be taken not to exceed a total dose of 2 mg/kg. Non-steroidal anti-inflammatory drugs (NSAIDs) are used extensively for relief of post-operative pain in veterinary species; their extensive hepatic metabolism may make toxic effects more likely in paediatric or neonatal animals and doses should be reduced by 50–75% in these patients.

Scant information exists on the use of epidural analgesia in such patients. Anecdotal sources historically used sacrococcygeal epidural analgesia for tail docking in neonates and have recommended a total dose of 1 mg/kg lidocaine and 0.1 mg/kg morphine. In patients under 3 months of age bupivacaine should probably be avoided due to its greater potential for cardiotoxicity.

Every effort should be made to restore normal feeding and behaviour as soon as possible after anaesthesia. Unweaned neonates should be returned to the dam as soon as they are able to maintain respiratory and cardiovascular function. Excessive surgical skin preparations should be removed because strong, unfamiliar odours may precipitate rejection of the neonate by its mother. Any surgical dressing or supports applied should not inhibit the patient's ability to feed or drink. Early nutritional support should be instituted if any evidence of a failure to feed within 24 hours of surgery is observed. Parenteral fluid administration should continue at maintenance rates until voluntary fluid intake has returned to normal levels.

References and further reading

Brown H and Kozlowski R (1997) *Physiology and pharmacology of the heart.* Blackwell Science, Oxford

Grundy SA (2006) Clinically relevant physiology of the neonate. *Veterinary Clinics of North America Small Animal Practice* **36(3)**, 443–459

Hosgood G (1998) *Small Animal Paediatric Medicine and Surgery.* Butterworth Heinemann, Oxford

Mathews KA (2005) Analgesia for the pregnant, lactating and neonatal to pediatric cat and dog. *Journal of Veterinary Emergency and Critical Care* **15(4)**, 273–284

Pascoe PJ and Moon PF (2001) Periparturient and neonatal anesthesia. *Veterinary Clinics of North America Small Animal Practice* **31(2)**, 315–340

28

Geriatric patients

Gina Neiger-Aeschbacher

Introduction

With improved veterinary care, the average age of dogs and cats has increased, thus augmenting the number of dogs and cats considered geriatric. The term 'geriatric' is most frequently used to define those animals that have reached 75–80% of their breed-specific expected lifespans. Some consider dogs older than 8 years and cats older than 12 years of age as geriatric. The chronological age may not match the physiological age as breed size, genetics, nutrition, environment and other factors influence the aging process. In general, smaller dogs live longer than large and giant-breed dogs. Geriatric patients now comprise one quarter and possibly up to one third of the total patient population in private veterinary practice. Aging in itself is not a disease, but geriatric patients are more vulnerable than younger animals and the likelihood of morbidity increases with age. Once maturity has been reached, age-related changes occur in all organ systems of otherwise healthy dogs and cats: geriatric patients show physiological regression in organ functions or in their mechanisms of compensation. These processes are progressive and irreversible. Their relevance for sedation and anaesthesia of *healthy* geriatric dogs and cats is discussed below. With improved technology and education, owners of geriatric dogs or cats will increasingly consent to sedation or anaesthesia for various procedures and interventions.

Comparative anatomy, physiology and pharmacology

A summary of the important physiological changes seen in geriatric dogs and cats is shown in Figure 28.1.

Organ system	Activity/performance reduced	Activity/performance increased	Clinical effect
Cardiovascular	Blood volume, cardiac output, baroreceptor activity, autoregulation of blood flow	Circulation time, vagal tone, vascular changes (thickened elastic fibres, increased wall collagen content, vessel wall calcification), cardiac arrhythmias (second-degree heart block, bundle branch block, ventricular premature contractions or atrial fibrillation)	Reduction in cardiac reserve capacity; decreased ability to maintain blood pressure under anaesthesia; longer circulation time (bolus injectable anaesthetic takes longer to effect); more rapid inhalational anaesthetic induction (reduced cardiac output)
Respiratory	Lung elasticity, respiratory rate, tidal volume, minute volume, oxygen consumption, carbon dioxide production, oxygen diffusion capacity, strength of muscles of respiration, chest wall compliance, elastic recoil, vital capacity, protective airway reflexes	Functional residual capacity	Decreased functional reserve, lower P_aO_2
Liver	Functional mass, blood flow (secondary to reduced cardiac output), microsomal enzyme activity, intrinsic metabolic activity (protein production, impaired clotting function)	Susceptibility to hypothermia and reduced ability to maintain blood glucose	Prolonged metabolism and excretion of drugs (hepatic conjugation); hypoproteinaemia; hypoglycaemia
Kidneys	Renal blood flow (secondary to reduced cardiac output), glomerular filtration rate, functional kidney mass (due to fewer functional nephrons), ability to concentrate urine and secrete hydrogen ions	Predisposition to acidosis	Less tolerant of dehydration and acute blood loss; overhydration (excessive fluid therapy) may lead to pulmonary oedema and compromised respiratory system; reduced renal clearance of drugs
Nervous	Cerebral perfusion; oxygen consumption, brain mass due to neural degeneration, myelin sheath, production of neurotransmitters, thermoregulation, sympathetic response to stress	Destruction of neurotransmitters	Enhanced effect of local and general anaesthetic drugs, increased susceptibility to cardiopulmonary depression and hypothermia when linked to anaesthesia; less resistance to stress, more anxiety

28.1 Overview of reported organ system changes in the otherwise healthy geriatric dog and cat.

Cardiovascular system

Several changes have been reported and all are considered significant. Together they lead to a reduction in cardiac reserve capacity. This can limit the patient's ability to compensate for cardiovascular changes that may occur during sedation and anaesthesia.

Progressive or degenerative cardiac diseases are common, with mitral regurgitation being the most important. Dilated cardiomyopathy, myocardial fibrosis and arterial hypertension are also frequently seen in the geriatric dog. In conjunction with changes in the conduction system, the likelihood of cardiac arrhythmias (second-degree heart block, bundle branch block, ventricular premature contractions or atrial fibrillation) increases. With stress and anxiety in the peri-anaesthetic period, pre-existing arrhythmias can be exacerbated. Certain anaesthetic agents also influence cardiac conduction in all dogs and cats, irrespective of age. Following the administration of alpha-2 adrenergic agonists (e.g. medetomidine), bradycardia and second-degree heart block can be observed; following thiopental, ventricular premature contractions or ventricular bigeminy; following ketamine, tachycardia.

Circulation time is increased and the responsiveness to circulating catecholamines is reduced.

Clinical implications

- Avoid extreme changes in heart rate (bradycardia, tachycardia), sudden changes in arterial blood pressure (hypotension, hypertension) and increased vascular resistance.
- Avoid or use with caution (reduce dose, titrate to effect) those sedative and anaesthetic drugs that may be arrhythmogenic.

Respiratory system

The changes in the respiratory system, listed in Figure 28.1, have all been reported in otherwise healthy geriatric patients. Collectively they result in decreased respiratory functional reserve, which can become significant when sedative or anaesthetic agents cause mild to moderate respiratory depression.

Clinical implications

- Avoid marked hypoxia and hypercapnia; oxygen supplementation (intubation, facemask, nasal cannula) should be used for both sedated and anaesthetized patients. Preoxygenation prior to induction is important, giving a decreased likelihood of hypoxia between induction of anaesthesia and endotracheal intubation.
- Pathological lung changes (e.g. pulmonary neoplasia, pneumonia, bullae) will have an intensified effect in geriatric patients.
- Avoid respiratory depression. Monitoring should include pulse oximetry, capnography and, ideally, blood gas analyses to assess ventilatory efficiency.

Liver

Liver function does not change in a clinically significant way with increasing age, although reduced microsomal enzyme activity can prolong drug metabolism and excretion of drugs, especially those that undergo conjugation. The reduction in cardiac output will decrease liver blood flow, which in turn will influence the rate of hepatic metabolism and drug excretion.

Clinical implications

- Prolonged recovery: there should be judicious use of drugs that have a long duration of action (e.g. acepromazine), that rely on hepatic conjugation for metabolism or that cannot be reversed.
- Pre-anaesthetic haematology and serum chemistry are recommended to assess hepatic function; clotting profiles are necessary before ultrasound-guided internal organ biopsy or surgery.
- Avoid or treat hypotension (assess plane of anaesthesia, fluid administration and the use of inotropic agents) to prevent reduction in liver blood flow, which will affect drug metabolism.

Kidney

Changes within the kidney lead to a reduction in functional reserve: the geriatric patient is predisposed to acidosis and the reduction in renal blood flow leads to reduced renal clearance of drugs. The extent of renal dysfunction should be properly assessed and a reduced clearance of parent drug or its metabolites normally excreted by the kidneys should be expected. Additional drug sensitivity can be caused through uraemic conditions.

Clinical implications

- Pre-anaesthetic biochemistry and electrolyte analysis are advised.
- Avoid hypovolaemia, hypotension, hypoxia and hypercapnia because of a possible effect on renal blood flow (i.e. reduction).
- Monitor urine production (1–2 ml/kg/h) during and after sedation and general anaesthesia. Reduced or non-existent urine output is a strong indicator of hypotension and inadequate renal perfusion and warns of impending renal damage caused by ischaemia.
- Be careful with drugs that depend on renal excretion (e.g. ketamine in the cat).

Nervous system

Cognitive, sensory, motor and autonomic nervous performance can be altered in the geriatric cat and dog. The changes within the central and peripheral nervous systems dictate a reduction in doses of all sedative and anaesthetic (volatile and injectable) drugs. The ability to process information is reduced (senility) and anxiety increases, especially in unfamiliar surroundings.

Pharmacology

The pharmacokinetic and pharmacodynamic properties of sedative and anaesthetic drugs change with age.

Decreased cardiac output results in reduced regional and organ blood flow, which in turn results in reduced drug absorption capacity, drug hepatic metabolism and renal clearance capacity. Preferential blood distribution in the geriatric dog and cat is to heart and brain, which can lead to a relative drug overdose. The process of aging also includes a change in body composition, with a decrease in lean body mass and an increase in body fat, thus decreasing total body water and cell mass. This affects plasma concentration of water-soluble and lipid-soluble drugs by changing their volumes of distribution and plasma elimination half-lives. The result is a prolongation of the drug's retention time in the body.

The number or density of receptors within the target tissue, the binding affinity to receptors and changes in homoeostatic mechanisms influence the response to a drug. This highlights the importance of tailoring drug dosage and dosing interval to the individual patient. However, pre-existing renal, hepatic and cardiac disease make it difficult to determine the actual safe and effective drug dosages for this age group. Reliable data in animals are rare and are mostly extrapolated from geriatric human patients.

The geriatric patient also frequently receives multiple drugs to treat other diseases; this increases the likelihood that one drug might affect the metabolism of one (or more) of the other drugs.

The free (non-protein-bound) portion of a drug is responsible for the pharmacodynamic (therapeutic) response. For highly protein-bound drugs, hypoproteinaemia leads to an increased concentration of free drug in the plasma and a lower dose is necessary to achieve the therapeutic effect.

Detailed knowledge of the drugs used for sedation and anaesthesia is necessary to provide appropriate care. The most frequently used drugs are described below and in Figure 28.2. No anaesthetic drug is absolutely contraindicated in the geriatric dog and cat, but there is no perfect anaesthetic for these patients. Desirable properties include:

- Fast and complete recovery (e.g. isoflurane, sevoflurane)
- Reversibility (e.g. opioids, benzodiazepines)
- Minimal or no metabolism required for drug elimination (e.g. etomidate, isoflurane, sevoflurane)
- Few adverse side effects (e.g. opioids, benzodiazepines)
- Clinically insignificant intrinsic toxicity (e.g. opioids, benzodiazepines, isoflurane, sevoflurane).

Drug	General properties	Specific effects in the geriatric patient	Precaution	Dose (mg/kg), route, dosing interval
Phenothiazine	Tranquillization Sedation Hepatic metabolism Hypotension via peripheral vasodilation Anti-arrhythmogenic Long duration of action Not reversible	↑ Tranquillization ↑ Recovery time ↑ Hypothermia (e.g. via peripheral vasodilation)	Volume expansion Blood pressure monitoring Use reduced dose, only once Avoid in case of dehydration, acute haemorrhage, liver dysfunction, major surgery	Acepromazine: 0.01–0.03 i.v./i.m./s.c. once, maximum total dose 0.5 mg
Benzodiazepine	Tranquillization Minimal cardiorespiratory effects Anticonvulsant Short duration of action Hepatic metabolism Reversible	More profound sedation ↑ Tranquillization and ↑ duration of effect in case of impaired hepatic metabolism	If required reverse effects with flumazenil (0.02–0.1 mg/kg i.v. to effect)	Diazepam: 0.1–0.4 i.v. Midazolam: 0.1–0.2 i.v./i.m.
Opioid	Tranquillization Drug-dependent mild to strong analgesic effect Minimal cardiovascular effects Drug- and dose-dependent bradycardia and respiratory depression Hepatic metabolism ↓ anaesthetic requirement Reversible Some are Controlled Drugs	Bradycardia can be prevented with the cautious use of anticholinergic drugs Respiratory depression can cause complications in geriatric patients with little functional respiratory reserve	Use with caution and titrate to the desired effect Oxygen supplementation Endotracheal intubation mandatory for general anaesthesia Be prepared to assist or control ventilation If required reverse all effects (including analgesia) with naloxone (0.02–0.1 mg/kg i.v. to effect) or preserve analgesia using e.g. butorphanol, nalbuphine or buprenorphine	Pethidine (meperidine): 3–5 i.m. q0.5–1h Morphine: 0.05–0.3 i.v./i.m. q2–4h Fentanyl: 0.005–0.01 i.v. q0.5h Hydromorphone: 0.05–0.1 iv/im q2–4h Methadone: 0.05–0.3 i.v./i.m. q2–4h Butorphanol: 0.1–0.5 i.v./i.m. q1–4h Buprenorphine: 0.005–0.02 i.v./i.m. q4–8h
Barbiturate (ultra short-acting)	Hypnosis Cardiovascular depression Cardiac arrhythmia Respiratory depression Initial apnoea Vasodilation Redistribution to lean/fat body compartments leads to arousal Hepatic metabolism	↑ Physiological drug effect (↓ plasma protein binding, ↓ lean body mass and water, ↑ fat depots, ↓ hepatic function) ↓ Margin of safety	Administer pre-anaesthetic sedative/analgesic medication for drug-sparing effect Titrate slowly to effect using dilute solution Use single dose only Start monitoring prior to induction phase and administer oxygen Protect airway by endotracheal intubation Be prepared to control ventilation	Thiopental: 5–12 slowly i.v. once

28.2 Overview of the most important injectable sedative, anaesthetic and analgesic substances and their use in the geriatric dog and cat (further details may be found in Chapters 9, 12 and 13). ↑ = Prolonged, increased, augmented; ↓ = Decreased, reduced, minimized. (continues) ▶

Drug	General properties	Specific effects in the geriatric patient	Precaution	Dose (mg/kg), route, dosing interval
Dissociative anaesthetic	Dissociative anaesthesia Stimulation of the sympathetic nervous system Tachycardia ↑ Secretions, e.g. airway Muscle rigidity Seizure potential Renal (cat) and hepatic (dog) metabolism	↑ Myocardial oxygen consumption ↑ Secretions may influence airway patency ↑ Recovery time if underlying renal/hepatic disease	Administer oxygen Protect airway by endotracheal intubation especially in cats Administer sedative/tranquillizer to ameliorate muscle stiffness and rigidity	Ketamine: 1–3 i.v. once with benzodiazepine
Propofol	Hypnosis Cardiovascular depression Respiratory depression, apnoea Redistribution to lean/fat body compartments leads to arousal Short duration of action Rapid, smooth recovery Rapid (mostly hepatic) metabolism No analgesic property	↓ Margin of safety ↑ Likelihood of respiratory depression and apnoea followed by haemoglobin desaturation and cyanosis	Administer pre-anaesthetic sedative/analgesic medication for drug-sparing effect Administer oxygen Titrate slowly (60–90 seconds) to effect Protect airway by endotracheal intubation Be prepared to control ventilation Provide adequate pain relief	Propofol: 2–6 slowly i.v. single bolus, multiple injections or infusion
Etomidate	Hypnosis Minimal cardiovascular effects Respiratory depression Short duration of action Rapid recovery Rapid hepatic metabolism Reduction of adrenal corticosteroid secretion Occasional retching and myoclonus during induction of unconsciousness	↓ Margin of safety	Administer pre-anaesthetic sedative/analgesic medication to further improve induction and recovery quality Administer oxygen Protect airway by endotracheal intubation Be prepared to control ventilation Provide adequate pain relief Avoid in patients with pre-existing adrenal corticosteroid deficiency	Etomidate: 0.5–3 i.v. single bolus
Non-steroidal anti-inflammatory drug	↓ Inflammation Relieve mild to moderate pain Comparably long duration of action Not controlled substances	↑ Likelihood of hepatic, renal and gastrointestinal side effects	Provide adequate fluid therapy and monitor/support systemic blood pressure to sustain satisfactory renal perfusion Observe for gastrointestinal and renal side effects as well as platelet dysfunction if used for several days postoperatively or in case of long-term preoperative administration Reduce length of therapy in the postoperative period to the minimum Avoid in patients with multiple problems such as dehydration, hypotension, hyponatraemia, hepatic disease, sepsis Judicious use in patients on angiotensin-converting enzyme (ACE) inhibitors	Carprofen: 2–4 i.v./s.c. Meloxicam: 0.2 s.c. Ketoprofen: 0.5–1 i.v./i.m./s.c.

28.2 (continued) Overview of the most important injectable sedative, anaesthetic and analgesic substances and their use in the geriatric dog and cat (further details may be found in Chapters 9, 12 and 13). ↑ = Prolonged, increased, augmented; ↓ = Decreased, reduced, minimized.

Dosage adjustment (either drug dose or interval of drug administration), especially of injectable sedative and anaesthetic drugs, is necessary for the geriatric patient. Some information is available from package inserts of human sedative or anaesthetic drugs but extrapolations need to be made carefully. Final adjustments need to be made following patient observation and assessment of clinical response.

Sedation or pre-anaesthetic tranquillization will help to reduce the anxiety and stress caused by separation from the owner, hospitalization, anaesthesia and treatment. The individual requirements for sedation or analgesia will be dictated by the patient (physical status, pre-existing disease, concurrent medication) and the planned diagnostic or surgical procedure. Indiscriminate use of drugs is not an option in this age group. A detailed description of sedative and anaesthetic drugs can be found elsewhere in this manual.

Anticholinergic agents

Anticholinergic agents (e.g. atropine, glycopyrronium) should be used with caution. They should only be used to treat bradyarrhythmias if the heart rate is too slow to maintain adequate arterial blood pressure and thus perfusion of vital organs. Routine use of anticholinergics can lead to tachycardia, which significantly increases myocardial oxygen demand and may cause myocardial hypoxia, followed by arrhythmias and cardiac failure. Their dose should be titrated to effect (e.g. to counterbalance the bradycardia caused by a pure opioid agonist), generally administering one half to two thirds of the normal drug dose to reduce the likelihood of tachycardia. Glycopyrronium, although not licensed for the dog and cat, is a better choice than atropine in the geriatric patient because it has fewer adverse effects.

Phenothiazines

Phenothiazines (e.g. acepromazine) should be used with care. The advantages and disadvantages of acepromazine have to be assessed in each individual, but low doses in combination with an opioid can provide excellent sedation.

Benzodiazepines

Benzodiazepines, such as diazepam and midazolam, are a better choice than acepromazine and cause more reliable sedation in the geriatric patient than they do in the younger patient. Reduced hepatic function will prolong the duration of action of benzodiazepines. When used alone, their cardiorespiratory side effects are minimal. However, depending on the individual patient and the requirements for sedation or anaesthesia, diazepam and midazolam are usually combined with other drugs, e.g. butorphanol (opioid) or ketamine, in selected patients.

Alpha-2 adrenergic agonists

Alpha-2 adrenergic agonists (e.g. medetomidine) are best avoided because of their profound effects on the cardiovascular, respiratory and central nervous systems. In geriatric patients with a healthy cardiovascular system, their advantages (reversibility) and disadvantages (bradycardia, atrioventricular conduction block, increased peripheral vascular resistance, hypertension) need to be carefully balanced against each other.

Opioids

Opioids provide sedation and analgesia with minimal cardiovascular effects. They reduce anaesthetic requirements for other drugs and can be helpful for induction and maintenance of anaesthesia. Respiratory depression is a side effect, which, in combination with other respiratory depressant drugs (e.g. isoflurane), can cause complications in geriatric patients with little functional respiratory reserve. A pure mu opioid agonist (e.g. morphine, fentanyl) provides better pain relief but also affects heart rate and the respiratory centre more than a partial agonist (e.g. buprenorphine or butorphanol). Advantages and disadvantages of opioid use need to be carefully considered in each individual.

Ultra short-acting barbiturates

Ultra short-acting barbiturates are best used only in healthy geriatric dogs and cats because the drug effects are enhanced and the margin of safety is decreased in patients of this age group (see Figure 28.2). Thiopental should be used as a single dose, titrated slowly to effect, to provide unconsciousness adequate for endotracheal intubation; this minimizes the likelihood of side effects and prolonged recovery.

Ketamine

Ketamine, together with a benzodiazepine, should be used with caution for induction and maintenance of anaesthesia. Myocardial hypoxia, an increased likelihood of airway and pulmonary complications (i.e. increased airway secretions) and, to a lesser extent, the possibility of seizure activity in the dog are the most important reasons for its judicious use. Because of its long duration of action, tiletamine (combined with zolazepam in commercially available preparations) is not recommended for geriatric patients.

Propofol and etomidate

Propofol and etomidate are useful as induction agents because of a short duration of action, a comparatively smooth onset of unconsciousness and relatively complete and rapid recovery. Nevertheless, appropriate patient care (e.g. oxygen supplementation) and monitoring (e.g. ventilation) remain very important.

Non-steroidal anti-inflammatory drugs

Non-steroidal anti-inflammatory drugs (NSAIDs) must be used with caution because many geriatric patients are on constant anti-inflammatory medication for osteoarthritis. Their use should be avoided in patients with hepatic, renal or gastrointestinal problems or those with platelet dysfunction.

Volatile anaesthetic agents

Volatile anaesthetic agents should be selected depending on their speed of uptake and elimination, their effect on cardiovascular function and extent of metabolism. Isoflurane and sevoflurane are appropriate choices for the geriatric patient because of:

- A fast induction of anaesthesia and recovery
- Compared with halothane, better preservation of cardiac output and splanchnic perfusion
- Clinically insignificant hepatic and renal metabolism.

Despite the administration of a high percentage of oxygen in the inspired gas mixture, a particularly critical period is the induction of anaesthesia using a facemask or a chamber, because a high concentration of anaesthetic vapour is inspired. The undesirable environmental pollution and exposure of personnel to anaesthetic vapours are other concerns during mask induction.

Important, dose-dependent effects (e.g. depth of anaesthesia, respiratory depression, vasodilation, hypotension) require careful monitoring in the anaesthetized geriatric patient. Pain relief is inadequate if volatile anaesthetics are used alone: halothane, isoflurane and sevoflurane are best used in a balanced, multimodal anaesthetic protocol.

Preoperative preparation

Evaluation of the geriatric dog and cat prior to sedation or anaesthesia needs to address all major organ systems and should include a complete account of all previously and currently administered medication (traditional and homoeopathic medication, vitamins, food supplements). It is advantageous if the patient is known to the veterinary surgeon, e.g. through earlier annual health checks and vaccinations. If a cardiac murmur or cardiac arrhythmia is auscultated, a cardiac work-up should be initiated to determine the causes and its effects on cardiac function. A thorough clinical examination should be followed by additional investigations such as haematology, serum biochemistry, urinalysis and diagnostic imaging. The extent of these additional diagnostic steps will depend on the history, the results of the clinical examination and the planned procedure. Depending on these findings, a modification of the sedative or anaesthetic technique might become mandatory. Owners must be kept informed about all intended actions and their consent (including for the use of non-licensed drugs) is, of course, essential.

Intravenous access is crucial for fluid and intravenous drug administration. Ideally, at least one peripheral intravenous catheter should be aseptically placed prior to administration of any sedative or anaesthetic drugs.

Intravenous fluid administration (5–10 ml/kg/h) using a balanced electrolyte solution is a reasonable choice. Glucose and electrolyte supplementation need to be addressed individually. The rate of fluid administration is governed by coexisting problems, such as hypoproteinaemia and cardiovascular disease, and needs to be adjusted accordingly. Fluid administration may be necessary for hours and even days following anaesthesia and surgery.

Pre-anaesthetic fasting should be kept to a minimum. In general, a period of 8 hours is sufficient. Water should be withdrawn 1 hour prior to premedication. If dehydration is of concern, fluid administration at maintenance rates can be started at this time.

Anaesthetic maintenance, monitoring and support

The advantages and disadvantages of sedation versus general anaesthesia need to be assessed individually. General anaesthesia incorporating a volatile anaesthetic offers particular advantages:

- A secure airway achieved by endotracheal intubation
- Ease of controlled ventilation
- Administration of 100% oxygen
- A high degree of control because of rapid drug uptake and elimination
- A low hepatic and renal burden because of minimal drug metabolism.

Isoflurane and sevoflurane have fewer side effects (e.g. better preservation of cardiac output and splanchnic perfusion) than halothane, which should only be used in healthy geriatric dogs and cats. Sevoflurane is the preferred agent when performing a mask induction technique.

It is important to understand that age itself is not a risk factor but ASA status (see Chapter 2), duration of anaesthesia and type of surgery will increase the likelihood of peri-anaesthetic complications and morbidity. Adequate pain relief, achieved either by using systemic analgesics or by local anaesthetic blocks, is essential. Carefully planned analgesia will not prolong but rather enhance the speed of recovery.

Both sedated and anaesthetized patients need careful monitoring. The extent of monitoring will depend on the general health status of the patient, the invasiveness of the procedure performed and the available equipment, but should be as complete and as continuous as feasible under practice conditions. Minimal monitoring should include:

- Pulse rate, rhythm and quality
- Respiratory rate, rhythm and estimation of tidal volume
- Arterial blood pressure (non-invasive: oscillometric method, Doppler)
- Core body temperature
- Capnography.

Further peri-anaesthetic monitoring (e.g. invasive arterial and central venous blood pressure measurement, arterial pH and blood gases, haematocrit and plasma total protein, electrolytes and blood glucose) needs to be chosen on an individual basis to improve patient care. In general, monitoring will be more intensive in geriatric compared with younger patients.

An important part of the sedative or anaesthetic protocol, especially for geriatric patients, is adequate preparation for critical situations and emergencies. The minimal and maximal tolerated values of all physiological parameters (e.g. heart rate, systolic, mean and diastolic arterial blood pressures and pain scoring) must be outlined to all staff involved and action for immediate correction or treatment needs to be established.

Duration of hospitalization should be kept to a minimum for geriatric patients because they tolerate stress less well than younger dogs and cats. In general they profit from attentive care, such as:

- Appropriate cage bedding to improve comfort
- Careful positioning during the intervention because of reduced joint flexibility
- Support and maintenance of normal body temperature (e.g. warm intravenous fluids, blankets, forced air warmer) because of a decreased thermoregulatory capacity. This helps to avert problems such as shivering, cardiac arrhythmias, reduced drug metabolism, prolonged recovery, increased infection risk and delayed wound healing
- Judicious fluid therapy to correct individual deficits and to maintain appropriate perfusion and oxygen delivery to tissues but avoiding volume overload
- Adequate nutrition, avoiding long pre-anaesthetic fasting and postoperative periods of food refusal and the risk of a catabolic state. The food should be palatable and may need to be individually prepared
- Appropriate time periods of restful sleep to enhance recovery and to minimize general fatigue.

Geriatric patients should be anaesthetized early in the day to allow for complete recovery under experienced staff observation.

Summary

Indiscriminate use of drugs should be avoided in this age group: appropriate drug selection is essential. There is no perfect sedative or anaesthetic drug. No anaesthetic drug is contraindicated absolutely and the mainstays of sedation and anaesthesia for the geriatric dog and cat are:

- Early oxygen supplementation
- Cautious drug selection: familiarity with the drug is more important than perfect drug pharmacology
- Administration of small doses of the selected drug titrated to a desired effect, whenever possible choosing the slow intravenous route
- Avoidance of any drug that is not absolutely necessary, i.e. 'keeping it simple'
- Rapid airway control and maintenance of airway patency
- Immediate treatment of undesirable changes and aberrations from preset cut-off points in physiological parameters
- Careful attention to detail in patient support, monitoring (including all drug effects) and care during the entire period of sedation/anaesthesia until complete recovery. Frequent postoperative check-ups in the weeks following a lengthy anaesthetic period may be required for geriatric patients with renal or hepatic disease.

Stress caused by separation from the owner, time spent in the hospital environment, the effects of sedation/anaesthesia and the diagnostic or surgical procedure can exacerbate pre-existing but normally covert pathology. Special care and constant observation during the entire peri-anaesthetic period are needed, but geriatric dogs and cats are not at a higher risk for complications than younger patients as long as age-related changes in physiology are understood. However, the ASA status *will* influence peri-anaesthetic morbidity and complications.

References and further reading

Fortney W (2005) Geriatrics. *Veterinary Clinics of North America: Small Animal Practice* **35(3)**

Harvey RC and Paddleford RR (1999) Management of geriatric patients – a common occurrence. *Veterinary Clinics of North America Small Animal Practice* **29(3)**, 683–699

Hosgood G and Scholl DT (1998) Evaluation of age as a risk factor for perianesthetic morbidity and mortality in the dog. *Journal of Veterinary Emergency and Critical Care* **8**, 222–236

Hosgood G and Scholl DT (2002) Evaluation of age and American Society of Anesthesiologists (ASA) physical status as a risk factor for perianesthetic morbidity and mortality in the cat. *Journal of Veterinary Emergency and Critical Care* **12**, 9–15

29

Anaesthetic complications, accidents and emergencies

Christine Egger

Introduction

- Some anaesthetic complications are common, and are caused by the central nervous system (CNS) and cardiopulmonary depressant effects of drugs used in anaesthesia, the procedure performed, or both.
- Many anaesthetic drugs decrease cardiac output, blood pressure, heart rate, tidal volume, respiratory rate and body temperature regulation.
- Complications arising from the surgical procedure itself may result in further depression of cardiac output and ventilation (i.e. haemorrhage, pneumothorax, head-up positioning).
- Human error is a frequent cause of problems encountered during anaesthetic management, stressing the importance of vigilance when monitoring patients during the peri-anaesthetic period.
- Correct calculation of anaesthetic drug dosages is critical to avoid absolute overdosage, as most anaesthetic drugs have a narrow therapeutic index.
- Careful titration of drugs to achieve the desired effect in each individual animal, according to its physical status, is particularly important in avoiding a relative overdose of anaesthetic drugs.
- Lack of pre-anaesthetic stabilization and peri-anaesthetic monitoring and vigilance can lead to an increased incidence of anaesthetic emergencies.
- When complications do occur, appropriate evaluation, management and documentation are critical to minimize or eliminate negative outcomes.
- Having a plan of action to deal with these events, should they occur, will result in improved patient outcome.

Anaesthetic complications

Respiratory complications

Respiratory complications, including hypoventilation, ventilation to perfusion mismatch, atelectasis and airway obstruction will ultimately result in hypoxaemia, hypercapnia, or both, if not recognized and corrected (Figure 29.1).

Clinical sign	Aetiology	Rule-outs	Treatment
Dyspnoea: Obstructive pulmonary disease	Upper airway (inspiratory dyspnoea)	Brachycephalics Soft palate entrapment Laryngeal or tracheal obstruction Laryngeal paralysis Head bandage too tight Kinked endotracheal tube	Oxygen Extend head and neck and pull tongue forward Suction airway Endotracheal intubation Steroids and diuretics ± Sedation
	Lower airway (expiratory dyspnoea)	Bronchospasm Asthma Anaphylaxis	Oxygen Bronchodilator Steroids, antihistamines
Restrictive pulmonary disease (rapid, shallow breaths)	Intrinsic: Extrinsic:	Pulmonary oedema, pneumonia, infiltrates, ARDS Pneumothorax, pleural effusion, increased intra-abdominal pressure	Oxygen Thoracocentesis Endotracheal intubation, IPPV Alveolar recruitment manoeuvre
Hypoxia	V/Q mismatch and right-to-left intrapulmonary shunting	Apnoea/hypoventilation Atelectasis Inadequate F_iO_2 Airway obstruction Restrictive lung disease Severe anaemia Severe hypotension Cardiac arrest	Oxygen Endotracheal intubation and IPPV Alveolar recruitment manoeuvre Reversal of CNS depressant drugs Thoracocentesis Bronchodilators, diuretics Haemoglobin transfusion Sympathomimetic support ± CPR

29.1 Common respiratory complications of general anaesthesia. ARDS = Acute respiratory distress syndrome; CNS = Central nervous system; CPR = Cardiopulmonary resuscitation; F_iO_2 = Fraction of inspired oxygen; FRC = Functional residual capacity; GI = Gastrointestinal; IPPV = Intermittent positive pressure ventilation; LOS = Lower oesophageal sphincter; RR = Respiratory rate; TV = Tidal volume; V/Q = Ventilation/perfusion. (continues) ▶

Clinical sign	Aetiology	Rule-outs	Treatment
Hypoventilation	Reduced FRC Reduced minute ventilation (RR or TV)	Positioning, relaxation of respiratory muscles Respiratory depressant drugs Abdominal distension Hypotension, hypothermia Airway obstruction	Endotracheal intubation, IPPV Reverse respiratory depressant drugs if effects are severe Reduce abdominal distension Correct hypotension, hypothermia Correct airway obstruction
Respiratory arrest	Depression of brainstem respiratory centres	Anaesthetics overdose Reflex apnoea Brainstem injury Cardiac arrest	Endotracheal intubation IPPV CPR
Hyperventilation	Increased minute ventilation (RR and/or TV)	Inadequate depth of anaesthesia Hypercapnia, hypoxaemia Hyperthermia	Check depth of anaesthesia and increase if required Check absorber granules, one-way valves, fresh gas flow and the breathing circuit
Aspiration	Aspiration of GI contents Aspiration of blood, saliva, mucus or pus	Drugs that decrease LOS tone Factors that delay gastric emptying (pain, fear, opioids) Increased intra-abdominal pressure (pregnancy, ascites, GI obstruction) Prolonged anaesthesia	Appropriate fasting Rapid intravenous induction and control of airway in fed patients Pre- or post-treatment with prokinetic drugs, H_2 blockers, or proton pump inhibitors Position head down to allow pharyngeal area to drain Suction and lavage of oesophagus Sucralfate

29.1 (continued) Common respiratory complications of general anaesthesia. ARDS = Acute respiratory distress syndrome; CNS = Central nervous system; CPR = Cardiopulmonary resuscitation; F_iO_2 = Fraction of inspired oxygen; FRC = Functional residual capacity; GI = Gastrointestinal; IPPV = Intermittent positive pressure ventilation; LOS = Lower oesophageal sphincter; RR = Respiratory rate; TV = Tidal volume; V/Q = Ventilation/perfusion.

Pathophysiological effects of hypoxaemia and hypercapnia

Effects of hypoxaemia on the cardiovascular system:

- The end products of aerobic metabolism (oxidative phosphorylation) are carbon dioxide and water, which are normally easily excreted.
- There is a cessation of oxidative phosphorylation when mitochondrial oxygen level falls below a critical level, resulting in anaerobic metabolism and the inefficient production of adenosine triphosphate (ATP).
- The main anaerobic metabolites are hydrogen and lactate ions, which are not easily excreted and accumulate in the circulation, resulting in acidosis and a base deficit.
- The clinical manifestations of hypoxaemia are usually related to symptoms arising from the most vulnerable organs: brain, heart, spinal cord, kidney or liver.
- The cardiovascular response to hypoxaemia is a product of neural and humoral reflexes and direct effects:
  - The reflex responses occur first and result from aortic and carotid chemoreceptors and baroreceptors and central cerebral stimulation
  - The humoral reflex effects result from catecholamine and renin–angiotensin release
  - These reflexes are excitatory and vasoconstrictive
  - The direct local vascular effects of hypoxaemia are inhibitory and vasodilatory, and occur later.
- The net response to hypoxaemia depends on the severity, which determines the magnitude and balance between the inhibitory and excitatory components.
- The balance may vary according to the type and depth of anaesthesia and the degree of pre-existing cardiovascular disease.
- *Mild arterial hypoxaemia* (saturation of haemoglobin with oxygen in arterial blood (S_aO_2) 80–90%) causes general activation of the sympathetic nervous system (SNS) and release of catecholamines:
  - Heart rate, stroke volume, myocardial contractility and cardiac output increase
  - Systemic vascular resistance increases slightly and mild hypertension may occur.
- With *moderate arterial hypoxaemia* (S_aO_2 60–80%) local vasodilation may predominate and systemic vascular resistance and blood pressure decrease:
  - Heart rate may continue to increase because of the baroreceptor reflex response to decreased blood pressure.
- With *severe hypoxaemia* (S_aO_2 <60%) local depressant effects dominate and blood pressure falls rapidly, the heart rate slows, shock develops and ventricular fibrillation or asystole follow.
- In sedated or anaesthetized patients, the early SNS reactivity to hypoxaemia may be reduced, and hypoxaemia may manifest clinically as bradycardia, severe hypotension and cardiovascular collapse.
- Hypoxaemia also promotes *cardiac arrhythmias*, as a result of a decrease in the myocardial oxygen supply:demand ratio:

- Arterial hypoxaemia may directly decrease myocardial oxygen delivery (decreased oxygen content)
- Hypoxaemia results in tachycardia, increasing myocardial oxygen consumption and allowing less time for diastolic filling and coronary artery perfusion, resulting in reduced oxygen supply
- Early increased systemic blood pressure causes an increased afterload on the left ventricle, which increases left ventricular oxygen demand
- Late systemic hypotension may decrease diastolic perfusion pressure, further decreasing oxygen supply
- If myocardial areas become hypoxic or ischaemic, ventricular premature contractions (VPCs), ventricular tachycardia and ventricular fibrillation can occur.

Effects of hypercapnia on the cardiovascular system:

- Hypercapnia, like hypoxaemia, can cause direct depression of both cardiac muscle and vascular smooth muscle, and at the same time cause reflex stimulation of the sympathoadrenal system.
- *Mild hypercapnia* (partial pressure of carbon dioxide in arterial blood (P_aCO_2) 45–59 mmHg (6–8 kPa)) results in mild SNS stimulation, tachycardia and mild hypertension.
- With *moderate to severe hypercapnia* (P_aCO_2 60–90 mmHg (8–11.3 kPa)) SNS stimulation first results in tachycardia and hypertension, increasing myocardial oxygen demand, and later results in decreased myocardial oxygen supply, due to tachycardia and late hypotension.
- Hypercapnia can also cause ventricular arrhythmias, including ventricular fibrillation.
- With *severe hypercapnia* (P_aCO_2 >90 mmHg (12 kPa)) severe CNS depression occurs.
- Hypercapnia can impair oxygenation due to displacement of oxygen in the alveolus by the high concentration of carbon dioxide, resulting in decreased alveolar and arterial oxygen concentration.
- Hypercapnia causes a shift in the oxyhaemoglobin dissociation curve to the right, facilitating oxygen off-loading and tissue oxygenation.
- Hypercapnia results in leakage of potassium from liver cells into plasma as a result of glucose release and mobilization in response to the increase in plasma catecholamines.

Effects of hypoxaemia and hypercapnia on the respiratory system:

- Both hypercapnia and hypoxaemia cause stimulation of respiration and an *increase in minute ventilation*, although this response is reduced with many anaesthetic drugs.
- At a P_aCO_2 of >100 mmHg (13.3 kPa), respiratory stimulation is reduced, and will eventually stop altogether, due to depression of the brainstem.
- In addition, severe hypoxaemia will result in inadequate supply of oxygen to the brainstem, resulting in depressed respiration and eventual apnoea.

General effects of anaesthesia on the respiratory system

- Ventilation/perfusion (alveolar ventilation to perfusion ratio) (V/Q) mismatch is a common complication of general anaesthesia.
- Air left within the lungs at end-expiration, called functional residual capacity, is reduced with general anaesthesia, particularly with the patient in dorsal recumbency, and this decrease in functional residual capacity leads to *V/Q mismatch* or *reduced alveolar ventilation* (hypoventilation).
- When the functional residual capacity is close to or less than the closing volume of the lung, the small airways begin to close, resulting in *atelectasis* and right-to-left shunting of blood in the pulmonary vasculature and consequent *hypoxaemia*.
- Causes of V/Q mismatch are atelectasis, patient positioning, accidental endobronchial intubation, bronchospasm, pneumonia, acute respiratory distress syndrome (ARDS), airway obstruction, hypoventilation and pulmonary arterial hypotension.
- Brainstem respiratory centres are depressed by general anaesthetics and mu agonist opioids, resulting in a shift in the carbon dioxide response curve (level of carbon dioxide at which inspiration is triggered), and reduced hypoxic respiratory drive.
- Reduced compliance and increased resistance of the thorax and lungs with general anaesthesia results in a change to a diaphragmatic breathing pattern.
- Cilial paralysis, mucosal drying and depressed airway reflexes (such as airway protective reflexes) also impair respiratory function during anaesthesia.

Obstructive pulmonary disease

Pathophysiology:

- During inspiration, work is done against elastic and resistive forces in the lungs, and any increase in resistance to airflow will increase the work of breathing.
- Obstruction of the upper or lower airways can have a marked effect on the resistance and the work of breathing, and animals will tend to ventilate in order to minimize this work.
- With obstructed airways, the animal will ventilate to minimize the resistance forces, resulting in a reduced respiratory rate and increased tidal volume to maintain minute ventilation.
- The ability to compensate for the increased work of breathing is reduced under the effects of many anaesthetic drugs, and many anaesthetics result in increased relaxation of tissues in the

pharyngeal area, causing further obstruction and increased resistance.
- Reduced minute ventilation can result in *hypercapnia* and *hypoxaemia*.

Upper airway obstruction (inspiratory dyspnoea):

- Partial obstruction will result in inspiratory stridor, with slow, deep breaths. Chest wall moving 'in' during inspiration may be observed.
- Full obstruction results in pronounced paradoxical breathing (abdomen expands and thorax contracts during inspiration) and hyperextension of head and neck.
- If inspiratory efforts are severe, the upper airway may undergo a dynamic inspiratory compression because of the marked pressure gradient in the upper airway.
- Prolonged obstruction and intense respiratory effort can result in pulmonary oedema and acute lung injury.

Causes:

- Soft palate entrapment (heavily sedated, non-intubated patients).
- Brachycephalic airway syndrome (breed predisposition).
- Laryngeal spasm (common during light levels of anaesthesia).
- Laryngeal paralysis (breed predisposition).
- Laryngeal or pharyngeal inflammation or oedema (trauma during intubation, or prolonged pressure of the endotracheal tube).
- Laryngeal or tracheal collapse (breed predisposition).
- Laryngeal, pharyngeal, tracheal or nasal obstruction (blood, mucus, vomitus, saliva, tumour, foreign body).
- Kinked or blocked endotracheal tube (over-inflation of endotracheal tube cuff).
- Too tight head and/or neck bandage (usually a problem after extubation).
- No gas flow into breathing circuit (rebreathing bag will be collapsed).

Treatment: See Figure 29.6 for drug doses.

- Extend head and neck and pull tongue forward to open airways, maintain in sternal recumbency.
- Provide supplemental oxygen (nasal cannula, mask, intratracheal oxygen).
- Suction airway, including the endotracheal tube, as required. A small amount of saline may help break up solid mucus, followed by suction.
- Endotracheal intubation or emergency tracheostomy may be necessary.
- Steroid and diuretic administration to reduce inflammation and oedema.
- Maintain intubation and general anaesthesia until swelling resolves, extubate early with supplemental oxygen (nasal cannula or mask).
- Maintain in sternal recumbency, with extended head and neck and the tongue pulled forward.
- Positive pressure ventilation may be required if the intrathoracic trachea or main stem bronchi are collapsed.
- Sedation may be helpful, but avoid heavy sedation in brachycephalic breeds, as relaxation of redundant pharyngeal tissue makes obstruction more likely.

Lower airway obstruction (expiratory dyspnoea):

Causes:

- Bronchospasm (usually occurs during light levels of anaesthesia).
- Bronchitis.
- Asthma.
- Chronic obstructive pulmonary disease (COPD).
- Anaphylactic or anaphylactoid reactions.

Treatment: See Figure 29.6 for drug dosages.

- Supplemental oxygen (nasal cannula, mask or endotracheal intubation).
- Deepen anaesthesia (ketamine and volatile agents are good bronchodilators).
- Bronchodilator administration:
  - Adrenaline, albuterol, clenbuterol, terbutaline
  - Aminophylline, theophylline.
- Steroids (methylprednisolone, dexamethasone).
- Antihistamines (diphenhydramine).
- Use a 'slow and deep' ventilation pattern, rather than 'fast and shallow'.

Restrictive pulmonary disease

Pathophysiology:

- Restrictive pulmonary diseases result in a tendency for the lungs to collapse and become less compliant.
- Decreased lung compliance and increased lung elastance can result from disease processes extrinsic to the lungs, such as intrathoracic disease, or intrinsic to the lungs, such as with a change in surfactant or bronchial mucus or an alteration of elastic tissue of the lungs (fibrosis, age).
- Decreased compliance results in increased work of breathing to overcome the elastic forces and expand the lungs.
- To minimize the work of breathing, a rapid shallow breathing pattern is adopted to minimize the elastic forces involved.
- Many anaesthetic agents decrease the respiratory rate, decreasing the ability of the patient to compensate.
- Hypoventilation and V/Q mismatch under anaesthesia will result in increased atelectasis, also reducing lung compliance.

Intrinsic restrictive pulmonary disorders:

- These disorders reduce surfactant and bronchial mucus, and increase lung water, reducing compliance.

- Causes include acute respiratory distress syndrome (ARDS), pulmonary oedema, pneumonia, lung consolidation, pulmonary infiltrates (infection, pulmonary disease, trauma, ventilator induced injury, endotoxaemia).

Extrinsic restrictive pulmonary disorders:

- These disorders alter gas exchange by interfering with normal lung expansion.
- Causes include pneumothorax, pleural effusions, mediastinal masses, neuromuscular disorders, and increased intra-abdominal pressure from ascites, pregnancy or gastrointestinal obstruction.

Treatment: See Figure 29.6 for drug dosages.

- Thoracocentesis to remove fluid or air (diagnostic and therapeutic).
- Placement of chest tubes may be required (see Chapter 21).
- Supplemental oxygen (nasal cannula, mask or endotracheal intubation).
- Treat cause (ARDS, endotoxaemia, pulmonary disease, infection; detailed treatments are beyond the scope of this book).
- Consider drugs such as furosemide, corticosteroids, antimicrobials, bronchodilators, surfactant therapy.
- Alveolar recruitment procedure (sigh): use reservoir bag to obtain a peak airway pressure of 30–40 cmH_2O for 40–60 seconds to reinflate atelectatic alveoli.
- Increase peak airway pressure during positive pressure ventilation to reinflate alveoli and reduce atelectasis.
- Positive end-expiratory pressure (PEEP) to reduce and prevent atelectasis.
- Try a 'fast and shallow' ventilation pattern, rather than 'slow and deep'.
- Long-term ventilator therapy using expensive, specially designed critical care ventilators may be required for some conditions. Details of patient management are found in books and articles on critical care.

Hypoxaemia

This is where arterial oxygen tension is <60 mmHg (<8 kPa).

- Early clinical signs of hypoxaemia include restlessness, dysphoria, tachycardia, cardiac irritability (arrhythmias) and hypertension.
- Cheyne-Stokes breathing pattern may be observed (increasing tidal volume followed by decreasing tidal volume separated by long expiratory pause).
- CNS depression, bradycardia, hypotension and cardiac arrest are late, often terminal, signs.
- Pulse oximetry is useful in place of arterial blood gas analysis:
  - A haemoglobin oxygen saturation of <90% is equivalent to P_aO_2 <60 mmHg (<8 kPa).
- Cyanotic mucous membrane colour occurs when 15 g/l of haemoglobin is not carrying oxygen. This colour change may be difficult to see in anaemic patients and under poor lighting conditions.
- Hypoxaemia is possible without hypercapnia (ventilated patient receiving low inspired oxygen).

Causes:

- Increased intrapulmonary shunting due to atelectasis is the most common cause of hypoxaemia during and following general anaesthesia:
  - Decreased functional residual capacity leads to V/Q mismatch and hypoventilation
  - When the functional residual capacity is close to or less than the closing volume of the lung, the small airways begin to close, resulting in atelectasis and right-to-left shunting of blood in the pulmonary vasculature and consequent hypoxaemia.
- Hypoventilation in a patient not receiving supplemental oxygen (on 'room air' or 21% fraction inspired O_2 (F_iO_2)) will result in hypoxaemia, even without the presence of atelectasis.
- Inadequate inspired oxygen:
  - Airway obstruction
  - Bronchoconstriction
  - Inadequate oxygen flow (low F_iO_2).
- Apnoea or respiratory arrest:
  - Induction apnoea secondary to thiopental, propofol or ketamine administration
  - Relative or absolute overdosage of anaesthetic drugs.
- Pulmonary parenchymal disease (oedema, pneumonia, parenchymal infiltrates).
- Intrathoracic disease (pneumothorax, pleural effusion).
- Severe anaemia and inadequate oxygen carrying capacity.
- Severe decrease in cardiac output (shock) or cardiac arrest.

Treatment: See Figure 29.6 for drug dosages.

- Preoxygenate with mask for 5 minutes prior to anaesthetic induction, particularly in patients with respiratory disease or in which difficult endotracheal intubation is anticipated. Placing patient in oxygen cage and then removing patient to induction area without continuing oxygen therapy is not adequate.
- Provide supplemental oxygen via nasal cannula, mask, or endotracheal intubation to increase F_iO_2 whenever hypoxaemia is observed or suspected.
- Intubate and provide oxygen and positive pressure ventilation to patients in which oxygen insufflation alone is inadequate to maintain oxygen saturation >91%.
- Increase peak airway pressure (up to 40 cmH_2O) during IPPV to re-expand atelectatic alveoli (alveolar recruitment manoeuvre) and consider the use of positive end-expiratory pressure (PEEP).

- Thoracocentesis to remove intrathoracic air or effusion (± chest tube placement).
- Treat pulmonary disease (diuretics, antibiotics, bronchodilators).
- Improve cardiac output, blood pressure and pulmonary perfusion (fluid therapy, sympathomimetic therapy).
- Cardiopulmonary resuscitation, as required.
- Increase oxygen-carrying capacity (haemoglobin) via transfusion of whole blood, packed red blood cells, or oxygen-carrying solutions (Oxyglobin®) (see Chapter 16).
- Decrease oxygen consumption due to pain, shivering or fever (analgesics, antipyretics).

Hypoventilation

This is reduced minute ventilation, reduced tidal volume and/or respiratory rate.

- Arterial pCO_2 >45 mmHg (6 kPa) is indicative of hypoventilation.
- End-tidal carbon dioxide monitoring is useful if arterial blood gas analysis is not available.
- Patients receiving 100% oxygen under anaesthesia are unlikely to become hypoxaemic during hypoventilation, but patients that are on room air (21% F_iO_2) will become hypoxaemic.

Causes:

- Induction of anaesthesia and dorsal recumbency can reduce functional residual capacity by more than 25%.
- Loss of normal end-expiratory diaphragmatic tone allows the abdominal contents to rise further up against the diaphragm, resulting in decreased lung volume and reduced chest and lung compliance.
- Decreased functional residual capacity leads to increased V/Q mismatch, alveolar hypoventilation and atelectasis and right-to-left shunting of blood in the pulmonary vasculature.
- Steep head-down position of greater than 30 degrees to horizontal can reduce functional residual capacity even more, as the intrathoracic blood volume increases and the abdominal organs impinge on the diaphragm.
- Use of mu agonist opioids, barbiturates, propofol and volatile agents, which directly depress the brainstem respiratory centres, can result in reduced minute ventilation.
- Abdominal distension (ascites, uroabdomen, pregnancy, gastrointestinal obstruction, haemoabdomen) will also contribute to hypoventilation.
- Severe hypotension, resulting in inadequate perfusion of CNS respiratory centres, will cause hypoventilation and possibly Cheyne-Stokes breathing pattern (repeated pattern of progressively increasing tidal volume, then progressively decreasing tidal volume followed by a long expiratory pause).
- Hypothermia will also cause depression of CNS respiratory centres and result in hypoventilation.
- The pain of thoracic injury (fractured ribs, flail chest) will contribute to hypoventilation.
- Partial obstruction of the airway and increased work of breathing:
  - Brachycephalic animals
  - Obstruction of the endotracheal tube with mucus, blood
  - Kinking of the endotracheal tube
  - Placement of inappropriately small endotracheal tube.

Treatment: See Figure 29.6 for drug dosages.

- Endotracheal intubation (or reintubation), oxygen therapy and positive pressure ventilation.
- Improve CNS perfusion with fluid therapy and sympathomimetic support.
- Lighten depth of anaesthesia.
- Warm patient to normothermia using warm intravenous and lavage fluids, circulating warm water blankets, and forced warm air blankets.
- Administer appropriate analgesics for chest trauma.
- Relieve abdominal distension.
- Consider reversing CNS depressant drugs where possible.

Apnoea/respiratory arrest

Causes:

- Rapid intravenous administration of propofol, thiopental or ketamine/benzodiazepine combination.
- Overdosage of barbiturates, propofol, volatile agents, opioids, ketamine.
- Reflex apnoea secondary to visceral traction or endotracheal intubation.
- Brainstem injury.
- Cardiac arrest.
- Equipment failure (closed pop-off valve, ventilator stopped).

Treatment:

- Endotracheal intubation.
- Positive pressure ventilation with oxygen supplementation.
- Lighten anaesthetic depth.
- Check anaesthetic equipment.
- Cardiopulmonary resuscitation.

Hyperventilation

- Increased minute ventilation (increased tidal volume and/or respiratory rate).

Causes:

- Inadequate anaesthetic depth and response to painful stimulation.
- Hypercapnia:
  - End-tidal carbon dioxide monitor extremely useful in this situation

- Increased inspired and expired carbon dioxide due to:
  - Exhausted absorber granules
  - Stuck or missing one-way valve(s)
  - Improper connection of the breathing circuit
  - Insufficient fresh gas flow with a non-rebreathing circuit.
- Hypoxaemia (hypoxic drive overrides carbon dioxide control of breathing).
- Panting due to opioid administration.
- Hyperthermia.
- Increased carbon dioxide production or administration (malignant hyperthermia, laparoscopy using carbon dioxide – will see increased expired carbon dioxide).

Treatment:

- Increase anaesthetic depth and/or administer additional analgesics if not due to hypercapnia or hypoxaemia.
- Ventilate lungs to remove carbon dioxide.
- Check anaesthetic circuit, one-way valves (quickly remove, dry, and replace; ensure correct size is used), and/or change absorber granules.
- Increase fresh gas flow if using a non-rebreathing circuit.
- See causes and correction of hypoxaemia earlier in the chapter.
- Turn off heating blankets, use cool intravenous fluids.

Aspiration

- Regurgitation and aspiration of stomach contents.
- Aspiration of saliva, blood or mucus.
- Can be silent (not observed).

Predisposing factors include:

- Drugs that relax the lower oesophageal sphincter, such as atropine, glycopyrronium, opioids, thiopental and volatile anaesthetics
- Factors that delay gastric emptying, such as fear, anxiety, pain, shock, opioids and anticholinergics
- Increased intra-abdominal pressure (pregnancy, obesity, abdominal effusion, gastrointestinal obstruction or head-down positioning)
- Prolonged anaesthesia (>2 hours).

Preventive measures:

- Appropriate pre-anaesthetic fasting.
- Rapid intravenous induction to allow rapid control of the airway. Use an endotracheal tube with a leak-tested inflated cuff that can provide a seal at 20 cmH_2O.
- Pretreatment with metoclopramide (prokinetic), which increases lower oesophageal sphincter tone, speeds gastric emptying and lowers gastric fluid volume.
- Pretreatment with H_2 blockers (famotidine, ranitidine), which decrease gastric volume and increase the pH of gastric contents.
- Pretreatment with proton pump inhibitors (omeprazole) to raise gastric pH.

Treatment once regurgitation occurs:

- Leave endotracheal tube in oesophagus if accidental oesophageal intubation triggers vomiting, to facilitate drainage away from pharyngeal and laryngeal areas. Place another endotracheal tube into trachea and inflate cuff, then remove first endotracheal tube.
- Check endotracheal cuff inflation and security of airway.
- Position with head down so that material flows out of the mouth.
- Suction to remove material from nasal and oral pharynx, oral cavity and oesophagus.
- Flush oesophagus with saline, possibly followed by sodium citrate (30 ml) in a large dog, or administer sucralfate to prevent oesophagitis and stricture formation.
- Leave stomach tube in place, to facilitate drainage away from pharyngeal and laryngeal areas. If patient has regurgitated once, it may do so again.
- Suction again prior to extubation and extubate with the cuff slightly inflated.

Barotrauma or volutrauma

- Trauma from pressure or sheer stress resulting in ruptured alveoli and pneumomediastinum and pneumothorax.
- Hypoxaemia and cardiac arrest will follow if it is not recognized and treated immediately.

Causes of barotrauma:

- Repetitive, excessive peak airway pressure with positive pressure ventilation (barotrauma).
- Repetitive collapse and re-expansion of normal or diseased lung during positive pressure ventilation (volutrauma).
- Closed pop-off valve will result in barotrauma, but will also result in decreased venous return and cardiac arrest.

Treatment of barotrauma:

- Avoid high peak airway pressures >40 cmH_2O in healthy lungs and >18 cmH_2O in diseased or compromised lungs.
- Use smaller tidal volume (5–8 ml/kg), lower peak airway pressures (10–14 cmH_2O), and faster rate (20–25 breaths/minute) to ventilate patients with compromised lungs.
- Thoracocentesis to correct pneumothorax.
- Administer oxygen.
- Check for a pulse.

Cardiovascular complications

For information on cardiovascular complications, see Figure 29.2.

Pathophysiology of cardiovascular complications

- Many anaesthetics (volatile and injectable) produce a dose-related:
  - Depression of left ventricular (LV), right ventricular (RV), and left atrial (LA) myocardial contractility (negative inotropy) by altering intracellular Ca^{2+} homeostasis
  - Decrease in LV diastolic function (negative lusitropy)
  - Decrease in LV afterload due to vasodilation and a reduction in systemic vascular resistance
  - Depression of baroreceptor reflex control of arterial pressure to varying degrees.
- These effects result in reduced venous return, hypotension, bradycardia and a decrease in cardiac output, and are exacerbated in a failing heart.
- Volatile anaesthetics and thiobarbiturates can sensitize the myocardium to the arrhythmogenic effects of adrenaline and can prevent or facilitate the development of atrial or ventricular arrhythmias during myocardial ischaemia or infarction, depending upon the volatile anaesthetic concentration and the extent of pre-existing myocardial disease.
- Volatile anaesthetics are relatively weak coronary vasodilators that are not capable of producing coronary steal at typically used clinical concentrations.

Clinical sign	Aetiology	Treatment
Bradyarrhythmias • Sinus bradycardia • Atrioventricular (AV) block (first and second degree) • Sinus arrest • Atrial standstill	Potent mu opioids High vagal tone Hypothermia CNS disease and increased ICP Hyperkalaemia Addisonian crisis	Anticholinergic Butorphanol or naloxone to reverse mu opioid effects Warm patient Decrease ICP Correct hyperkalaemia
Tachyarrhythmias • Sinus tachycardia • Atrial tachycardia • Atrial fibrillation	Drug-induced (atropine) SNS stimulation: pain, hypoxaemia, awareness, hyperthermia, anaemia, hypotension, hypovolaemia Myocardial disease	Rule out or treat underlying cause Beta blockers (esmolol or propranolol)
Ventricular arrhythmias • Ventricular premature contractions • Ventricular tachycardia • Ventricular fibrillation	Hypoxia, myocardial ischaemia, traumatic myocarditis, GDV, splenic disease, hypercapnia, acid–base imbalance, electrolyte imbalance, drug effects (thiobarbiturates)	Rule out or treat underlying cause Lidocaine, procainamide, mexiletine Magnesium sulphate CPR
Hypotension	**Decreased venous return:** • Vasodilation • Hypovolaemia • IPPV • Pericardial effusion • Tension pneumothorax • Closed pop-off valve • Surgical packing and retraction of organs • Severe bradycardia	Increase intravascular volume with balanced, isotonic crystalloid or colloid administration Thoracocentesis Pericardiocentesis Open pop-off valve Reduce surgical traction Reduce mean airway pressure and the I:E ratio with IPPV
	Vasodilation (volatile anaesthetics, propofol and thiopental cause vasodilation)	Administer a vasoconstrictor: • Dopamine • Ephedrine • Adrenaline • Vasopressin
	Ventricular dysfunction	Administer a positive inotrope: • Dobutamine • Dopamine • Ephedrine • Adrenaline
Hypertension	Pain Hypoxaemia Hypercapnia Metabolic acidosis Underlying renal or cardiac disease	Rule out or treat underlying cause Beta blockers ACE inhibitors

29.2 Common cardiovascular complications of general anaesthesia. ACE = Angiotensin converting enzyme; CNS = Central nervous system; CPR = Cardiopulmonary resuscitation; GDV = Gastric dilatation–volvulus; ICP = Intracranial pressure; I:E = Inspired:expired; IPPV = Intermittent positive pressure ventilation; SNS = Sympathetic nervous system.

- Volatile anaesthetics exert important cardioprotective effects against reversible and irreversible myocardial ischaemia in experimental animals by activating intracellular signal transduction pathways.

Cardiac arrhythmias

Bradyarrhythmias

- Severe bradyarrhythmias can greatly reduce cardiac output and tissue perfusion, particularly if there is limited ability to increase stroke volume by either increased contractility or vasoconstriction and increased venous return.
- Severe bradyarrhythmias can result in syncope in awake animals, and severe hypotension in anaesthetized animals.
- Bradyarrhythmias seen under anaesthesia include:
  - Sinus bradycardia
  - Atrioventricular (AV) block (first and second degree)
  - Sinus arrest
  - Atrial standstill.

Causes:

- Drug effects (high dose mu agonist opioids, alpha-2 adrenergic agonists).
- CNS disease, particularly if there is increased intracranial pressure (ICP).
- Hypothermia.
- High vagal tone.
- Vagal stimulation (i.e. during surgery).
- Hyperkalaemia.

Treatment: See Figure 29.6 for drug dosages.

- Anticholinergic (atropine or glycopyrronium).
- Use naloxone to reverse opioids.
- Reduce ICP (mannitol).
- Warm patient.
- Correct hyperkalaemia (dextrose, sodium bicarbonate, insulin; see Chapter 23).
- Cardiopulmonary resuscitation (ventricular standstill):
  - Atropine
  - Adrenaline
  - Isoproterenol (if bradycardia refractory to adrenaline or atropine).

Atrial tachyarrhythmias

- Severe tachyarrhythmias greatly reduce cardiac output and tissue perfusion due to decreased time for diastolic filling, reduced ejection time and reduced time for coronary perfusion, resulting in myocardial ischaemia.
- Types of tachyarrhythmia seen under anaesthesia include:
  - Sinus tachycardia
  - Atrial tachycardia
  - Atrial fibrillation.

Causes:

- Drug-induced (anticholinergics, particularly atropine).
- Sympathetic nervous system stimulation due to:
  - Pain
  - Awareness
  - Hyperthermia
  - Hypotension
  - Hypovolaemia
  - Hypoxaemia
  - Hypercapnia
  - Hypoglycaemia
  - Hyperthyroidism
  - Anaemia
  - Phaeochromocytoma
  - Myocardial disease.

Treatment: See Figure 29.6 for drug dosages.

- Correct underlying problem (pain, awareness, hypovolaemia, anaemia, hypoxaemia, hypercapnia, hypoglycaemia).
- Treat with beta blockers (propranolol or esmolol) if tachycardia is resulting in decreased time for diastolic filling and for myocardial perfusion, cardiac output is decreased and the underlying cause cannot be found.

Ventricular arrhythmias

- The specialized conduction system of the heart is responsible for:
  - Initiating cardiac depolarization
  - Coordinating the electrical impulses throughout the atria and ventricles
  - Coordinating ventricular contractions, essential for effective cardiac output from the ventricles.
- It is critical that excitation and contraction be coordinated, to maintain adequate cardiac output and tissue perfusion.
- Common types of ventricular arrhythmias seen under anaesthesia:
  - Ventricular premature contractions (VPCs)
  - Ventricular tachycardia
  - Ventricular fibrillation.

Causes:

- Gastric dilatation and volvulus (GDV).
- Splenic trauma, torsion, tumour, splenomegaly.
- Traumatic myocarditis.
- Hypoxaemia and myocardial ischaemia (hypotension, severe anaemia).
- Hypercapnia and acid–base imbalance.
- Electrolyte imbalance (hypokalaemia, hypomagnesaemia).
- Drug effects (thiobarbiturates, halothane, ketamine).

Treatment: See Figure 29.6 for drug dosages.

- Treat underlying problem (hypoxaemia, hypercapnia, electrolyte or acid–base imbalance, surgical correction).

- Supplemental oxygen.
- Alter anaesthetic protocol or stop anaesthetic drug administration.
- Lidocaine bolus injection ± continuous rate infusion.
- Procainamide.
- Cardiopulmonary resuscitation (ventricular fibrillation).

Electrolyte abnormalities observed with electrocardiography

- Hyperkalaemia results in peaked T waves, QRS widening, P-R prolongation, loss of P waves, loss of R wave amplitude, ST depression.
- Hypokalaemia results in T wave flattening/ inversion, prominent U wave, increased P wave, P-R prolongation, ST depression.
- Hypercalcaemia results in shortening of Q-T interval, shortened ST segment.
- Hypocalcaemia results in prolongation of Q-T interval.
- Hypermagnesaemia results in prolonged P-R interval, widened QRS.
- Hypomagnesaemia results in increased P-R and Q-T intervals, myocardial irritability, potentiation of digoxin toxicity.

Hypotension

Pathophysiology

- Blood pressure is a measure of the force driving tissue perfusion.
- A mean arterial blood pressure of at least 60 mmHg is necessary for perfusion of vital organs, such as the brain, heart and kidneys.
- Hypoperfusion of vital organs and the extremities results in inadequate tissue delivery of oxygen and removal of waste products, and clinical signs of shock and subsequent organ dysfunction.

Causes

- Hypovolaemia:
  - Haemorrhage
  - Pre-existing fluid deficits
  - Fluid loss due to evaporation and 'third spacing'
  - Relative hypovolaemia due to vasodilation
  - Inadequate intraoperative fluid administration.
- Vasodilation:
  - Anaesthetic drug-induced – barbiturates, propofol, volatile agents, epidural administration of local anaesthetics
  - Severe metabolic or respiratory acidosis
  - Severe hypoxaemia
  - Endotoxaemia
  - Septicaemia
  - Anaphylactic or anaphylactoid reactions.
- Myocardial depression (decreased contractility):
  - Drug-induced (thiopental, halothane)
  - Hypoxaemia or ischaemia-induced
  - Acid–base disturbance (respiratory or metabolic acidosis)
  - Endotoxaemia
  - Electrolyte imbalance
  - Cardiomyopathy
  - Catecholamine depletion.
- Cardiac arrhythmias that decrease cardiac output:
  - Bradycardia
  - AV block
  - Tachycardia
  - Atrial fibrillation
  - Ventricular tachycardia.
- Obstruction of venous return:
  - IPPV – increased intrathoracic pressure will decrease venous return to the heart, reducing cardiac output
  - Pericardial effusion
  - Tumours (especially mediastinal)
  - Tension pneumothorax
  - Surgical packing
  - Retraction of organs (cranial abdominal surgery).
- Reflex hypotension (vagal reflex):
  - Excessive traction or pressure on the eye or viscera.

Treatment

See Figure 29.6 for drug dosages.

- Reduce amount of injectable or inhalational anaesthetics by administering additional analgesics with anaesthetic-sparing effects (mu agonist opioids, ketamine, lidocaine).
- Correct absolute and relative hypovolaemia and provide for ongoing losses with crystalloids, colloids or blood products.
- Administer an infusion of balanced, crystalloid, isotonic solution during anaesthesia and surgery at 5–10 ml/kg/h.
- Bolus intravenous administration of 20–30 ml/kg of balanced, isotonic, crystalloid solution, or 5–20 ml/kg of colloid solution (maximum 20 ml/kg/ 24 hours) to increase intravascular volume.
- Attempt crystalloid fluid bolus up to twice in patients without underlying cardiac disease or oliguric or anuric renal failure.
- Correct hypoxaemia, hypercapnia, acid–base and electrolyte disturbances.
- Treat bradyarrhythmias (anticholinergics), and tachyarrhythmias (treat cause of sympathetic nervous system stimulation, or beta blocker therapy) that may be affecting cardiac output.
- Stop surgical retraction of viscera or the globe if a vagal reflex occurs, and administer an anticholinergic.
- Reduce tidal volume and peak airway pressure with positive pressure ventilation and maintain an inspiration:expiration ratio of 1:2 or 1:3 to minimize the negative haemodynamic effects of positive pressure ventilation.

- Provide sympathomimetic support:
  - Anticholinergics (chronotropic)
  - Dobutamine (a beta-1 adrenergic agonist and a positive inotrope)
  - Dopamine (D_1, D_2, beta and alpha adrenergic agonist causing positive inotropy, chronotropy, and vasoconstriction to increase venous return)
  - Ephedrine (alpha and beta adrenergic agonist, provides inotropic and chronotropic support, as well as vasoconstriction of great veins to increase venous return)
  - Noradrenaline (mainly an alpha adrenergic agonist, providing arterial vasoconstriction). Short-term treatment for refractory hypotension with endotoxaemia
  - Phenylephrine (alpha adrenergic agonist providing arterial vasoconstriction). Treatment for excessive alpha adrenergic blockade and vasodilation. Short-term use only (<20 minutes)
  - Adrenaline (alpha and beta agonist and provides inotropic and chronotropic support, as well as arterial vasoconstriction (vasodilation in the muscle beds). Excessive vasoconstriction will decrease splanchnic perfusion). Useful for cardiopulmonary arrest or refractory hypotension with endotoxaemia
  - Vasopressin (causes arterial vasoconstriction and venoconstriction to increase venous return). Used for cardiopulmonary resuscitation or vasodilatory shock in patients that do not respond to dopamine, noradrenaline or adrenaline (i.e. septic shock).

Hypertension

- Arterial blood pressure is the most important determinant of left ventricular afterload and cardiac work.
- Hypertension results in increased myocardial work and increased myocardial oxygen demand, which could result in myocardial ischaemia and cardiac arrhythmias.
- Hypertension can result in retinopathy, blindness and renal failure.
- Sudden hypertension during anaesthesia is an indication of SNS stimulation, and possible causes must be ruled out.

Causes

- Pain.
- Mild hypoxaemia.
- Hypercapnia.
- Metabolic acidosis.
- Underlying renal or cardiac disease.
- Phaeochromocytoma.
- Stimulation of adrenal glands during surgery.
- Use of phenylephrine during ophthalmic surgery.

Note that early stages of hypoxaemia, hypercapnia, and metabolic acidosis result in sympathetic nervous system stimulation, tachycardia, peripheral vasoconstriction and hypertension. As the hypoxaemia and acid–base disturbances become more severe, myocardial depression and vasodilation result in hypotension and reduced cardiac output.

Treatment

See Figure 29.6 for drug dosages.

- Treat underlying cause, if possible.
- Beta adrenergic blockers (esmolol, propranolol) or ACE inhibitors (enalapril) may be required.
- Temporary increase in isoflurane or sevoflurane levels during catecholamine release (phaeochromocytoma or adrenal gland stimulation) or magnesium sulphate
- Acepromazine to treat hypertension from phenylephrine use as a local vasoconstrictor (see Chapter 17).

Haemorrhage

- Haemorrhage results in a decrease in plasma volume and haemoglobin concentration, reducing the oxygen carrying capacity of the blood.
- As the haemoglobin concentration declines, the body responds by:
  - Increasing cardiac output (increased heart rate, increased systemic vascular resistance, increased contractility and stroke volume)
  - Increasing uptake of oxygen (increased tidal volume and respiratory rate)
  - Increasing extraction of oxygen within the tissues (increased extraction ratio).
- Once maximal increases in ventilation, cardiac output and oxygen extraction have occurred, delivery of oxygen to the tissues becomes compromised, in spite of an increase in SNS tone and cardiac output in response to haemorrhage, oxygen content must be increased or signs of inadequate tissue delivery of oxygen (shock) will develop.
- Total blood volume can be estimated as 60–70 ml/kg in cats and 80–90 ml/kg in dogs.
- Replace blood lost with blood products (whole blood, packed red blood cells or artificial haemoglobin solutions) when there has been a loss of ≥20% of total blood volume in relatively healthy patients, and ≥10% of total blood volume in debilitated patients.
- Blood loss of less than 20% in healthy animals and 10% in debilitated animals can be treated with crystalloid or colloid solutions to restore intravascular volume.
- Replace estimated lost blood volume with balanced electrolyte solution (e.g. lactated Ringer's (Hartmann's)) at three times the volume lost.
- Replace the lost volume with colloid solution (etherified starch, dextrans, whole blood) at equal the volume lost.
- Hypertonic saline (7.5%) at 4 ml/kg.
- See Chapter 16 for details of blood transfusion.

Miscellaneous complications

For information on miscellaneous complications, see Figure 29.3.

Excitement or dysphoria on recovery

Causes

- Pain.
- Full urinary bladder.
- Hypoxaemia.
- Hypotension.
- Metabolic or respiratory acidosis.
- Central cholinergic syndrome (excessive use of atropine).
- Ketamine-induced psychotomimetic effects.
- Opioid-induced dysphoria (most common with mu agonists and butorphanol).

Treatment

See Figure 29.6 for drug dosages.

- Determine and treat underlying problem.
- Sedation with acepromazine, a benzodiazepine or alpha-2 agonist.
- Naloxone reversal if opioid-induced dysphoria is suspected.

Complication	Causes	Treatment
Excitement or dysphoria on recovery	Pain Hypoxaemia Hypotension Full urinary bladder Metabolic or respiratory acidosis Drug-induced (mu agonist opioids, ketamine)	Treat underlying problem Sedation or tranquillization: • Acepromazine (0.01–0.05 mg/kg) • Diazepam or midazolam (0.2–0.5 mg/kg) • Medetomidine (1–5 µg/kg) • Butorphanol or naloxone to reverse mu opiate effects
Prolonged recovery	Hypoventilation Hypothermia Hypotension Hypoxaemia Hypercarbia Metabolic acidosis Reduce renal or hepatic function	Correct underlying problems of hypothermia, hypotension, hypoxaemia Reverse mu agonist opiates with butorphanol or naloxone Administer intravenous fluids to improve renal and hepatic perfusion
Hypothermia	Redistribution of heat from body core to periphery with vasodilation Cold anaesthetic gases Cold ambient temperature Cold intravenous and surgical lavage fluids Open body cavities CNS depression Reduced muscle tone resulting in reduced muscle heat generated Prolonged anaesthesia	Provide supplemental heat to keep patients warm during the premedication, induction, surgery and recovery periods Use circulating warm water or warm air blankets Use warm intravenous and lavage fluids Reduce surgery time Increase ambient temperature of surgery and recovery areas Provide supplemental oxygen in recovery to meet metabolic oxygen requirements that can greatly increase due to shivering
Hyperthermia	Thyroid storm Heavy-coated dog breeds Heavy drapes, heating blankets, heat lamps Tiletamine/zolazepam	Turn off supplemental heat Administer room temperature or slightly cooler fluids Alcohol to inguinal and axillary regions Cool with a fan Administer acepromazine
Hypoglycaemia	Neonates and paediatrics Well controlled diabetics Sepsis Insulinoma	Supplement glucose in at-risk patients. Monitor blood glucose every 30–60 minutes during anaesthesia and treat hypoglycaemia as it occurs Check for hypoglycaemia in all cases of prolonged recovery from anaesthesia
Oliguria or anuria (urine production <0.5 ml/kg)	Pre-existing renal disease Inadequate replacement of fluid deficits and ongoing losses Hypotension Use of anti-prostaglandin drugs in the face of hypotension and renal hypoperfusion Mu opioid agonists (morphine)	Fluid challenge with balanced, isotonic crystalloid (20–30 ml/kg) or colloid (5–20 ml/kg) to replace fluid deficits Diuretic administration (i.e. furosemide) Dextrose or mannitol to cause an osmotic diuresis Dopamine or dobutamine to increase cardiac output and renal perfusion
Myopathy Neuropathy	Poor positioning during surgery Inadequate padding of muscles and nerves on hard tables Prolonged duration of anaesthesia Prolonged, severe hypotension	Appropriate padding and positioning, particularly with large and giant-breed dogs Reduce anaesthesia time Monitor blood pressure and maintain normal blood pressure during anaesthesia

29.3 Miscellaneous anaesthetic complications.

Hypothermia

Pathophysiology

- Hypothermia results in CNS depression, bradycardia, hypotension, hypoventilation, decreased basal metabolic rate, decreased urine production, decreased anaesthetic drug requirements and decreased oxygen requirements.
- Hypothermia results in slowed metabolism of drugs and hypoventilation, delaying recovery from injectable and volatile anaesthetics.
- Hypothermia can result in a coagulopathy by decreasing the activity of the enzymes associated with the clotting cascade and decreasing platelet function.
- Hypothermia results in intense shivering in the recovery period, increasing metabolic activity and tissue oxygen demand, and can result in hypoxaemia, myocardial ischaemia, hypercapnia, metabolic acidosis and cardiac arrhythmias.
- Hypothermia contributes to increased postoperative infection rates, by suppressing immune function and by causing thermoregulatory vasoconstriction, decreasing oxygen delivery to the wound.
- Hypothermia results in 'thermal discomfort' in the recovery period, which is an additional stressor for the animal.
- Hypothermia is neuroprotective and cardioprotective and mild hypothermia can reduce intracranial pressure.

Causes

- Common anaesthetic complication due to redistribution of heat from the body core to the periphery with vasodilation.
- Cold ambient temperature of operating room and recovery areas and exposure of body cavities to room air.
- Using cool fluids intravenously or for surgical lavage.
- All volatile anaesthetics decrease the normal vasoconstrictive response to hypothermia and promote heat loss.

Treatment

- Use circulating warm water or warm air blankets during surgery and recovery.
- Insulate patient with bubble packing, aluminium foil and towels.
- Surgical lavage with warm fluids.
- Reduce surgical time.
- Increase ambient temperature of the operating room and recovery room.
- Warm intravenous fluids prior to administration.
- Reduce dose of volatile agent to avoid relative overdosage as hypothermia decreases anaesthetic requirements.
- Use heat and moisture exchangers (see Chapter 5).

Hyperthermia

- Hyperthermia results in disruption of enzyme activity, denaturation of proteins, coagulopathy and cell death.
- Organs most susceptible to damage from hyperthermia are the brain, heart, kidneys and liver.
- Hyperthermia can be passive (due to excessive patient heating from external sources) or active (fever, thyroid storm, malignant hyperthermia).

Causes

- Thyroid storm.
- Heavy-coated breeds.
- Use of tiletamine/zolazepam (Telazol, Zoletil).
- Warm ambient temperature.
- Large dogs and rebreathing systems that maintain humidity.

Treatment and prevention

- Monitor body temperature, especially with forced arm air blankets, since over-heating is possible.
- To prevent accidental skin burns provide insulation between warm water heating blankets and exposed skin.
- Turn down or turn off heating blankets.
- Administer room temperature or slightly cooler fluids.
- Apply alcohol to inguinal and axillary regions.
- Cool with a fan.
- Regularly service and maintain heating devices.

Hypoglycaemia

Because the CNS requires glucose as a major energy source, hypoglycaemia during anaesthesia can result in an unexplained increase in depth of anaesthesia, tachycardia and hypertension, prolonged recovery or failure to recover from anaesthesia, and seizures or muscle tremors during recovery.

Causes

Hypoglycaemia is common in neonatal and paediatric patients, but can also occur with well controlled diabetics during fasting, and in patients with septicaemia or insulinoma.

Treatment

- Supplement glucose in neonates, paediatrics and insulinoma patients by administering 5% dextrose in sterile water (D5W) (not a volume replacement fluid); or add 50 ml 50% dextrose to 1 l lactated Ringer's (Hartmann's) to provide a 2.5% dextrose solution for volume replacement.
- Monitor blood glucose during anaesthesia and recovery in patients predisposed to hypoglycaemia and supplement glucose as necessary.

Myopathy or neuropathy

Pathophysiology

The main mechanism for development of myopathy (myositis) under anaesthesia is hypoperfusion and ischaemic damage due to prolonged compression, inadequate padding and/or prolonged hypotension.

- The main mechanisms for perioperative peripheral neuropathies include:
  - Stretch
  - Compression
  - Generalized ischaemia
  - Metabolic derangement (diabetes mellitus, severe anaemia)
  - Surgical resection.
- Axonal reactions to injury of nerves during anaesthesia include:
  - Transient ischaemic nerve block – no structural nerve damage and lasts only minutes
  - Neuropraxia – demyelination of peripheral fibres of the nerve trunk, recoverable in 4–6 weeks
  - Axonotmesis – complete disruption of the axons within an intact nerve sheath, recovery depends on regeneration of the distal nerve and complete recovery is unlikely
  - Neurotmesis – complete nerve disruption, surgical repair, if possible, will return only partial function.

Causes

- Poor positioning on surgical table (limbs in hyperextension).
- Inadequate padding of muscles and nerves.
- Prolonged duration of anaesthesia.
- Prolonged or severe hypotension.
- Most common in large-breed dogs.

Treatment and prevention

- Prevention with adequate padding, careful positioning, reduced duration of anaesthesia and prevention of hypotension.
- Treat with intravenous fluids, anti-inflammatory drugs (steroids or non-steroidal anti-inflammatory drugs (NSAIDs)), analgesics, sedatives, vasodilators.

Oliguria or anuria

Pathophysiology of oliguria and anuria under anaesthesia

- Urine production of <0.5 ml/kg/h is considered inadequate.
- The primary mechanism for oliguria or anuria under anaesthesia is reduced perfusion of the kidneys, and a reduction in glomerular filtration rate.

Causes

- Pre-existing renal disease.
- Inadequate fluid replacement for deficits and ongoing losses.
- Hypotension, particularly if severe or prolonged.
- Use of anti-prostaglandin drugs in the face of hypotension and renal hypoperfusion.

Treatment

- Balanced, isotonic, crystalloid intravenous fluid challenge of 20–30 ml/kg/h if no underlying cardiac disease.
- Colloid administration at 5–20 ml/kg/h (maximum of 20 ml/kg/24 hours).
- Diuretic administration.
- Dextrose or mannitol to create an osmotic diuresis.
- Dopamine or dobutamine to increase cardiac output and improve renal perfusion.

Prolonged recovery

Causes

- Hypoventilation will prolong recovery from volatile anaesthetics that are dependent upon exhalation for termination of effect.
- Hypercapnia, hypoxaemia, metabolic acidosis and hypoglycaemia will cause CNS depression and delay recovery.
- Hypotension results in decreased perfusion of liver and kidneys, resulting in delayed metabolism of anaesthetic drugs.
- Hypothermia results in hypoventilation, and also slowed metabolism of other anaesthetic drugs.
- Hepatic and renal disease can slow metabolism and excretion of drugs.

Treatment

See Figure 29.6 for drug doses.

- Correct hypercapnia, hypoxaemia, acidosis, hypoglycaemia and hypothermia.
- Reverse respiratory depressant effects of mu agonist opioids with butorphanol titrated to effect.
- Maintain on intravenous fluids to maintain renal and hepatic perfusion.

Anaesthetic mishaps and accidents

Anaesthetic mishaps can be categorized as preventable and unpreventable. Unpreventable mishaps include idiosyncratic drug reactions. The vast majority of accidents are preventable, and commonly due to human error, or equipment malfunctions.

Common human errors

- Unrecognized breathing circuit disconnection.
- Anaesthesia machine not set up properly:

  - Lack of adequate training and familiarity with anaesthetic equipment
  - No machine check prior to inducing anaesthesia.
- Administration errors:
  - Drug interactions with concurrent medications
  - Wrong dose (underdosage, relative or absolute overdosage)
  - Wrong route of administration
  - Wrong syringe (always label syringes)
  - Wrong drug.
- Airway mismanagement:
  - Inadequate ventilation (wrong IPPV setting)
  - Unrecognized oesophageal or endobronchial intubation
  - Premature extubation
  - Inadequate oxygen flowmeter settings
  - Laryngeal injuries – vocal fold paralysis, granuloma, arytenoid dislocation
  - Tracheal perforation
  - Chemical tracheitis (inadequately rinsed tubes after cleaning with a chemical disinfectant)
  - Tracheal ischaemic necrosis or rupture.
- Fluid mismanagement:
  - Fluid overloading
  - Wrong type of fluid
  - Intravenous line disconnection
  - Not priming administration set and fluid line.
- Burns:
  - Heating pads (never use electrical heating pads or push any heating blanket into body with positioning pads)
  - Radiant heat lamps
  - Airway burns (some types of lasers).
- Corneal abrasions or ulcers.
- Post-anaesthetic blindness or renal failure secondary to hypotension and inadequate cardiopulmonary support:
  - Most common causes are hypotension during anaesthesia and inadequate perfusion of the optic nerve or kidneys.

Common equipment malfunction

- Breathing circuit disconnected or not set up correctly.
- Oxygen flowmeter turned off.
- Monitoring device failure.
- Ventilator failure.
- Unfilled or overfilled volatile anaesthetic vaporizers.
- Exhausted absorber granules.
- Stuck or missing one-way valves.

Anaesthetic emergencies

Anaphylactic or anaphylactoid reactions (type I – immediate)

For information on anaphylactic reactions see Figure 29.4.

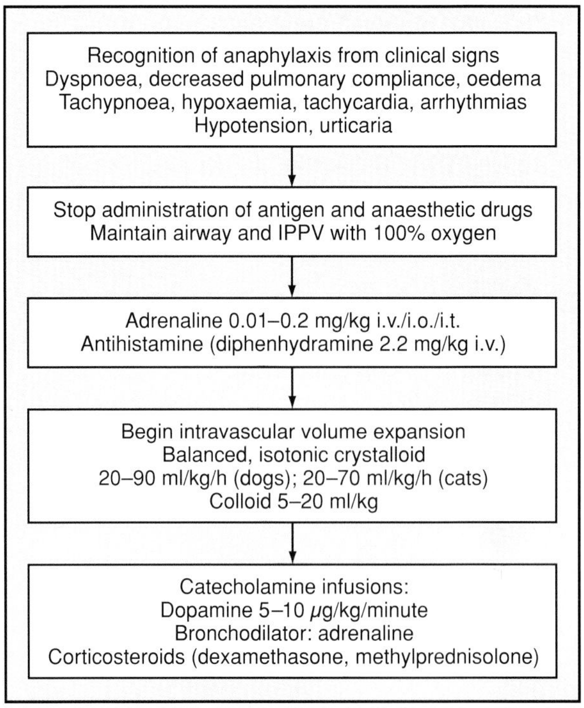

Recognition of anaphylaxis from clinical signs
Dyspnoea, decreased pulmonary compliance, oedema
Tachypnoea, hypoxaemia, tachycardia, arrhythmias
Hypotension, urticaria
Stop administration of antigen and anaesthetic drugs
Maintain airway and IPPV with 100% oxygen
Adrenaline 0.01–0.2 mg/kg i.v./i.o./i.t.
Antihistamine (diphenhydramine 2.2 mg/kg i.v.)
Begin intravascular volume expansion
Balanced, isotonic crystalloid
20–90 ml/kg/h (dogs); 20–70 ml/kg/h (cats)
Colloid 5–20 ml/kg
Catecholamine infusions:
Dopamine 5–10 μg/kg/minute
Bronchodilator: adrenaline
Corticosteroids (dexamethasone, methylprednisolone)

29.4 Algorithm for anaphylaxis during anaesthesia. i.o. = Intraosseous; i.t. = Intratracheal; i.v. = Intravenous.

Hypersensitivity reactions are divided into four types:

- Type I (immediate)
- Type II (cytotoxic)
- Type III (immune complex)
- Type IV (delayed, cell-mediated).

Type I (immediate) hypersensitivity reactions are the most common and life-threatening hypersensitivity reactions that occur in the peri-anaesthetic period. An example of a type II hypersensitivity reaction that might occur during anaesthesia is haemolytic transfusion reactions.

Anaphylaxis (type I hypersensitivity) reaction (mediated by IgE)

- Anaphylaxis is an exaggerated response to an allergen and appears within minutes of exposure to the antigen in a sensitized patient; it is most commonly seen with antibiotic administration in the peri-anaesthetic period.
- Previous exposure results in production of allergen-specific IgE antibodies which cause mast cell and basophil activation and the release of chemical mediators, including leukotrienes, histamine, prostaglandins, kinins and platelet-activating factor, on subsequent exposure.
- Anaphylaxis manifests as urticaria, angioedema, laryngeal oedema, pulmonary oedema, bronchoconstriction, hypoxaemia, vasodilation, increased membrane permeability, hypovolaemia, hypotension, tachycardia, arrhythmias, shock and death.

Anaphylactoid (type I hypersensitivity) reaction (not mediated by IgE or other antigen/antibody interactions)

- Anaphylactoid reactions manifest similarly to anaphylactic reactions, and urticaria, angioedema, laryngeal oedema, pulmonary oedema, bronchoconstriction, hypoxaemia, vasodilation, increased membrane permeability, hypovolaemia, hypotension, tachycardia, arrhythmias, shock and death can occur.
- Anaphylactoid reactions do not require previous exposure to the antigen.
- Anaphylactoid reactions are more common than anaphylactic reactions in the peri-anaesthetic period.
- The triggering drug directly causes mast cell degranulation or causes activation of complement.
- This can occur with any drug, but has been reported to occur with opioids, muscle relaxants, NSAIDs, dextrans, thiopental, propofol and radiocontrast agents.

Treatment of anaphylactoid and anaphylactic reactions

See Figure 29.6 for drug dosages.

- Anaphylactic and anaphlylactoid reactions are clinically indistinguishable, both life-threatening, and treated in the same way.
- Discontinue drug administration and all anaesthetic agents.
- Administer supplemental oxygen in order to maintain normal oxygen saturation (endotracheal intubation and 100% F_iO_2 may be required to maintain oxygenation).
- Intravenous fluids up to shock rate (see Chapter 16).
- Adrenaline for bronchodilation and vasoconstriction.
- Antihistamine: diphenhydramine.
- Aminophylline for bronchodilation.
- Steroids: methylprednisolone or dexamethasone.
- Sodium bicarbonate 0.5–1 mmol/kg for severe metabolic acidosis.

Cardiopulmonary arrest

See Figures 29.5 and 29.6 for information on cardiopulmonary arrest (CPA).

What is cardiopulmonary arrest?

- Sudden, unexpected cessation of *functional* ventilation and circulation.
- Cardiac arrest and respiratory arrest may occur simultaneously, but if respiratory arrest occurs first, cardiac arrest will immediately follow unless there is rapid resuscitative intervention to restore circulation and ventilation.

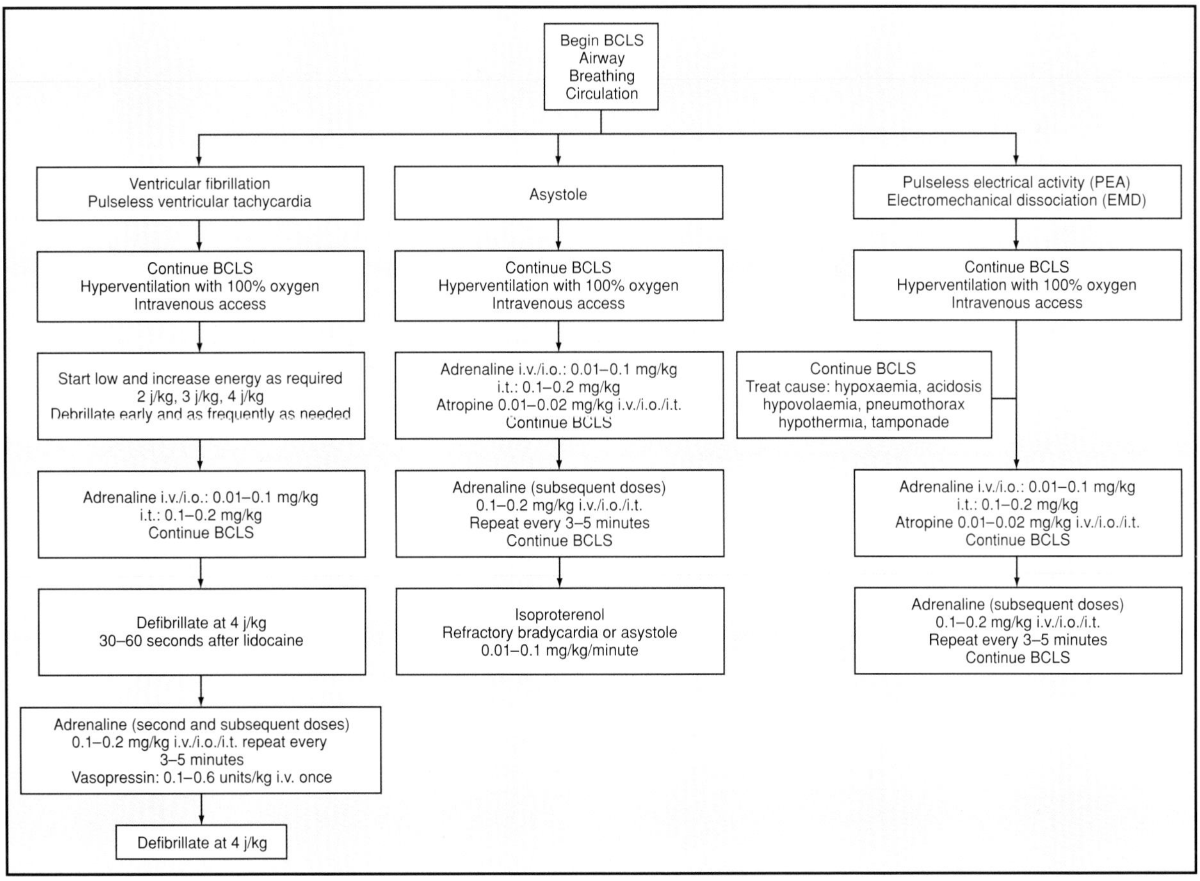

29.5 CPR algorithm for pulseless cardiopulmonary arrest. BCLS = Basic cardiac life support; i.o. = Intraosseous; i.t. = Intratracheal; i.v. = Intravenous.

Drug	Indications	Dose	Possible side effects
Atropine	Bradycardia Atrioventricular (AV) block Sinus arrest Ventricular asystole	0.01–0.02 mg/kg i.v.	Tachycardia Central cholinergic syndrome
Aminophylline	Bronchospasm Asthma Anaphylaxis	Dogs: 2–6 mg/kg i.m., s.c., or slowly i.v. (over 15 minutes) Cats: 2–4 mg/kg i.m., s.c. only	Tachycardia Arrhythmias Hypotension
Albuterol	Bronchospasm Asthma Anaphylaxis	0.15 mg/kg inhaled	Tachycardia Arrhythmias Hypotension
Calcium	Known hypocalcaemia Calcium channel blocker overdosage	0.1–0.3 ml/kg 10% CaCl, slowly i.v. 0.5–1 ml/kg of 10% calcium gluconate, slowly i.v.	Bradycardia Arrhythmias
Corticosteroids	Anti-inflammation Stabilization of blood vessels Analgesia	Dexamethasone: 0.5–1 mg/kg i.v. Methylprednisolone: 20 mg/kg i.v.	Infection Gastrointestinal or renal ischaemia
Diphenhydramine	Antihistamine	2.2 mg/kg i.v. or i.m.	Hypotension if given rapidly intravenously
Dobutamine	Hypotension Myocardial dysfunction	2–10 µg/kg/minute i.v.	Tachycardia Arrhythmias
Dopamine	Renal failure Hypotension Myocardial dysfunction Vasodilation	2–20 µg/kg/minute i.v.	Tachycardia Arrhythmias
Ephedrine	Hypotension	0.03–0.06 mg/kg i.v.	Tachycardia Arrhythmias
Adrenaline	Hypotension Refractory bradycardia Anaphylaxis Cardiopulmonary arrest	0.01–0.2 mg/kg i.v./i.o./i.t. 0.01–0.03 µg/kg/minute	Tachycardia Arrhythmias
Esmolol	Beta blocker Hypertension Tachycardia	50–200 µg/kg/minute i.v.	Hypotension
Furosemide	Diuretic Pulmonary oedema Cerebral oedema Laryngeal oedema	1–2 mg/kg i.v.	Excessive diuresis Hypokalaemia
Glycopyrronium	Bradycardia	0.01 mg/kg i.v.	Tachycardia
Isoproterenol	Refractory bradycardia Ventricular asystole	0.01–0.1 µg/kg/minute i.v.	Hypotension
Lidocaine	Ventricular premature contractions Ventricular tachycardia	Dogs: 1–2 mg/kg i.v.; 20–100 µg/kg/minute i.v. Cats: 0.25–0.75 mg/kg, slowly i.v.	Bradycardia Hypotension Seizures
Magnesium sulphate	Given with prolonged cardiopulmonary arrest or intractable ventricular fibrillation	30 mg/kg i.v. over 10 minutes	Hypotension CNS depression
Procainamide	Ventricular premature contractions Ventricular tachycardia Ventricular fibrillation	Dogs: 10–20 mg/kg i.v; 25–50 µg/kg/minute i.v. Cats: 8–20 mg/kg i.m. or s.c.	Bradycardia Hypotension Seizures
Terbutaline	Bronchospasm Asthma Anaphylaxis	Dogs: 0.01 mg/kg i.v. Cats: 0.01 mg/kg s.c.	Tachycardia Hypotension Arrhythmias
Sodium bicarbonate	Metabolic acidosis During CPR: • If pre-existing metabolic acidosis • >10 minutes of CPR	0.5 mmol/kg i.v. over 20–30 minutes	Metabolic alkalosis Respiratory arrest if given too quickly Hyperosmolality
Vasopressin	Vasodilatory shock (sepsis) Patients in ventricular fibrillation unresponsive to defibrillation or adrenaline	0.1–0.6 IU/kg once i.v.	Severe vasoconstriction Arrhythmias

29.6 Emergency drugs used during general anaesthesia in cats and dogs. CPR = Cardiopulmonary resuscitation; i.m. = Intramuscular; i.o. = Intraosseous; i.t. = Intratracheal; i.v. Intravenous; s.c. = Subcutaneous.

- CPA results in decreased delivery of oxygen to the tissues and decreased removal of carbon dioxide. The anaerobic conditions result in increased production of lactate and hydrogen ions. A severe oxygen debt and mixed respiratory and metabolic acidosis quickly develop.
- Irreversible neurological damage will occur within 3 minutes of depriving the brain of oxygen ('three minute emergency').
- Multiple organ failure (cardiac, renal, hepatic, etc.) is possible.
- Reperfusion injury is an inevitable sequela to cardiopulmonary resuscitation (CPR), and can worsen damage to vital tissues.

Goals of CPR

- Restore and maximize *coronary* and *cerebral* perfusion.
- Restore normal cardiac rhythm.
- Restore effective respiratory exchange.
- Prevent irreversible neurological damage.
- Prevent irreversible damage to heart, kidneys and other vital organs.
- Prevent further arrest.
- CPR and emergency cardiac care should be considered at any time a patient cannot adequately oxygenate or perfuse vital organs.

Common causes of cardiopulmonary arrest in the peri-anaesthetic period

- Hypoxaemia.
- Hypercapnia.
- Electrolyte abnormalities (hyperkalaemia).
- Acid–base abnormalities.
- Hypotension, hypovolaemia, shock.
- Hypothermia.
- Autonomic nervous system (ANS) imbalance (vagal stimulation).
- Sensitization of the myocardium to catecholamines (xylazine, halothane).
- Pre-existing cardiac disease.
- Anaesthetic agent overdose.
- Severe trauma, systemic or metabolic disease.
- Significant underlying cardiac or respiratory disease.

Signs of impending cardiac arrest
These include:

- Changes in respiratory rate, depth and pattern, such as bradypnoea or agonal gasping
- Weak, irregular pulses, tachycardia, ventricular premature contractions
- Bradycardia, particularly in patients who are hypoxaemic prior to CPA
- Hypotension, as well as poor response to sympathomimetic agents
- Cyanotic or grey mucous membranes
- Hypothermia, despite attempts to warm the patient
- Sudden and unexplained increase in depth of anaesthesia.

Signs of cardiopulmonary arrest
These include:

- Collapse, loss of consciousness, no skeletal muscle tone
- Loss of palpable central pulses, such as the femoral pulse
- Lack of heart sounds detectable by auscultation
- Agonal gasping or absent ventilation
- Fixed, dilated pupils (occurs within 45 seconds of arrest)
- Cyanotic or pale mucous membranes (capillary refill time and mucous membrane colour can remain normal for up to 2 minutes after cardiac arrest, depending on the underlying cause)
- Abnormal ECG
  - *Note:* pulseless electrical activity (PEA) can look 'normal' for several minutes after arrest has occurred.

Prevention and readiness

- Monitoring and prevention of hypoxaemia, hypercapnia, hypovolaemia, hypotension and hypothermia of patients in the intensive care unit (ICU) and patients under anaesthesia.
- Fully stocked emergency cart.
- Dosage wall chart.
- *Equipment:* airway suction, endotracheal tubes and laryngoscope, tracheotomy kit, 100% oxygen, means of ventilation, intravenous or intraosseous catheters, fluids, chest tube placement kit, thoracotomy kit and electrical defibrillator.

Basic cardiac life support
The ABCs of CPR are the procedures required to sustain artificial ventilation and coronary and cerebral perfusion while you correct the underlying problem and include:

- Airway management
- Breathing
- Circulation.

Airway management (A):

- Endotracheal intubation is the most common technique to obtain control of the airway.
- Use of a laryngoscope will greatly facilitate visualization of the glottis and will avoid oesophageal intubation.
- Suction may be required to remove blood, saliva, gastrointestinal contents, mucus, pus.
- After assuring that the endotracheal tube has been correctly placed, secure in place and inflate the cuff to ensure there is an airtight seal between the tracheal mucosa and the endotracheal tube.
- When attempting intubation of an animal when working alone, place the animal in dorsal recumbency to aid visualization and endotracheal tube placement.
- A tight-fitting facemask can be used in animals that are difficult or impossible to intubate orotracheally, or if you are awaiting help.

- Laryngeal mask airways, used commonly in humans, can aid in ventilation of animals difficult to intubate.
- Tracheotomy is sometimes necessary in patients that cannot be intubated due to anatomical difficulties or obstructions blocking the airway (e.g. bones, balls).
- Percutaneous tracheal cannulation:
  - Used to provide oxygen when endotracheal intubation or tracheotomy cannot be performed
  - Involves inserting a long, over-the-needle catheter between the tracheal rings, and insufflation of oxygen through the catheter during chest compressions
  - This technique does not allow positive pressure ventilation; it does provide some oxygenation during resuscitation.
- If positive pressure ventilation is not possible during resuscitation, oxygenation may still be adequate as long as effective chest compressions are administered, along with supplemental oxygen.

Breathing (B):

- Assess pulse after giving two breaths; if no pulse, continue ventilation and begin chest compressions.
- Ideally, intermittent positive pressure ventilation (IPPV) is administered with 100% oxygen whenever possible, to maximize oxygen delivery to the tissues.
- Commonly performed using an anaesthetic circuit and reservoir bag.
- The reservoir bag should be 6–10 times the patient's tidal volume; tidal volume is 10–15 ml/kg.
- Bag-valve devices (paediatric and adult sizes), also called 'Ambu' bags, can be used along with supplemental oxygen (can deliver up to 100% oxygen).
- IPPV should be administered at a rate of 20–40/minute (1:1 ratio with compressions).
- Airway pressure during IPPV should be <30 cmH_2O to avoid barotrauma and excessive decreases in venous return to the heart, but may need to be higher in patients with poor pulmonary and thoracic compliance.
- Efficacy of ventilation is assessed by observing the degree of chest expansion, mucous membrane colour improvement and airway resistance.
- An end-tidal carbon dioxide of >14 mmHg indicates good CPR technique. Pulse oximetry may not function because of poor quality or non-existent pulse.
- Jugular vein blood gas analysis is more indicative of body state compared with arterial gas analysis during CPA.

Circulation (C):

- Reassess circulation after intubation and a few seconds of IPPV in order to ascertain if the patient is still in cardiac arrest.
- Chest compressions must be begun as early as possible and should not be stopped, if possible, during resuscitation.
- External chest compressions are attempted at a rate of 60–120/minute.
- Effective perfusion of the heart and brain are best achieved when chest compression consumes 50% of the duty cycle, with the remaining 50% devoted to the relaxation phase, allowing blood to flow into the chest and heart.
- The goal of chest compressions is to maximize vital organ perfusion by maximizing the force and rate of compressions.

Mechanism of blood flow during CPR: Two theories have been proposed as the mechanism that creates forward blood flow with external chest compressions in CPR.

Cardiac pump theory:

- Compression of the chest wall over the heart directly compresses the heart chambers to create forward blood flow.
- This technique involves placing the patient in right lateral recumbency and compressing the chest wall directly over the heart.
- This technique is most likely to be important in animals <10 kg with compliant chest walls (cats, small dogs, rabbits, ferrets).
- This technique is not as effective in patients with non-compliant chest walls (e.g. patients with pneumothorax or hydrothorax), obese animals or animals with barrel-shaped chests (e.g. Bulldogs). Placing these patients in dorsal recumbency and compressing the sternum will improve the efficacy of this method.

Thoracic pump theory:

- According to this theory, positive intrathoracic pressure created with chest wall compression increases pressure in all intrathoracic structures (including the heart and major arteries), creating forward blood flow.
- The great veins collapse and the atrioventricular valves close to prevent retrograde blood flow.
- This technique is most important in animals ≥10 kg and animals with poorly compliant chest walls.
- This technique also becomes more important than the cardiac pump techniques as CPR continues, as the heart becomes less compliant during prolonged CPR.
- When using this technique, it is important to maximize high intrathoracic pressure using the following:
  - Place the patient in dorsal recumbency, support with sandbags and compress over sternum.
  - Place the patient in lateral recumbency and compress the chest wall at the widest point of the ribs.
  - Use simultaneous chest compressions and IPPV.
  - Restrict abdominal movement with continuous abdominal compression or by using abdominal wrapping.

- Keep airway pressure low between chest compressions (i.e. no IPPV between compressions) to aid venous return.

Determinants of vital organ perfusion during CPR:

- During conventional (closed chest) CPR, cerebral and myocardial flows are less than 5% of the pre-arrest values and renal and hepatic blood flow is 1–5% of pre-arrest values.
- Cerebral perfusion pressure and cerebral blood flow are dependent on the gradient between the carotid arterial pressure and the intracranial pressure during systole (during thoracic compression).
- The greater the pressure generated during chest compression, the greater the cerebral perfusion pressure, resulting in improved cerebral perfusion.
- Myocardial perfusion pressure and myocardial blood flow are dependent on the pressure gradient between the aorta and right atrium during diastole (release phase of thoracic compression), so allowing adequate time for venous return is critical.
- Force, rate and duration of chest compression during CPR will determine the effectiveness of organ perfusion during CPR.
- Irrespective of the mechanism of forward blood flow during CPR, increasing the force and rate of chest compressions will significantly increase the arterial pressure.
- Detection of a central pulse, end-tidal carbon dioxide >14 mmHg (1.9 kPa), pupil constriction, return of reflexes and flow on Doppler probe placed on the eye are signs of good CPR technique.

Advanced cardiac life support

These (DEF) are the procedures that specifically treat the cause of arrest and restore normal cardiac function:

- Drugs
- Electrocardiography
- Fluid therapy.

Drugs (D): See Figure 29.6 for drug doses.

Adrenaline:

- For asystole and bradycardia unresponsive to anticholinergics.
- Causes vasoconstriction, offsetting the vasodilation and pooling of blood that occurs with cardiac arrest.
- Positive inotrope increases cardiac contractility.
- Improves cerebral and cardiac perfusion, due to beta-2 agonist effects.
- Positive chronotrope and stimulates sinoatrial node.

Vasopressin:

- Indicated in patients with vasodilatory shock, and patients in ventricular fibrillation who are unresponsive to defibrillation or adrenaline.
- Dosage is unknown for animals, but the standard human dosage is approximately 0.1–0.6 units/kg i.v., once only.

Atropine:

- For severe bradycardia or asystole.
- Blocks vagal reflexes.

Isoproterenol:

- For refractory bradycardia or asystole.

Dopamine:

- For shock, hypotension.
- If patient has bradycardia unresponsive to anticholinergics.

Dobutamine:

- For shock, hypotension.

Sodium bicarbonate:

- Not routinely used during CPR, unless it is used to treat a pre-existing metabolic acidosis, hyperkalaemia or Addisonian crisis.
- $NaHCO_3$ is also administered after 10 minutes of CPR, since the patient is almost certainly acidotic at this point.

Calcium:

Not routinely used during CPR unless there is a pre-existing hypocalcaemia, hyperkalaemia or calcium channel blocker toxicity.

Magnesium sulphate:

- Given with prolonged CPA or intractable ventricular fibrillation.

Lidocaine:

- For ventricular tachycardia.
- Cats may be more sensitive to lidocaine and are usually given low doses.
- Lidocaine is also a free radical scavenger, and may offset some of the reperfusion injury.

Mannitol:

- Osmotic diuretic sometimes given during and after CPR to help offset the development of cerebral oedema in the resuscitated patient.

Steroids:

- Occasionally given after resuscitation to prevent the development of cerebral oedema and offset the effects of shock and reperfusion injury.

Routes of administration:

Central venous catheter:

- A cranial vena cava or jugular catheter is the best route for administration of drugs in an arrested patient, as this results in delivery of the drug close to the heart.

Intratracheal:

- Several drugs, such as adrenaline, atropine, vasopressin and lidocaine, can be given via the endotracheal tube.
- The dose used is doubled and it is administered into the distal trachea via a sterile canine urinary catheter.
- Once the breathing system is reattached and IPPV begins, the drug is rapidly dispersed throughout the lungs, and is rapidly absorbed.

Intraosseous catheter (tibia, radius or ulna):

- Administration of drugs via this route can be as fast as through a central venous catheter. The medullary cavity does not collapse during CPA.

Peripheral venous catheter:

- It can take up to 2 minutes for drugs administered via a peripheral catheter to reach the heart during CPR.
- A flush of 10–30 ml of saline may be necessary for the drug to reach the heart.
- Occasionally, surgical cut-down to the vein may be attempted in order to isolate and catheterize the vein.

Intracardiac:

- Direct injection of drugs into the heart chamber is always indicated during open-chest CPR.
- During closed-chest CPR, this technique is only used if there is no existing venous catheter or if intratracheal administration has failed.
- This technique is associated with several disadvantages:
  - Chest compressions must be terminated while the intracardiac injection is attempted
  - Risk of laceration of coronary arteries or lung tissue
  - Injection of drug into the heart wall, rather than the heart chamber, can result in intractable ventricular fibrillation.

Intralingual:

- The intralingual technique is often used in very small mammals (mice, rats) and in neonates (puppies and kittens).
- There is a rich vascular plexus at the base of the tongue, and drugs injected at this site can be rapidly absorbed.

Electrocardiography (E): Placement of ECG leads is important for identification of the arrhythmia that has resulted in CPA in order to initiate appropriate therapy. Common arrest arrhythmias in veterinary patients include:

- Pulseless electrical activity (PEA) (also know as electromechanical dissociation (EMD) or pulseless idioventricular rhythm)
- Ventricular asystole
- Ventricular fibrillation.

Pulseless electrical activity: This occurs when there is electrical activity without sufficient mechanical activity to cause adequate cardiac output.

Causes of PEA include:

- Predisposing factors: hypovolaemia, hypoxaemia, acidosis, hypothermia, hyper- or hypokalaemia, tension pneumothorax, cardiac tamponade
- There may be a depletion of myocardial oxygen and ATP stores, resulting in inability of the heart muscle to contract.

Treatment of PEA involves:

- Basic cardiac life support (Airway, Breathing, Circulation)
- Adrenaline
- Atropine
- Dexamethasone
- Electrical defibrillation.

Ventricular asystole: This is the absence of electrical and mechanical cardiac activity – the 'flat-line' on the ECG. Causes of ventricular asystole include:

- Increased vagal tone
- Oculocardiac reflex
- Vasovagal response to manipulation of abdominal viscera
- Hyperkalaemia
- Severe hypoxaemia.

Treatment of ventricular asystole involves:

- Basic cardiac life support
- Adrenaline
- Atropine.

Ventricular fibrillation:

- Chaotic, disorganized, ectopic ventricular activity resulting in sustained systole.
- Because the activity is disorganized, no effective cardiac output occurs.
- Since there is no diastolic period in ventricular fibrillation, no myocardial perfusion can occur and the myocardium is very rapidly depleted of its ATP stores.

Causes of ventricular fibrillation include:

- Predisposing factors: hypovolaemia, hypoxaemia, acidosis, hypothermia, hyper- or hypokalaemia
- Frequently the end result of severe multisystem dysfunction.

Treatment of ventricular fibrillation involves:

- Basic cardiac life support
- Electrical DC countershock with a defibrillator, as soon as ventricular fibrillation is identified; apply countershocks very closely together
- Fibrillation results in rapid depletion of cardiac ATP stores, so rapid correction will be more likely to result in a successful outcome

- Defibrillate during expiration, when lungs are at their smallest, to minimize the chance of burning lung tissue and decrease resistance to flow of the countershock
- Pharmaceutical treatment can include:
  - Adrenaline (may change 'fine' fibrillation to 'coarse' fibrillation, which is easier to convert)
  - Atropine
  - Lidocaine.

Fluid administration (F):

- Shock volumes are only administered if CPA was due to or preceded by severe volume depletion (haemorrhage, severe dehydration, anaphylactic or distributive shock):
  - 90 ml/kg/h in dogs
  - 60 ml/kg/h in cats.
- CPA results in a relative vascular volume loss as severe vasodilation results in pooling of blood in the periphery and decreased venous return. Fluid rates used during CPR are:
  - 30 ml/kg/h in dogs
  - 20 ml/kg/h in cats.
- Many types of fluids commonly found in veterinary practice can be used, including lactated Ringer's solution, 0.9% NaCl, other crystalloids, colloids or whole blood.
- Avoid fluids containing glucose (such as D5W) as these have been associated with poorer neurological recovery and outcome.

Open-chest CPR* versus *closed-chest CPR: Closed-chest CPR will, at most, generate approximately 20–30% of the normal cardiac output, while open-chest CPR will generate 60–80% of the normal cardiac output.

Indications for open-chest CPR:

- No palpable femoral pulses within 5–10 minutes of beginning basic cardiac life support with external chest compressions.
- No return of spontaneous cardiac contraction after 10 minutes of basic and advanced CPR, despite generating good palpable pulses.
- Chest cavity or abdomen already exposed (thoracotomy or laparotomy).
- Any conditions that interfere with generation of high intrathoracic pressure, such as:
  - Pneumothorax, pleural effusion, or any severe chest pathology
  - Diaphragmatic hernia
  - Flail chest
  - Very large or obese animals (very non-compliant chests)
  - Severe pericardial effusion
  - Tracheal or bronchial disruption
  - Conditions associated with low systemic arterial and venous pressures (poor venous return):
    - Severe haemorrhage
    - Septic, anaphylactic or distributive shock
    - Severe hypotension due to drug overdosage.

Signs of successful resuscitation include the following:

- Decreased pupil size (from fixed and dilated)
- Return of the pupillary light reflex and palpebral reflex
- Return of spontaneous ventilation
- Return of airway protective reflexes.

Post-resuscitative life support

- Post-resuscitative life support measures are undertaken to optimize cardiac output, blood volume, blood pressure, tissue perfusion, oxygenation, oxygen-carrying capacity, acid–base and electrolyte balance and organ function.
- Monitor electrolytes, acid–base status, central venous pressure, body temperature and urine output and provide supportive measures to maintain homeostasis of these parameters.
- Administer supplemental oxygen: the successfully resuscitated patient is likely to have pulmonary contusions, pulmonary oedema, pneumothorax, cerebral oedema and/or cardiac arrhythmias. Oxygen will help to offset some of these problems.
- Maximize oxygen-carrying capacity and tissue delivery of oxygen by maintaining normovolaemia, normotension and adequate haemoglobin concentration.
- Maintenance of adequate blood pressure may require inotropic support agents: dobutamine, dopamine, adrenaline infusions may be indicated in the post-resuscitation period.
- Nutritional support should always be considered in the post-resuscitation period.

Cerebral resuscitation

- Rapid restoration of cerebral perfusion and oxygenation is critical for effective cerebral resuscitation.
- Cerebral oedema, hypoxaemia, hypoventilation and increased ICP are all possible sequelae to CPA due to prolonged cerebral hypoxia and post-resuscitation reperfusion injury.
- Maximizing mean arterial pressure while minimizing increases in intracranial pressure is necessary to maintain adequate cerebral perfusion pressure.
- A high-normal perfusion pressure can augment collateral cerebral blood flow and has been shown to result in improvement in neurological function.
- Mean arterial pressure should be maintained between 70 and 80 mmHg, but higher mean arterial pressure may be required to maintain cerebral perfusion if there is a pre-existing increased ICP (i.e. trauma, tumour).

- Adequate volume loading and sympathomimetic support may be required to maintain cerebral perfusion.
- Maintaining a normal haemoglobin concentration and oxygen saturation is critical post-CPA. It is imperative to avoid global tissue hypoxia and worsening of the increased ICP and neurological damage.
- Slight hyperventilation may also be indicated for 24–48 hours, as mild hypocarbia will decrease cerebral blood flow, offsetting elevations in ICP.
- Steroids and mannitol are administered to offset the reperfusion injury and decrease any cerebral oedema.
- Furosemide may be administered to offset cerebral oedema.
- Keep head slightly elevated and avoid jugular compression to avoid increased ICP.
- Monitor for and control seizures.

References and further reading

Beale RJ, Hollenberg SM, Vincent JL and Parrillo JE (2004) Vasopressin and inotropic support in septic shock: an evidence based review. *Critical Care Medicine* **32(11)**, S455–465

Cole SG, Otto CM and Hughes D (2002) Cardiopulmonary cerebral resuscitation in small animals – a clinical practice review (part 1). *Veterinary Emergency and Critical Care* **12(4)**, 261–267

Cole SG, Otto CM and Hughes D (2003) Cardiopulmonary cerebral resuscitation in small animals – a clinical practice review (part 2). *Veterinary Emergency and Critical Care* **13(1)**, 13–23

Den Ouden DT and Meinders AE (2005) Vasopressin: physiology and clinical use in patients with vasodilatory shock: a review. *The Netherlands Journal of Medicine* **63(1)**, 4–13

Holmes CL, Patel RM, Russell JA and Walley KR (2001) Physiology of vasopressin relevant to management of septic shock. *Chest* **120**, 989–1002

Macintire DK, Drobatz KJ, Haskins S and Saxon WD (2004) *Manual of Small Animal Emergency and Critical Care Medicine.* Blackwell Publishers, Ames, Iowa

Stoelting RK (1999) *Pharmacology & Physiology in Anesthetic Practice, 3rd edn.* Lippincott Williams & Wilkins, Philadelphia

Tranquilli, WJ (2006) *Lumb and Jones Veterinary Anesthesia and Analgesia, 4th edn.* Blackwell Publishers, Ames, Iowa

Wingfield WE and Raffe MR (2002) *The Veterinary ICU Book.* Teton NewMedia, Jackson, Wyoming

Index

Page numbers in *italics* indicate figures

Index

Index

Index

Index